Muscular Dystrophy

Muscular Dystrophy

Edited by **Carsten Cooper**

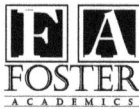

FOSTER
ACADEMICS

New Jersey

Published by Foster Academics,
61 Van Reypen Street,
Jersey City, NJ 07306, USA
www.fosteracademics.com

Muscular Dystrophy
Edited by Carsten Cooper

International Standard Book Number: 978-1-63242-281-1 (Hardback)

Printed in the United States of America.

Contents

Preface

Every book is a source of knowledge and this one is no exception. The idea that led to the conceptualization of this book was the fact that the world is advancing rapidly; which makes it crucial to document the progress in every field. I am aware that a lot of data is already available, yet, there is a lot more to learn. Hence, I accepted the responsibility of editing this book and contributing my knowledge to the community.

With over 30 distinct types as well as subtypes known and several more to be recognized and sorted, muscular dystrophy is an extremely heterogeneous group of inherited neuromuscular disorders. The book presents an elaborative analysis of the different types of muscular dystrophies, genes related to each subtype, disease diagnosis, management as well as available treatment options. Though every distinct type and subtype of muscular dystrophy is related to a distinct causative gene, most of them have overlapping clinical presentations, making molecular diagnosis certain for both patient management as well as disease diagnosis. Discussions regarding the presently available diagnostic approaches that have revolutionized clinical research are presented in this profound book along with the pathophysiology of the various muscular dystrophies, all-round functions of the involved genes as well as efforts towards efficient patient management and diagnosis.

While editing this book, I had multiple visions for it. Then I finally narrowed down to make every chapter a sole standing text explaining a particular topic, so that they can be used independently. However, the umbrella subject sinews them into a common theme. This makes the book a unique platform of knowledge.

I would like to give the major credit of this book to the experts from every corner of the world, who took the time to share their expertise with us. Also, I owe the completion of this book to the never-ending support of my family, who supported me throughout the project.

Editor

Section 1

Introduction to Muscular Dystrophies

Alpha-Dystroglycanopathy

Mieko Yoshioka

Department of Pediatric Neurology, Kobe City Pediatric
and General Rehabilitation Center for the Challenged,
Japan

1. Introduction

Alpha-dystroglycanopathies are a clinically and genetically heterogenous group of muscular dystrophies characterized by the reduced or absent glycosylation of alpha-dystroglycan (Muntoni et al., 2002). The hypoglycosylation of alpha-dystroglycan leads to decreased binding of its ligands, including laminin, agrin and perlecan in skeletal muscle and neurexin in the brain. The only known target for this type of glycosylation is alpha-dystroglycan, and together with other proteins of the dystrophin-glycoprotein complex it forms a link between extracellular matrix proteins and actin cytoskeleton. The clinical manifestations of alpha-dystroglycanopathies are extremely variable, leading to a broad spectrum of phenotypes with limb-girdle muscular dystrophy (LGMD) without mental retardation delineating the milder end, and Walker-Warburg syndrome (WWS), muscle-eye-brain disease (MEB) and Fukuyama type congenital muscular dystrophy (FCMD) the severe end (Muntoni & Voit, 2004) (Fig. 1). In most of the severe disorders, the eyes and the brain are affected in addition to congenital muscular dystrophy (CMD). Here, CMD is defined as onset of weakness prenatally or within the first 6 months of life, and LGMD is defined by later onset weakness, specifically after having acquired ambulation. The brain abnormalities are described as cobblestone lissencephaly; available pathological studies have demonstrated breeches of the glia limitans and over-migration of cortical neurons into the pial spaces. In WWS, the life-span of patients is severely reduced and brain and eye abnormalities extremely severe (Dobyns et al., 1989); MEB and FCMD patients generally survive beyond infancy, ocular manifestations are usually milder in FCMD than in MEB (Fukuyama et al., 1981, Santavuori et al., 1989). To date, mutations in six genes which encode putative or confirmed glycosyltransferases have been identified in these autosomal recessively inherited disorders: *Protein-O-mannosyl transferase 1 and 2 (POMT1* and *POMT2), Protein-O-mannose 1,2-N-acetylglucosaminyltransferase 1 (POMGnT1), Fukutin-related protein (FKRP), Fukutin (FKTN),* and *LARGE.* Initially, each gene was associated with one syndrome (original phenotype) : *POMT1* and *POMT2* mutations giving rise to WWS; *POMGnT1* mutations in patients with MEB; *FKRP* mutations in patients with congenital or late-onset muscular dystrophies (MDC1C and LGMD 2I); *FKTN* mutations in patients with FCMD; *LARGE* mutations in a patient with congenital muscular dystrophy type 1D (MDC 1D). Subsequently, mutation analysis in patients with milder or more severe syndromes within the dystroglycanopathy spectrum demonstrated allelic heterogeneity for different mutations in each of the dystroglycanopathy genes (Fig. 1). Null mutations in *POMT1, POMT2, POMGnT1, FKRP,*

FKTN and *LARGE* are associated with the most severe end of the clinical spectrum (WWS) of dystroglycanopathy, although not an absolute rule.

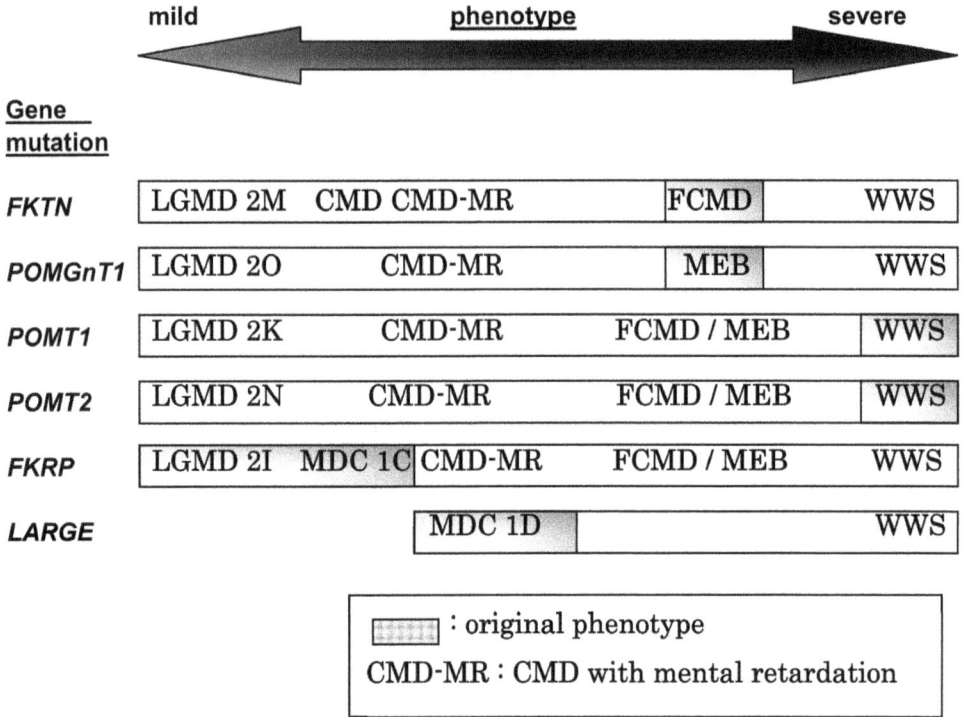

Fig. 1. Gene mutations and clinical phenotypes of alpha-dystroglycanopathy

2. Broader clinical spectrum and worldwide distribution of *FKTN* mutations

A wide clinical spectrum is also evident for the *FKTN* mutations that were first reported in patients with FCMD and later in patients with WWS and in patients with LGMD 2M without mental retardation. FCMD is the second most common form of muscular dystrophy in Japanese population after Duchenne muscular dystrophy, but is seen very rarely in other population. The incidence of FCMD is 3-10 per 100,000 or nearly half that of Duchenne muscular dystrophy in the Japanese population, with a carrier frequency of one in 80 and is one of the most common autosomal recessive disorder in Japan (Fukuyama & Ohsawa,1984). FCMD patients have muscular dystrophy with severe mental retardation and a neuronal migration abnormality. Epilepsy and eye abnormalities are also frequently associated with FCMD. Toda et al. (1993) localized the FCMD locus to chromosome 9q31-33 using genetic linkage analysis. They further defined the FCMD locus within a much smaller segment and also found evidence for strong linkage disequilibrium. Haplotype analysis using the markers D9S2105, 2107, and D9S172 indicated that most FCMD-bearing chromosomes in Japanese pedigrees were derived from a single ancestral founder (Toda et al., 1996). Most Japanese FCMD patients are homozygous for an ancestral founder mutation in FCMD gene, which arose from the insertion of a 3 kb retrotransposon element into the 3' untranslated region (UTR). Some patients are compound heterozygous, carrying another mutation in addition to the founder insertion, and leading to a more severe FCMD variant (Kobayashi et al., 1998a). The absence of patients with two non-founder mutations in Japan led to the hypothesis that this may be lethal, however since 2003 compound heretozygosity for many different mutations have been described in non-Japanese populations, including homozygosity for nonsense mutations. To date, at least 24 different *FKTN* mutations have been described in non-Japanese patients and phenotypes of these patients cover the entire range of alpha-dystroglycanopathies (Yis et al., 2011).

We performed clinical studies in 41 families with FCMD examined between 1972 and 1992 (Yoshioka & Kuroki, 1994). These patients were diagnosed on the standard criteria of FCMD described by Fukuyama et al. (1960). After the discovery of FCMD gene, we investigated gene mutations of these FCMD families (Yoshioka et al., 2008). Here, we at first describe the clinical studies performed until 1992 and later analysis of the genotype-phenotype relationship in FCMD. We then present Japanese CMD patients with alpha-dystroglycanopathy with other gene mutations than *FKTN* and without any known gene mutation. In addition, we describe *FKTN* mutations outside Japan and compare them with Japanese FCMD patients.

2.1 Japanese FCMD patients diagnosed on standard criteria between 1972 and 1992

We performed clinical and genetic studies in 41 families with FCMD examined by us between 1972 and 1992 (Table 1) (Yoshioka & Kuroki, 1994). The diagnosis in these patients was established according to standard criteria described by Fukuyama et al. in 1960, which were, briefly, early onset hypotonia, joint contractures, severe mental retardation with occasional convulsions, and dystrophic abnormalities detected in the muscle biopsy specimen. Nine families (22%) had multiple affected children ("familial" FCMD). Unfortunately, two siblings in nine families had already died at the time of examination, and detailed clinical data other than their clinical diagnosis were therefore not available. The other 32 families had only one affected child ("sporadic" FCMD). Parental consanguinity was documented in 5 sporadic FCMD families and none of the familial cases. In total, 48 patients, including 7 sib pairs, were evaluated with regard to maximum motor ability, mental and convulsion states, cranial CT or MRI findings, and EEG and ophthalmological data.

	Total	Familial	Sporadic
Number of families	41	9	32
Consanguineous marriage	5	0	5
Number of patients	50	18	32
Male : female	22 : 28	5 : 13	17 : 15

Table 1. Patients with Fukuyama-type Congenital Muscular Dystrophy (FCMD) [diagnosed according to standard criteria between 1972 and 1992, reproduced from Yoshioka & Kuroki, 1994]

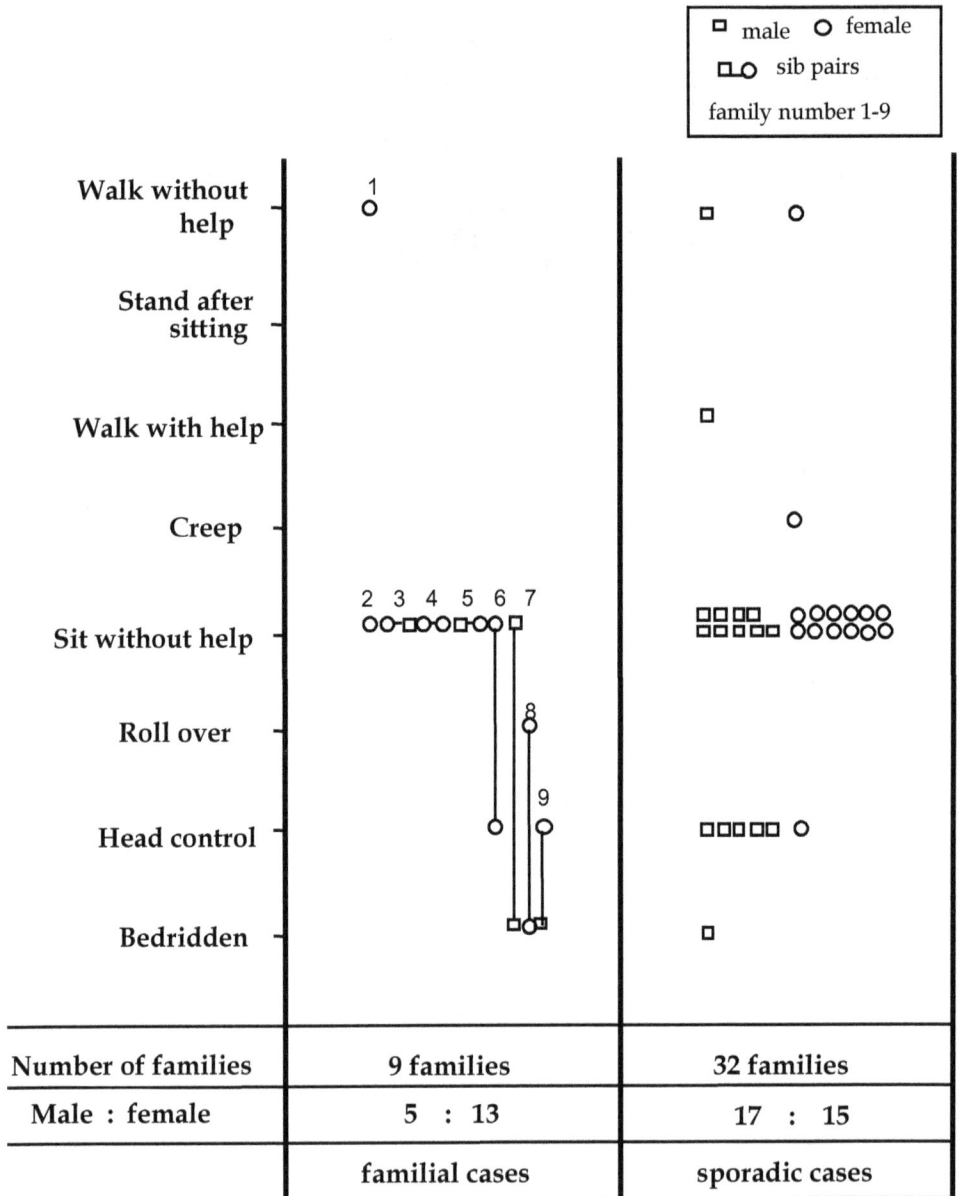

Fig. 2. Maximum motor ability in sib pairs and in familial and sporadic FCMD cases. The familial cases are numbered from 1 to 9. The members of each sib pair are connected by a line (Reproduced from Yoshioka & Kuroki, 1994).

Three patients in our familial group but only one in our sporadic group showed no head control ("bedridden"), whereas a few ambulatory patients were seen in both groups (Fig. 2).

The familial FCMD patients showed relatively more severe motor disability than that in the sporadic FCMD patients. The maximum motor ability in most patients in both groups consisted of sitting without help. Although the speech ability varied between sibs and between families (Fig. 3), all patients showed moderate to severe mental retardation. As for convulsion states, about half of the patients had febrile or afebrile convulsions in both familial and sporadic groups. The convulsion state in 7 sib pairs was the same; both sibs in 3 families had afebrile or febrile convulsions, while in 4 other families neither had convulsion. EEG showed paroxysmal discharges in three sibling pairs with convulsions, while in two of the other sibling pairs without convulsion a difference between siblings in EEG findings was apparent. Ophthalmologically, myopia, weakness of the orbicularis oculi, nystagmus, and optic nerve atrophy were common findings.

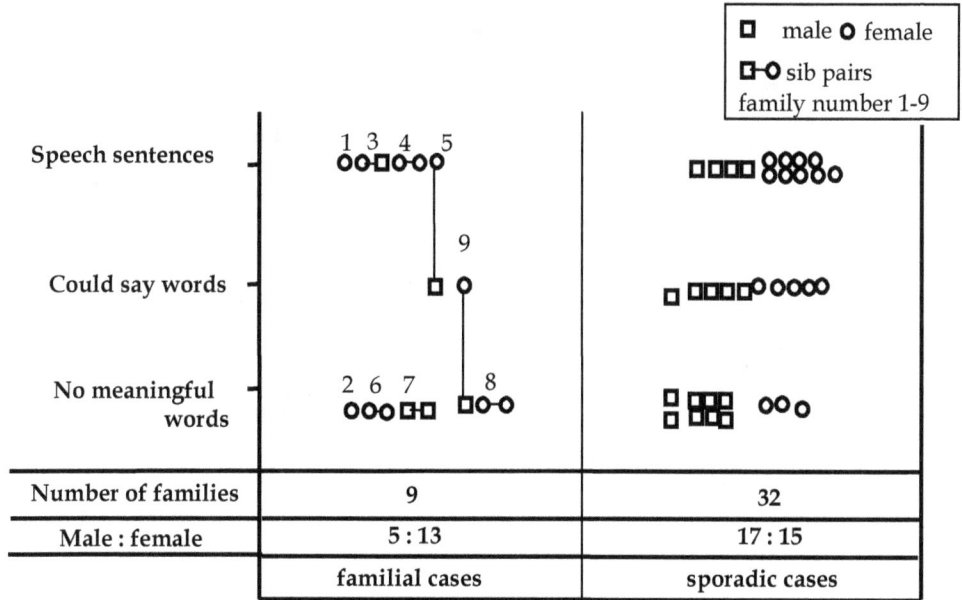

Fig. 3. Speech ability in sib pairs and in familial and sporadic FCMD cases. Familial cases are numbered from 1 to 9, and the members of each sib pair are connected by a line (Reproduced from Yoshioka & Kuroki, 1994).

Typical CT or MRI findings seen in FCMD were pachygyria or polymicrogyria of the fronto-temporo-occipital regions, moderate dilatation of the lateral ventricles, especially posteriorly (colpocephaly), the abnormal signal in the cerebral white matter, and cerebellar cysts closely related to polymicrogyria (Fig. 4). However, in one family (S-family), the elder brother had the typical CT findings of FCMD, while the younger brother had marked dilatation of the lateral ventricles and an occipital encephalocele (Fig. 5). In addition, retinal detachment was present in the younger brother at birth, whereas in the elder brother it developed at 3 years. Our study revealed that FCMD patients ranged from ambulatory to bedridden, and some were able to form sentences while others uttered no meaningful words. Convulsions were found in about half of the patients. Hydrocephalus, encephalocele and retinal detachment were rare but true findings in FCMD.

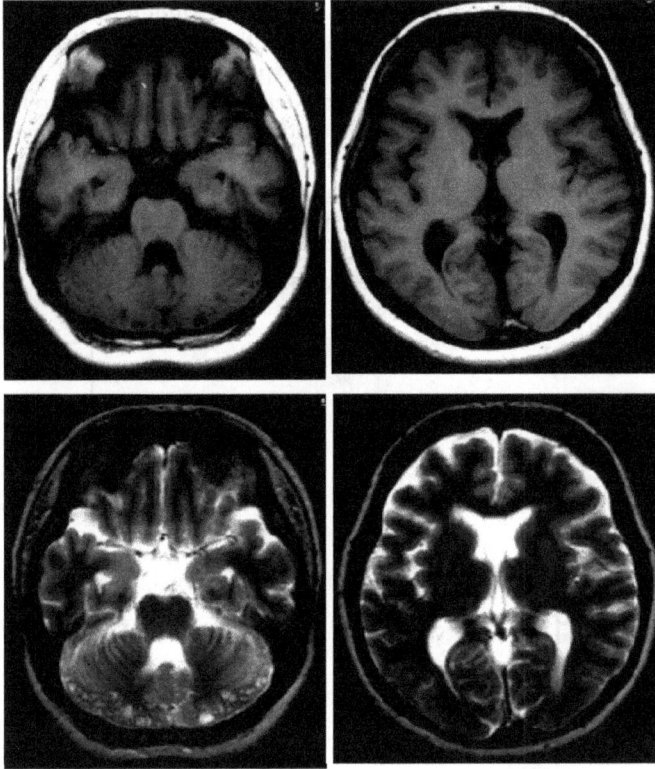

Fig. 4. Typical MR imaging in a FCMD patient aged 16 years. T1-(upper) and T2-(lower) weighted axial magnetic resonance images of the cerebellum (left) and cerebrum (right). Cerebral cortical dysplasia is mild, and numerous cysts closely related to polymicrogyria are seen in the cerebellum (Reproduced from Yoshioka et al., 2008).

Based on these observations, we considered the clinical spectrum of FCMD to be much broader than previously described and to overlap with that of "mild" WWS and of MEB.

2.2 Genetic study of S-family and further analyses of FCMD haplotype

The FCMD locus was initially localized to chromosome 9q31-33 by genetic linkage analysis and homozygosity mapping (Toda et al., 1993, 1994).

We analyzed one Japanese family (S-family) in which three siblings were affected with severe cerebral malformations in association with ocular anomalies and muscle disease (Yoshioka et al., 1992). Both parents were healthy and nonconsanguineous. The elder brother showed pachygyria on computed tomographic scan (Fig.5), retinal detachment in both eyes at the age of three years and dystrophic findings on a muscle biopsy. He was diagnosed clinically as having FCMD. The second pregnancy resulted in a male infant with anencephaly who survived for five minutes. Anencephaly was regarded as WWS with extreme brain abnormality. The third son exhibited at birth such characteristic features as pachygyria, encephalocele, hydrocephalus, retinal detachment in both eyes, elevated serum creatine kinase activity, and arthrogryposis multiplex congenita which were consistent with WWS (Fig.5).

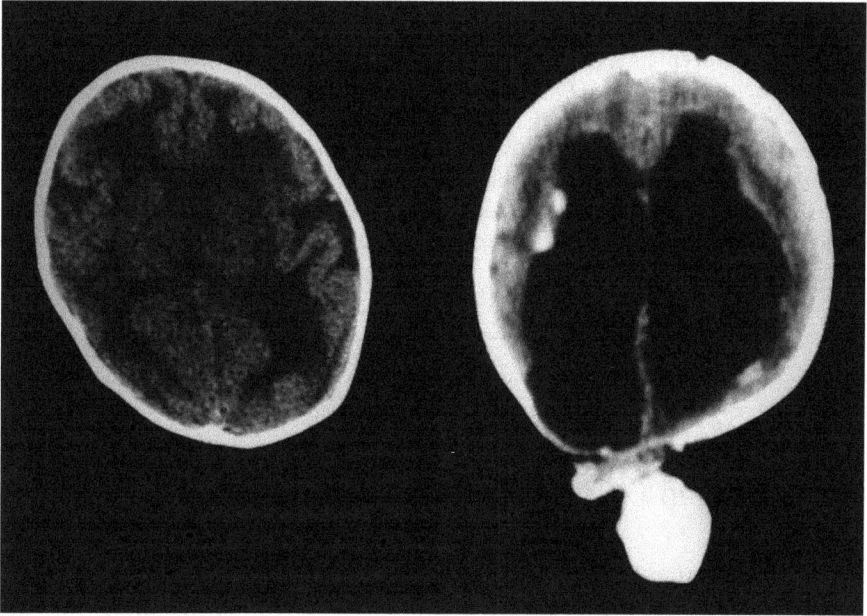

Fig. 5. Cranial computed tomographic scans of two siblings of S-family. Left: the first son at the age of 5 months. Moderate dilatation of the lateral ventricles, especially posteriorly (colpocephalic) and pachygyria in the temporo-parietal region are shown. The low density area in the white matter is apparent. Right: the third son at birth. Marked dilatation of lateral ventricles and occipital encephalocele are evident (Reproduced from Yoshioka & Kuroki, 1994).

Genetic analysis of this family was performed using polymorphic microsatellite markers flanking the FCMD locus (Toda et al., 1995). Genomic DNA was extracted from peripheral blood leukocytes of the parents, the first and the third siblings. Both patients (FCMD and WWS) shared exactly the same haplotype at seven marker loci spanning 16 cM and surrounding the FCMD locus. This suggests that both affected siblings should carry the same combination of FCMD alleles, each with a mutation. Since the patients of FCMD and WWS carry the identical combination of mutations on either allele of the FCMD locus, these clinical conditions are caused by the mutations in the same gene. The difference in clinical manifestations between FCMD and WWS may reflect the pleiotropy or variation of expressivity of the FCMD gene.

Later, it was found that one specific haplotype was shared by 82% of FCMD chromosomes (Kobayashi et al., 1998b). These data supported the hypothesis of a single founder of this disease in the Japanese population. Moreover, eight haplotypes different from the founder's were observed in FCMD chromosomes, indicating that eight different FCMD mutations in addition to the founder's have occurred in Japan. Thereafter, it was clarified that a retrotransposal insertion exists within this candidate-gene interval in all FCMD chromosomes carrying the founder haplotype. Two independent point mutations confirm that a mutation of this gene is responsible for the condition (Kobayashi et al., 1998a).

Using new polymorphic microsatellite markers, we genotyped five CMD patients from four families including the S-family who had severe eye and brain anomalies, such as retinal dysplasia and hydrocephalus (Yoshioka et al., 1999). All patients were heterozygous for the founder haplotype of the FCMD gene. In S-family, the Japanese founder haplotype of the FCMD gene was derived from the patients' mother and the haplotype, which cosegregate with nonsense mutation on exon 3 of the FCMD gene, was derived from their father (Fig. 6). Thus, two siblings were compound heterozygotes for FCMD. This showed severe eye anomalies such as retinal dysplasia or detachment and hydrocephalus could be included in the clinical spectrum of FCMD. The clinical spectrum of FCMD is much broader than previously presumed.

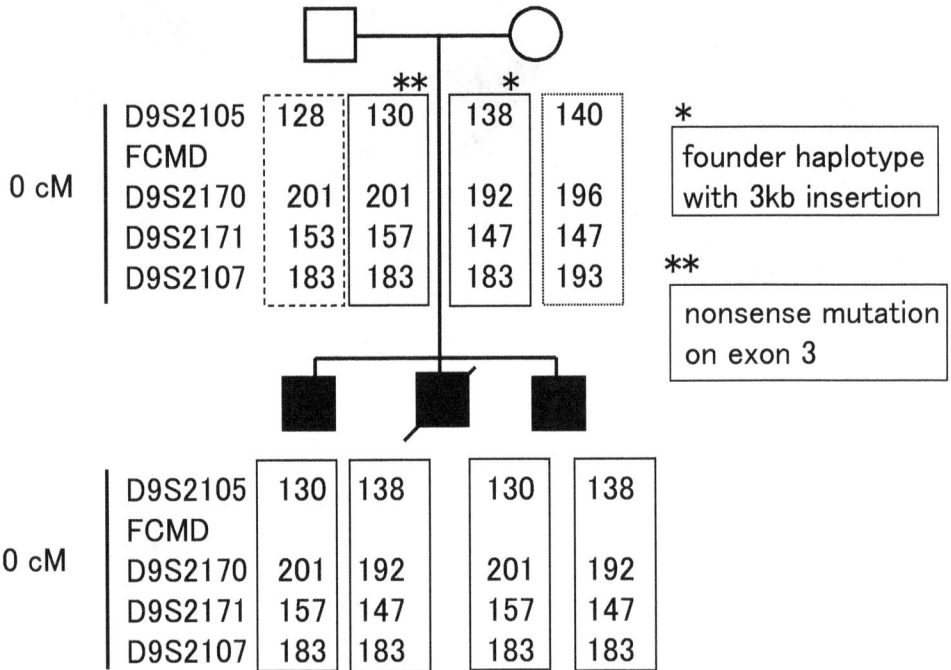

Fig. 6. Genotypes of S-family including two brothers at polymorphic microsatellite loci flanking the FCMD locus. This family is heterozygous for the founder insertion allele. The founder haplotype 138-192-147-183 for markers D9S2105-D9S2170-D9S2171-D9S2107 was derived from the patients' mother and the haplotype 130-201-157-183, which cosegregated with nonsense mutation on exon 3 of the FCMD gene, was derived from their father. Thus, two brothers are compound heterozygotes for the disease (Reproduced from Yoshioka et al., 1999).

To investigate the distribution and origin of the founder insertion of FCMD, Watanabe et al. (2005) screened a total of 4,718 control DNA samples from Japanese and other Northeast

Asian population. Fifteen founder chromosomes were detected among 2,814 Japanese individuals. Heterozygous carriers were found in various regions throughout Japan, with an averaged ratio of 1 in 188, although previous reports have estimated the carrier frequency to be as high as 1 in 80 and the incidence to be 3-10/100,000 births (Fukuyama & Ohsawa, 1984). In Korean populations, they detected one carrier in 935 individuals. However, they were unable to detect any heterozygous alleles in 203 Mongolians and 766 Mainland Chinese populations. These data largely rule out the possibility that a single ancestor bearing an insertion-chromosome immigrated to Japan from Korea or Mainland China and appear to confirm that FCMD carriers are rare outside of Japan.

2.3 Phenotype-genotype relationship in FCMD after discovery of FCMD gene, *FKTN*

Between 1994 and 2006, we diagnosed thirty-five patients with FCMD because they had the founder mutation homozygously or heterozygously, in Kobe City Pediatric and General Rehabilitation Center for the Challenged, Utano National Hospital, Shiga Medical Center for Children and Shizuoka Childrens's Hospital (Yoshioka et al., 2008). Among these 35 patients, we found 18 patients (eight boys and 10 girls) carrying a homozygous founder mutation (homozygous patients or homozygotes) and 17 patients (eight boys and nine girls) with a compound heterozygous mutation (heterozygous patients or heterozygotes). The range of follow-up was between one and 30 years (average 16.5 years) in homozygotes and between two and 19 years (average 12.8 years) in heterozygotes (Table 2).

	Homozygous patients	Heterozygous patients
Number of patients	18	17
Male : Female	8 : 10	8 : 9
Follow-up period : mean	16.5 years	12.8 years
Range : years : months	1 : 2~30 : 8	2 : 5~19 : 5
Maximum motor ability		
Bedridden	2	8
Head control	0	3
Sit without help	15	4
Walk without help	1	2
Mental status		
No meaningful words	2	11
Speak single words	5	5
Speak in sentences	11	1
Radiological findings		
Pachygyria/polymicrogyria	16	16
Hydrocephalus	0	2
Cephalocele	0	1
Ophthalmological findings		
Retinal dysplasia	0	7
Retinal detachment	0	5

Table 2. Clinical characteristics of FCMD patients diagnosed between 1994 and 2006 (Reproduced from Yoshioka et al., 2008)

Genomic DNA was extracted from patients' peripheral blood leukocytes. After digestion of genomic DNA with *Pvu*II, Southern hybridization was performed using fEco8-1 as a probe to detect the 3 kb founder insertion in the DNA. If a patient had only one founder insertion (compound heterozygotes), we then screened all exons and flanking introns of the *FKTN* gene by polymeraze chain reaction direct sequencing to detect nonsense or missense mutations. Some members had been genotyped with polymorphic microsatellite markers as described previously (Kobayashi et al., 1998b). Each chromosome containing the 3 kb retrotransposal insertion was concordant with the founder haplotype represented as 138-192-147-183 for markers D9S2105-D9S2170-D9S2171-D9S2107.

Clinical characteristics in both groups are summarized in Table 2. Most homozygotes could sit without help and speak in sentences, while half of the heterozygotes were bedridden and most spoke no meaningful words. Typical CT or MRI findings of FCMD were seen in almost all cases. These included polymicrogyria within the cerebral cortex that was primarily in the frontal lobes (Figs.4 and 5). In the cerebellum, numerous intraparenchymal cysts closely related to the polymicrogyria were seen at the hemispheres (Fig.4). More severe cortical dysplasia was usually found in heterozygotes than in homozygotes. Hydrocephalus and cephalocele were found only in heterozygotes. In particular, ophthalmological findings showed a clear difference between the two groups; retinal dysplasia and detachment were only found in heterozygotes.

In comparison with our study, systematic analysis of the FCMD gene in 107 unrelated patients by Kondo-Iida et al. (1999) revealed that 80 probands (75%) were homozygous for the 3 kb insertion, 25 (23%) were heterozygous, and two did not show the 3 kb insertion on either allele. In our study, however, the number of homozygotes and heterozygotes was almost the same. Although both groups included some sib pairs in our study, the number of probands was 16 for the homozygotes and 15 for the heterozygotes, which was also almost the same number. This result might be due to the small number of patients examined or a regional inclination in our study, as most of our patients lived in the western part (Kansai district) of Japan.

According to the report by Kondo-Iida et al. (1999), among patients homozygous for the founder mutation, 91.5% showed milder (stand or walk with or without support) or typical (able to sit unassisted or to slide on buttocks) phenotypes, and only 2.5% of cases were classified as severe (could sit only with support or had no head control), while among patients with heterozygous for the founder mutation, 92% showed severe phenotypes. This was true in our study, as most homozygotes could sit without help, while half of the heterozygotes were bedridden. It was speculated that because the 3'-UTR of a gene affects the stability of its mRNA, the 3 kb sequence inserted in that portion of the FCMD gene may alter the secondary structure of FCMD mRNA and render it unstable. This notion is supported by RT-PCR analysis that revealed low levels of the expected amplification product occurred in patients who were homozygous for the founder mutation and lower than normal in patients heterozygous for the insertion and another mutation. In other words, chromosomes carrying the 3 kb insertion may merely produce a lower level of mature fukutin than normal and generate a relatively mild phenotype. On the other hand, nonfounder mutations, which include nonsense and missense mutations within the coding region, cause major structural changes in the fukutin protein and thus are likely to produce severe effects.

2.4 Seizure-genotype relationship in FCMD patients diagnosed between 1994 and 2006

Mutational analysis of 35 patients with FCMD is shown in Table 3. Each chromosome containing the 3 kb retrotransposal insertion was concordant with the founder haplotype represented as 138-192-147-183 for markers D9S2105-D9S2170-D9S2171-D9S2107. Eighteen patients were homozygous for the 3 kb insertion and 17 were heterozygous. Mutations other than the 3 kb insertion were identified seven of the 12 heterozygous patients examined. These included five patients with a nonsense mutation in exon 3, one patient with a missense mutation in exon 5 and one patient with a nonsense mutation in exon 8. Among five patients with mutation in exon 3, afebrile seizures were found in three patients. One of them showed intractable seizures and the other developed infantile spasms at age six months. Two of five patients with a mutation in exon 3 had no seizures during follow-up as they died at ages 2 and 5 years, respectively, raising the possibility that seizures could

Haplotype	Location	Mutation	Type of mutation	No. of patients	Seizure status No. of patients
Homozygous for the founder haplotype (138-192-147-183)	3′ Untranslated region	3 Kb insertion	Instability of mRNA	18	Afebrile seizures : 8 Febrile seizures : 3 No seizure : 7
Heterozygous for the founder haplotype*				17	Afebrile seizures : 9 Febrile seizures : 5 No seizure : 3
130-201-157-183	Exon 3	R47X	Nonsense	5	Afebrile seizures : 3 (Intractable : 1, infantile spasms : 1) No seizure : 2 (died aged 2 and 5 years)
Not examined	Exon 5	M133T	Missense	1	Afebrile seizures : 1 (Intractable : 1)
Not examined	Exon 8	R307X	Nonsense	1	Febrile seizures : 1
139-201-155-183	Unknown**	Unknown	Unknown	4	Afebrile seizures : 3 (Intractable : 2) Febrile seizures : 1
148-196-153-183	Unknown	Unknown	Unknown	1	Febrile seizures : 1
128-199-155-183	Not done***	Not done	Not done	1	Afebrile seizures : 1
138-194-155-183	Not done	Not done	Not done	1	Febrile seizures : 1
138-199-147-191	Not done	Not done	Not done	1	No seizure : 1
138-196-147-191	Not done	Not done	Not done	1	Febrile seizures : 1
Not examined	Not done	Not done	Not done	1	Afebrile seizures : 1

* Haplotypes other than the founder's haplotype are shown below.
** Sequence analyzed, but no mutation found
*** Sequence analysis was not done yet.

Table 3. Relationship between genotypes and seizures in FCMD patients (Reproduced from Yoshioka et al., 2008).

develop later. All five patients also showed severe clinical manifestations suggestive of WWS. One patient with a missense mutation in exon 5 had intractable complex partial seizures and severe psychomotor retardation. However, one patient aged six years with a nonsense mutation in exon 8 developed a febrile seizure at the age of four years four months and he had no EEG paroxysmal discharges. On the other hand, five of twelve patients who underwent sequence analysis of chromosome without the 3 kb insertion revealed no mutation within the coding region of *FKTN*. It is probable that the mutations in these alleles lie in regulatory regions such as promoter sequences or intronic sequences critical for alternative splicing. Among them, four patients showed the same haplotype, 139-201-155-183, for markers D9S2105-D9S2170-D9S2171-D9S2107 and showed severe phenotypes. In addition, two of them had intractable seizures.

It is interesting that in this study seven of 18 (39%) homozygous and three of 17 (18%) heterozygous patients had no seizures during follow-up. Although two of our heterozygotes without seizures died at ages 2 and 5 years, respectively, all homozygotes without seizures were older than four years and two patients were over 30 years of age.

In addition, some had only febrile seizures throughout their life. Antiepileptic drugs were prescribed for half of the FCMD patients and no intractable seizures were observed in homozygotes. These facts showed that seizures occurring in FCMD patients were not always severe. Milder cortical dysplasia was suggested in FCMD, especially in homozygotes.

From these observations, it was concluded that mutational analysis of the FCMD gene could predict seizure prognosis. Heterozygotes usually developed seizures earlier than homozygotes and some heterozygotes showed intractable seizures. Special attention is necessary when treating epilepsy in heterozygotes. Mutational analysis other than the 3 kb insertion and haplotype analysis may also help to predict seizure prognosis.

2.5 Worldwide distribution of *Fukutin* mutation

A Turkish geneticist who had read our paper (Yoshioka et al., 1999) asked us to analyze her CMD patient. This Turkish boy had characteristics of WWS. Parents were first cousins, and their first son was unaffected. The infant was born by cesarean section and weighed 2,700 gm (25th percentile); his height was 50cm (50th percentile), and head circumference was 47 cm (>97th percentile). Physical examination showed respiratory difficulties, central cyanosis, generalized hypotonia, hydrocephaly, bilateral buphthalmus, and cataracts. Rieger's anomaly with iris atrophy and peripheral corneal adhesions was noticed. After cataract extraction of the right eye, ocular examination showed that the optic disc and the retina were hypoplastic. Cranial computed tomography showed hydrocephalus and cortical atrophy. After birth, this patient was supported by mechanical ventilation and died on the 10th day. Neuropathological examination showed agyric hemispheres with polymicrogyria in several cortical segments and severe cortical disorganization in other segments. The ventricles released 600ml of cerebrospinal fluid. CMD was also seen, with variation in fiber size, and fibrosis. Immunohistochemical analysis showed greatly reduced staining for alpha-dystroglycan, but normal immunoreactivity for beta-dystroglycan in the skeletal muscle membrane. Serum creatine kinase levels were greatly elevated.

Genetic analysis of this family was performed. As expected, the patient had no Japanese founder insertion. We then screened all exons and flanking introns of the fukutin gene in the patient by polymerase chain reaction direct sequencing. We detected a homozygous 1bp insertion mutation, nt504(insT), in exon 5 of *FKTN*. This mutation causes a frameshift, resulting in a premature termination at codon 157. Both parents and the brother were heterozygous for this mutation. This is the first case worldwide in which a *FKTN* mutation has been found outside the Japanese population (Silan et al., 2003).

Later, another Turkish boy with WWS phenotype was found to have a homozygous nonsense mutation in *FKTN* by the research group in the Netherlands (Beltran-Valero de Bernabe et al., 2003). The homozygous nonsense mutations within the coding region identified in two Turkish patients are predicted to cause a total loss of *FKTN* and are likely to produce a more severe phenotype which closely resembles WWS.

Manzini et al. (2008) assembled a large cohort of patients with typical WWS (43 affected individuals from 40 families), drawn from Middle Eastern consanguineous families (16 patients from 14 families) and from consanguineous and nonconsanguineous families from Europe and the Americas (27 cases). They found that 40% (16/40 families) of patients in their cohort carried mutations in the coding sequence of *POMT1*, *POMT2*, *FKRP* or *FKTN* with no *POMGnT1* or *LARGE* mutations detected. *FKTN* and *FKRP* mutations in particular were much more common than previously suggested and were mostly identified in non-consanguineous patients of European descent (6/27 cases). All Ashkenazi Jewish patients in their group shared an identical haplotype at the *FKTN* locus and the same homozygous mutation c.1167_1168insA in exon 9 suggesting a founder effect in this population. They identified the carrier frequency of this mutation to be 0.7% in the Ashkenazi population in Israel, which will be extremely informative for genetic testing. A striking difference was observed in the geographic distribution of mutations, as Middle East families were mostly carriers of *POMT1* mutations (35.7%, 5/14 families), while the most common cause of European/American cases was *FKTN* mutations (18.5%, 5/27 cases). An additional four USA Ashkenazi Jewish families with WWS were found to have a founder mutation in *FKTN* in this population (Chang et al., 2009).

The cohort consisted of 92 unrelated individuals who showed hypoglycosylation of alpha-dystroglycan at the sarcolemma by immunolabelling of skeletal muscle sections (80 patients) or had the clinical phenotype being highly suggestive of a alpha-dystroglycanopathy (12 patients) was analyzed the mutation of genes related to alpha-dystroglycanopathy (Godfrey et al., 2007). Homozygous and compound heterozygous mutations were detected in a total of 31 probands (34 individuals from 31 families). Mutations in *FKTN*, typically associated with FCMD in Japan were found in six patients, none of whom are of Japanese origin. Only two of these patients had structural brain involvement; one patient affected by WWS and one by a MEB-FCMD phenotype. The remaining patients had no structural brain involvement; one case had CMD-no mental retardation and never acquired the ability to walk but has normal IQ and five individuals from three families have entirely normal intellect and a mild LGMD phenotype (LGMD 2M). Interestingly in the latter two of these families, a dramatic response to steroid therapy was noted (Godfrey et al., 2006).

Vuillaumier-Barrot et al. (2009) reported four newly diagnosed Caucasian patients with *FKTN* mutations with a broad spectrum of phenotypes ranging from CMD associated with mental retardation to LGMD without central nervous system involvement. Two patients (two sisters) presented with CMD, mental retardation, and posterior fossa malformation including cysts, and brain atrophy at brain MRI. The other two patients had normal intelligence and brain MRI. Sequencing of the *FKTN* gene identified three previously described mutations and two novel misssense mutations.

In contrast to studies in Middle East families and European/American cases, a 10-year-old Korean boy with clinical features of FCMD was found to have homozygous Japanese insertion mutation (Lee et al., 2009). His parents were heterozygous carriers of the same mutation. He is the first genetically confirmed FCMD patient in Korea and the first non-Japanese patient carrying homozygous Japanese founder mutation. According to a large northeast Asian population study (Watanabe et al., 2005), the carrier frequency of 3-kb insertion mutation in Korean population is 1 in 935. Based on this observation, the incidence of FCMD by 3-kb insertion mutation is as low as 1 in 3,496,900 in Korea. On the other hand, the Japanese founder mutation was not detected in 766 mainland Chinese individuals (Watanabe et al., 2005). However, the first FCMD case was reported in the Chinese population with a Japanese founder 3-kb insertion and the other copy with a known c.139C>T mutation (Xiong et al., 2009). These Asian case reports emphasize the importance of considering the *FKTN* founder mutation for diagnostic purposes outside of Japan and suggest that segments of the Chinese, Korean and Japanese populations may have a recent common ancestor.

2.6 Milder phenotype of FCMD

The first indication that *FKTN* mutations may also cause a much less severe phenotype came from Murakami et al. (2006). They reported that six Japanese patients, all of whom were compound heterozygotes for *FKTN* founder mutation and a point mutation, had minimal muscle weakness, normal intellect and dilated cardiomyopathy. No mutation was found in the other responsible genes for alpha-dystroglycanopathy including *FKRP*, *POMGnT1*, *POMT1*, *POMT2*, and *LARGE* in these patients. Pathological findings in the biopsied skeletal muscles showed only minimal dystrophic changes, but have altered glycosylation of alpha-dystroglycan and reduced laminin binding ability. Cardiac involvement is the most remarkable finding in these patients. All the patients showed dilated cardiomyopathy, and two of them had life-threatening, rapidly progressive cardiac insufficiency. Cardiac involvement is rarely described in patients with alpha-dystroglycanopathy except for some patients with LGMD 2I.

Recently, milder cases of muscular dystrophy associated with *FKTN* mutations have also been reported in non-Japanese populations. Godfrey et al. (2006, 2007) reported on five non-Japanese children from three families with normal intelligence and limb-girdle phenotype, caused by heterozygous point mutations in the *FKTN* gene. Puckett et al. (2009) reported an additional two brothers with a LGMD phenotype due to compound heterozygous *FKTN* mutation. These two brothers had elevated CK, mild muscle weakness and normal cognition. They lack any cardiac or ocular abnormalities. In addition to their mild clinical presentation, patients were also unique from an ethnic and molecular standpoint. Their father was of European descent and their mother, Japanese. The children, however, did not possess the common Japanese founder mutation. Rather, the brothers had two *FKTN* missense mutations, one of which, c527T>C, had not been previously reported. This is significant, as the vast majority of patients reported have been either homozygous or heterozygous for the common retrotransposon insertion. Despite the milder skeletal muscle phenotype of these patients and those reported by Murakami et al. (2006), muscle biopsies show a reduction in fully glycosylated alpha-dystroglycan similar to severe forms of CMD, such as FCMD and MEB. This emphasizes that immunophenotype may correlate poorly with clinical severity.

3. Japanese patients with alpha-dystroglycanopthy with other gene mutations than *FKTN*

In Japan, FCMD is the most common form of CMD, whereas MEB, WWS, MDC1C and MDC1D were rarely seen. WWS has been observed in many population groups with a worldwide distribution (Dobyns et al., 1989). In contrast, both MEB and FCMD show striking founder effects. MEB was first described in Finland, where it is most prevalent, owing to a strong founder effect following by genetic drift (Santavuori et al., 1989, Haltia et al., 1997). Consequently, most MEB patients have come from a small, geographically isolated population in Finland, with few Caucasian exceptions. Taniguchi et al. (2003) examined 30 patients from various countries, including Japan and Korea, who were diagnosed as WWS, severe FCMD or MEB. Two Japanese patients were identified as compound heterozygotes of *POMGnT1* mutations. Severe hydrocephalus was observed prenatally by an ultrasonograph in both patients, and in one of them hydrocephalus required a ventriculo-peritoneal shunt at one year of age. Therefore, MEB patients may exist with a broader distribution than previously expected. Later, Matsumoto et al. (2005) performed detailed genetic and clinico-pathological analyses on 62 Japanese patients whose limb-muscle specimens showed altered glycosylation of alpha-dystroglycan. *FKTN* mutations were found in 54 patients (86%) examined, reflecting the most common form of CMD in Japan. In this study, the first patient with MDC1C (*FKRP* mutation) in oriental countries was found. Clinically, this patient showed severe muscle weakness from early infancy, marked elevation of serum CK level, calf hypertrophy, and normal intelligence; those are consistent with MDC1C. Further, the structural abnormality in the cerebellum was seen on brain MRI including disorganized folia and multiple cysts, those are commonly observed in FCMD/MEB. In addition, two MEB (*POMGnT1* mutations) and one WWS (*POMT1* mutation) were genetically confirmed. These studies show that patients with alpha-dystroglycanopathy in Japan have not only *FKTN* mutations but also have mutations of other genes such as *POMT1*, *POMT2*, *POMGnT1* and *FKRP*. Molecular genetic studies have been helpful in defining subgroups of CMD.

4. CMD patients without known gene mutations of alpha-dystroglycanopathy

We studied a Japanese CMD patient with brain abnormalities without *FKTN* mutation using immunohistochemical analysis of dystrophic muscle and full mutational analysis of *POMGnT1* and *FKRP* genes (Yoshioka et al., 2004).

Hypotonia and generalized muscle weakness became apparent during the first year of life. Consanguineous marriage was not noted. He obtained head control at 4 months, rolled over at 9 months, learned to sit unsupported at 12 months, crept at 19 months and stood with support at 26 months of age. At 4 years he could walk with the short leg braces using walker and speak two-word's sentences. Serum creatine kinase levels were markedly elevated (2,776 IU/L, normal range < 130 IU/L). Brain MRI showed thick and bumpy cortices with shallow sulci and abnormal white matter changes (Fig. 7). Ophthalmologically, he had no abnormalities. Immunohistochemical analysis showed reduced staining of alpha-dystroglycan, while expression of merosin and beta-dystroglycan was normal (Fig. 8). Sequence analysis of *POMGnT1* and *FKRP* revealed no mutation.

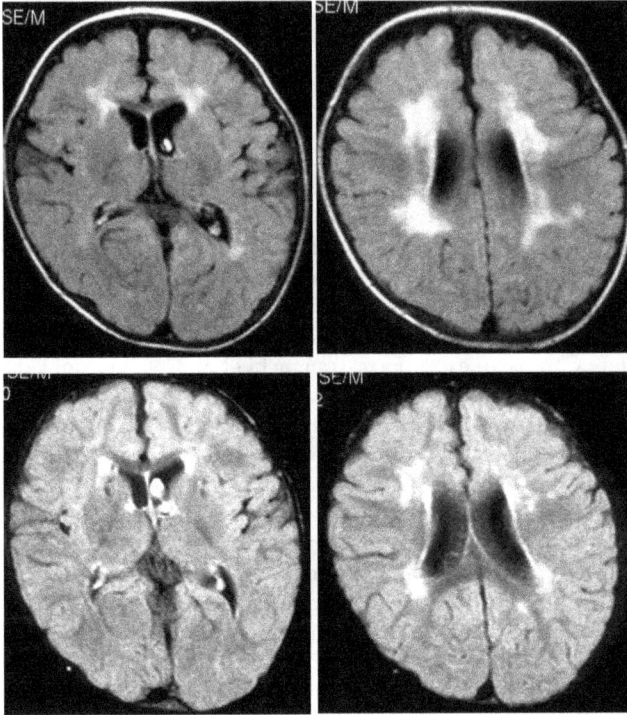

Fig. 7. MR imaging at 15 months of age (the upper line) and 26 months of age (the lower line) on T2-weighted sequences. The cerebral white matter shows symmetric high intensity, which decreases with age (Reproduced from Yoshioka et al. , 2004).

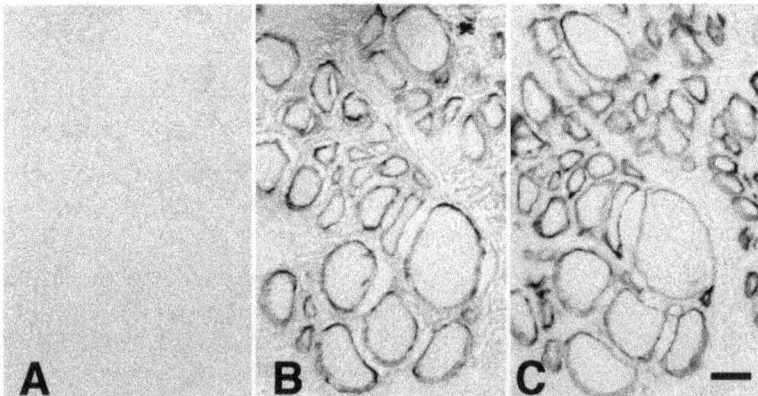

Fig. 8. Immunohistochemistry. Transverse serial frozen sections of skeletal muscle biopsies from the patient were immunostained with antibodies against alpha-dystroglycan (A), beta-dystroglycan (B), and laminin alpha-2 (merosin) (C). Note that beta-dystroglycan and laminin alpha-2 were present but alpha-dystroglycan was absent in sarcolemma of muscle fibers. Scale bar=20 micrometer (Reproduced from Yoshioka et al.,2004).

From these observations, this CMD patient seemed to belong to alpha-dystroglycanopathy. However, sequence analysis of *FKTN, POMGnT1 and FKRP* showed no mutations. Although analyses of *POMT1, POMT2* and *LARGE* are necessary, there seems to be still many CMDs whose causative genes are unknown. We previously reported these patients including this case as a variant of CMD (Yoshioka et al., 2002).

Among their 62 Japanese patients with alpha-dystroglycanopathy, Matsumoto et al. (2005) found four patients with no mutation in the known genes associated with glycosylation defects of alpha-dystroglycan. They were clinically diagnosed to have MEB or WWS. All four patients showed severe mental retardation, hypotonia from early infancy, and eye involvements. Brain MRI displayed type II lissencephaly, enlarged lateral ventricles, and hypoplastic brainstem and cerebellum. In the skeletal muscles, three patients who were clinically diagnosed as WWS showed severe dystrophic changes with marked fibrous tissue involvement. However, one patient who was clinically diagnosed as MEB showed only mild myopathic changes in his muscle.

It was true in non-Japanese patients with alpha-dystroglycanopathy. Although 31 among 92 probands (34%) with alpha-dystroglycanopathy had homozygous and compound heterozygous mutations in the known genes, a large number of remaining patients with clinico-pathological features indistinguishable from the ones with mutations were not found to have mutations in any of the genes studied (Godfrey et al., 2007). More, as yet undefined, genes are likely to be involved in the pathogenesis of the alpha-dystroglycanopathies. The identification of these genes may provide additional information on the pathway of glycosylation of alpha-dystroglycan.

5. Conclusion

Defects in genes responsible for altered glycosylation of alpha-dystroglycan cause a group of muscular dystrophies that are variably associated with central nervous and eye abnormalities, known as alpha-dystroglycanopathies. These comprise FCMD, MDC1C and 1D, WWS, and MEB. Mutations have been reported in six putative or demonstrated glycosyltransferases; *FKTN, FKRP, LARGE, POMT1, POMT2,* and *POMGnT1.* Although each disorder was initially associated with one gene, it has recently been shown that the spectrum of phenotypes is broader than previously thought, and all these syndromes can be associated with mutations in any of the six genes known to be involved in alpha-dystroglycan glycosylation (Fig. 1).

A wide clinical spectrum is also evident for the *FKTN* mutations that were first reported in patients with FCMD, and later also in patients with WWS, and in patients with LGMD. FCMD is most frequent in Japan, and relatively homogenous phenotype. The strikingly high prevalence of FMD among the Japanese appears to result from the initial founder effect, whose expansion occurred in relative isolation. Most FCMD-bearing chromosomes in Japan are derived from a single ancestral founder who lived a few thousands years ago. Seventy-five percent of Japanese patients are homozygous for the ancestral mutation and have a relatively milder phenotype than patients who are compound heterozygous for the ancestral mutation and another mutation. The Japanese founder 3′ insertion mutation is therefore regarded as a relatively mild mutation. The most common form of FCMD in Japan presents clinically with a combination of generalized muscle weakness, congenital structural brain malformations, seizures, decreased vision, and cardiomyopathy. Most patients are never able to walk independently and have moderate to severe cognitive delay. Japanese patients, who are compound heterozygous for the founder and another mutation, have much more severe WWS-like manifestations including hydrocephalus and microphthalmia.

However, an increasing number of *FKTN* mutations are being reported outside Japan. To date, at least 24 different *FKTN* mutations have been described in non-Japanese patients and phenotypes of these patients cover the entire range of alpha-dystroglycanopathies (Yis et al., 2011). Among 23 patients with CMD and mutations in the *FKTN* gene in non-Japanese populations, 10 patients had a WWS-like phenotype including severe brain and eye abnormalities, the remainder had a milder FCMD, MEB or LGMD phenotype. In addition to the Japanese founder mutation, the mutation c.1167insA in exon 9 has been found to be homozygous in seven non-consanguineous Ashkenazi Jewish families, with an estimated carrier frequency of the mutation of 0.7% in the Ashkenazi population in Israel. Affected patients in these Jewish families all had a severe WWS-like phenotype.

The WWS phenotype caused by *FKTN* mutations is associated with the presence of two loss-of-function mutations, although not an absolute rule. The relatively few reports of *FKTN* mutations in patients with mild phenotypes may be a result of ascertainment bias and the recent increase in the number of reports of such findings may result in increased mutation analysis in *FKTN* for such patients in the future.

In summary, these results confirm that outside Japan, muscular dystrophy due to *FKTN* mutations is not as rare as initially supposed, and could be associated with a large spectrum of phenotypes, compared to the relatively homogenous phenotype in the Japanese population.

Although alpha-dystroglycanopathy is still largely unknown, comprehensive mutation analysis in patients and genotype/phenotype correlation across the spectrum of disease caused by these genes may provide clues to gene function. Functional analysis in animal models will determine how these mutations affect the proteins.

6. References

Beltran-Valero de Bernabe D, van Bokhoven H, van Beusekom E, van den Akker W, Kant S, Dobyns WB, Cormand B, Currier S, Hamel B, Talim B, Topaloglu H & Brunner HG. (2003) A homozygous nonsense mutation in the fukutin gene causes a Walker-Warburg syndrome phenotype. *Journal of Medical Genetics* Vol.40, No.11, (November 2003), pp.845-848, ISSN 0022-2593

Chang W, Winder TI, LeDuc CA, Simpson LL, Millar WS, Dungan J, Ginsberg N, Plaga S, Moore SA & Chung WK. (2009) Founder *Fukutin* mutation causes Walker-Warburg syndrome in four Ashkenazi Jewish families. *Prenatal Diagnosis* Vol.29, No.6 (June 2009), pp.560-569, ISSN 0197-3851

Dobyns WB, Pagon RA, Armstrong D, Curry CJR, Greenberg F, Grix A, Holmes LB, Laxova R, Michels VV, Robinow M & Zimmerman RL. (1989) Diagnostic criteria for Walker-Warburg syndrome. *American Journal of Medical Genetics* Vol. 32, No. 2 (February 1989), pp.195-210, ISSN 0148-7299

Fukuyama Y, Kawazura M & Haruna H. (1960) A peculiar form of congenital progressive muscular dystrophy. Report of fifteen cases. *Paediatria Universitatis Tokyo* Vol. 4, No.4, (April 1960) pp.5-8, ISSN 0030-9303

Fukuyama Y, Osawa M & Suzuki H. (1981) Congenital progressive muscular dystrophy of the Fukuyama type --- clinical, genetic and pathological considerarions----. *Brain & Development* Vol.3, No.1, pp.1-29, ISSN 0387-7604

Fukuyama Y & Ohsawa M. (1984) A genetic study of the Fukuyama type congenital muscular dystrophy. *Brain&Development* Vol. 6, No. 4 , pp373-390, ISSN 0387-7604

Godfrey C, Escolar D, Brockington M, Clement EM, Mein R, Jimenez-Mallebrera C, Torelli S, Feng L, Brown SC, Sewry CA, Rutherford M, Shapira Y, Abbs S & Muntoni F. (2006) Fukutin gene mutations in steroid-responsive limb girdle muscular dystrophy. *Annals of Neurology* Vol. 60, No.5 (November 2006), pp.603-610, ISSN 0364-5134

Godfrey C, Clement E, Mein R, Brockington M, Smith J, Talim B, Straub V, Robb S, Quinlivan R, Feng L, Jimenez-Mallebrera C, Mercuri E, Manzur AY, Kinali M, Torelli S, Brown SC, Sewry CA, Bushby K, Topaloglu H, North K, Abbs S & Muntoni F. (2007) Refining genotype-phenotype correlations in muscular dystrophies with defective glycosylation of dystroglycan. *Brain* Vol. 130, No. 10, (October 2007), pp.2725-2735, ISSN 0006-8950

Haltia M, Leivo I, Somer H, Pihko H, Paetau A, Kivela T, Tarkkanen A, Tome F, EngvallE & Santavuori P. (1997) Muscle-eye-brain disease: A neuropathological study. *Annals of Neurology* Vol. 41, No. 2, (February 1997), pp.173-180, ISSN 0364-5134

Kobayashi K, Nakahori Y, Miyake M, Matsumura K, Kondo-Iida E, Nomura Y, Segawa M, Yoshioka M, Saito K, Osawa M, Hamano K, Sasakihara Y, Nonaka I, Nakagome Y, Kanazawa I, Nakamura Y, Tokunaga K & Toda T. (1998a) An ancient retrotransposal insertion causes Fukuyama-type congenital muscular dystrophy. *Nature* Vol. 394, No. 6691, (July 1998), pp. 388-392, ISSN 0028-0836

Kobayashi K, Nakahori Y, Mizuno K, Miyake M, Kumagai Y, Honma A, Nonaka I, Nakamura Y, Tokunaga K & Toda T. (1998b). Founder-haplotype analysis in Fukuyama-type congenital muscular dystrophy (FCMD). *Human Genetics* Vol. 103, No.3, (September 1998), pp. 323-327, ISSN 0340-6717

Kondo-Iida E, Kobayashi K, Watanabe M, Sasaki J, Kumagai T, Koide H, Saito K, Osawa M, Nakamura Y & Toda T. (1999) Novel mutations and genotype-phenotype relationships in 107 families with Fukuyama-type congenital muscular dystrophy (FCMD). *Human Molecular Genetics* Vol. 8, No. 12, (November 1999), pp.2303-2309, ISSN 0964-6906

Lee J, Lee BL, Lee M, Kim JH, Kim JW & Ki CS. Clinical and genetic analysis of a Korean patient with Fukuyama congenital muscular dystrophy. (2009) *Journal of the Neurological Sciences* Vol. 281, No. 1−2, (June 2009), pp. 122-124, ISSN 0022-510X

Manzini MC, Gleason D, Chang BS, Hill S, Barry BJ, Partlow JN, Poduri A, Currier S, Galvin-Parto P, Shapiro LR, Schmidt K, Davis JG, Basel-Vanagaite L, Seidahmed MZ, Salih MAM, Dobyns WB & Walsh CA. (2008) Ethnically diverse causes of Walker-Warburg syndrome (WWS): FCMD mutations are a more common cause of WWS outside of the Middle East. *Human Mutation* Vol. 29, No.11, (November 2008) E231-241, ISSN 1098-1004

Matsumoto H, Hayashi YK, Kim DS, Ogawa M, Murakami T, Noguchi S, Nonaka I, Nakazawa T, Matsuo T, Futagami S, Campbell KP & Nishino I. (2005) Congenital muscular dystrophy with glycosylation defects of alpha-dystroglycan in Japan. *Neuromuscular Disorders* Vol. 15, No. 5, (May 2005), pp.342-348, ISSN 0960-8966

Muntoni F, Brockington M, Blake DJ, Torelli S & Brown SC. (2002) Defective glycosylation in muscular dystrophy. *Lancet* Vol.360, No.9343, (November 2002), pp 1419-21, ISSN 0140-6736

Muntoni F & Voit T. (2004) The congenital muscular dystrophies in 2004: a century of exciting progress. *Neuromuscular Disorders* Vol. 14, No. 10, (October 2004), pp.635-649, ISSN 0960-8966

Murakami T, Hayashi YK, Noguchi S, Ogawa M, Nonaka I, Tanabe Y, Ogino M, Takada F, Eriguchi M, Kotooka N, Campbell KP, Osawa M & Nishino I. (2006) Fukutin gene mutations cause dilated cardiomyopathy with minimal muscle weakness. *Annals of Neurology* Vol. 60, No. 5, (November 2006), pp.597-602, ISSN 0364-5134

Puckett RL, Moore SA, Winder TL, Willer T, Romansky SG, Covault KK, Campbell KP & Abdenur JE. (2009) Further evidence of Fukutin mutations as a cause of childhood onset limb-girdle muscular dystrophy without mental retardation. *Neuromuscular Disorders* Vol. 19, No. 5, (May 2009), pp. 352-356, ISSN 0960-8966

Santavuori P, Somer H, Sainio K, Rapola J, Kruus S, Nikitin T, Ketonen L & Leisti J. (1989) Muscle-eye-brain disease (MEB). *Brain & Development* Vol. 11, No. 3, pp.147-153, ISSN 0387-7604

Silan F, Yoshioka M, Kobayashi K, Simsek E, Tunc M, Alper M, Cam M, Guven A, Fukuda Y, Kinoshita M, Kocabay K & Toda T. (2003) A new mutation of the fukutin gene in a non-Japanese patient. *Annals of Neurology* Vol. 53, No.3, (March 2003), pp.392-396, ISSN0364-5134

Taniguchi K, Kobayashi K, Saito K, Yamanouchi H, Ohnuma A, Hayashi YK, Manya H, Jin DK, Lee M, Parano E, Falsaperla R, Pavone P, Coster RV, Talim B, Steinbrecher A, Straub V, Nishino I, Topaloglu H, Voit T, Endo T & Toda T. (2003) Worldwide distribution and broader clinical spectrum of muscle-eye-brain disease. *Human Molecular Genetics* Vol.12, No.5, (March 2003), pp.527-534, ISSN 0964-6906

Toda T, Segawa M, Nomura Y, Nonaka I, Mastuda K, Ishihara T, Suzuki M, Tomita I, Origuchi Y, Ohno K, Sasaki Y, Takada K, Kawai M, Otani K, Murakami T, Saito K, Fukuyama Y, Shimizu T, Kanazawa I & Nakamura Y. (1993) Localization of a gene for Fukuyama type congenital muscular dystrophy to chromosome 9q31-33. *Nature Genetics* Vol. 5, No. 3, (November 1993) , pp 283-286, ISSN 1061-4036

Toda T, Ikegawa S, Okui K, Kondo E, Saito K, Fukuyama Y, Yoshioka M, Kumagai T, Kanazawa I & Nakamura Y. (1994) Refined mapping of a gene responsible for Fukuyama-type congenital muscular dystrophy: evidence for strong linkage disequilibrium. *American Journal of Human Genetics* Vol. 55, No.5, (November 1994), pp 946-950, ISSN 0002-9297

Toda T, Yoshioka M, Nakahori Y, Kanazawa I, Nakamura Y & Nakagome Y. (1995) Genetic identity of Fukuyama-type congenital muscular dystrophy and Walker-Warburg syndrome. *Annals Neurology* Vol. 37, No. 1, (January 1995), pp 99-101, ISSN 0364-5134

Toda T, Miyake M, Kobayashi K, Mizuno K, Saito K, Osawa M, Nakamura Y, Kanazawa I, Nakagome Y, Tokunaga K & Nakahori Y. (1996) Linkage-disequilibrium mapping narrows the Fukuyama-type congenital muscular dystrophy (FCMD) candidate region to <100 kb. *American Journal of Human Genetics* Vol. 59, No.6 , (December 1996), pp 1313-1320, ISSN 0002-9297

Vuillaumier-Barrot S, Quijano-Roy S, Bouchet-Seraphin C, Maugenre S, Peudenier S, Van den Bergh P, Marcorelles P, Avila-Smirnow D, Chelbi M, Romero NB, Carlier RY, Estournet B, Guicheney P & Seta N. (2009) Four Caucasian patients with mutations in the fukutin gene and variable clinical phenotype. *Neuromuscular Disorders* Vol. 19, No. 3, (March 2009), pp.182-188, ISSN 0960-8966

Watanabe M, Kobayashi K, Jin F, Park KS, Yamada T, Tokunaga K & Toda T. (2005) Founder SVA retrotransposal insertion in Fukuyama-type congenital muscular dystrophy and its origin in Japanese and northeast Asian populations. *American Journal of Medical Genetics* A Vol.138, No. 4, (November 2005), pp. 344-348, ISSN 0148-7299

Xiong H, Wang S, Kobayashi K, Jiang Y, Wang J, Chang X, Yuan Y, Liu J, Toda T, Fukuyama Y & Wu X. (2009) *Fukutin* gene retrotransposal insertion in a non-Japanese Fukuyama congenital muscular dystrophy [FCMD] patient. *American Journal of Medical Genetics Part A* Vol. 149A, No. 11, (November 2009), pp.2403-2408, ISSN 0148-7299

Yis U, Uyanik G, Heck PB, Smitka M, Nobel H, Ebinger F, Dirik E, Feng L, Kurul SH, Brocke K, Unalp A, Ozer E, Cakmakci H, Sewry K, Cirak S, Muntoni F, Hehr U & Morris-Rosendahl DJ. (2011) Fukutin mutations in non-Japanese patients with congenital muscular dystrophy: Less severe mutations predominate in patients with non-Walker-Warburg phenotype. *Neuromuscular Disorders* Vol. 21, No.1, (January 2011), pp.20-30, ISSN 0960-8966

Yoshioka M, Kuroki S, Nigami H, Kawai T & Nakamura H. (1992) Clinical variation within sibships in Fukuyama-type congenital muscular dystrophy. *Brain & Development* Vol. 14, No. 5 (September 1992), pp.334-337, ISSN 0387-7604

Yoshioka M & Kuroki S. (1994) Clinical spectrum and genetic studies of Fukuyama congenital muscular dystrophy. *American Journal of Medical Genetics* Vol. 53, No. 3, (November 1994), pp.245-250, ISSN 0148-7299

Yoshioka M, Toda T, Kuroki S & Hamano K. (1999) Broader clinical spectrum of Fukuyama-type congenital muscular dystrophy manifested by haplotype analysis. *Journal of Child Neurology* Vol. 14, No. 11, (November 1999), pp.711-715, ISSN 0883-0738

Yoshioka M, Kuroki K, Sasaki H & Baba T. (2002) A variant of congenital muscular dystrophy. (2002) *Brain & Development* Vol.24, No.1, (January 2002), pp.24-29, ISSN 0387-7604

Yoshioka M, Sugie K, Nishino I & Toda T. (2004) Immunohistochemical studies of a variant of congenital muscular dystrophy. *No to Hattatsu* (Japanese) Vol.36, No.1, (January 2004), pp.55-59, ISSN 0029-0831

Yoshioka M, Higuchi Y, Fujii T, Aiba H & Toda T. (2008) Seizure-genotype relationship in Fukuyama-type congenital muscular dystrophy. *Brain & Development* Vol. 30, No. 1 (January 2008), pp.59-67, ISSN 0387-7604

2

Nuclear Poly (A)-Binding Protein and Oculopharyngeal Muscular Dystrophy

Jnanankur Bag*, Quishan Wang and Rumpa Biswas Bhattacharjee
University of Guelph, Department of Molecular and Cellular Biology, Guelph, Ontario,
Canada

1. Introduction

Oculopharyngeal muscular dystrophy (OPMD) is an autosomal-dominant late-onset human genetic disease (Brais et. al, 1998). The symptoms usually appear around the age of fifty, and are characterized by drooping of the eyelid and swallowing difficulties. Both conditions may progress until the eyelid nearly or completely covers the eyeball (ptosis) and the ability to swallow is lost (dysphagia). In addition, patients suffer from proximal limb weakness; muscles of the shoulder and hip girdles may also gradually become weak. OPMD is highly prevalent amongst the French Canadian population of the Quebec province where almost one in every one thousand people is a carrier. In contrast only one in 100,000 people in Europe, including France is a carrier of OPMD. All cases of OPMD in Quebec could be traced to a single ancestor in the 15th century (Brunet et. al., 1990). OPMD is also more common amongst Bukhara Jews (Blumen et. al., 200). Possibly due to mass immigration during the 16th to 17th century, OPMD spread from Europe to many parts of the world (Hill et. al, 2001). OPMD patients have also been reported in Mexico, Thailand, Japan and China (Rivera et. al., 2008; Uyama et. al., 2000; Witoonpanich et.al., 2004; Ye et. al., 2011). A de novo germ line mutation has also been found in a Swiss OPMD patient (Gurtler et. al., 2006).

The mutation causing OPMD has been mapped to the gene encoding the nuclear poly (A) - binding protein PABPN1 at the short arm of chromosome 14 (14q11) of the human genome (Brais et. al., 1998). The human PABPN1 gene contains six GCG repeats following the AUG initiation codon. In OPMD patients expansion of the six GCG repeats to between 8-13 repeats have been found. A short poly alanines tract consisting of ten alanines is present at the N-terminal end of normal PABPN1. Six of these ten alanines are encoded by GCG while the last four alanines are coded by GCA. Compared to other trinucleotide expansion mutations such as the CAG expansion in Huntington's disease, the GCG expansion in OPMD is very modest and genetically stable. Mutations introducing two or more alanines are dominant whereas a single additional alanine expansion is recessive. Generally, the homozygous mutations exhibit more severe phenotypes than the heterozygotes. The severity of the disease increases with the increasing length of the GCG expansion, and also results in earlier onset of the disease (Messaed & Rouleau, 2009). The precise mechanism of trinucleotide repeat expansion in OPMD and other neurodegenerative diseases such as the

---

* Corresponding Author

Huntington is not clear. A slippage model, where the newly synthesized DNA strand dissociates and translocates to a new pairing position during DNA replication has been proposed. Perhaps this misalignment of the nascent strand in the repetitive tract results in the addition or deletion of repeats. Because of the stable nature of the GCG trinucleotide repeats of PABPN1 gene this model may not be applicable for the generation of mutation in OPMD patients. Unequal cross over during DNA replication may be the underlying mechanism for (GCG) repeat.

2. Structure and cellular function of PABPN1

Mammalian PABPN1 is a highly conserved nuclear RNA binding protein of 32.8 kDa with specificity for the poly (A) tract of eukaryotic mRNAs (Figure 1). It consists of one typical RRM domain with consensus RNP1 and RNP2 motifs in the central region of the polypeptide, separating the acidic glutamine rich N-terminal domain from the more basic arginine rich C- terminal domain (Kuhn et. al., 2003). The RNP domain and the C-terminal region of PABPN1 are required for binding to both RNA and its polypeptide partners. Interestingly the RNP domain of PABPN1 has no sequence similarity with the RNA binding domain of the cytoplasmic poly (A) - binding protein PABPC1 or other RNA binding proteins (Kuhn et. al., 2003). Recent crystal structure analyses of human PABPN1 suggest that PABPN1 RRM adopts a fold similar to canonical RRM structure consisting of a four stranded antiparallel β-sheet structure spatially arranged as β4β1β3β2. However, the fold of the third loop and dimerization of the crystal are distinct features of PABPN1 (Ge et. al., 2008).The nuclear localization signal is located between amino acids 289-306 and overlaps with the oligomerization domain (Abu-Baker et.al., 2005; Calado et.al., 2000). Due to the presence of the alanine tract PBPN1 is prone to aggregate formation. However, the polyalanine tract is not conserved, and is absent in Drosophila without any detectable loss of cellular function (Shinchuk et.al., 2005).

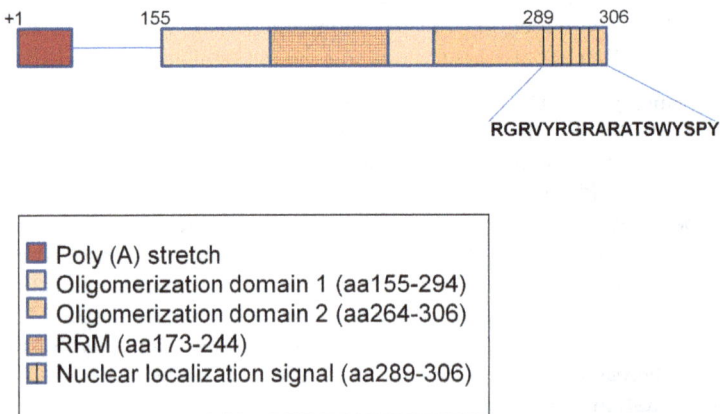

Fig. 1. Schematic diagram of various domains of PABPN1

The main cellular function of PABPN1 is to stimulate the elongation of poly (A) tract of eukaryotic mRNA, and at the same time control its length (Wahle, 1995). After the first ten adenine residues have been added PABPN1 binds to it as a monomer, and as the length of the poly (A) tract increases additional PABPN1 assembles on the tract at a packing density of 15 adenines per PABPN1 molecule (Bienroth et. al., 1993; Kuhn & Wahle, 2004; Wahle, 1995). Both cleavage and poly adenylation specific factor (CPSF) and PABPN1 stimulate the activity of poly (A) polymerase by mutually stabilizing their interaction with mRNA in a transient complex. Although both CPSF and PABPN1 alone can stimulate the polyadenylation by poly (A) polymerase but the extension of the 3` end is much faster when both are present. When the poly (A) tail length has reached 250-300 nucleotides, further extension of the poly (A) tract becomes very slow (Wahle, 1995). The oligomerization of PABPN1 is functionally important and may serve as a molecular ruler to determine the length of the poly (A) tract (Keller et. al., 2000). The wild type PABPN1 exists in equilibrium as monomers, dimmers and oligomers and filamentous complexes (Nemeth et. al., 1995). Expansion of the poly alanine tract in OPMD mutant PABPN1 enhances its aggregation property. However, no loss of cellular function due to this mutation has been detected (Messaed & Rouleau, 2009). In addition, PABPN1 can associate with RNA polymerase II along the chromatin axis before or shortly after the transcription initiation, and the assembly of PABPN1 on the poly (A) tract may be coupled to transcription (Bear et. al., 2003). Studies have shown that PABPN1 remains associated with the released mRNA-protein complex (mRNP) until it reaches the cytoplasmic side of the nuclear pore. Very little PABPN1 is present in the cytoplasmic side of the nuclear envelope suggesting perhaps during or shortly after passage through the nuclear pore PABPN1 is displaced by PABPC1 (Abu-Baker et. al., 2005; Afonia et. al, 1998; Calado et. al., 2000; Kraus et.al., 1994) . PABPN1 has also been shown to interact with the SKI-binding polypeptide (SKIP) transcription factor and stimulate myogenesis (Kip et. al., 2001). Depletion of PABPN1 in myoblasts prevents myogenesis and reduces the length of the poly (A) tract of mRNAs (Apponi et. al., 2010). Because, of the vital role of PABPN1 in mRNA metabolism it is not certain that whether the observed effect on myogenesis was related to a specific effect on myogenesis or due to impairment of global mRNA metabolism. The poly A extension mutant of PABPN1 appears to function normally in pol(A) tail elongation process. Since PABPN1 can interact with both RNA and polypeptide partners, like other RNA binding proteins additional interacting partners such as micro RNAs and signaling polypeptides may soon be detected to suggest additional cellular functions for PABPN1 .

3. Pathology of OPMD

The most distinctive feature of OPMD is the presence of intranuclear filamentous inclusions in skeletal muscle fibers. The inclusions are composed of aggregates of mutant PABPN1 and several additional proteins which will be discussed later. The filaments are less than 0.25 nm long tubular in structures with an average outer diameter of 8.5 nm and an inner diameter of 3 nm. Approximately 2-5% of nuclei of skeletal muscle cells of OPMD patients show the presence of nuclear inclusions (Tome et. al., 1997). The myo-pathological patterns of OPMD, which progress with age include variations in the diameter of muscle fibers; increase in the number of internal nuclei; and increased presence of endomysical connective tissues. Also, a variable number of typical rimmed vacuoles are found in OPMD muscle fibers (Uyama et. al., 2000). Recently, neuro-pathological abnormalities have also been described in some OPMD patients (Boukriche et. al., 2002). Recent studies using a transgenic mouse model of OPMD severe muscular atrophy of the fast glycolytic muscles were observed. Transcrsiptome analyses of the OPMD mouse muscle showed deregulation of a large number of genes by expression of OPMD mutant PABPN1 but not by the wild type PABPN1, and approximately one third of the affected genes were associated with muscle atrophy (Trollet et. al., 2010). There is a strong correlation between the presence of intra nuclear inclusions (INI) and the PABPN1 mutation. All patients whose muscle biopsy showed 8.5nm intranuclear filaments have expanded PABPN1 alleles (Bao et. al., 2002). This view was further supported by the formation of large mutant PABPN1 aggregates similar to the INI in cell culture models ectopically expressing human PABPN1. In cell culture models over expression of both wild type and mutant PABPN1 resulted in aggregate formation (Tavanez et. al., 2005). However, the wild type PABPN1 formed aggregates more slowly than what was observed with the poly alanine expanded mutant PABPN1 (Schinchuk et.al., 2005). More apoptotic cell death was also observed in cells with mutant PABPN1 aggregates (Bao et. al., 2002; Fan et. al., 2001; Tavanez et. al., 2005).

4. Misfolded protein aggregates

Misfolding of proteins may lead to formation of protein aggregates. This process could be triggered by many factors including oxidative and temperature stresses. In addition, point mutations and expansion of poly alanine or poly glutamine tracts may increase aggregation by favoring the assembly of the unfolded or partly folded monomers into the early pre-fibrillar species which can turn into aggregates with more distinctive morphologies called protofilaments or protofibrils. The protofibrils may act as seeds where other misfolded polypeptides are recruited to form insoluble fibrillar aggregates (Chiti et. al., 2003). For many years it was believed that the ability to form amyloid fibrils is limited to small number of proteins. However, more recent studies have uncovered that for some proteins the fibrillar aggregates represent a biochemically active form. For examples the aggregated fibers known as curli produced by *E. coli is* important for cell adhesion (Chapman et. al., 2002); yeast prion Sup35, a translation termination factor (eRF3) forms aggregates (Tuite et. al., 2011). Many studies support a role of Aβ amyloid aggregates in sealing capillaries following traumatic injuries (Atwood et. al., 2003). Studies have shown that *Aplysia* cytoplasmic poly adenylation element binding protein (CPEB) exists in two different structural isoforms, one being the soluble isoform and the other as a prion like protein aggregates, and interestingly the CPEB prion is involved in stimulating synaptic growth and long term memory (Si et. al., 2003). It is therefore, conceivable that the poly alanine expansion of PABPN1 results in a gain of function(s). Most RNA binding polypeptides, are capable of participating in a variety of cellular processes, thus it is likely that the OPMD mutation of PABPN1 results in the loss of some cellular functions while gaining one or more new biological activity. Future research needs to be directed towards unraveling additional cellular functions for both mutant and the wild type PABPN1.

Studies using synthetic peptides consisting of varying lengths of the homopolymeric alanines were used to determine the length of the alanines tract that leads to inclusions. Conformational transition to insoluble aggregates was found to depend on the length as well as concentration, temperature, and incubation time. No β sheet complex was detected with less than 8 alanines while ala 10- 15 showed significant conversion of monomeric peptides to β-sheet aggregates. Homopolymers of 15 or more alanines residues showed the highest conversion to aggregates under all conditions examined (Schinchuk et. al., 2005). These results agree with the in vivo observations that the OPMD mutant PABPN1 is more prone to form aggregates than the wild type PABPN1. *In vitro* studies also showed that fibril formation can be induced by low amounts of both mutant and wild type fibrils serving as seeds. Atomic force microscopy revealed morphlogic differences between wild type and mutant fibrils. In addition, the wild type fibrils were less resistant to solubilization by chaotropic agent guanidinium thiocyanate than what was observed for the mutant fibrils. Examination of the kinetics of fibril formation with PABPN1 fragments containing the polyalanine tract in real time using tryptophan fluorescence suggest that fibril formation coincides with the burial of the tryptophans in the fibrillar core. These studies did not detect any soluble pre-fibrillar intermediates suggesting that the unfolded soluble form directly converts into folded insoluble structure (Schinchuk et. al., 2005).

5. Cellular stress and PABPN1 aggregates

A variety of cellular stresses results in the formation of misfolded proteins, and in order to maintain cell viability and subsequent recovery when physiologically favorable conditions return most organisms produce a family of chaperones known as the heat shock proteins (HSPs) which helps the proper folding process (Daugaard et. al., 2007). It appears that the presence of mutant PABPN1 aggregates but not the wild type cohort in the nuclei produces a modest stress response resulting in the increase of HSP70 expression. Treatment of cells with indomethacin or $ZnSO_4$ augmented the stress response and further induction of HSP70 expression was observed (Figure 2). In addition, expression of HSP27, HSP40 and HSP105 also increased. Both ibuprofen and $ZnSO_4$ treated cells showed reduced level of protein aggregates and apoptotic cell death. Furthermore, in the drug treated cells all four HSPs were colocalized with the PABPN1 (Wang & Bag, 2008). These results suggest that HSPs interact with misfolded PABPN1 and are able to dissociate the aggregates by refolding it into its native form. Similar results were obtained by heat shock treatment of cells and over

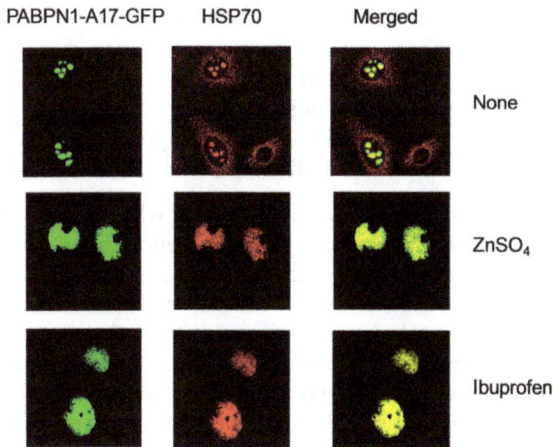

Fig. 2. Effect of different agents on aggregate formation by PABPN1-A17–GFP. HeLa cells were transfected with the PABPN1-A17–GFP expression vector and 48 hours after transfection, cells were treated with the indicated agents for 6 h and following a 24 h recovery period cells were examined for green fluorescence by confocal microscopy. HSP70 was detected by immunofluorescence with Texas red conjugated secondary antibody.

expression of HSP70 alone (Bao et. al., 2002' Wang et. al., 2005; Wang & Bag, 2008). Studies in our laboratory showed that deletion of the ATPase domain of HSP70, which is important for its chaperone function abolishes its ability to dissociate the mutant PABPN1 aggregates (unpublished).

6. Effect of PABPN1 on myogenesis

Despite the essential cellular function of PABPN1 in biogenesis of mRNA the pathologic symptoms are only seen in a restricted group of skeletal muscles such as the extraocular and pharyngeal muscles. Therefore, in addition to its role in mRNA biogenesis PABPN1 may be needed for proper differentiation of myogenic cells, which may be lost in mutant PABPN1 due to expansion of the poly alanine tract. Studies using a myoblast cell culture model showed that over expression of PABPN1 facilitates differentiation of myoblasts into myotubes (Kim et. al., 2001). PABPN1 has been shown to interact with SKIP which share significant homology to several transcriptional co activators such as Bx42 of *Drosophila melanogaster* (Wieland et. al., 1992), and mammalian NcoA-62 (Baudino et. al., 1998). SKIP appears to co-operate with PABPN1 in stimulating E box mediated tarnscription in presence of myoD by forming a hetero trimeric complex (Kim et. al., 2001. The N terminal domain of PABPN1 alone is necessary for interacting with SKIP. The C terminal domain including the RNA binding domains of PABPN1 are dispensable for its role in myogenesis (Kim et.al 2001). Although the poly alanine expanded PABPN1 also binds to SKIP *in vitro* (Tavanez et. al., 2009) it is not clear whether it can cooperate with MyoD to stimulate E box regulated transcription. However, this prospect is conceivable because of the location of poly alanines expansion is within the SKIP binding domain of PABPN1.

In addition to a loss of function in myogenesis the mutant PABPN1 may also gained a function albeit fortuitously, by trapping essential myogenic factors. Studies from our laboratory have indeed supports this hypothesis. We have shown that both myf 5 and Pax 3 co-localize with mutant PABPN1 aggregates but not with the wild type PABPN1 (Figure 3). Ectopic expression of wild type PABPN1 in C2C12 mouse myoblasts had a small beneficial effect on the expression level of various muscle specific proteins including myoD, myogenin, muscle creatine kinase, α-actin and slow troponin C. In contrast, expression of mutant PABPN1 reduced the abundance of those proteins (Figure 4) (Wang & Bag 2006).

The experimental results discussed above may explain why skeletal myogenesis could be affected but very little is known regarding specific targeting of the craniofacial muscles. To address this issue it has been proposed that continuous remodeling of the extraocular myofibers could result in selective loss of this muscle cells (Wirtschafter et. al., 2004). Since *in vivo* myonuclei of most skeletal muscles are post mitotic, therefore, continuous myofiber remodeling in extraocular muscle will require upregulation of genes in cell cycling and renewal of differentiated muscle cells (Wirtschafter et. al., 2004). The negative effect of mutant PABPN1 on myogenesis would show more pronounced effect on muscles that require more frequent rejuvenation than the other skeletal muscles over many years.

7. Protein aggregates and cell death

A direct connection between protein aggregation and cell death is controversial (Andrew et. al., 2000; Fan & Rouleau, 2003; Rubinsztein, 2002). Studies using live cell imaging have

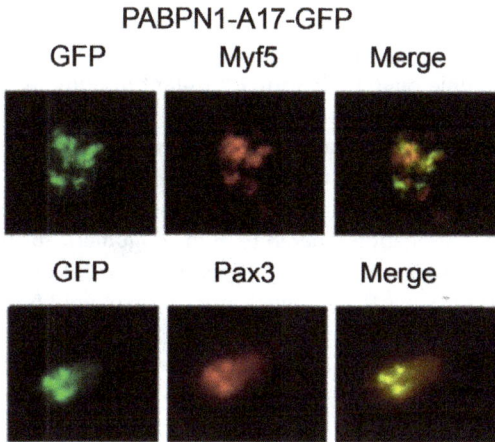

Fig. 3. Co-localization of Pax3/7 and Myf-5 in PABPN1-A17-GFP-transfected cells. Cells grown on coverslips were transfected and 48 h after transfection cells were fixed in methanol and incubated with the appropriate antibody. The green fluorescence of PABPN1-GFP and the red fluorescence of Texas red-conjugated secondary antibody were observed by fluorescence microscopy.

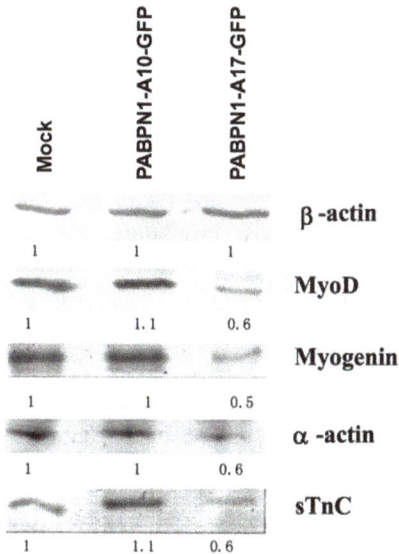

Fig. 4. Expression of muscle-specific proteins in PABPN1-A10 (or A17)-GFP-transfected cells. Cells were transfected with the appropriate Plasmid DNA after 2 days in the 2 days inthe differentiation medium, cells were lysed and the levels of various muscle proteins, were determined by Western blotting using jappropriate antibodies The Western blots were scanned and the levels of muscle proteins in transfected cells were determined and corrected for the difference in loading and transfection efficiency. The polypeptide levels in PABPN1-A17-GFP-transfected cells relative to that of the PABPN1-A10-GFP expressing cells are given at the bottom of each lane.

shown that cells expressing poly glutamine expanded huntingtin survives better than those without aggregates. It is believed that aggregation sequesters this protein and improves cell survival whereas the soluble oligomeric form of mutant huntingtin is more toxic to the cell (Arresate et. al., 2004). Whether the same is true for PABPN1 is not clear. The wild type PABPN1 naturally exists in a functional oligomeric form and is also present as aggregates in the speckles but these are not known to cause cell death. Two overlapping oligomerization domains are found within the C-terminal region of PABPN1. These domains are necessary for oligomerization and aggregation. Therefore, if the oligomeric form of mutant PABPN1 is toxic to the cell it must assume a different structure than that of the wild type protein. Indeed this may be the case since the sub nuclear location of wild type and mutant PABPN1 are different. The wild type PABPN1 was shown by immuno fluorescent microscopy to co-localize with the splicing factor SC35 and the nuclear matrix associated protein PML while the mutant PABPN1 did not (Messaed et. al., 2007; Tavanez et. al., 2005). However, this observation is paradoxical since both proteins seems to function normally in the poly adenylation process, and presence of wild type PABPN1 in the speckles is related to its role in transcription and splicing coupled polyadenylation. In contrast to the pro-apoptotic effect of mutant PABPN1 the wild type PABPN1 demonstrated anti-apoptotic function in mammalian cells. The wild type PABPN1 apparently up regulates the translation of anti apoptotic protein X-linked inhibitor of apoptosis (XIAP) which prevents activation of caspase 3 by inhibiting caspase 9 (Davies & Rubinsztein, 2011). Thus a loss of anti-apoptotic function of mutant PABPN1 may be responsible for cell death in OPMD muscles.

Several studies using cultured non-muscle cells as experimental models showed that strategies that reduced protein misfolding also decreased aggregate formation and cell death. Ectopic expression of the molecular chaperones HSP40 and HSP70 in cells transfected with the mutant PABPN1 reduce aggregate formation and cell death (Abu_Baker et. al., 2003; Bao et. al., 2002; 2004). Also anti-amyloid compounds such as Congo red and doxycyclin can reduce PABPN1 aggregate formation and cell death in a cell culture model (Bao et. al., 2004). We have shown that $ZnSO_4$, 8-hydroxyquinoline, indomethacin and ibuprofen induced HSP 70 expression, and nuclear localization of both HSP70 and the constitutive chaperone HSC 70 in mutant PABPN1 expressing HeLa cells, and reduced the formation of mutant PABPN1 aggregates and cell death (Wang et. al., 2005)

In several chronic neurodegenerative disorders including Alzheimer's, Huntington's, and Parkinson's, caused by the formation of protein aggregates, there is evidence that programmed cell death (apoptosis) may be involved (Desjardins & Ledoux, 1998). Apoptotic cell death has also been observed in cell models and transgenic mouse models of OPMD (Fan & Rouleau, 2003; Hino et. al., 2004; Dion et. al., 2005). However, the molecular mechanisms causing apoptosis remain elusive. Many studies suggest that in the aggregate containing cells, apoptosis proceeds through the up regulation of the tumor suppressor protein p53 (Bae et. al., 2005; Biswas et. al., 2005; Hooper et. al., 2007). Stabilization of p53 within the cell further leads to the activation of down stream proteins like PUMA (p53-upregulated modulator of apoptosis), Bax (Bcl-2-associated X protein) and Bad (Bcl-2-associated death promoter) that change the permeability of mitochondrial and endoplasmic reticulum membranes (Biswas et. al., 2005; Mattson, 2004). These events lead to the release of cytochrome C from mitochondria and calcium from the ER, which further activates the enzyme called caspase (Mattson, 2004). The cascades of proteolytic activities initiated by caspases are believed to trigger various morphological and biochemical aspects of the cell death process. Furthermore, in Huntington's disease, the GAPDH-Siah1 apoptotic pathway (Hara et. al., 2005) facilitates nuclear translocation of mHtt protein and the resultant neurotoxicity (Bae et. al., 2006). In addition to mitochondrial alterations, ER stress, due to the presence of misfolded polyglutamine has also been linked to the cell death in Huntington's and Alzheimer's disease models (Zhao & Ackerman, 2006).

We have demonstrated that although in OPMD cell death is restricted to a sub class of skeletal muscles, non muscle cells in culture also underwent apoptosis. This was not unexpected since PABPN1 is ubiquitously expressed. We found that in HeLa cells aggregation of the poly alanine expansion mutant PABPN1, favors apoptosis over necrosis or ER stress as cell death pathway. At the molecular level, cascades of biochemical events lead to apoptotic cell death due to the accumulation of mutant PABPN1 aggregates. Our results suggest that the apoptotic response to the accumulation of mutant PABPN1 aggregates was initiated by nuclear translocation of the glycolytic enzyme GAPDH. In the last decade several studies have shown that GAPDH is a multi-functional protein (Chuang et. al., 2005). This enzyme usually resides in the cytoplasm as a tetrameric active enzyme. As a response to cellular stress, the catalytic cysteine 150 of GAPDH is S-nitrosylated by nitric oxide, generated by the induction of inducible nitric oxide synthase (iNOS). It has been shown that Nitrosylated GAPDH binds to Siah1, an E3 ubiquitin ligase, and is transported to the nucleus as an inactive enzyme by piggy backing Siah1 (Hara et. al., 2005). The downstream target of GAPDH in the nucleus is p53 (Sen et. al., 2008). In our study, following ectopic expression of mutant PABPN1, we observed that the abundance of total as well as phosphorylated p53 was increased (Figure 5). p53 a tumor suppressor protein with wide ranging biological function including cell cycle arrest, apoptosis, and its abundance is known to increase in response to a variety of cellular damage (Green & Kroemer, 2009). In cells under stress, post translational modifications, especially phosphorylation and acetylation contribute to p53 stabilization and hence its activation (Sakaguchi et. al., 1998). It has been proposed that phosphorylation of p53 at ser 46 modulate the p53 gene promoter selection thereby dictating the fate of the cell to undergo p53 mediated apoptosis and/or growth arrest (Mayo et. al., 2005). The importance of phosphorylation in p53 mediated apoptosis was further underlined, by demonstrating that mutation of Ser46 to Ala decreases the ability of p53 to induce apoptosis (Oda et. al., 2000). It is known that p53 mediated apoptosis can be carried out by both transcription dependant and independent manner (Chuang et. al., 2005; Pietsch et. al., 2008). We found that in mutant PABPN1 cells, abundance of p53 and its phosphorylated isoform (p-p53) increases (Figure 5). Furthermore we also observed a redistribution of p53 in the nucleus and the mitochondria of mutant PABPN1 transfected cells (Figure 6). There was also a concomitant rise in the p53 transcription targeted pro apoptotic protein: Puma (Figure 5).

Thus, it appears that in mutant PABPN1 cells, activated p53 could be translocated to the nucleus and triggered the transcription dependant apoptosis (Wang et. al., 2007). This might be the reason why we did not observe acetylation of p53, since p53 acetylation occurs predominantly in transcription independent apoptosis (Yamaguchi et. al., 2009). However, both the transcription dependant and independent pathways are not necessarily mutually

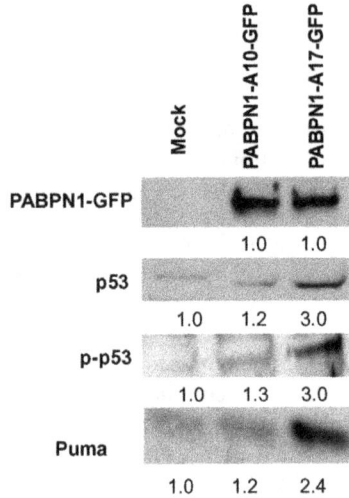

Fig. 5. PABPN1-A17 upregulates p53 and p53 mediated transcription: Following transfection, cells were harvested after 72 hours in SDS loading buffer. Whole cells extracts from PABPN1-A10, 17–GFP and mock-transfected HeLa cells were analyzed for apoptosis related proteins by western blotting. β-actin and GAPDH were used as loading controls.

exclusive. In fact, it has been suggested that the transcription dependent nuclear action of p53 cooperates with its transcription-independent, cytosolic/ mitochondrial action through activation of the *PUMA* gene (Chipuk et. al., 2005). Upon activation, Puma triggers apoptosis by releasing the p53 from its association with Bcl2 to activate Bax (Uo et. al., 2007;Wang et. al., 2007; Zhang et. al., 2009). Puma may also directly interact with Bax, promoting its mitochondrial translocation (Chipuk et. al., 2004; Zhang et. al., 2009). Puma may release p53 from its complex with Bcl2. The released p53 then could oligomerize the monomeric Bax in the cytosol causing the latter to induce mitochondrial outer membrane permeabilization (MOMP) (Dewson et. al., 2003; Jurgensmeier et. al., 1998). The activation of Bax by p53 is known to occur by a 'hit and run' style transient molecular associations (Chipuk et. al., 2004; Moll et. al., 2006; Green & Kroemer, 2009; Pietsch et. al., 2008).

It will be important to examine if a similar apoptotic signal contributes to cell death in muscle cells. In a recent study with the OPMD mouse model over-expression of Bcl2 rescued muscle weakness and apoptosis (Davies & Rubinsztein, 2011), therefore suggesting a similar Bax/Bcl2 pathway for apoptosis in both muscle and non-muscle cells. However, in the OPMD mouse the effect of Bcl2 on muscle weakness was transient, thus other cell death pathways may also contribute to cell death when Bax is inactivated by Bcl2. It is conceivable in the light of our observations in HeLa cells that increase in p53 level might eventually release Bax from Bcl2 mediated inactivation by sequestering Bcl2.

There are several pathways for apoptosis. The precise mechanism of apoptosis depends on developmental programs and the nature of the inducer (Green & Kroemer, 2009; Pietsch et. al., 2008). The Puma/Bax dependent pathway is usually triggered by a variety of cellular stress such as heat shock and oxygen stress (Uo et. al., 2007; Zhang et. al., 2009). The results of our study suggest that accumulation of misfolded protein aggregates also induces stress related apoptosis. In this context it is interesting to note that as discussed in a previous section a small but reproducible induction of a number of heat shock proteins including HSP70, HSP27, HSP40, and HSP105 was observed in mutant PABPN1 expressing cells (Wang & Bag 2008). Furthermore, all of these HSPs were found to be translocated to the cell nucleus and co-localize with the mutant PABPN1 aggregates. Further induction of HSPs using ibuprofen or indomethacin was shown to reduce the aggregate burden and apoptosis in mutant PABPN1 expressing cells (Wang & Bag 2008). HSP 70 has been shown to prevent heat stress induced apoptosis in cultured cells by preventing Bax translocation without directly interacting with Bax (Stankiewicz et. al., 2005). The mechanism how HSP70 induction with ibuprofen in mutant PABPN1 expressing cells prevents cell death will be of interest for further investigation.

The accumulated evidence supports a biochemical catastrophe model where loss of function combined with adventitious gain of function due to poly alanine expansion leads to cell death. The gain of function includes but not limited to increased aggregate formation, interaction with HSPs, trapping of various transcription factors and mRNAs. In studies using mtHtt aggregate formation in *C. elegans* it was shown that presence of mtHtt aggregates interferes with proper folding of normal cellular proteins and cell death could result from not only the aggregate burden of the mutant protein but also by the misfolding of many normal proteins which results in at the least reduction in the abundance of biologically active important cellular proteins (Gidalevitz et. al 2006). Since most studies measured protein abundance using western blotting techniques which does not measure the level of biological activity of the protein these changes has remained under explored.

The following hypotheses might explain the late onset and specificity of cellular targets *in vivo* of OPMD mutation: I) although aggregates can be cleared through proteasome degradation pathway, this pathway is not sufficient to completely prevent accumulation of aggregates; ii) aging is also associated with collapse of protein homeostasis resulting in accumulation of misfolded normal cellular proteins (Taylor & Dillin, 2011) and when this is combined with a mutation in an aggregate prone protein such as the PABPN1, it greatly increases accumulation of both mutant PABPN1 and many normal nuclear proteins in the intranuclear aggregates; iii) aging may also affect the ability to clear the aggregates through proteasome mediated decay; iv) although both muscle and non muscle cells undergo apoptosis, non-muscle cells are renewed through stem cells, in contrast since myogenesis is affected due to loss of function of mutant PABPN1, regeneration of differentiated muscle cells are affected; iv) skeletal muscles in adults are renewed only when injury occurs but in contrast the adult extraocular muscles undergo continuous remodeling (Wirtschafter et. al., 2004), therefore, extraocular muscles are more susceptible to the loss of myogenic role of mutant PABPN1.

8. Novel therapies for OPMD

Mouse and Drosophila models have been used to develop new therapies to treat OPMD. Administration of anti-amyloid agent doxycyclin to OPMD mice significantly reduced aggregate formation in muscle cells. In addition to its anti-amyloid properties doxycyclin also acts as an anti apoptotic agent to protect muscle cells (Davies et. al., 2006; 2008). In another study cystamine protected against the cytotoxicity of mutant PABPN1 in the OPMD mouse. Cysatmine inhibits transglutaminase 2 which is elevated in OPMD muscle cells (Davies et. al., 2010). Studies using the Drosophila model of OPMD single chain antibody against PABPN1 also produced nearly complete rescue of OPMD muscles and restored muscle gene expression (Chartier et. al., 2009). In a nematode model of OPMD the inhibitor of Sir2 sitinol also showed promising results in protecting muscle cells from apoptosis (Catoire et. al., 2008). Gene therapy approach using Bcl2 over expression also rescued OPMD mouse from muscle degeneration (Davies & Rubinsztein, 2011).

Several anti amyloid agents such as the disaccharide trehalose, and Congo red also worked in cell culture models of OPMD (Davies et. al., 2006). In our laboratory we have used ibuprofen, indomethacin, 8-hydroxy quinoline and $ZnSO_4$ to induce HSP 70 expression in HeLa cells. All of these agents significantly reduced the aggregate burden and cell death (Wang et.al., 2005). However these compounds have not been tested in an animal model yet. Ibuprofen's effectiveness was tested in a mouse model of Alzheimer disease without success. However, its conjugation with glutathione greatly improved its effectiveness in reducing aggregate formation and cell death in Alzheimer rats (Pinnen et. al., 2010). Zn^+ is an essential mineral nutrient and many people supplement their diet with it, as such, it is potentially a desirable treatment option. Similarly 8-hydroxy quinoline is also an approved agent used in animal feed as antimicrobial and antparasitic agent (Raether & Hanel, 2003). Its effective dose in the cultured cell is within the range of non-toxic dose. Various derivatives of this drug demonstrated their ability in reducing amyloid plaques in clinical trials on Alzheimer patients (Gouras & Beal 2001; Di Vaira et. al., 2004). In addition to the use of various pharmacological approaches in developing new therapies for OPMD, *in situ* myoblasts transfer by local administrations (Mouly et. al., 2006) or localized gene therapy of affected muscles using Bcl2 or HSP 70 gene expression should be considered.

9. References

Abu-Baker, A., Messaed, C., Laganiere, J., Gasper, C., Brais, B. & Rouleau, G. (2003). Involvement of the ubiquitin-proteasome pathway and molecular chaperones in oculopharyngeal muscular dystrophy. *Hum Mol Genet*, Vol. 12, No. 20, (October), pp. 2609–2623

Afonina, E., Stauber, R. & Pavlakis, G.N. (1998). The human poly(A)-binding protein 1 shuttles between the nucleus and the cytoplasm. *J Biol Chem, Vol.* 273, No. 21, (May), pp. 13015-21.

Andrew, P., Lieberman, M. & Fischbeck, KH. (2000). Triplet repeat expansion in neuromuscular disease. *Muscle Nerve*, Vol. 23, No. 6, (June). pp. 843–850

Apponi, LH., Leung, SW., Williams, KR., Valentini, SR., Corbett, AH. & Pavlath, GK. (2010). Loss of nuclear poly(A)-binding protein 1 causes defects in myogenesis and mRNA biogenesis. *Hum Mol Genet*, Vol. 19, No. 6, (December). pp. 1058-65

Arresate, M., Mitra, S., Schweitzer, E.S., Regal, M.R. & Finkbeiner, S. (2004). Inclusion body formation reduces levels of mutant Huntingtin and the risk of neuronal death. *Nature*, Vol. 431, No. 7010,(October), pp. 805–810

Atwood, CS., Bowen, RL., Smith, MA. & Perry, G. (2003). Cerebrovascular requirement for sealant, anti-coagulant and remodeling molecules that allow for the maintenance of vascular integrity and blood supply. *Brain Res Brain Res Rev*, Vol. 43, No. 1, (September), pp. 164-78

Bae, B-I., Xu, H., Igarashi, S., Fujimuro, M., Agrawal, N., Taya, Y., Hayward, S.D. & Sawa, A. (2005). p53 mediates cellular dysfunction and behavioral abnormalities in Huntington's disease. *Neuron*, Vol. 47, No.1, (July), pp. 29-41

Bao, Y., Cook, LJ., O'Donovan, D., Uyama, E. & Rubinsztein, DC. (2002). Mammalian, yeast, bacterial and chemical chaperones reduce aggregate formation and death in a cell model of oculopharyngeal muscular dystrophy. *J Biol Chem*, Vol. 277, No.14, (April), pp. 12263–12269

Bao, YP., Sarkar, S, Uyama, E. & Rubinsztein, DC. (2004). Congo red, doxycycline, and HSP70 over expression reduce aggregate formation and cell death in cell models of oculopharyngeal muscular dystrophy. *J Med Genet*, Vol. 41, No. 1, (January), pp. 47–51.

Bates, GP., Mangiarini, L., Mahal, A. & Davis, SW. (1997). Transgenic models of Huntington's disease. *Hum Mol Genet*, Vol. 6, No.10, (June), pp. 1633–1637.

Baudino, TA., Kraichely, DM., Jefcoat, SCJr., Winchester, SK., Partridge, NC. & MacDonald, PN. (1998). Isolation and characterization of a novel coactivator protein, NCoA-62, involved in vitamin D-mediated transcription. *J Biol Chem*, Vol. 273, No.26, (June), pp.16434-16441

Bear, DG., Fomproix, N., Soop, T., Björkroth, B., Masich, S. & Daneholt, B. (2003). Nuclear poly(A)-binding protein PABPN1 is associated with RNA polymerase II during transcription and accompanies the released transcript to the nuclear pore. *Exp Cell Res*, Vol. 286, No.2, (June), pp. 332–344

Behrouz, F., Enrique, P., Richard, AH. & Sylvie, E. (1995). Formation of an extremely stable polyalanine ß-sheet macromolecule. *Biochem Biophys Res Commun*, Vol. 211, No.1, (June), pp. 7–13

Bermano, G., Shepherd, RK., Zehner, ZE. & Hesketh, JE. (2001). Perinuclear mRNA localization by vimentin 3'-untranslated region requires a 100 nucleotide sequence and intermediate filaments. *FEBS Lett*, Vol. 497, No.2 ,(May), pp. 77–81

Bhushan, S., Malik, F., Kumar, A., Isher, HK., Kaur, IP., Taneja, SC. &. Singh, J. (2009). Activation of p53/p21/PUMA alliance and disruption of PI-3/Akt in multimodal targeting of apoptotic signaling cascades in cervical cancer cells by a pentacyclic triterpenediol from *Boswellia serrata*. *Mol Carcinog*, Vol.43, No.12, (December), pp.1093-108

Bienroth, S., Keller, W. & Wahle, E. (1993). Assembly of a processive messenger RNA polyadenylation complex. *EMBO J*, Vol. 12, No. 2, (February), pp. 585-594

Biswas, SC., Ryu, E., Park, C., Malagelada, C. & Greene, LA. (2005). Puma and p53 play required roles in death evoked in a cellular model of Parkinson disease. *Neurochem Res*, Vol. 30, No. 6-7, (June-July), pp. 839–845

Blasutig, IM., New, LA., Thanabalasuriar, A., Dayarathna, TK., Goudreault, M., Quaggin, SE., Li, SS-C., Gruenheid, S., Jones, N. & Pawson, T. (2008). Phosphorylated YDXV motifs and Nck SH2/SH3 adaptors act cooperatively to induce actin reorganization. *Mol Cell Biol*, Vol. 28, No.6, (January), pp.2035-2046

Blumen, SC., Nisipeanu, P., Sadeh, M., Asherov, A., Tome, FM. & Korczyn, AD. (1993). Clinical features of oculopharyngeal muscular dystrophy among Bukhara Jews. *Neuromuscul. Disord*, Vol. **3**, No. 5-6, (September-November), pp. 575-577

Boukriche Y, Maisonobe T. & Masson C. (2002) Neurogenic involvement in a case of oculopharyngeal muscular dystrophy. *Muscle Nerve*, Vol. 25, No.1, (January), pp. 98-101

Brais, B., Bouchard, JP., Xie, YG., Rochefort, DL., Chretien N., Tome, F.M., Lafrenier, R.G., Rommens, J.M., Uyama, E. & Nohira, O. (1998) Short GCT expansions in the PABPN1 gene cause oculopharyngeal muscular dystrophy. *Nat. Genet*, Vol. 18, No. 2, (February), pp. 164-166.

Brown, LY. & Brown, SA. (2004). Alanine tracts: the expanding story of human illness and trinucleotide repeats. *Trends Genet*, Vol. 20, No. 1, (January), pp.51-58

Brunet, G., Tome, FM., Samson, F., Robert, JM. & Fardeau, M. (1990). Oculopharyngeal muscular dystrophy: a census of French families and genealogic study. *Rev. Neurol*, Vol. 146, No.6-7,pp. 425–429

Burdon, RH. (1982). The human heat shock proteins: their induction and possible intracellular functions. In Schlesinger, M.J., Ashburner, M. and Tissieres, A. (eds), *Heat Shock from Bacteria to Man*, Cold Spring Harbor Laboratory, New York, USA

Calado, A., Tome, FMS., Brais, B., Rouleau, GA, Kuhn, U., Wahle, E. & Fonseca-Carmo, M. (2000). Nuclear inclusions in oculopharyngeal muscular dystrophy consist of poly(A) binding protein 2 aggregates which sequesters poly(A) RNA. *Hum Mol Genet*,Vol. 9, No. 15, (September), pp. 2321–2328

Carmichael, J., Chatellier, J., Woolfson, A., Milstein, C., Fersht, AR. & Rubinsztein, DC. (2000). Bacterial and yeast chaperones reduce both aggregate formation and cell death in mammalian cells models of Huntington's disease. *Proc Natl Acad Sci USA*,Vol. 97, No. 17, (August) pp.9701–9705

Catoire, H., Pasco, MY., Abu-Baker, A., Holbert, S., Tourette, C., Brais, B., Rouleau, GA., Parker, JA. & Néri, C. (2008). Sirtuin inhibition protects from the polyalanine muscular dystrophy protein PABPN1. *Hum Mol Genet*, Vol.17, Vol.14, (July), pp. 2108-2117

Chapman, MR., Robinson, LS., Pinkner, JS., Roth, R., Heuser, J., Hammar, M., Normark, S. & Hultgren, SJ. (2002). Role of Escherichia coli curli operons in directing amyloid fiber formation.*Science*, Vol.295, No.5556, (February), pp.851-855

Chartier, A., Raz, V., Sterrenburg, E., Verrips, CT., van der Maarel, SM. & Simonelig, M.(2009). Prevention of oculopharyngeal muscular dystrophy by muscular expression of Llama single-chain intrabodies in vivo. *Hum Mol Genet*,Vol. 18, No. 10, (May), pp. 1849-1859

Chen, S., Berthelier, V., Yang, W. & Wetzel, R. (2001). Polyglutamine aggregation behavior *in vitro* support a recruitment mechanism of cytotoxicity. *J Mol Biol*, Vol. 311, No. 1, (August) pp.173–182

Chen, Z., Li, Y. and Krug, R. (1999). Influenza A virus NS1 protein targets poly(A)-binding protein II of the cellular 3' end processing machinery. *EMBO J*, Vol. 18, No.8, (April), pp. 2273–2283

Chipuk, JE., Kuwana, T., Bouchier-Hayes, L., Droin, NM., Newmeyer, DD., Schuler, M. & Green, DR. (2004). Direct activation of Bax by p53 mediates mitochondrial membrane permeabilization and apoptosis. *Science*, Vol. 303, No.5660, pp. 1010–1014

Chipuk, JE., Bouchier-Hayes, L., Kuwana, T., Newmeyer, DD. & Green, DR. (2005). PUMA couples the nuclear and cytoplasmic proapoptotic function of p53. *Science*, Vol. 309, No. 5741, (September), pp. 1732–1735

Chiti, F., Stefani, M., Taddei, N., Ramponi, G. & Dobson CM. (2003). Rationalization of the effects of mutations on peptide and protein aggregation rates.*Nature*, Vol.424, No.6950, (August), pp.805-808

Chuang, DM., Hough, C. & Senatorov, VV. (2005). Glyceraldehyde-3-phosphate dehydrogenase, apoptosis, and neurodegenerative diseases. *Annu Rev Pharmacol Toxicol*, Vol.45, pp.269-290

Corbeil-Girard, LP., Klein AF., Sasseville, AM., Lavoie, H., Dicaire, MJ., Saint-Denis A., Page, M., Duranceau, A., Codere, F., Bouchard, JP., Karpati, G., Rouleau, GA., Massie, B., Langelier, Y. and Brais, B. (2005). PABPN1 overexpression leads to upregulation of genes encoding nuclear proteins that are sequestered in oculopharyngeal muscular dystrophy nuclear inclusions. *Neurobiol Dis*, Vol. 18, No. 3 (April), pp. 551–567.

Cumming, CJ., Reinstein E., Sun Y., Antalify B., Jiang, Y., Ciechanovert, A., Orr, HT., Beaudet, AL. & Zoghbi, HY. (1999). Mutation of the E6-AP ubiquitin ligase reduces nuclear inclusion frequency while accelerating polyglutamine-induced pathology in SCAI mice. *Neuron*, Vol. 24, No. 4, (December), pp. 879–892

Daugaard, M., Rohde, M. & Jäättelä, M. (2007). The heat shock protein 70 family: Highly homologous proteins with overlapping and distinct functions. *FEBS Lett*, Vol. 581, No.19, (July), pp.3702-10.

Davies, JE., Wang, L., Garcia-Oroz, L., Cook, LJ., Vacher, C., O'Donovan, DG. & Rubinsztein, DC. (2005). Doxycycline attenuates and delays toxicity of the oculopharyngeal muscular dystrophy mutation in transgenic mice. *Nat Med*, Vol. 11, No.6, (June), pp. 672-677

Davies, JE. & Rubinsztein, DC. (2006). Polyalanine and polyserine frameshift products in Huntington's disease. *J Med Genet*, Vol.43, No.11, (June), pp.893-896

Davies, JE., Sarkar, S. & Rubinsztein, DC. (2008). Wild-type PABPN1 is anti-apoptotic and reduces toxicity of the oculopharyngeal muscular dystrophy mutation. *Hum Mol Genet*, Vol. 17, No. 8, (April), pp.1097-1108

Davies JE, Rose C, Sarkar S. & Rubinsztein DC. (2010). Cystamine suppresses polyalanine toxicity in a mouse model of oculopharyngeal muscular dystrophy. *Sci Transl Med*, Vol. 2, No. 34, (June), pp. 34ra40

Davies, JE. & Rubinsztein, DC. (2011). Over-expression of BCL2 rescues muscle weakness in a mouse model of oculopharyngeal muscular dystrophy. *Hum Mol Genet*, Vol. 20, No. 6, (March), pp.1154-1163

Desjardins, P. & Ledoux, S. (1998). The role of apoptosis in neurodegenerative diseases. *Metab Brain Dis*, Vol. 13, No. 2, ( ),pp. 79–96

Dewson, G., Snowden, RT., Almond, JB., Dyer, MJS. & Cohen, GM.(2003). Conformational change and mitochondrial translocation of Bax accompany proteosome inhibitor-induced apoptosis of chronic lymphocytic leukemic cells. *Oncogene*, Vol. 22, No.17, (May), pp. 2643-2654

Dhar, SK. & St Clair, DK. (2009). Nucleophosmin Blocks Mitochondrial Localization of p53 and Apoptosis. *J Biol Chem*, Vol. 284, No. 24, (June), pp. 16409–16418

Di Vaira, M., Bazzicalupi, C., Orioli, P., Messori, L., Bruni, B. & Zatta, P. (2004). Clioquinol, a drug for Alzheimer's disease specifically interfering with brain metal metabolism: structural characterization of its zinc(II) and copper(II) complexes. *Inorg Chem*, Vol. 43, No. 13, (May), pp. 3795–3797

Dion, P., Shanmugam, V., Gaspar, C., Messaed, C., Meijer, I., Toulouse, A., Laganiere, J., Roussel, J., Rochefort, D., Laganiere, S., Allen, C., Karpati, G., Bouchard, JP., Brais, B. & Rouleau, GA. (2005). Transgenic expression of an expanded (GCG) (13) repeat PABPN1 leads to weakness and coordination defects in mice. *Neurobiol. Dis*, Vol. 18, No.3, (April),pp. 528–536

Dreyfuss, G., Adams, S. & Choi, YF. (1984). Physical changes in cytoplasmic messenger ribonucleoproteins in cells treated with inhibitors of mRNA transcription. *Mol Cell Biol*, Vol. 4, No. 3,(March),pp. 415–423

Fan, X. & Rouleau, GA. (2003). Progress in understanding the pathogenesis of oculopharyngeal muscular dystrophy. *Can J Neurol Sci*, Vol. 30, No. (1), (February), pp. 8–14

Fan, XP., Dion, P., Laganiere, J., Brais, B. & Rouleau, GA. (2001). Oligomerization of polyalanine expanded PABPN1 facilitates nuclear protein aggregation that is associated with cell death. *Hum Mol Genet*, Vol. 10, No. 21, (October), pp. 2341–2351

Ge, H., Zhou, D., Tong, S., Gao, Y., Teng, M. & Niu, L. (2008). Crystal structure and possible dimerization of the single RRM of human PABPN1.Proteins, Vol. 71, No. 3, (May), pp.1539-1545

Gidalevitz, T., Ben-Zvi, A., Ho, KH. & Brignull, HR. (2006). Morimoto RI. Progressive disruption of cellular protein folding in models of polyglutamine diseases. *Science*, Vol. 311, No. 5766, (March) pp. 1471-1474

Gouras, GK. & Beal, MF. (2001). Metal chelator decreases Alzheimer ß-amyloid plaques. *Neuron*, Vol. 30, No.3, (June), pp. 641–642

Green, DR. & Kroemer, G. (2009). Cytoplasmic functions of the tumour suppressor p53. *Nature*, Vol. 458, No.7242, (April), pp. 1127-1130

Gürtler, N., Plasilova, M., Podvinec, M., Boesch, N., Müller, H. & Heinimann, K . (2006). A de novo PABPN1 germline mutation in a patient with oculopharyngeal muscular dystrophy. *Laryngoscope*, Vol.116, No.1, (January), pp.11-14

Hara, MR., Agrawal, N., Kim, SF., Cascio, MB., Fujimuro, M., Ozeki, Y., Takahashi, M., Cheah, JH., Tankou, SK., Hester, LD., Ferris, CD., Hayward, SD., Snyder, SH. & Sawa, A. (2005). S-nitrosylated GAPDH initiates apoptotic cell death by nuclear translocation following Siah1 binding. *Nat Cell Biol*, Vol. 7, No.7, (July), pp. 665–674

Heiser, V., Engemann, S., Brocker, W., Dunkel, I., Boeddrich, A., Waelter, S., Nordhoff, E., Lurz, R., Schugardt, N., Rautenberg, S. Herhaus, C., Barnickel, G., Böttcher, H., Lehrach, H. & Wanker, EE. (2002). Identification of benzothiazoles as potential polyglutamine aggregation inhibitors of Huntington's disease by using an automated filter retardation assay. *Proc Natl Acad Sci USA*, Vol.99, No.4, (December),pp. 16400-16406

Hill, ME., Creed, GA., McMullan, TF., Tyers, AG., Hilton-Jones, D., Robinson, DO. & Hammans, SR. (2001). Oculopharyngeal muscular dystrophy. Phenotypic and genotypic studies in a UK population. *Brain*, Vol. 124, No.3, (March), pp. 522-526

Hino, H., Araki, K., Uyama, E., Takeya, M., Araki, M., Yoshinobu, K., Mike, K., Kawazoe, Y., Maeda, Y., Uchino, M. & Yamamura, K. (2004). Myopathy phenotype in transgenic mice expressing mutated PABPN1 as a model of oculopharyngeal muscular dystrophy. *Hum Mol Genet*, Vol. 13, No. 2, (Jan), pp. 181–190

Hooper, C., Meimaridou, E., Tavassoli, M., Melino, G., Lovestone, S &, Killick, R. (2007). p53 is upregulated in Alzheimer's disease and induces tau phosphorylation in HEK293a cells. *Neuroscience Letters*, Vol. 418, No. 1, (May), pp. 34-37

Hyun, TH., Barreet-Connor, E. & Milne, DB. (2004). Zinc intakes and plasma concentrations in men with osteoporosis: The Rancho Bernardo study. *Am J Clin Nutr*, Vol. 80, No.3, (September), pp. 715–721

Jurgensmeier, JM., Xie, .Z, Deveraux, Q., Ellerby, L., Bredesen, D. & Reed, JC. (1998). Bax directly induces release of cytochrome *c* from isolated mitochondria. *Proc Natl Acad Sci USA*, Vol.95, No.9, (April), pp.4997–5002

Keller,RW., Kühn, U., Aragón, M., Bornikova, L., Wahle, E. & Bear, DG. (2000). The nuclear poly(A) binding protein, PABP2, forms an oligomeric particle covering the length of the poly(A) tail. *J Mol Biol*. Vol. 297, No.3, (March), pp. 569-583

Kelley, PM. & Schlesinger, M. (1978). The effect of amino acid analogues and heat shock on gene expression in chicken embryo fibroblasts. *Cell*, Vol. 15, No.4,(December), pp. 1277–1286.

Kerwitz, Y., Kuhn, U., Lilie, H., Knoth, A., Scheuermann, T., Friedrich, H., Schwarz, E. & Wahle, E. (2003). Stimulation of poly(A) polymerase through a direct interaction with the nuclear poly(A) binding protein allosterically regulated by RNA. *EMBO J*, Vol. 22, No.14, (July), pp. 3705–3714

Kim, YJ., Noguchi, S., Hayashi, YK., Tsukahara, T., Sahimizu, T. & Arahata, K. (2001). The product of an oculopharyngeal muscular dystrophy gene, poly(A)-binding protein 2, interacts with SKIP and stimulates muscle-specific gene expression. *Hum Mol Genet*, Vol. 10, No.11,(May), pp. 1129–1139.

Klein, AF., Ebihara, M., Alexander, C., Dicaire, MJ., Sasseville, AM., Langelier, Y., Rouleau, GA. & Brais B. (2008). PABPN1 polyalanine tract deletion and long expansions modify its aggregation pattern and expression. *Exp Cell Res*, Vol.314, No.8, (May), pp.1652–1666

Knights, CD., Catania, J., Giovanni, DD., Muratoglu, S., Perez, R., Swartzbeck, A., Quong, AA., Zhang, X., Beerman, T., Pestell, TR. & Avantaggiati, ML. (2006). Distinct p53 acetylation cassettes differentially influence gene-expression patterns and cell fate. *J Cell Biol*, Vol. 173, No.4, (May), pp.533–544

Krause, S., Fakan, S., Weis, K. & Wahle, E. (1994). Immunodetection of poly(A) binding protein II in the cell nucleus. *Exp Cell Res*, Vol.214, No.1, (September), pp.75-82

Kühn U, Nemeth A, Meyer S, Wahle E. (2003). The RNA binding domains of the nuclear poly(A)-binding protein. *J Biol Chem*, Vol. 278, No. 19, (May), pp. 16916-16925

Kühn, U. & Wahle, E. (2004). Structure and function of poly(A) binding proteins. *Biochim Biophys Acta*, Vol. 1678, No.2-3, (May), pp.67-84

Lagunas, L., Bradbury, CM., Laszlo, A., Hunt, CR. & Gius, D. (2004). Indomethacin and ibuprofen induce hsc70 nuclear localization and activation of the heat shock response in Hela cells. *Biochem Biophys Res Commun*, Vol. 313, No.4, (January), pp. 863–870.

Lee, BS., Chen, J., Angelidis, C., Jurivich, DA. & Morimoto, RI. (1995). Pharmacological modulation of heat shock factor 1 by antiinflammatory drugs resulted in protection against stress-induced cellular damage. *Proc Natl Acad Sci USA*, Vol. 92, No.16, (August), pp. 7207–7211.

Lenk, R., Ransom, L., Kaufmann, Y. & Penman, S. (1977). A cytoskeletal structure with associated polyribosomes from HeLa cells. *Cell*, Vol. 10, No.1, (January), pp.67–78

Li, P., Nijhawan, D., Budihardjo, I., Srinivasula, SM., Ahmad, M., Alnemri, ES. & Wang, X. (1997). Cytochrome C and dATP- dependant formation of Apaf-1/caspase-9 complex initiates an apoptotic protease cascade. *Cell*, Vol.91, No.14, (November), pp. 479-489

Mattson, MP. (2004). Pathways towards and away from Alzheirmer's disease. *Nature*, Vol.430, No.7000, (August), p.631-639

Mayo, LD., Seo, YR., Jackson, MW., Smith, ML., Rivera, GJ., Korgaonkar, CK. & Donner, DB. (2005). Phosphorylation of human p53 at serine 46 determines promoter selection and whether apoptosis is attenuated or amplified. *J Biol Chem*, Vol.280, No.28, (July), pp. 25953–25959

Messaed, C., Dion, PA., Abu-Baker, A., Rochefort, D., Laganiere, J., Brais, B. & Rouleau, GA. (2007). Soluble expanded PABPN1 promotes cell death in oculopharyngeal muscular dystrophy. *Neurobiol Dis*. Vol.26, No.3, (June), pp.546-57

Messaed, C. & Rouleau, GA. (2009). Molecular mechanisms underlying polyalanine diseases. *Neurobiol Dis*, Vol.34, No.3, (June), pp.397-405

Moll, UM., Marchenko, N. & Zhang, XK. (2006). p53 and Nur77/TR3-transcription factors that directly target mitochondria for cell death induction. *Oncogene*, Vol.25, No.34, (August), pp. 4725-4743

Mosser, DD., Caron, AW., Bourget, L., Denis-Larose, C. and Massie, B. (1997). Role of the human heat shock protein hsp70 in protection against stress-induced apoptosis. *Mol Cell Biol*, Vol.17, No.9, (September), pp.5317–5327

Mosser, DD. and Morimoto, RI. (2004). Molecular chaperones and the stress of oncogenesis. *Oncogene*, Vol.23, No.16, (April), pp. 2907–2918

Nakano, K. & Vousden, KH. (2001). PUMA, a novel proapoptotic gene, is induced by p53. *Mol Cell*, Vol. 7, No.3, (March), pp. 683-694

National Toxicology Program (1985) NTP toxicology and carcinogenesis studies of 8-hydroxyquinoline (CAS No: 1482-24-3) in F3441 N rats and B6C3F1 mice (feed studies). *Natl Toxicol., Program Tech. Rep. Ser*, Vol.276, (April) 1–170

Nemeth, A., Krause, S., Blank, D., Jenny, A., Jenö, P., Lustig, A. & Wahle, E. (1995). Isolation of genomic and cDNA clones encoding bovine poly(A) binding protein II. *Nucleic Acids Res*, Vol.23, No.20, (October), pp.4034-4041

Oda, E., Ohki, R., Murasawa, H., Nemoto, J., Shibue, T., Yamashita, T., Tokino, T., Taniguchi, T. & Tanaka, N. (2000). Noxa, a BH3-only member of the Bcl-2 family and candidate mediator of p53-induced apoptosis. *Science*, Vol.288, No.5468, (May), pp. 1053-1058

Oda, K., Arakawa, H., Tanaka, T., Matsuda, K., Tanikawa, C., Mori, T., Nishimori, H., Tamai, K., Tokino, T., Nakamura, Y. & Taya, Y. (2000). p53AIP1, a potential mediator of p53-dependent apoptosis, and its regulation by Ser-46-phosphorylated p53. *Cell*, Vol.102, No. 6, (September), pp. 849–862

Pallepati, P. & Averill-Bates, D. (2010). Mild thermotolerance induced at 40 degrees C increases antioxidants and protects HeLa cells against mitochondrial apoptosis induced by hydrogen peroxide: Role of p53. *Arch Biochem Biophys*, Vol.495, No.2, (March) pp.97-111

Pietsch, EC., Sykes, SM., McMahon, SB. & Murphy, ME. (2008). The p53 family and programmed cell death. *Oncogene*, Vol.27, No.50, (October), pp. 6507–6521

Pinnen, F., Sozio, P., Cacciatore, I., Cornacchia, C., Mollica, A., Iannitelli, A., D Aurizio, E., Cataldi, A., Zara, S., Nasuti, C. & Di Stefano A. (2011). Ibuprofen and Glutathione Conjugate as a Potential Therapeutic Agent for Treating Alzheimer's Disease. Arch Pharm (Weinheim). Vol.22, No. , *Arch Pharm Chem Life Sci*, Vol. 11, pp.139-148

Poirier, MA., Li, H., Macosko, J., Cai, S., Amzel, M. & Ross, CA. (2002). Huntingtin spheroids and protofibrils as precursors in polyglutamine fibrilization. *J Biol Chem*, Vol. 277, No.43, (October), pp. 41032–41037

Raether, W. & Hanel, H. (2003). Nitroheterocyslic drugs with broad spectrum activity. *Parasitol. Res*, Vol. 90, No.S1, (June) S19–S39

Rankin, J., Wyttenbach, A. & Rubinsztein, DC. (2000). Intracellular green fluorescent protein-polyalanine aggregates are associated with cell death. *Biochem J*, Vol.348, No.1, (May) 15–19.

Rivera, D., Mejia-Lopez, H., Pompa-Mera, EN., Villanueva-Mendoza, C., Nava-Castañeda, A., Garnica-Hayashi, L., Cuevas-Covarrubias, S. & Zenteno, JC. (2008). Two different PABPN1 expanded alleles in a Mexican population with oculopharyngeal muscular dystrophy arising from independent founder effects. *Br J Ophthalmol*, Vol. 92, No.7, (July), pp. 998-1002

Rubinsztein, DC. (2002) Lessons from animal models of Huntington's diseases. *Trends Genet*, Vol.18, No.4, (April),pp. 202–209

Sakaguchi, K., Herrera, JE., Saito, S., Miki, T., Bustin, M., Vassilev, A., Anderson, CW. & Appella, E. (1998). DNA damage activates p53 through a phosphorylation-acetylation cascade. *Genes Dev*. Vol.12, No. 18, (September),pp. 2831–2841

Sakahira, H., Breuer, P., Hayer-Hartl, MK. & Hartl, FU. (2002). Molecular chaperones as modulators of polyglutamine protein aggregation and toxicity. *Proc Natl Acad Sci USA*, Vol.99, No. Suppl 4, (June), pp.16412–16418

Saudou, F., Finkbeiner, S., Devys, D. & Greenberg, ME. (1998). Huntingtin acts in the nucleus to induce apoptosis but death does not correlate with the formation of intranuclear inclusions. *Cell*, Vol.95, No.1, (October), pp. 55–66

Schaffar, G., Breuer, P. & Botera, R. (2004). Cellular toxicity of polyglutamine expansion proteins: mechanism of transcription factor deactivation. *Mol Cell*, Vol.15, No.1, (July), pp.95–105

Scheffner, M., Huibregtse, JM., Vierstra, RD. & Howley, PM. (1993). The HPV-16 E6 and E6-AP complex functions as a ubiquitin-protein ligase in the ubiquitination of p53. *Cell*, Vol.75, No.3, (November) pp.495-505

Sen, N., Hara, MR., Kornberg, MD., Cascio, MM., Bae, B., Shahani, N., Thomas, B., Dawson, TM., Dawson, VL., Snyder, SH. & Akira, S. (2008). Nitric oxide-induced nuclear GAPDH activates p300/CBP and mediates apoptosis. *Nat Cell Biol*, Vol. 10, No. 7, (July), pp. 866–873

Shinchuk, LM., Sharma, D., Blondelle, SE., Reixach, N., Inouye, H. & Kirschner. DA. (2005). Poly-(L-alanine) expansions form core beta-sheets that nucleate amyloid assembly. *Proteins*, Vol. 61. No.3, (November), pp.579-589

Si, K., Giustetto, M., Etkin, A., Hsu, R., Janisiewicz, AM., Miniaci, MC., Kim, JH., Zhu, H. & Kandel, ER. (2003). A neuronal isoform of CPEB regulates local protein synthesis and stabilizes synapse-specific long-term facilitation in aplysia. *Cell*, Vol.115, No.7, (December), pp.893-904

Song, S. & Finkel, F. (2007). GAPDH and the search for alternative energy. *Nature Cell Biology*, Vol. 9, No. 8, (August) pp. 869 – 870

Stankiewicz, AR., Lachapelle, G., Foo, CP., Radicioni, SM. & Mosser, DD. (2005). Hsp70 inhibits heat-induced apoptosis upstream of mitochondria by preventing Bax translocation. *J Biol Chem*. Vol. 280, No.46, (November), pp. 38729-38739

Tavanez, JP., Calado, P., Braga, J., Lafarga, M. & Carmo-Fonseca, M. (2005). In vivo aggregation properties of the nuclear poly(A)-binding protein PABPN1. *RNA*, Vol.11, No.5, (May), pp.752-762

Tavanez, JP., Bengoechea, R., Berciano, MT., Lafarga, M., Carmo-Fonseca, M. & Enguita, FJ. (2009). Hsp70 chaperones and type I PRMTs are sequestered at intranuclear inclusions caused by polyalanine expansions in PABPN1. *PLoS One*, Vol. 4, No.7, (July), pp. e6418

Taylor, RC. & Dillin, A. (2011). Aging as an event of proteostasis collapse. *Cold Spring Harb Perspect Biol*. 2011 , Vol. 3, No.5, (May), pii: a004440. doi: 10.1101/cshperspect.a004440

Tomé, FM., Chateau, D., Helbling-Leclerc, A. & Fardeau M. (1997). Morphological changes in muscle fibers in oculopharyngeal muscular dystrophy. *Neuromuscul Disord*, Vol.7, No.Suppl 1, (October), pp.:S63-69.

Towbin, H. & Gordon, J. (1984). Immunoblotting and dot immunobinding: current status and outlook. *J Immunol Methods*, Vol.72, No. 2, (September), pp. 313-340

Trollet, C., Anvar, SY., Venema, A., Hargreaves, IP., Foster, K., Vignaud, A., Ferry, A., Negroni, E., Hourde, C., Baraibar. MA., 't Hoen, PA., Davies, JE., Rubinsztein, DC., Heales, SJ., Mouly, V., van der Maarel, SM., Butler-Browne, G., Raz, V. & Dickson, G. (2010). Molecular and phenotypic characterization of a mouse model of oculopharyngeal muscular dystrophy reveals severe muscular atrophy restricted to fast glycolytic fibres. *Hum Mol Genet*, Vol.19, Vol.11, (June), pp.2191-207

Trottier, Y., Devys, D., Imbert, G., Saudou, F., An, I., Lutz, Y., Weber, C., Agid, Y., Hirsch, EC. & Mandel, JL. (1995). Cellular localization of the Huntington's disease protein and discrimination of the normal and mutated form. *Nat Genet*, Vol.10, No1, (May), pp.104-110

Tuite, MF., Marchante, R. & Kushnirov, V. (2011). Fungal Prions: Structure, Function and Propagation. *Top Curr Chem*, Vol.30, (June) [Epub ahead of print]

Uyama, E., Tsukahara, T., Goto, K., Kurano, Y., Ogawa, M., Kim, YJ., Uchino, M. & Arahata, K. (2000). Nuclear accumulation of expanded PABP2 gene product in oculopharyngeal muscular dystrophy. *Muscle Nerve*, Vol. 23, No.10, (October), pp.1549-1554

van der Sluijs, BM., van Engelen, BG. & Hoefsloot, LH.(2003). Oculopharyngeal muscular dystrophy (OPMD) due to a small duplication in the PABPN1 gene. *Hum Mutat*, Vol. 21, No.5, (May), pp.553

Wahle, E. (1991) A novel poly(A)-binding protein acts as a specificity factor in the second phase of messenger RNA polyadenylation. *Cell*, Vol. 66, No.4, (August), pp. 759–768

Wahle, E., Listig, A., Jeno, P. & Maurer, P. (1993). Mammalian poly(A)-binding protein II. *J Biol Chem*, Vol. 268, No.4, (February), pp. 2937–2945

Wahle, E. (1995) Poly(A) tail length control is caused by termination of processive synthesis. *J Biol Chem*, Vol.270, No.6, (February), pp. 2800–2808

Wang, C. & Chen, J. (2003). Phosphorylation and hsp90 binding mediate heat shock stabilization of p53. *J Biol Chem*, Vol. 278, No.3, (January), pp. 2066–2071

Wang, P., Yu, J. & Zhang, L. (2007). The nuclear function of p53 is required for PUMA-mediated apoptosis induced by DNA damage. *Proc Natl Acad Sci USA*, Vol.104, No.10, (March), pp. 4054–4059

Wang, Q., Mosser, DD. & Bag, J. (2005). Induction of HSP70 expression and recruitment of HSC70 and HSP70 in the nucleus reduce aggregation of a polyalanine expansion mutant of PABPN1 in HeLa cells. *Hum Mol Genet*, Vol. 14, No.23, (October), pp. 3673-3684

Wang, Q. & Bag, J. (2006). Ectopic expression of a polyalanine expansion mutant of poly(A)-binding protein N1 in muscle cells in culture inhibits myogenesis. Vol. 340, No.3, (February), pp. 11-15

Wang, Q. & Bag, J. (2008). Induction of expression and co-localization of heat shock polypeptides with the polyalanine expansion mutant of poly(A)-binding protein N1 after chemical stress. *Biochem Biophysical Res Commun*, Vol. 370, No.1, (May), pp. 11-15

Wieland, C., Mann, S., von Besser, H. & Saumweber, H. (1992). The Drosophila nuclear protein Bx42, which is found in many puffs on polytene chromosomes, is highly charged. *Chromosoma*, Vol.101, No.8, (June), pp.517-525.

Wirtschafter, JD., Ferrington, DA. & McLoon, LK. (2004). Continuous remodeling of adult extraocular muscles as an explanation for selective craniofacial vulnerability in oculopharyngeal muscular dystrophy. *J Neuroophthalmol*, Vol.24, No.1, (March), pp.62-76

Witoonpanich, R., Phankhian, S., Sura, T., Lertrit, P., Phudhichareonrat, S. (2004). Oculopharyngodistal myopathy in a Thai family. *J Med Assoc Thai*, Vol. 87, No.12, (March), pp. 1518-21

Wolter, KG., Hsu, YT., Smith, CL., Nuchushtan, A., Xi, XG. & Youle, RJ. (1997) Movement of Bax from the cytosol to mitochondria during apoptosis. *J Cell Biol*, Vol. 139, No. 5, (December), pp. 1281-1292

Yamaguchi, H., Woods, NT., Piluso, LG., Lee, HH., Chen, J., Bhalla, KN., Monteiro, A., Liu, X., Hung, MC. & Wang, HG. (2009). p53 acetylation is crucial for its transcription-independent proapoptotic functions. *J Biol Chem*, Vol.284, No.17, (April), pp. 11171-11183

Ye, J., Zhang, H., Zhou, Y., Wu, H., Wang, C. & Shi, X. (2011). A GCG expansion (GCG)$_{11}$ in polyadenylate-binding protein nuclear 1 gene caused oculopharyngeal muscular dystrophy in a Chinese family. *Mol Vis*, Vol. 17, (May), pp.1350-1354

Zhang, Y., Xing, D. & Liu, L. (2009). PUMA promotes Bax translocation by both directly interacting with Bax and by competitive binding to Bcl-X L during UV-induced apoptosis. *Mol Biol Cell*, Vol.30, No. 13, (July), pp. 3077–3087

Zhao, L. & Ackerman, SL. (2006). Endoplasmic reticulum stress in health and disease. *Curr Opin Cell Biol*, Vol.18, No.4, (August), pp. 444–452

3

Possible Diverse Roles of Fukutin: More Than Basement Membrane Formation?

Tomoko Yamamoto[1], Atsuko Hiroi[1], Yoichiro Kato[1],
Noriyuki Shibata[1], Makiko Osawa[2] and Makio Kobayashi[1]
[1]*Department of Pathology, Tokyo Women's Medical University,*
[2]*Department of Pediatrics, Tokyo Women's Medical University,*
Japan

1. Introduction

Fukutin is a gene responsible for Fukuyama-type congenital muscular dystrophy (FCMD) (Kobayashi et al. 1998). FCMD is associated with ocular and central nervous system (CNS) malformation characterized by cobblestone lissencephaly (Fukuyama et al. 1960; Osawa et al. 1997), and is included in α-dystroglycanopathy, one of the groups of muscular dystrophy. α-dystroglycan (α-DG) is one of the components of dystrophin-glycoprotein complex (DGC) linking extracellular and intracellular proteins (Fig. 1). O-linked glycosylation is a characteristic of α-DG, which is necessary for binding of extracellular matrix proteins to form the basement membrane. Causative genes of α-dystroglycanopathy are related to the glycosylation of α-DG, and hypoglycosylation of α-DG is involved in the pathogenesis of α-dystroglycanopathy (Martin 2005; Michele & Campbell 2003; Schessl et al. 2006).

The pathomechanism of muscular, ocular and CNS lesions of FCMD has gradually been elucidated, and the sequence of the *fukutin* gene is also known [GenBank: AB008226] (Kobayashi et al. 1998). Like other α-dystroglycanopathy diseases, reduced glycosylation of α-DG is observed at the cellular/basement membrane of the striated muscle, eye and CNS of FCMD patients (Hayashi et al. 2001; Yamamoto et al. 2010). Although fukutin is related to the glycosylation of α-DG, its actual role in the glycosylation is unknown. Moreover, post-transcriptional regulation of fukutin still remains to be elucidated. Interestingly, besides basement membrane formation, fukutin seems to have additional functions.

2. Diseases included in α-dystroglycanopathy

FCMD, muscle-eye-brain disease (MEB), Walker-Warburg syndrome (WWS), and some other types of muscular dystrophies such as MDC (congenital muscular dystrophy) 1C, MDC1D, limb girdle muscular dystrophy (LGMD) 2I and LGMD2K are in the disease category of α-dystroglycanopathy. FCMD is a congenital disease characterized by muscular dystrophy associated with CNS and ocular lesions. It is the second most common muscular dystrophy in Japan and was first described in 1960 by Fukuyama et al. (Fukuyama et al. 1960). MEB was initially reported in Finland, and ocular anomalies are especially conspicuous compared with FCMD (Pihko & Santavuori 1997). WWS is a severe disease and most of the patients die in infancy (Dobyns 1997). The CNS and eye are severely affected. The CNS lesions of FCMD, MEB and WWS are characterized by cobblestone lissencephaly, traditionally known as type II lissencephaly or polymicrogyria. Severe cases exhibit pachygyria. MDC1C (Brockington et al. 2001), MDC1D (Longman et al. 2003), LGMD2I (Brockington et al. 2001) and LGMD2K (Yis et al. 2011) are milder forms of α-dystroglycanopathy, in which CNS and eye lesions are less severe or absent. The clinical onset of LGMDs is late compared with that of congenital ones. Examples of animal models of α-dystroglycanopathy are fukutin chimeric mice (Chiyonobu et al. 2005; Masaki & Matsumura 2010), large[myd] mice (Lee et al. 2005; Masaki & Matsumura 2010), large[vls] mice (Lee et al. 2005; Masaki & Matsumura 2010), POMGnT1 knockout mice (Yang et al. 2007) and P0-DG null mice (Masaki & Matsumura 2010).

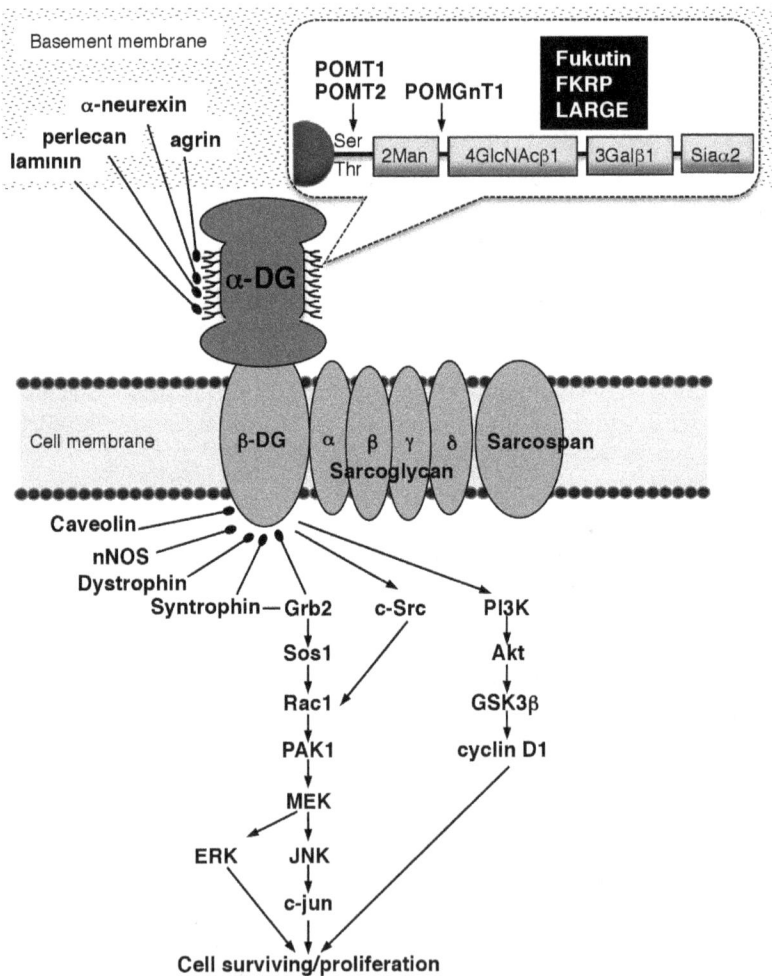

Fig. 1. A model of the dystrophin-glycoprotein complex in the skeletal muscle.

α-dystroglycanopathy shows the reduced glycosylation of α-DG at the cell/basement membrane. α-DG is a component of the DGC linking extracellular matrix and intracellular proteins (Fig. 1). It is a heavily glycosylated protein involved in the basement membrane formation by binding extracellular matrix proteins (Martin 2005; Michele & Campbell 2003; Schessl et al. 2006). Gene products involved in the glycosylation of α-DG include protein-O-mannosyltransferase 1 (POMT1), POMT2, O-linked mannose β1,2-N-acetylglucosaminyltransferase (POMGnT1), fukutin, fukutin-related protein (FKRP) and LARGE. α-dystroglycanopathy is caused by mutations of each gene. A wide spectrum of clinical disorders can be produced by mutations of one causative gene, especially *fukutin* and *FKRP* (Beltrán-Valero de Bernabé et al. 2003; Godfrey et al. 2007; Martin 2005; Schessl et al. 2006; Yis et al. 2011).

A common gene mutation of FCMD patients is homozygous founder mutation of *fukutin* (Kobayashi et al. 1998). However, a severe phenotype resembling WWS appears with heterozygous founder mutations and/or mutations that affect much of the coding protein (Beltrán-Valero de Bernabé et al. 2003; Cotarelo et al. 2008, Saito et al. 2000a), and milder phenotypes like LGMD have been reported (Godfrey et al. 2006; Godfrey et al. 2007; Murakami et al. 2006; Yis et al. 2011). *FKRP* mutations also produce clinical disorders over a wide spectrum covering most of the clinical phenotypes of α-dystroglycanopathy (Brockington et al. 2001; Martin 2005; Mercuri et al. 2006b; Schessl et al. 2006). *POMGnT1* is known as a gene responsible for MEB (Kano et al. 2002; Manya et al. 2003; Yoshida et al. 2001), but WWS is also associated with mutations of *POMGnT1* (Martin 2005; Schessl et al. 2006; Taniguchi et al. 2003). Major genes responsible for WWS are *POMT1* (Akasaka-Manya et al. 2004; Beltrán-Valero de Bernabé et al. 2002; Kim et al. 2004; Sabatelli et al. 2003) and *POMT2* (van Reeuwijk 2005), but milder phenotypes can occur as a result of their mutations (Balci et al. 2005; Biancheri et al. 2007; Mercuri et al. 2006a).

3. The glycosylation of α-DG for basement membrane formation, with regard to the pathogenesis of α-dystroglycanopathy

In striated muscle, glycosylated α-DG binds to several extracellular matrix proteins, such as laminin, agrin and neurexin, to form the basement membrane (Fig. 1) (Masaki & Matsumura 2010; Michele and Campbell 2003). After translation, DG is cleaved into α-and β-DG (Ibraghimov-Beskrovnaya et al. 1992; Michele and Campbell 2003). The C-terminal region of α-DG binds to the N-terminus of β-DG, a transmembrane protein. α-DG undergoes N-linked and O-linked glycosylation, and Sia-α-2,3-Gal-β-1,4-GlcNAc-β-1,2-Man-Ser/Thr in the mucin-like domain is involved in the interaction with laminin (Masaki & Matsumura 2010; Michele and Campbell 2003; Yoshida-Moriguchi et al. 2010). POMT1 together with POMT2 is required for the addition of mannose to a Ser/Thr residue (Manya et al. 2004), and POMGnT1 for the next step (Takahashi et al. 2001). These proteins possess glycosyltransferase activities (Manya et al. 2004; Takahashi et al. 2001). Although fukutin, FKRP and LARGE are related to the glycosylation of α-DG, it has not been fully elucidated how they work during the α-DG glycosylation (Martin 2005; Schessl et al. 2006). Recently, it has been clarified that phosphorylation on the O-linked mannose is required of α-DG for laminin binding, and this modification is mediated by LARGE (Yoshida-Moriguchi et al. 2010).

In α-dystroglycanopathy, epitopes recognized by monoclonal antibodies, IIH6 and VIA4-1 (Ervasti & Campbell 1993; Martin 2005; Michele and Campbell 2003), are reduced in the sarcolemma of the striated muscle, immunohistochemically. In western blotting, the hypoglycosylation is exhibited by a reduction of the molecular weight: a band of about 156 kDa in normal skeletal muscles shifts to a lower weight in muscles in cases of α-dystroglycanopathy. This hypoglycosylation is considered to cause a loss of α-DG function as a receptor for extracellular matrix proteins, which results in muscular dystrophy.

DGC similar to that of the skeletal muscle is observed in the peripheral and central nervous systems. In the CNS, the glia limitans is covered with the basement membrane where the glcosylated α-DG is observed. Morphological abnormalities of the basement membrane and the glia limitans have been reported in the CNS of FCMD (Fig. 2) (Nakano et al. 1996; Takada et al. 1987; Yamamoto et al. 1997; Yamamoto et al. 2010) and WWS (Beltrán-Valero de Bernabé 2002; Miller et al. 1991) patients and in mouse models of FCMD (Chiyonobu et al. 2005) and MEB (Yang et al. 2007). Fragile basement membrane caused by hypoglycosylation

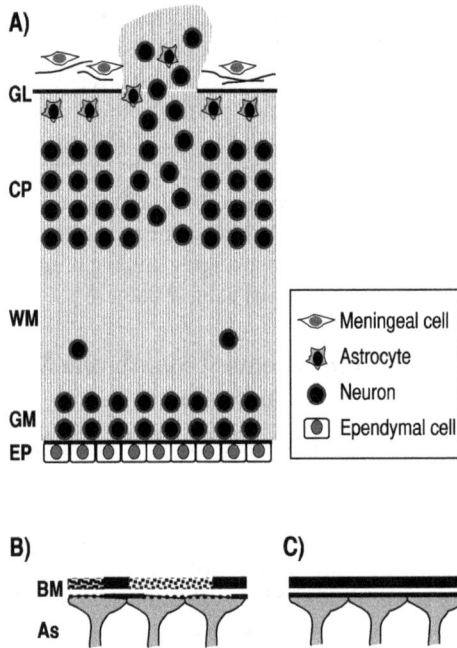

GL: glia limitans, CP: cortical plate, WM: white matter, GM: germinal matrix, EP: ependymal cells, BM: basement membrane, As: endfeet of astrocytes

Fig. 2. Schemas of the glia limitans of fetal FCMD cerebrum. A) Immature neurons and glia over-migrate into the leptomeninges through disruption of the glia limitans. B) The glia limitans is composed of astrocytic endfeet covered with the basement membrane. In the glia limitans of FCMD, both cell and basement membranes of astrocytes become ambiguous, even in the area without disruption, electron microscopically. Distribution of the abnormality is irregular. C) The cell and basement membranes are linear in controls.

of α-DG induces disruption of the glia limitans in the fetal period, which is considered to result in cobblestone lissencephaly. The glia limitans is formed by endfeet of astrocytes, and reduction of laminin binding has been observed in an astrocytoma cell line by knockdown of fukutin (data not shown). Astrocytes are considered to play an important role in the pathogenesis of the CNS lesion of α-dystroglycanopathy.

Thus, hypoglycosylation of α-DG at the basement membrane is involved in the pathogenesis of α-dystroglycanopathy. However, a wide clinical spectrum of disorders due to mutations of each causative gene might not be explained only by the abnormal basement membrane (Jiménez-Mallebrera et al. 2009).

4. Clinicopathological characteristics of FCMD

Generally, FCMD patients are found as a floppy infant, achieve peak motor function between 2 and 8 years, and die before 30 years old. They are mentally retarded, and more than 50% of patients have seizure. Abnormal eye movement and myopia are frequently seen, and cardiac symptoms may also be present (Fukuyama et al. 1960; Osawa et al. 1997). However, clinical manifestations of FCMD vary widely from mild to severe: patients of mild type can walk and talk meaningfully to some extent, while severe ones are very retarded and some cases may die *in utero*.

In the skeletal muscle, muscle fibers markedly decrease in number, which is associated with interstitial fibrosis and fatty infiltration. Myocardial fibrosis of varying degrees is observed in patients, particularly those more than 10 years old (Osawa et al. 1997). In eyes, retinal dysplasia with discontinuity of the inner limiting membrane is observed (Hino et al. 2001). In the cobblestone lissencephaly of post-natal patients, disorganization of cortical neurons, heterotopic glioneuronal tissues and surface fusions are seen, histologically (Kamoshita et al. 1976; Takada et al. 1984). Generally, the cerebral cortical lesion is extensive, but the cerebellum and brainstem are partially or mildly affected. Pachygyria and migration arrest are clear in severe cases mimicking WWS. On the other hand, a portion of the cerebral cortex shows an almost normal-looking appearance in mild cases. In fetal cases, the glia limitans formed by astrocytic endfeet in the CNS surface is disrupted, through which the glioneuronal tissues over-migrate into the leptomeninges (Fig. 2) (Nakano et al. 1996; Takada et al. 1987; Yamamoto et al. 1997; Yamamoto et al. 2010). Even in non-disrupted areas, both cell and basement membranes are abnormal, electron microscopically (Yamamoto et al. 1997; Yamamoto et al. 2010). The degree of disruption varies from case to case and even from area to area in a single patient (Takada et al. 1987; Yamamoto et al. 1997).

5. Functions of fukutin

5.1 *Fukutin* gene

Fukutin gene [GenBank, Accession AB038490] spans more than 100 kb of genomic DNA on chromosome 9q31 (Kobayashi et al. 1998; Toda et al. 1994). Fukutin mRNA composed of 10 exons is 7,349 bp with an open reading frame of 1,383 bp, beginning at base 112 (Kobayashi et al. 1998). Fukutin protein has 461 amino acids and the calculated molecular weight is 53.6 kDa, containing a hydrophobic signal sequence in the N-terminal (Kobayashi et al. 1998).

Retrotransposal 3-kb insertion of tandemly repeated sequences in the 3'-untranslated region is a common gene abnormality in FCMD patients and was determined as the ancestral founder haplotype (Kobayashi et al. 1998). Other mutations such as missense and nonsense mutations have been found (Beltrán-Valero de Bernabé 2003; Kobayashi et al. 1998). Japanese FCMD patients carry at least one copy of a founder mutation (Yoshioka 2009).

5.2 Functions of fukutin besides basement membrane formation in the nervous system

Fukutin is involved in basement membrane formation via the glycosylation of α-DG as described above. From the standpoint of CNS malformation, the most important component in the CNS is astrocytes that form the glia limitans. However, from the standpoint of total CNS function, the roles of fukutin in other components should be kept in mind during and after development (Fig. 3).

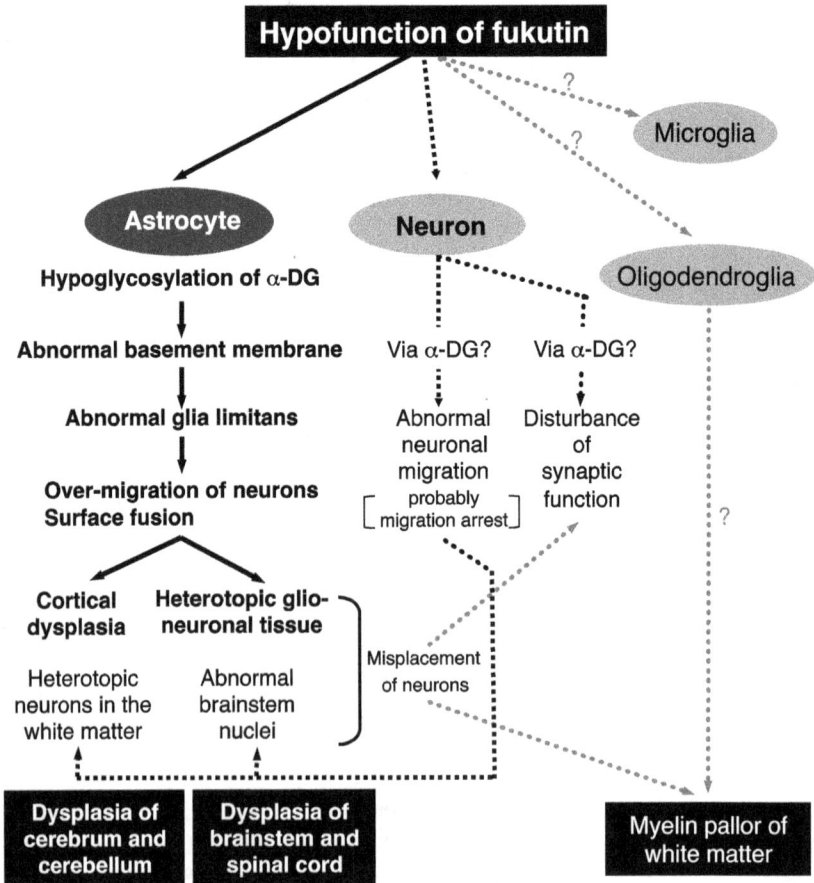

Fig. 3. Hypothesis for the CNS lesion of FCMD.

Fukutin is expressed in mature and immature neurons (Saito et al. 2000b; Sasaki et al. 2000; Yamamoto et al. 2002; Yamamoto et al. 2010). Mature neurons express α-DG detected by the antibody of VIA4-1, but not IIH6C4 (Hayashi et al. 2001; Hiroi et al. 2011; Saito et al. 2006). α-DG is considered to be involved in post-synaptic function (Moore et al. 2002; Satz et al. 2010). Since fukutin and the glycosylated α-DG are co-expressed in mature neurons, fukutin may be involved in synaptic function via the glycosylation of α-DG (Hiroi et al. 2011; Saito et al. 2006).

In the fetal cerebral and cerebellar cortex, fukutin and the glycosylated α-DG detected by VIA4-1 are co-expressed in immature neurons, especially in cells before and during migration (Hiroi et al. 2011). Fukutin may be involved in neuronal migration via the glycosylation of α-DG. However, this function appears to be minimal or immediately compensated for by other molecules because migration arrest in the FCMD brain is slight (Saito et al. 2003; Yamamoto et al. 2010), and forebrain histogenesis is preserved in mice with a neuron-specific deletion of DG (Satz et al. 2010).

The expression and function of fukutin in oligodendroglia and microglia are unclear. However, in the peripheral nerve, the DGC is found in Schwann cells, a counterpart of oligodendroglia, and is related to myelination and myelin maintenance (Masaki and Matsumura 2010). Fukutin-deficient chimeric mice exhibit a loss of myelination in the peripheral nerve (Masaki and Matsumura 2010; Saito et al. 2007), so that a function of oligodendroglia may be impaired.

Thus, fukutin is considered to have functions in neurons and glia, presumably mediated by the glycosylation of α-DG, which are not restricted to basement membrane formation. Interestingly, since neither mature nor immature neurons are positive for IIH6C4, the glycosylation of α-DG may be different between astrocytes and neurons (Hiroi et al. 2011). An experiment using mice genetically treated to lose DG in various patterns demonstrated a difference between glial and neuronal DG (Satz et al. 2010). Difference in DG glycosylation in different types of cells may be one of the reasons for the broad spectrum of CNS lesions of cobblestone lissencephaly (Satz et al. 2010).

5.3 Possible involvement of fukutin in neuroglial differentiation

The adult human cerebrum and cerebellum show less expression of fukutin than fetal ones, on immunohistochemistry and *in situ* hybridization (Saito et al. 2000b; Yamamoto et al. 2002). Fukutin expression is reduced after differentiation of cultured neuronal cells (Hiroi et al. 2011). Neuroblastoma cells extend neurites after knockdown of fukutin by RNAi (Fig. 4) (Hiroi et al. 2011). In an astrocytoma cell line, cells elongate cytoplasmic processes with increased expression of glial fibrillary acidic protein after knockdown of fukutin, and cells become epithelioid with an increase of Musashi-1 protein by transfection of fukutin (data not shown). Fukutin may be involved in neuroglial differentiation. In neurons, fukutin appears to prevent neuronal differentiation during migration. Although it is not clear whether this process is mediated by the glycosylation of α-DG, this seems very reasonable because immature neurons begin to differentiate after settlement in an appropriate site of the cortex.

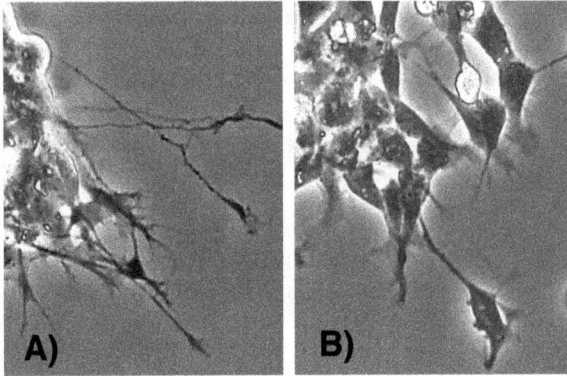

Fig. 4. RNAi in neuroblastoma cell line, IMR-32. After knockdown of fukutin, cells elongate neurites more (A) than in a control (B).

5.4 Functions of fukutin in somatic cells

Fukutin is expressed in various somatic organs (Kobayashi et al. 1998; Yamamoto et al. 2010). The DGC exists in epithelial cells, and DG plays a role in regulating cytoskeletal organization, cell polarization and cell growth in epithelial cells (Sgambato & Brancaccio 2005). Decrease of glycosylated α-DG has been reported in various cancers, and DG may act as a cancer suppressor (Sgambato & Brancaccio 2005). In a human non-tumorigenic mammary cell line, the percentage of cells in G_0/G_1 phase of the cell cycle is increased by DG overexpression (Sgambato et al. 2004). Since the DGC is linked to the cell signaling pathway (Oak et al. 2003) the glycosylation of α-DG can influence cell proliferation. At the C-terminus, β–DG binds to dystrophin and other intracellular proteins connecting to cell signaling pathways, such as growth factor receptor bound protein 2 (Grb2) involved in the MAPK/ERK cascade (Fig. 1) (Oak et al. 2003; Masaki and Matsumura 2010), with c-jun in the downstream region of the pathway (Oak et al. 2003). Tyrosine phosphorylation of the C-terminus of β-DG is dependent on c-src (Oak et al. 2003, Sotiga et al. 2001), and a signaling pathway is activated by laminin binding initiated by src family kinase (Zhou et al. 2007). The PI3K/AKT pathway is also involved (Langenbach et al. 2002).

Participating in the glycosylation of α-DG in epithelial cells as well (Yamamoto et al. 2008), fukutin may affect various epithelial cellular functions via the glycosylated α-DG. Fukutin may suppress cell proliferation/survival in epithelial cells because knockdown of fukutin in cancer cell lines made them proliferate more, at least in the short term (Yamamoto et al. 2008). There is a possibility of unknown functions of fukutin without intervention of the glycosylation of α-DG because nuclear localization of fukutin is suggested in cancer cell lines (Yamamoto et al. 2008). Involvement of fukutin in an immunological system is also supposed because fukutin is expressed in lymphoblast (Kobayashi et al. 1998).

The effects of fukutin might be different in different kinds of cells since cellular proliferation showed no change or rather a reduction after knockdown of fukutin in astrocytoma cells (data not shown). More experiments are required to clarify this point because there might have been some technical problems and alternative splicing has been reported in fukutin (Kobayashi et al. 2001).

5.5 Characteristics of fukutin mRNA with regard to neuroglial functions

In the CNS, synaptic plasticity is an important mechanism to adapt neurons to varying circumstances. Quick responses are needed at dendrites. Plasticity may also be required in astrocytes. Astrocytic endfeet are components of the blood-brain barrier (BBB), which maintains the CNS function by regulating transportation of water and various molecules. In the BBB, the basement membrane, positive for antibodies against glycosylated α-DG, VIA4-1 and IIH6C4, is formed between capillary and astrocytic endfeet. Moreover, the glycosylated α-DG is a receptor for some microorganisms (Cao et al. 1998; Kunz et al. 2005; Masaki and Matsumura 2010; Rambukkana et al. 1998). The glycosylation of α-DG should be prompt to adapt to varying circumstances at the most peripheral part of a cell.

There is a special type of mRNA called localized mRNA that is related to the maintenance of cell polarity, asymmetrical segregation and synaptic plasticity (López de Heredia and Jansen 2004; Ule and Darnell 2006). Localized mRNA has a binding site of an RNA-binding protein in the 3'-UTR region. A complex composed of mRNA and proteins is transported to peripheral areas of a cell such as dendrites, using a molecular motor like dynein and kinesin (López de Heredia and Jansen 2004). After reaching an appropriate site, the mRNA starts to be translated. mRNA of Arc, the immediate early gene product related to synaptic plasticity, is one of the localized mRNAs. A complex consisting of Arc mRNA and several proteins is transported along the microtubules and the mRNA undergoes local translation at a site of synaptic activity (Bramham et al. 2010). Kinesin is a motor of this complex. The transcription of Arc is regulated by cyclic AMP response element binding protein (CREB) (Bramham et al. 2010). A CRE-like sequence has been found in the fukutin gene promoter, and the transcription of fukutin may be regulated by CREB (Fang et al. 2005). Taking account of the possible functions of fukutin at the synapse and the BBB, it seems reasonable that fukutin mRNA is a localized mRNA. In the experiment using an astrocytoma cell line, Musashi-1 protein, one of the RNA-binding proteins, may bind to the 3'-UTR region of fukutin mRNA, suggesting that fukutin is a localized mRNA (data not shown).

6. Therapeutic strategies

From a therapeutic standpoint, many new strategies are underway for muscular dystrophy, particularly Duchenne muscular dystrophy (Collins & Bönnemann 2010; Cossu & Sampaolesi 2007; Muntoni et al. 2007; Odom et al. 2007). For α-dystroglycanopathy, full restoration of α-DG glycosylation might not be required (Kanagawa et al. 2009). Gene delivery using adeno-associated virus vectors may be applicable because causative genes of α-dystroglycanopathy are small enough to be packaged into this vector (Collins & Bönnemann 2010; Odom et al. 2007). Gene therapy using LARGE may be one of the candidates because gene transfer of LARGE restores α-DG receptor function not only in Large^myd mice but also in cultured cells from FCMD, MEB and WWS patients (Barresi et al. 2009). Transgenic overexpression of T-cell GalNAc transferase (GALgt2) in the skeletal muscle increases glycosylation of α-DG (Collins & Bönnemann 2010; Yoon et al. 2009). Transfer of fukutin restores glycosylation of α-DG in knock-in mice carrying the retrotransposal insertion in the mouse fukutin ortholog (Kanagawa et al. 2009).

However, there is a big underlying problem in patients with CNS malformation. Strategies might have to be different between muscle and CNS. The complicated structure of the CNS composed of several components should be noted. On FCMD, fukutin is expressed at least in astrocytes and neurons in the CNS. If the functions of fukutin in these cells are compensated for by other molecules after development, a therapy during the critical period *in utero* might be sufficient. In contrast, if fukutin continues to play important roles after development, lifelong therapy should be applied. In terms of future advances and applications of gene therapy for FCMD, it may be necessary to determine its precise roles to achieve an effective method while avoiding unprecedented side effects as much as possible. Since fukutin has several isoforms derived from alternative splicing (Kobayashi et al. 2001), investigations of each isoform may also be required.

7. Conclusion

Fukutin is related to the glycosylation of α-DG, which is involved in the pathogenesis of muscular dystrophy and ocular and CNS malformation of FCMD. Besides the basement membrane formation, fukutin has more diverse roles in other cells, including synaptic function and neuronal migration. Determination of the precise roles of fukutin seems to be important for further understanding of the disease and for future gene therapy.

8. Acknowledgement

The authors wish to thank Mr. Mizuho Karita, Mr. Hideyuki Takeiri, Mr. Fumiaki Muramatsu, Mrs. Noriko Sakayori and Mr. Shuichi Iwasaki for their excellent technical assistance and help in the preparation of this paper.

9. References

Akasaka-Manya, K.; Manya, H.; Endo T. (2004). Mutations of the *POMT1* gene found in patients with Walker-Warburg syndrome lead to a defect of protein O-mannosylation. *Biochem Biophys. Res. Commun.* 325, 75-79

Balci, B.; Uyanik, G.; Dincer, P.; Gross, C.; Willer, T.; Talim, B.; Haliloglu G.; Kale G.; Hehr U.; Winkler J.; Topaloglu H. (2005). An autosomal recessive limb girdle muscular dystrophy (LGMD2) with mild mental retardation is allelic to Walker-Warburg syndrome (WWS) caused by a mutation of the *POMT1* gene. *Neuromusc. Disord.* 15, 271-275

Barresi, R.; Michele, D.E.; Kanagawa, M.; Harper, H.A.; Dovico, S.A.; Satz, J.S.; Moore, S.A.; Zhang, W.; Schachter, H.; Dumanski, J.P.; Cohn, R.D.; Nishino I.; Campbell, K.P. (2004). LARGE can functionally bypass *a*-dystroglycan defects in distinct congenital muscular dystrophies. *Nat. Med.* 10, 696-703

Beltrán-Valero de Bernabé, D.; Currier, S.; Steinbrecher, A.; Celli, J.; van Beusekom, E.; van der Zwaag, B.; Kayserili, H.; Merlini, L.; Chitayat, D.; Dobyns, W.B.; Cormand, B.; Lehesjoki, A.-E.; Cruces, J.; Voit, T.; Walsh, C.A.; van Bokhoven, H.; Brunner, H.G. (2002). Mutations in the *O*-mannosyltransferase gene *POMT1* give rise to the severe neuronal migration disorder Walker-Warburg syndrome. *Am. J. Hum. Genet.* 71, 1033-1043

Beltrán-Valero de Bernabé, D., van Bokhoven H., van Beusekom E., van den Akker, W.; Kant, S.; Dobyns, W.B.; Cormand, B.; Currier, S.; Hamel, B.; Talim, B.; Topaloglu,

H.; Brunner, H.G. (2003). A homozygous nonsense mutation in the *fukutin* gene causes a Walker-Warburg syndrome phenotype. *J. Med. Genet.* 40, 845-848

Biancheri, R.; Falace, A.; Tessa, A.; Pedemonte, M.; Scapolan, S.; Cassandrini, D.; Aiello, C.; Rossi, A.; Broda, P.; Zara, F.; Santorelli, F.M.; Minetti, C.; Bruno, C. (2007). POMT2 gene mutation in limb-girdle muscular dystrophy with inflammatory changes. *Biochem. Biophys. Res. Commun.* 363, 1033-1037

Bramham, C.R.; Alme, M.N.; Bittins, M.; Kuipers, S.D.; Nair, R.R.; Pai, B.; Panja, D.; Schubert, M.; Soule, J.; Tiron, A.; Wibrand, K. (2010). The Arc of synaptic memory. *Exp. Brain. Res.* 200, 125-140

Brockington, M.; Yuva, Y.; Prandini, P.; Brown, S.C.; Torelli, S.; Benson, M.A.; Herrmann, R.; Anderson, L.V.B.; Bashir, R.; Burgunder, J.-M.; Fallet, S.; Romero, N.; Fardeau, M.; Straub, V.; Storey, G.; Pillitt, C.; Richard, I.; Sewry, C.A.; Bushby, K.; Voit, T.; Blake, D.J.; Muntoni, F. (2001). Mutations in the fukutin-related protein gene (*FKRP*) identify limb girdle muscular dystrophy 2I as a milder allelic variant of congenital muscular dystrophy MDC1C. *Hum. Mol. Genet.* 10, 2851-2859

Cao, W.; Henry, M.D.; Borrow, P.; Yamada, H.; Elder, J.H.; Ravkov, E.V.; Nichol, S.T.; Compans, R.W.; Campbell, K.P.; Oldstone, M.B. (1998). Identification of alpha-dystroglycan as a receptor for lymphocytic choriomeningitis virus and Lassa fever virus. *Science* 282, 2079-2081

Chiyonobu, T.; Sasaki, J.; Nagai, Y.; Takeda, S.; Funakoshi, H.; Nakamura, T.; Sugimoto, T.; Toda, T. (2005). Effects of fukutin deficiency in the developing brain. *Neuromusc. Disord.* 15, 416-426

Collins, J.; Bönnemann, C.G. (2010). Congenital muscular dystrophies: toward molecular therapeutic interventions. *Curr. Neurol. Neurosci. Rep.* 10, 83-91

Cossu, G.; Sampaolesi, M. (2007). New therapies for Duchenne muscular dystrophy: challenges, prospects and clinical trials. *Trends Mol. Med.* 13, 520-526

Cotarelo, R.P.; Valero, M.C.; Prados, B.; Peña, A.; Rodríguez, L.; Fano, O.; Marco, J.J.; Martínez-Frías, M.L.; Cruces, J. (2008). Two new patients bearing mutations in the *fukutin* gene confirm the relevance of this gene in Walker-Warburg syndrome. *Clin. Genet.* 73, 139-145

Dobyns, W.B. (1997). Walker-Warburg and other cobblestone lissencephaly syndromes: 1995 update. In: *Congenital Muscular Dystrophies*, Fukuyama Y., Osawa M., Saito K. (eds), pp89-98, Elsevier, Amsterdam

Ervasti, J.M.; Campbell, K.P. (1993). A role for the dystrophin-glycoprotein complex as a transmembrane linkder between laminin and actin. *J. Cell Biol.* 122, 809-823

Fang, H.; Sodja, C.; Chartier, J.; Desbois, A.; Lei, J.; Walker, P.R.; Sikorska, M. (2005). Identification of a functional CRE in the promoter of Fukuyama congenital muscular dystrophy gene *fukutin*. *Mol. Brain Res.* 136, 1-11

Fukuyama, Y.; Kawazura, M.; Haruna, H. (1960). A peculiar form of congenital progressive muscular dystrophy. *Paediatr. Univ. Tokyo* 4, 5-8

Godfrey, C.; Escolar, D.; Brockington, M.; Clement, E.M.; Mein, R.; Jimenez-Mallebrera, C.; Torelli, S.; Feng, L.; Brown, S.C.; Swery, C.A.; Rutherford, M.; Shapira, Y.; Abbs, S.; Muntoni, F. (2006). *Fukutin* gene mutations in steroid-responsive limb girdle muscular dystrophy. *Ann. Neurol.* 60, 603-610

Godfrey, C.; Clement, E.; Mein, R.; Brockington, M.; Smith, J.; Talim, B.; Straub, V.; Robb, S.; Quinlivan, R.; Feng, L.; Jimenez-Mallebrera, C.; Mercuri, E.; Manzur, A.Y.; Kinali,

M.; Torelli, S.; Brown, S.C.; Swery, C.A.; Bushby, K.; Topaloglu, H.; North, K.; Abbs, S.; Muntoni, F. (2007). Refining genotypa-phenotype correlations in muscular dystrophies with defective glycosylation of dystroglycan. *Brain* 130, 2725-2735

Hayashi, Y.K.; Ogawa, M.; Tagawa, K.; Noguchi, S.; Ishihara, T.; Nonaka, I.; Arahata, K. (2001). Selective deficiency of α-dystroglycan in Fukuyama-type congenital muscular dystrophy. *Neurology* 57, 115-121

Hino, N.; Kobayashi, M.; Shibata, N.; Yamamoto, T.; Saito, K.; Osawa, M. (2001). Clinicopathological study on eyes from cases of Fukuyama type congenital muscular dystrophy. *Brain Dev.* 23 , 97-107

Hiroi, A.; Yamamoto, T.; Shibata, N.; Osawa, M.; Kobayashi, M. (2011). Roles of fukutin, the gene responsible for Fukuyama-type congenital muscular dystrophy, in neurons: possible involvement in synaptic function and neuronal migration. *Acta Histochem. Cytochem.* 44, 91-101

Ibraghimov-Beskrovnaya, O.; Ervasti, J.M.; Leveille, C.J; Slaughter, C.A.; Sernett, S.W.; Campbell, K.P. (1992). Primary structure of dystrophin-associated glycoproteins linking dystrophin to the extracellular matrix. *Nature* 355, 696-702

Jiménez-Mallebrera, C.; Torelli, S.; Feng, L.; Kim, J.; Godfrey, C.; Clement, E.; Mein, R.; Abbs, S.; Brown, S.C.; Campbell, K.P.; Kröger, S.; Talim, B.; Topaloglu, H.; Quinlivan, R.; Roper, H.; Childs, A.M.; Kinali, M.; Sewry, C.A.; Muntoni, F. (2009). A comparative study of α-dystroglycan glycosylation in dystroglycanopathies suggest that the hypoglycosylation of α-dystroglycan dose not consistently correlate with clinical severity. *Brain Pathol.* 19, 596-611

Kamoshita, S.; Konishi, Y.; Segawa, M.; Fukuyama Y. (1976). Congenital muscular dystrophy as a disease of the central nervous system. *Arch. Neurol.* 33, 513-516.

Kanagawa M.; Nishimoto A.; Chiyonobu T.; Takeda S.; Miyagoe-Suzuki Y.; Wang F.; Fujikake N; Taniguchi M.; Lu Z,; Tachikawa M.; Nagai Y.; Tashiro F.; Miyazaki J.; Tajima Y.; Takeda S.; Endo T.; Kobayashi K.; Campbell KP.; Toda T. (2009). Residual laminin-binding activity and enhanced dystroglycan glycosylation by LARGE in novel model mice to dystroglycanopathy. *Hum. Mol. Genet.* 18, 621-631

Kano, H.; Kobayashi, K.; Herrmann, R.; Tachikawa, M.; Manya, H.; Nishino, I.; Nonaka, I.; Straub, V.; Talim, B.; Voit, T.; Topaloglu, H.; Endo, T.; Yoshikawa, H.; Toda, T. (2002). Deficiency of α-dystroglycan in Muscle-Eye-Brain disease. *Biochem. Biophys. Res. Commun.* 291, 1283-1286

Kim, D.-S.; Hayashi, Y.K.; Matsumoto, H.; Ogawa, M.; Noguchi, S.; Murakami, N.; Sakuta, R.; Mochizuki, M., Michele, D.E.; Campbell, K.P.; Nonaka, I.; Nishino, I. (2004). POMT1 mutation results in defective glycosylation and loss of laminin-binding activity in α-DG. *Neurology* 62, 1009-1011

Kobayashi, K.; Nakahori, Y.; Miyake, M.; Matsumura, K.; Kondo-Iida, E.; Nomura, Y.; Segawa, M.; Yoshioka, M.; Saito, K.; Osawa, M.; Hamano, K.; Sakakihara, Y.; Nonaka, I.; Nakagome, Y.; Kanazawa, I.; Nakamura, Y.; Tokunaga, K.; Toda, T. (1998). An ancient retrotransposal insertion causes Fukuyama-type congenital muscular dystrophy. *Nature* 394, 388-392

Kobayashi, K.; Sasaki, J.; Kondo-Iida, E.; Fukuda, Y.; Konoshita, M.; Sunada, Y.; Nakamura, Y.; Toda, T. (2001). Structural organization, complete genomic sequences and mutational analyses of the Fukuyama-type congenital muscular dystrophy gene, *fukutin. FEBS Lett* 489, 192-196

Kunz, S.; Rojek, J.M.; Kanagawa, M.; Spiropoulou, C.F.; Barresi, R.; Campbell, K.P.; Oldstone, M.B.A. (2005). Posttranslational modification of α-dystroglycan, the cellular receptor for arenaviruses, by the glycosyltransferase LARGE is critical for virus binding. *J. Virol.* 79, 14282-14296

Langenbach, K.J.; Rando, T.A. (2002). Inhibition of dystroglycan binding to laminin disrupts the PI3K/Akt pathway and survival signaling in muscle cells. *Muscle Nerve.* 26, 644-653

Lee, Y.; Kameya, S.; Cox ,G.A.; Hsu, J.; Hicks, W.; Maddatu, T.P.; Smith, R.S.; Naggert, J.K.; Peachey, N S.; Nishina, P.M. (2005). Ocular abnormalities in *Large*[myd] and *Large*[vls] mice, spontaneous models for muscle, eye and brain diseases. *Mol. Cell Neurosci.* 30, 160-172

Longman C.; Brockington, M.; Torelli, S.; Jimenez-Mallebrera, C.; Kennedy, C.; Khalil, N.; Feng, L.; Saran, R.K.; Voit, T.; Merlini, L.; Sewry, C.A., Brown, S.C., Muntoni, F. (2003). Mutations in the human LARGE gene cause MDC1D, a novel form of congenital muscular dystrophy with severe mental retardation and abnormal glycosylation of α-dystroglycan. *Hum Mol. Genet.* 12, 2853-2861

López de Heredia, M.; Jansen R.-P. (2004). mRNA localization and the cytoskeleton. *Curr. Opin. Cell Biol.* 16, 80-85

Manya, H.; Sakai, K.; Kobayashi, K.; Taniguchi, K.; Kawakita, M.; Toda, T.; Endo, T. (2003). Loss-of-function of an N-acetylglucosaminyltransferase, POMGnT1, in muscle-eye-brain disease. *Biochem. Biophys. Res. Commun.* 306, 93-97

Manya, H.; Chiba, A.; Yoshida, A.; Wang, X.; Chiba, Y.; Jigami, Y.; Margolis, R.U.; Endo T. (2004). Demonstration of mammalian protein O-mannosyltransferase activity: Coexpression of POMT1 and POMT2 required for enzymatic activity. *Proc. Natl. Acad. Sci. USA* 101, 500-505

Martin, P.T. (2005). The dystroglycanopathies: The new disorders of O-linked glycosylation. *Semin Pediatr. Neurol.* 12, 152-158

Masaki T.; Matsumura K. (2010). Biological role of dystroglycan in schwann cell function and its implication in peripheral nervous system diseases. *J Biomed Biotech* doi:10.1155/2010/740403

Mercuri, E.; D'Amico, A.; Tessa, A.; Berardineli, A.; Pane, M.; Messina, S.; van Reeuwijk, J.; Bertini, E.; Muntoni, F.; Santorelli, F.M. (2006). POMT2 mutation in a patient with 'MEB-like' phenotype. *Neuromusc. Disord.* 16, 446-448a

Mercuri, E.; Topaloglu, H.; Brockington, M.; Berardenelli, A.; Pichiecchio, A.; Santorelli, F.; Rutherford, M.; Talim, B.; Ricci, E.; Voit, T.; Muntoni, F. (2006). Spectrum of brain changes in patients with congenital muscular dystrophy and *FKRP* gene mutations. *Arch. Neurol.* 63, 251-257b

Michele, D.E.; Campbell, K.P. (2003). Dystrophin-glycoprotein complex: post-transcriptional processing and dystroglycan function. *J. Biol. Chem.* 278, 15457-15460

Miller, G.; Ladda, R.L.; Towfighi, J. (1991). Cerebro-ocular dysplasia-Muscular dystrophy (Walker Warburg) syndrome. Findings in 20-week-old fetus. *Acta Neuropathol.* 82, 234-238

Moore, S.A.; Saito, F.; Chen, J.; Michele, D.E.; Henry, M.D.; Messing, A.; Cohn, R.D.; Ross-Barta, S.E.; Westra, S.; Williamson, R.A.; Hoshi, T.; Campbell, K.P. (2002). Deletion of brain dystroglycan recapitulates aspects of congenital muscular dystrophy. *Nature* 418, 422-425

Muntoni, F.; Wells, D. (2007). Genetic treatments in muscular dystrophies. *Curr. Opin. Neurol.* 20, 590-594

Murakami, T.; Hayashi, Y.K.; Noguchi, S.; Ogawa, M.; Nonaka, I.; Tanabe, Y.; Ogino, M.; Takada, F.; Eriguchi, M.; Kotooka, N.; Campbell, K.P.; Osawa, M.; Nishino, I. (2006). Fukutin gene mutations cause dilated cardiomyopathy with minimal muscle weakness. *Ann. Neurol.* 60, 597-602

Nakano, I.; Funahashi, M.; Takada, K.; Toda, T. (1996). Are breaches in the glia limitans the primary cause of the micropolygyria in Fukuyama-type congenital muscular dystrophy (FCMD)? Pathological study of the cerebral cortex of an FCMD fetus. *Acta Neuropathol.* 91, 313-321

Oak, S.A.; Zhou, Y.W.; Jarrett, H.W. (2003). Skeletal muscle signaling pathway through the dystrophin glycoprotein complex and Rac1. *J. Biol. Chem.* 278, 39287-39295

Odom, G.L.; Gregorevic, P.; Chamberlain, J.S. (2007). Viral-mediated gene-therapy for the muscular dystrophies: successes, limitations and recent advances. *Biochim. Biophys. Acta* 1772, 243-262

Osawa M.; Sumida S.; Suzuki N.; Arai Y., Ikenaka H., Murasugi H., Shishikura K., Suzuki H., Saito K., Fukuyama Y. (1997). Fukuyama type congenital muscular dystrophy, In: *Congenital Muscular Dystrophies*, Fukuyama Y., Osawa M., Saito K. (Eds.), pp. 31-68, Elsevier, Amsterdam

Pihko, H.; Santavuori, P. (1997). Muscle-eye-brain (MEB) disese — a review. In: *Congenital Muscular Dystrophies*, Fukuyama Y., Osawa M., Saito K. (eds), pp99-104, Elsevier, Amsterdam

Rambukkana, A.; Yamada, H.; Zanazzi, G.; Mathus, T.; Salzer, J.L.; Yurchenco, P.D.; Campbell, K.P.; Fischetti, V.A. (1998). Role of α-dystroglycan as a Schwann cell receptor for *Mycobacterium leprae*. *Science* 282, 2076-2079

Sabatelli, P.; Columbaro, M.; Mura, I.; Capanni, C.; Lattanzi, G.; Maraldi, N.M.; Baltrán-Valero de Bernabé, D.; van Bokoven, H.; Squarzoni, S.; Merlini, L. (2003). Extracellular matrix and nuclear abnormalities in skeletal muscle of a patient with Walker-Warburg syndrome caused by *POMT1* mutation. *Biochim. Biophys. Acta* 1638, 57-62

Saito, F.; Masaki, T.; Saito, Y.; Nakamura, A.; Takeda, S.; Shimizu, T.; Toda, T.; Matsumura, K. (2007). Defective peripheral nerve myelination and neuromuscular junction formation in fukutin-deficient chimeric mice. *J. Neurochem.* 101, 1712-1722

Saito, K.; Osawa, M.; Wang, Z.-P.; Ikeya, K.; Fukuyama, Y.; Kondo-Iida, E.; Toda, T.; Ohashi, H.; Kurosawa, K.; Wakai, S.; Kaneko, K. (2000). Haplotype-phenotype correlation in Fukuyama congenital muscular dystrophy. *Am. J. Med. Genet.* 92, 184-190a

Saito, Y.; Mizuguchi, M.; Oka, A.; Takashima, S. (2000). Fukutin protein is expressed in neurons of the normal developing human brain but is reduced in Fukuyama-type congenital muscular dystrophy brain. *Ann. Neurol.* 47, 756-764b

Saito, Y.; Kobayashi, M.; Itoh, M.; Saito, K.; Mizuguchi, M., Sasaki, H., Arima K., Yamamoto T., Takashima S., Sasaki M., Hayashi K., Osawa M. (2003). Aberrant neuronal migration in the brainstem of Fukuyama-type congenital muscular dystrophy. *J. Neuropathol. Exp. Neurol.* 62, 497-508

Saito, Y.; Yamamoto, T.; Mizuguchi, M.; Kobayashi, M.; Saito, K.; Ohno, K.; Osawa, M. (2006). Altered glycosylation of α-dystroglycan in neurons of Fukuyama congenital muscular dystrophy brains. *Brain Res.* 1075, 223-228

Sasaki, J.; Ishikawa, K.; Kobayashi, K.; Kondo-Iida, E.; Fukayama, M.; Mizusawa, H.; Takashima, S.; Sakakihara, Y.; Nakamura, Y.; Toda, T. (2000). Neuronal expression of the fukutin gene. *Hum. Mol. Genet.* 9, 3083-3090

Satz, J.S.; Ostendorf, A.P.; Hou, S.; Turner, A.; Kusano, H.; Lee, J.C.; Turk, R.; Nguyen, H.; Ross-Barta, S.E.; Westra, S.; Hoshi, T.; Moore, S.A.; Campbell, K.P. (2010). Distinct functions of glial and neuronal dystroglycan in the developing and adult mouse brain. *J Neurosci* 30, 14560-14572

Schessl, J.; Zou, Y.; Bönnemann, C.G. (2006). Congenital muscular dystrophies and the extracellular matrix. *Semin. Pediatr. Neurol.* 13, 80-89

Sgambato, A.; Camerini, A.; Faraglia, B.; Pavoni, E.; Montanari, M.; Spada, D.; Losasso, C.; Brancaccio, A.; Cittadini, A. (2004). Increased expression of dystroglycan inhibits the growth and tumorigenicity of human mammary epithelial cells. *Cancer Biol. Ther.* 3, 967-975

Sgambato, A.; Brancaccio, A. (2005). The dystroglycan complex: From biology to cancer. *J. Cell Physiol.* 205, 163-169

Sotgia, F.; Lee, H.; Bedford, M.T.; Petrucci, T.; Sudol, M.; Lisanti, M.P. (2001). Tyrosine phosphorylation of β-dystroglycan at its WW domain binding motif, PPxY, recruits SH2 domain containing proteins. *Biochemistry* 40, 14585-14592

Takada, K.; Nakamura, H.; Tanaka J. (1984). Cortical dysplasia in congenital muscular dystrophy with central nervous system involvement (Fukuyama type). *J. Neuropathol. Exp. Neurol.* 43, 395-407

Takada, K.; Nakamura, H.; Suzumori, K.; Ishikawa, T.; Sugiyama, N. (1987). Cortical dysplasia in a 23-week fetus with Fukuyama congenial muscular dystrophy (FCMD). *Acta Neuropathol.* 74, 300-306

Takahashi, S.; Sasaki, T.; Manya, H.; Chiba, Y.; Yoshida, A.; Mizuno, M.; Ishida, H.; Ito, F.; Inazu, T.; Kotani, N.; Takasaki, S.; Takeuchi, M.; Endo, T. (2001). A new β1,2-*N*-acetylglucosaminyltransferase that may play a role in the biosynthesis of mammalian *O*-mannosyl glycans. *Glycobiology* 11, 37-45

Taniguchi, K.; Kobayashi, K.; Saito, K.; Yamanouchi, H.; Ohnuma, A.; Hayashi, Y.K.; Manya, H.; Jin D.K.; Lee, M.; Parano, E.; Falsaperla, R.; Pavone, P.; Coster, R.V.; Talim, B.; Steinbrecher, A.; Straub, V.; Nishino, I.; Topaloglu, H.; Voit, T.; Endo, T.; Toda, T. (2003). Worldwide distribution and broder clinical spectrum of muscle-eye-brain disease. *Hum. Mol. Genet.* 12, 527-534

Toda, T.; Ikegawa, S.; Okui, K.; Kondo, E.; Saito, K.; Fukuyama, Y.; Yoshioka, M.; Kumagai, T.; Suzumori, K.; Kanazawa, I.; Nakamura, Y. (1994). Refined mapping of a gene responsible for Fukuyama-type congenital muscular dystrophy: Evidence for strong linkage disequilibrium. *Am. J. Hum. Genet.* 55, 946-950

Ule, J.; Darnell, R.B. (2006). RNA binding proteins and the regulation of neuronal synaptic plasticity. *Curr. Opin. Neurobiol.* 16, 102-110

van Reeuwijk, J.; Janssen, M.; van den Elzen, C.; Beltrán-Valero de Bernabé, D.; Sabatelli, P.; Merlini, L.; Boon, M.; Scheffer, H.; Brockington, M.; Muntoni, F.; Huynen, M.A.; Verrips, A.; Walsh, C.A.; Barth, P.G.; Brunner, H.G.; van Bokhoven, H. (2005). *POMT2* mutations cause α-dystroglycan hypoglycosylation and Walker-Warburg syndrome. *J. Med. Genet.* 42, 907-912

Yamamoto, T.; Toyoda, C.; Kobayashi, M.; Kondo, E.; Saito, K.; Osawa, M. (1997). Pial-glial barrier abnormalities in fetuses with Fukuyama congenital muscular dystrophy. *Brain Dev.* 19, 35-42

Yamamoto, T.; Kato, Y.; Karita, M.; Takeiri, H.; Muramatsu, F.; Kobayashi, M.; Saito, K.; Osawa, M. (2002). Fukutin expression in glial cells and neurons: implication in the brain lesions of Fukuyama congenital muscular dystrophy. *Acta Neuropathol.* 104, 217-224

Yamamoto, T.; Kato, Y.; Shibata, N.; Sawada, T.; Osawa, M.; Kobayashi, M. (2008). A role of fukutin, a gene responsible for Fukuyama type congenital muscular dystrophy, in cancer cells: a possible role to suppress cell proliferation. *Int J Exp Pathol* 89, 332-341

Yamamoto, T.; Shibata, N.; Saito, Y.; Osawa, M.; Kobayashi M. (2010). Functions of fukutin, a gene responsible for Fukuyama type congenital muscular dystrophy, in neuromuscular and other somatic organs. *Cent. Nerv. Syst .Agents Med. Chem.* 10, 169-179

Yang, Y.; Zhang, P.; Xiong, Y.; Li, X.; Qi, Y.; Hu H. (2007). Ectopia of meningeal fibroblasts and reactive gliosis in the cerebral cortex of the mouse model of muscle-eye-brain disease. *J Comp Neurol* 505, 459-477

Yis, U.; Uyanik, G.; Heck, P.B.; Smitka, M.; Nobel, H.; Ebinger, F.; Dirik, E.; Feng, L.; Kurul, S.H.; Brocke, K.; Unalp, A.; Özer, E.; Cakmakci, H.; Sewry, C.; Cirak, S.; Muntoni, F.; Hehr, U.; Morris-Rosendahl, D.J. (2011). *Fukutin* mutations in non-Japanese patients with congenital muscular dystrophy: less severe mutations predominate in patients with a non-Walker-Warburg phenotype. *Neuromusc. Disord.* 21, 20-30

Yoon, J.H.; Chandrasekharan, K.; Xu, R.; Glass, M.; Singhal, N.; Martin, P.T. (2009). The synaptic CT carbohydrate modulates binding and expression of extracellular matrix proteins in skeletal muscle: Partial dependence on utrophin. *Mol. Cell Neurosci.* 41, 448-63

Yoshida, A.; Kobayashi, K.; Manya, H.; Taniguchi, K.; Kano, H;, Mizuno, M.; Inazu, T.; Mitsuhashi, H.; Takahashi, S.; Takeuchi, M.; Herrmann, R.; Straub, V.; Talim, B.; Voit, T.; Topaloglu, H.; Toda, T.; Endo, T. (2001). Muscular dystrophy and neuronal migration disorder caused by mutations in a glycosyltransferase, POMGnT1. *Dev. Cell* 1, 717-724

Yoshida-Moriguchi, T.; Yu, L.; Stalnaker, S.H.; Davis, S.; Kunz, S.; Madson, M.; Oldstone, M.B.A.; Schachter, H.; Wells, L.; Campbell, KP. (2010). *O*-mannosyl phosphorylation of alpha-dystroglycan is required for laminin binding. *Science* 327, 88-92

Yoshioka, M. (2009). Phenotypic spectrum of fukutinopathy: most severe phenotype of fukutinopathy. *Brain Dev.* 31, 419-422

Zhou, Y.; Jiang, D.; Thomason, D.B.; Jarrett, H.W. (2007). Laminin-induced activation of Rac1 and JNKp46 is initiated by src family kinases and mimics the effects of skeletal muscle contraction. *Biochemistry* 46, 14907-14916

4

Myotonic Dystrophy Type 1 (DM1): From the Genetics to Molecular Mechanisms

Jonathan J. Magaña[1] and Bulmaro Cisneros[2]
[1]Genetics Department, Genomic Medicine Laboratory, National Rehabilitation Institute;
[2]Genetics and Molecular Biology Department, CINVESTAV-IPN,
Mexico

1. Introduction

For a long time, the human genome was considered an intrinsically stable entity; however, it is currently known that our human genome contains many unstable elements consisting of tandem repeat elements, mainly Short tandem repeats (STR), also known as microsatellites or Simple sequence repeats (SSR) (Ellegren, 2000). These sequences involve a repetitive unit of 1-6 bp, forming series with lengths from two to several thousand nucleotides. STR are widely found in pro- and eukaryotes, including humans. They appear scattered more or less evenly throughout the human genome, accounting for ca. 3% of the entire genome (Sharma et al., 2007). STR are polymorphic but stable in general population; however, repeats can become unstable during DNA replication, resulting in mitotic or meiotic contractions or expansions. STR instability is an important and unique form of mutation that is linked to >40 neurological, neurodegenerative, and neuromuscular disorders (Pearson et al., 2005). In particular, abnormal expansion of trinucleotide repeats (CTG)n, (CGG)n, (CCG)n, (GAA)n, and (CAG)n have been associated with different diseases such as fragile X syndrome, Huntington disease (HD), Dentatorubral-pallidoluysian atrophy (DRPLA), Friedreich ataxia (FA), diverse Spinocerebellar ataxias (SCA), and Myotonic dystrophy type 1 (DM1).

In 1909, Hans Gustav Wilhelm Steinert, as well as Frederick Eustace Batten and H.P. Gibb, described for the first time a muscular dystrophy characterized by progressive muscle weakness and myotonia (involuntary muscle contraction and delayed relaxation due to muscle hyperexcitability) denominated Myotonic dystrophy or Steinert disease (Schara and Schoser, 2006). Currently, two distinct mutations are known that lead to the clinical syndrome of DM: Myotonic dystrophy type 1 (DM1), caused by expansion of CTG repeats within the 3' untranslated region of the Dystrophia myotonica-protein-kinase gene (*DMPK*) on chromosome 19 (Brook et al., 1992), and Myotonic dystrophy type 2, due to expansion of CCTG repeats in intron 1 of the Zinc finger protein gene (*ZNF9*) on chromosome 3 (Liquori et al., 2001). DM1 is an autosomal dominant inherited disease that represents the most common form of muscular dystrophy in adults with a prevalence of 1 in 8,000 individuals worldwide. In addition to muscular pathology, DM1 symptomatology includes cardiac conduction defects, insulin resistance, and cognitive alterations in the congenital form of the disease (Harper et al., 2002). For some time, it was difficult to decipher the manner in which a repeat expansion in the *DMPK* gene causes a multisystemic disease with dominant inheritance pattern. However, the fact that such a mutated region is transcribed but untranslated implies that mutant RNA might play a significant role in the disease process. Supporting this hypothesis, growing pieces of evidence obtained over the past 10 years have established that DM1- mutant RNA accumulates in the nuclei, disturbing RNA splicing and gene expression through sequestering of splicing and transcription factors, respectively (Day & Ranum, 2005; Ebralidze et al., 2004).

In this chapter, the clinical features of DM1 and the scientific pathway that allowed elucidation of the molecular basis of DM1 pathogenesis are described in detail. In addition, a discussion of recent developments in molecular therapy for fighting DM1 is provided.

2. Clinical aspects

DM1 is one of the most frequent genetic diseases and is also one of the most variable disorders. Symptoms and severity vary greatly among family members and between generations. Patients may even remain undiagnosed or be misdiagnosed for years, if not recognized as being a member of a family with DM1. However, within the broad spectrum of clinical symptoms, there are some distinct phenotypes according to age-of-onset and number of CTG repeats.

2.1 Multisystemic symptomatology

Clinical manifestations of DM1 involve a great number of organs and tissues and vary from the pre-/post-natal period to adulthood. Skeletal muscle pathology is the most characteristic feature of DM1. Impaired muscle relaxation from myotonia can lead to stiffness and cramping, especially in distal muscles of the hands, but it is rarely a significant complaint registered by patients. Muscle weakness and wasting start distally on distal limbs, neck, and face, and progress proximally over time, often leading to severe disability as the disease progresses (Schara and Schoser, 2006). Respiratory muscle involvement is common, and respiratory failure, either from the primary muscle process or from cardiopulmonary involvement, is a significant contributor to patient mortality (Machuca-Tzili L et al., 2005). A less well-defined but important disease feature is its effect on the Central nervous system (CNS) and cognition, which can be manifested by psychological dysfunction, mental retardation, excessive diurnal sleepiness, and neuropathological abnormalities (Rubinsztein et al., 1998; Laberge et al., 2009). Recent work has demonstrated global deficits with neuropsychological testing, as well as radiographic changes in the brains of affected individuals, including increased white matter lesion burden, decreased gray matter mass (especially in hippocampal and thalamic regions), and hypometabolism in frontal lobes (Di Constanzo et al., 2002a, 2008b; Ono et al., 2001). Alterations of personality associated with DM1 include avoidant personality, obsessive-compulsive, passive-aggressive, and schizotypic traits, whose occurrence is not attributable to the patients' disabling condition (Delaporte 1998; Winblad et al., 2005). Other studies have found severe impairment in all measurements of general intelligence and verbal fluency (Rubinsztein et al., 1997).

In addition to the effects on the CNS, 90% of patients with DM1 could develop cardiac abnormalities at some point of disease development. First-degree atrioventricular block and intraventricular conduction disorders are observed commonly in subjects with DM1, followed by lethal arrhythmias and occasional signs of cardiomyopathy. Echocardiograph findings include prolapsed mitral valve, depressed left ventricular systolic function, reductions in ejections fraction, fractional shortening, and reduced stroke volume (Melacini et al., 1995). In fact, sudden cardiac failure is one of the main causes of death in these patients and occurs with a high incidence of 30%. In the ocular system of these patients, the incidence of lens opacities is very high and manifests as posterior subcapsular, iridescent, multicolored cataracts. Moreover, changes in the Retinal pigment epithelium (RPE), known as Pigment pattern dystrophy (PPD), could be present in the peripheral retina or in macula, mimicking retinitis pigmentosa (Grover et al., 2002; Kim et al., 2009; Louprasong et al., 2010). The ocular muscles are also affected, resulting in external ophthalmoplegia, bilateral motility disturbance, obicularis oculi and levator muscle weakness, and ptosis. Other ocular defects include decreased vision and decreased intraocular pressure (Rosa et al., 2011). Patients with DM1 could also present endocrine defects including insulin resistance and gonadal atrophy (García de Andoin et al., 2005; Matsumura et al., 2009), as well as smooth muscle dysfunction, the clinical effects of which are observed mainly in the gastrointestinal tract and result in disordered esophageal and gastric peristalsis (Machuca-Tzili L et al., 2005).

2.2 Adult-onset and congenital myotonic dystrophy

Based on the clinical findings as well as age-at-onset and disease course, DM1 has been categorized into two main and somewhat overlapping phenotypes: adult-onset, and Congenital myotonic dystrophy (CDM). A rough correlation exists between CTG repeat tract size and these two main forms of DM1 (see Genetics of DM1 section).

Adult-onset presents the classical manifestations of DM1, including myotonia, muscle weakness, cardiac rhythm abnormalities, and endocrine and gonadal abnormalities. The disease progresses insidiously but can become debilitating in the fifth and sixth decades of life. Some authors have classified adult-onset in into two subtypes (mild and classic DM1) according to age-at-onset. Mild DM1 could be asymptomatic or may have only cataracts, mild myotonia, and/or diabetes mellitus. It usually begins in old age and patients may have fully active lives and normal or minimally shortened life span. Classic DM1 is the most common presentation of DM1. The predominant symptom is distal muscle weakness, leading to foot drop disturbance and difficulty with performing tasks requiring fine manual dexterity. Myotonia may interfere with daily activities and the typical face of the patients is principally caused by weakness of facial and levator palpebrae muscles; however, expressivity can be variable, and the presentation could include one or several DM1 features, including cardiac abnormalities, respiratory failure, endocrine abnormalities, smooth muscle dysfunction, cataracts, and hypersomnolence. Age-at-onset for classic DM1 is typically in the third of fourth decades of life, and presents uncommonly after 40 years of age. Nevertheless, in some cases, the pathology begins in the childhood stage (first decade of life), exhibiting evident facial weakness and myotonia, and more severe evolution characterized by low IQ, psychiatric alteration, and early cardiac abnormalities.

CDM is the most severe form of the disease and is usually inherited maternally (Harley et al., 1993). Prenatal stage is characterized by polyhydramnios and reduced fetal movement, all caused by muscle action failure. The main features of congenital DM1 include generalized hypotonia and weakness, pharyngeal weakness, and arthrogryposis, involving predominantly the lower limbs. Less constant features include facial diplegia, diaphragmatic paralysis, respiratory failure, decreased gastrointestinal-tract motility, congenital cataracts, and electrocardiographic abnormalities. Surviving infants exhibit delayed motor development and are often mentally retarded. Typically, affected infants have an inverted V-shaped upper lip, which is characteristic of significant bilateral facial weakness. It is noteworthy that myotonia is not observed in the first years of life (Schara and Schoser, 2006).

2.3 Prognosis and diagnosis of DM1

Life expectancy appears to be reduced in patients with DM1 and is variable depending on the clinical phenotype presented. Subjects with adult-onset DM1 have a nearly normal Quality of life (QOL) during childhood and early adulthood. Nevertheless, many patients become severely disabled by the fifth or sixth decades of life. Chest infections partly due to aspiration and diaphragm weakness are common and may precipitate respiratory failure. Sudden cardiac death is not uncommon, even in younger patients, but it may be preventable by cardiac pacemaker implantation (Machuca-Tzili L et al., 2005). In addition, treatment for diabetes mellitus including annual measurement of serum glucose and glycosylated hemoglobin concentration is indicated to improve the QOL of these patients. Approximate average age of death for patients with adult-onset disease is between 50 and 60 years, and when symptoms begin in the childhood stage, life expectancy is not necessarily reduced, but complications are more common.

In congenital DM1, stillbirths are seldom reported. In severe cases, mortality is high in the first hours and days of life, caused by respiratory insufficiency despite active resuscitation. After the neonatal period, prognosis is more favorable, and despite retarded motor development, all patients become able to walk independently at different ages. Death is frequent in these patients before the age of 30 years, which is caused suddenly by cardiomyopathy and cardiac arrhythmias (Harper, 2001). In the second decade of life, myotonia becomes a more prominent feature, in addition to classical symptoms observed in the adult-onset form, such as infertility and gastrointestinal problems.

An accurate diagnosis of DM1 is important, not only to enable a differential diagnosis among neurological diseases, but also to predict disease severity and to assist patients with appropriate medical monitoring and symptom management. For some time, clinical features were employed to establish the diagnosis of DM1; however, the disease's multisystemic and variable symptomatology caused misdiagnosis in some instances. For example, congenital DM1 could be clinically confused with several other congenital neuromuscular disorders, including myotonia congenita, congenital myopathies, spinal muscular atrophy type 1 or -2, congenital myasthenic syndromes, Möbius syndrome, Spinal muscular atrophy with respiratory distress (SMARD1), the congenital form of glycogenosis type 2, or anoxic brain damage (Harper, 2001; Harper & Monckton, 2004). In adults, Myotonic dystrophy type 2 (DM2) is the condition that is most similar to DM1; the symptoms are practically the same in both dystrophies. Other hereditary distal myopathies, such as hereditary myofibrillar myopathy, hereditary inclusion body myositis, distal muscular dystrophy (Miyoshi, Nonaka, Welander, Markesbery-Griggs), or limb-girdle muscular dystrophies could be confused (Bird, 2011). Currently, diagnosis of DM1 disease is based on DNA testing in individuals who are clinically suspected of having DM1. Patients may have had an electromyography and occasionally muscle biopsy and other tests prior to clinical suspicion of the diagnosis. Electromyography was the most helpful laboratory study prior to the availability of genetics. The combination of myotonic discharges and myopathic- appearing motor units, predominantly in distal muscles and the face, is highly suspicious of DM1. Because electrical myotonic discharges are not usually observed during infancy and many other disorders are associated with myotonia, including myotonia and congenital parmyotonia, this particular test should be taken only as a suggestive finding of DM1. Muscle biopsy is histologically grossly abnormal in clinically affected individuals. Features include variability in fiber size, fibrosis, rows of internal nuclei, sarcoplasmic masses, and an increased number of intrafusal muscle fibers. However, it should be emphasized that there is no clinical indication for performing a muscle biopsy to conducting the diagnosis of DM1 (The International Myotonic Dystrophy Consortium [IDMC], 2000). If clinical features suggest DM1 but DM1 genetic testing is negative, then DM2 testing should be performed. Finally, serum creatine kinase concentration may be mildly elevated in patients with DM1, but it is often normal in asymptomatic individuals.

The DNA test for DM1 is highly relevant because, it confirms the diagnosis in cases with clinically uncertain symptoms, eliminating the need for invasive muscle biopsy. Currently, molecular diagnosis identifies the DM1 mutations in 100% of affected subjects (IDMC, 2000). In addition, determination of insert sizes of CTG repeats aids relatively in predicting disease severity (see Table 1), which is especially useful in young asymptomatic subjects. Despite several advances in the field of DNA analytic techniques, identification of DM1 expanded alleles continues to represent a challenge because of the immense length and variability of expanded alleles and due to the extremely stable secondary structure formed by repetitive, CG-rich sequences. Mutation analysis is based on detection of expanded DMPK alleles, usually by Southern blot analysis. The use of Field-inversion gel electrophoresis (FIGE) and Pulsed-field gel electrophoresis (PFGE), as well as digoxigenin-labeled short CAG-repeat-specific, locked nucleic acid probes have increased the resolution of this technique (Jakubicza et al., 2004). However, Southern blot analysis is not suitable for routine clinical use because it is a time-consuming technique that requires large amounts of genomic DNA and the use in the majority of instances of radioactive probes. Moreover, Southern blot fails to detect premutated alleles and alleles with small expansions. PCR-based assays have been developed to replace Southern blot. PCR utilizing flanking primers allows for amplification up to approximately 100 CTG repeats, but it is unreliable above this size; thus, amplification of alleles with very large numbers of CTG repeats (>100) continue to require Southern blot analysis (Falk, 2006; Tishkoff, 1998; Warner, 1996). Certain improvements in amplification of alleles with large numbers of repeats have been obtained by adding highly stable Taq DNA polymerases, and PCR-enhancing agents, such as glycerol, betaine, and 7-deaza-dGTP to the master reaction (Cheng et al., 1996; Kakourou et al., 2010; Magaña et al., 2011a; Skrzypczak-Zielinska et al., 2009). Currently, identification of DM1 expanded alleles is performed through fluorescent PCR and capillary electrophoresis. The use of a fluorescently labeled primer permits detection of the amplified products by an Argon lasser, and its comparison with a molecular size marker allows sizing of alleles of <100 CTG repeats. Interestingly, a simple fluorescent PCR system that can rapidly identify the largest alleles for any disorder with CTG/CAG repeat expansion was developed (Warner et al., 1996). This method utilizes a fluorescently labeled locus-specific primer flanking the CTG repeat together with paired primers amplifying from multiple priming sites within the CTG repeat. Triplet repeat primed (TP-PCR) gives a characteristic ladder on the fluorescent trace, enabling rapid identification of large, pathological CTG repeats that cannot be amplified employing flanking primers. Although TP-PCR detects expanded alleles of all lengths, it does not allow for their sizing. In fact, samples with large CTG expansions identified by TP-PCR will require Southern blotting if accurate estimation of size is required (Magaña et al., 2011a). Therefore, there is no single method available yet that can reliably identify and size all ranges of expanded alleles in the DM1 locus.

3. Genetics of DM1

DM1 is the most common type of myotonic dystrophy in adults and it belongs to a growing group of genetic diseases caused by expansion of unstable microsatellite repeats. In 1992, DM1 was shown to be caused by an expanded CTG repeat in the 3'-Untranslated region (3'UTR) of the Dystrophy myotonic-protein kinase (DMPK) gene in chromosome 19q (Brook et al., 1992) (Figure 1). This gene is composed of 15 exons that encode several alternatively spliced isoforms of a serine/threonine protein kinase that range from 60-70 kDa. The number of CTG repeats in the DMPK gene is polymorphic. In unaffected individuals, length of the CTG expansion ranges from 5-34 repeats; this range of repeats is stably inherited and possesses a relatively low mutation rate. DM1 alleles present a range of intermediate alleles that is known as the "premutation range" and that includes between 35 and 49 CTG repeats (Table 1); this range is not clinically significant, but it is genetically unstable, which may cause the expansion of repeats in subsequent generations to reach the pathological range (IDMC, 2000), whereas affected individuals with as few as 50 repeats can exhibit symptoms of the disease in adulthood (Table 1).

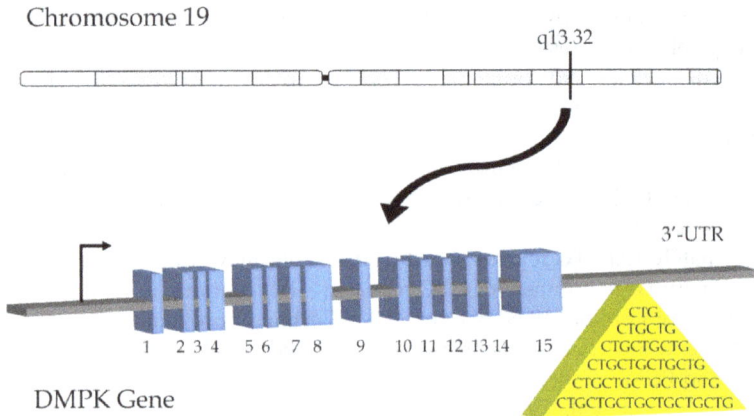

Fig. 1. DMPK gene. The DMPK gene is located in chromosome 19 at the q13.32 band. Blue rectangles indicate exons and the straight gray line, introns. The CTG repeat tract is located in the 3'unstranslated region of the gene.

In DM1, puzzling genetic phenomena, such as anticipation and the congenital form, which were difficult to explain by conventional Mendelian genetics, are largely attributable to the "dynamic" mutation. Expanded repeat size correlated inversely with age-at-onset, and repeat size increases in successive generations in DM1, providing the molecular basis for anticipation (Harper et al., 1992; Harley et al., 1992; Ashizawa et al., 1992). Paternal mutant alleles usually do not exceed 1,000 CTGs in offspring, whereas maternal transmission frequently gives rise to further expansions of mutant repeats beyond 1,000 CTGs in children with congenital myotonic dystrophy (Lavedan et al., 1993; Ashizawa et al., 1994). Premutation alleles tend to expand into the full-mutation range more frequently with paternal than with maternal transmission (Martorell et al., 2001; 2004). This accounts for the paternal origin of the *de novo* mutations of myotonic dystrophy. The terminal event of anticipation in DM1 is the congenital form, which accompanies severely compromised nuptial and reproductive capability. Consequently, anticipation is expected to deplete the population of patients with DM1 in gradual fashion. However, the prevalence of the disease has been relatively steady; in part, this can be explained by the considerable pool of normal individuals who have permutation alleles who can act as a reservoir for the future origin of new cases through genetic instability (Martorell et al., 2001).

Phenotype	CTG repeat size	Age-at-onset (years)
Normal	5-34	NA
Premutation	35-49	NA
Adult-onset (Mild)	50-150	60-70
Adult-onset (Classic)	100-1,000	10-30
Congenital	>1,000	From birth to 10

Table 1. Correlation between CTG repeat length and phenotype in DM1. NA, Not applicable.

3.1 Origin and distribution of the CTG repeat polymorphism

Myotonic dystrophy is one of the most common inherited neuromuscular disorders and has been described in global populations except for the majority of sub-Saharan ethnic populations (Krahe et al., 1995; Ashizawa & Epstein, 1991). Prevalence varies but generally ranges from 1/8,000-1/50,000 in European and Japanese populations (Harper et al., 2002). High prevalence has been reported in different regions of the world, such as Northeastern Quebec, Canada (Bouchard et al., 1989), and Istria, Croatia (Medica et al., 2004), with a founder effect. Based on the paucity of DM1 in sub-Saharan ethnic populations, it was postulated that the DM1 mutation occurred after human migration out of Africa (Ashizawa & Epstein, 1991). When the $(CTG)_n$ DM1 mutation was identified, it was found to be in complete linkage disequilibrium with the Alu 1-kb insertion (Alu+) allele located 5 kb upstream of the $(CTG)_n$ repeat within the *DMPK* gene (Zerylnick et al., 1995). Since then, $(CTG)_n$ repeat expansion has always been found on the Alu+ background in European and Asian populations (Krndija et al., 2005; Pan et al., 2001), with the exception of a Nigerian Yoruba family (Krahe et al., 1995). Subsequent analyses of $(CTG)_n$ and the Alu+/‐ polymorphism in populations worldwide appears to point to the consensus that $(CTG)_5$ Alu+ is the ancestral haplotype for all observed haplotypes and that $(CTG)_n$ expansion alleles have derived from this ancestral haplotype through expansion in successive generations of larger normal alleles with >18 CTG repeats (Tishkoff et al., 1998). Supporting this hypothesis, African-Negroid, African-American, and Taiwanese populations all exhibit low frequency of (CTG) >18 alleles and low DM1 prevalence (Acton et al., 2007; Goldman et al., 1994; Hsiao et al., 2003; Pan et al., 2001), whereas the relatively high frequency of (CTG) >18 alleles observed in Japanese, Yugoslav and European populations appears to be associated with moderate-to-high incidence of DM1 (Leifsdottir et al., 2005; Mladenovic et al., 2006). Thus, in the absence of epidemiological data for DM1, frequency estimation of $(CTG)_n$ alleles with >18 repeats in healthy population could be an indirect estimator of DM1 prevalence (Magaña et al., 2011).

Analysis of haplotypes of the DMPK region demonstrated that the majority of European and Asian DM1 $(CTG)_n$ expanded alleles are on one haploytpe (haplotype A) background, while the Nigerian DM1 mutation was found to be on a different haplotype background (Krahe, et al., 1995). Therefore, $(CTG)_5$ repeats in the *DMPK* gene is the most common allele in the majority of the populations; however, allelic distribution of other alleles is different among populations by means of the genetic drift effect on these populations or due to the genic flow caused by the emergence of new populations.

3.2 Expansion and Instability of CTG repeats

The molecular mechanism underlying repeat instability has yet to be completely elucidated. However, remarkable progress has been achieved through research done not only in patient-derived tissues and cells, but also in a variety of experimental systems, including *in vitro*, bacteria, yeast, and transgenic animal models. The use of these experimental models has recapitulated the expansion-prone instability of the expanded $(CTG)_n$ repeat, with degree of repeat instability in correlation with repeat size.

Age-dependent, tissue-specific somatic CTG repeat instability is observed in patients with DM1, with a strong bias toward expansions. The first wave of somatic instability has been suggested to occur between 13 and 16 weeks of gestation, and the second, which is less than the first, could continue throughout adulthood (Jansen et al., 1994). Likewise, a high degree of instability is detected in germ cells. In male gametes, smaller repeats are highly unstable, tending to enlarge significantly during spermatogenesis, while in female gametes, high instability is exhibited mainly in larger repeats (Martorell et al., 2004). It is thought that CTG repeats have already expanded in DM1-affected oocytes, leading to the conclusion that the initial CTG expansion occurs prior to completion of meiosis II of oogenesis (De Temmerman et al., 2004). In transgenic mice, the expanded $(CTG)_n$ repeat exhibits the majority of the characteristics of the expanded repeat in patients' tissues, including expansion bias, the parental gender effect, intergenerational instability, age-dependent increase, and inter-tissue variability of the repeat size (Fortune et al., 2000; Gourdon et al., 1997; Monckton et al., 1997; Seznec et al., 2000; 2001). Characterization of transgenic mice with expanded CTG-CAG repeats in the background of mismatch repair-gene deficiencies revealed that *Msh2*, *Msh3*, *Msh6*, and *Pms2* play important roles in repeat instability (Savouret et al., 2004; Van den Broek et al., 2002). Studies *in vitro* provide evidence that CTG-CAG repeats form non-B DNA structures during DNA replication (Wojciechowska et al., 2005); it is thought that the aberrant repair of these DNA intermediates is a source for development of the triplet repeat expansions. In *Escherichia coli*, CTG repeats are unstable by deletion prone, although expansions do occur depending on repeat length and direction of replication; the mechanism of instability includes slippage of the strands at the replication fork, gene conversion-like events, and recombination (Hashem et al., 2002). Analysis of CTG-CAG repeat instability in yeast has revealed the participation of molecules involved in DNA replication and repair (Shimizu et al., 2001). Although studies in bacteria and yeasts have provided insights into the mechanism of CTG repeat instability, their extrapolation to humans should be carefully considered due to obvious interspecies differences. Figure 2 depicts the major contributors to CTGG instability schematically. It is noteworthy that identification of the molecular mechanism causing expansion of CTG repeats might allow the design of therapeutic strategies against DM1, aimed at inducing deletions of the already expanded CTG repeats or preventing expansion from occurring.

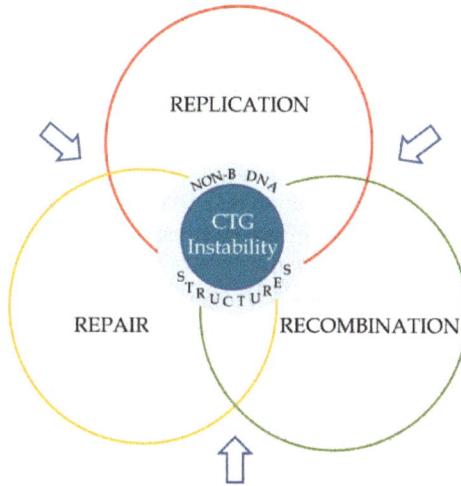

Fig. 2. Major contributors factor to CTG instability *in vivo*. Studies performed on cells and tissues from subjects with DM1, as well as on organism models including transgenic mice, bacteria, and yeast, have revealed that DNA segments containing expanded CTG repeats form unusual DNA structures that, in conjunction with alterations in the replication, recombination and repair processes, lead to CTG instability.

4. RNA-mediated mechanisms of pathogenesis

The mechanism by which the expanded CTG repeat leads to the multisystemic clinical phenotype of DM1 is not fully understood. Because of the location of $(CTG)_n$ in the 3' UTR, the gene's coding region remains intact in the mutant *DMPK* gene; however, the $(CTG)_n$ repeat is transcribed into the messenger RNA (mRNA) as a $(CUG)_n$ repeat. Recent studies have led to three major models of the disease mechanism for DM1 as follows: a) DMPK haploinsufficiency; b) loss-of-function of genes in the vicinity of the CTG repeat, and c) a toxic gain-of-function by the expanded CUG repeat in mutant *DMPK* mRNA.

a.   Due to decreased levels of *DMPK* mRNA and protein in adult DM1 tissue (Fu et al., 1993), DMPK deficiency was proposed as the pathogenic mechanism of DM1 soon after identification of the DM1 mutation. The functional implications of a reduction in *DMPK* expression were genetically tested with the generation of knockout mice. *DMPK-/-* mice develop mild, late-onset, progressive skeletal myopathy, which suggested that DMPK might be necessary for the maintenance of skeletal muscle structure (Reddy et al., 1996). Subsequent divulged showed that DMPK-deficient mice also exhibited some cardiac-conduction abnormalities (Berul et al., 2000) and metabolic impairment such as abnormal glucose tolerance, reduced glucose uptake, and impaired insulin-dependent GLUT4 trafficking in muscle (Llagostera et al., 2007). However, the fact that *DMPK-/-* mice demonstrated solely a mild phenotype for only some DM symptoms and that no *DMPK* point mutations have been associated with a DM1 phenotype strongly suggested that the multi systemic features of DM1 were not caused by simply DMPK haploinsufficiency.

b. A second mechanism proposed to explain the pathogenesis of DM1 is based on the effect exerted by CTG expanded repeats on chromatin structure (Otten & Tapscott, 1995), which in turn might lead to partial silencing of neighboring *DMWD* (Dystrophia myotonica-containing WD repeat motif) and *SIX5* (Sine oculis homeobox homolog 5) genes (Alwazzan et al., 1999; Klesert et al., 1997; Sarkar et al., 2000). This hypothesis is supported by the fact that *DMWD* expression levels are reported as decreased in repeat expansion-bearing patients (Alwazzan et al., 1998; Gennarelli et al., 1999). Moreover, mutant analysis in *Drosophila* has shown that *D-Six4*, the closest *Six5* homolog in flies, is required for normal development of gonad muscle and mesodermal components. This suggested that human *Six5* could participate in muscle-wasting and testicular-atrophy phenotypes in DM1 (Kirby et al., 2001). However, *Six5* knockout mice only develop cataracts that lacked the distinctive iridescent opacities characteristic of cataracts of patients with DM1 (Klesert et al., 2000).

c. Data from patients as well as from transgenic mice and cell lines developed for DM1 modeling have offered compelling evidence in support of the third model, which proposes that CUG repeats in the pathogenic range fold into RNA hairpins that are not exported from the nucleus but that, instead, accumulate within ribonuclear foci, acquiring a new toxic function by trapping essential cellular RNA-binding proteins including alternative-splicing modulators and transcription factors, thus disturbing the gene-expression and alternative- splicing processes, respectively (Davis et al., 1997; Ebralidze et al., 2004; Ranum & Cooper 2006; Taneja et al., 1995).

4.1 Nuclear retention of mutant *DMPK* RNA

Preferential accumulation of mutant *DMPK* mRNA in nuclear foci has been observed by the Fluorescent *in situ* hybridization (FISH) technique in fibroblasts, myoblasts, and neurons from different nerve tissues (cerebral cortex, hippocampus, dentate gyrus, thalamus, substantia nigra, and brainstem) of subjects with DM1 (Davis et al., 1997; Day & Ranum, 2005; Machuca-Tzili et al., 2005). These findings have also been corroborated in muscle tissue of patients with DM1 by Northern blot analysis (Davis et al., 1997; Klesert et al., 2000; Wang et al., 1994). Furthermore, electron microscopy examination has revealed that the CUG-repeat RNA forms double-stranded RNA (Michalowski et al., 1999), which might impede its export to the cytoplasm. It has been demonstrated that nuclear accumulation of mutant transcripts increases in proportion to the number of CUG repeats, suggesting that the length of the (CUG)n tract strongly determines the formation of nuclear aggregates (Klesert et al., 2000). Furthermore, the number and morphology of ribonuclear foci in DM1 are also quite variable in different cell types and tissues; in proliferating DM1 cells in culture, these RNA-rich accumulations range from a few small foci in fibroblasts to dozens of larger foci in myoblasts. In contrast, only a few nuclear foci are observed in postmitotic cells, such as myofibers and cortical neurons.

Interestingly, mutant *DMPK* RNA is able to form ribonucleoprotein complexes by binding to certain RNA-binding proteins (Miller et al., 2000) including modulators of alternative-splicing and transcription factors, which are correspondingly depleted from their normal subcellular localizations (for review, see Llamusi & Artero, 2008). This aberrant event causes alteration in the normal expression of numerous muscular and neuronal proteins, supporting the multisystemic phenotype of the disease (see later). Given the fact that nuclear accumulation of mutant *DMPK* RNA is the basis for its toxic function, definition of the steps at which mutant mRNA transport is blocked would aid in improving the definition of the molecular basis of the pathology and eventually, in designing a therapeutic treatment (Mastroyiannopoulos et al., 2005).

4.2 Alternative-splicing misregulation

Accumulation of mutant *DMPK* mRNA in nuclei of muscle and nerve cells facilitates its aberrant union with proteins that participate in the regulation of nuclear processes, such as splicing modulators and transcription factors; thus, the normal function of a number of proteins might be impaired. Mutant mRNA of DM1 is able to interact and form aggregates with proteins that participate in the alternative splicing of pre-mRNAs, such as the Muscleblind-like family (MBNL1, MBNL2, and MBNL3), the CUG-binding protein 2 (ETR-3), the Protein kinase RNA-activated (Protein kinase R) PKR enzyme, and the heterogeneous nuclear ribonucleoprotein H (hnRNP H), which results in interference in developmentally regulated alternative splicing of defined pre-mRNAs (Fardaei et al., 2002; Jiang et al., 2004; Kanadia et al., 2003; Kuyumcu-Martínez & Cooper 2006; Mankodi et al., 2001; Miller et al., 2000). Furthermore, DM1 mutation cells activate CUG triplet repeat RNA-binding protein 1 (CUG-BP1), also denominated CUGBP1/Elav-like family member 1 (CELF1), through hyperphosphorylation and stabilization in the cell nucleus (Ho et al., 2005; Philips et al., 1998; Savkur et al., 2001; 2004; Timchenko et al., 2001). It is known that up to 74% of human genes undergo alternative splicing, during which exons or parts of exons can be skipped during pre-mRNA processing, resulting in the expression of multiple variant mRNAs; therefore, alternative-splicing misregulation could be the best explanation for the multisystemic characteristics of DM1 pathology. The function of these splicing regulators determines the tissue- and developmental phase- specific expression of certain protein isoforms (Taneja et al., 1995). Within this group of splicing regulators, CELF1 and MBNL are those that are best understood. CELF1 and MBNL1 play opposite roles in exon selection in several pre-mRNA transcripts; while MBNL1 promotes the transition of splicing from fetal to adult exons, CELF1 aids in retaining fetal exons. According to current evidence, the abnormal length of the (CUG)n segment determines the entrapment of muscle-bound MBNL proteins in ribonuclear aggregates and in the stabilized expression of CELF1, which in turn causes aberrant pre-mRNA splicing that results in abnormal expression of fetal splice isoforms in the tissues of adult subjects with DM1 (Figure 3).

To date, alterations in at least 14 pre-mRNA alternative-splicing events have been reported (Ranum & Day, 2006; Magaña et al., 2009), seven of which have been found in skeletal and cardiac muscle, affecting the following genes: *TNNT2* (cardiac Troponin T gene); *IR* (Insulin receptor gene); *MTMR1* (Myotubularin-related protein 1); *TNNT3* (skeletal muscle Troponin T gene); *RyR* (Ryanodine receptor gene); *SERCA2* (Sarco/endoplasmic reticulum calcium ATPase 2 gene), and *ClCN-1* (muscle-specific Chloride Channel) (Charlet et al., 2002; Ho et al., 2005; Kimura et al., 2005; Mankodi et al., 2002; Philips et al., 1998; Savkur et al., 2001). Moreover, alterations in the transcript processing of *Tau*, *NMDAR1* (N-methyl-D-aspartate receptor 1), and *APP* (Amyloid protein precursor) genes have been observed to occur in the brain of subjects with DM1 (De León & Cisneros, 2008; Jiang et al., 2004) (Figure 3).

It is noteworthy that utilization of transgenic mice and cellular models together with the information obtained in clinical trials has enabled correlation of alterations in transcript maturation with DM1 symptomatology. In subjects with DM1, the presence of an *IR* gene-derived mRNA that lacks exon 11 has been described, which results in the synthesis of an insulin-resistant receptor isoform (Savkur et al., 2001). This phenomenon could explain the development of diabetes in these individuals. Likewise, several studies have reported the expression of immature transcripts of *RyR* and *SERCA2* genes in skeletal muscle of patients with DM1; the products of these genes regulate calcium homeostasis during sarcolemma depolarization: at the beginning of muscle contraction, Ca^{2+} is released from the sarcoplasmic reticulum through ion channels formed by RyR, while SERCA2 pumps the former back to the lumen of the sarcoplasmatic reticulum to restore cytoplasmic Ca^{2+} levels, consequently inducing muscle relaxation. Thus, alterations in this process could be related with the muscle weakness observed in DM1. With respect to the employment of transgenic mice for studying DM1-associated mis-splicing, it has been reported that a transgenic mouse over-expressing CELF1 exhibits production of alternative TNNT2 gene mRNA with the inclusion of exon 5, which is exclusively observed in fetal tissues (Ho et al., 2005; Timichenko et al., 2001). Troponin T forms part of a protein complex that regulates actin-myosin interactions during muscle contraction. The fetal isoform is less sensitive to Ca^{2+}, resulting in a weaker cardiac-muscle contraction. Based on these observations, it has been proposed that aberrant processing of the Troponin T gene transcript might be the cause of the development of arrhythmia and the loss of myocardial function described in patients with DM1. Characterization of a second transgenic mouse that over-expressed CELF1 showed the presence of mRNA from the *ClCN-1* gene with inclusion of exon 7 in muscle tissue. The presence of exon 7 generates higher degradation of the transcript, with the consequent decrease in levels of the protein, a chloride-channel component (Charlet et al., 2002; Mankodi et al., 2002), which ultimately results in decreased transmembranal conductance of chloride ions in muscle fibers. This physiological alteration correlates with the classic clinical sign of DM1: myotonia. Supporting the crucial role of mis-splicing in the development of DM1, the knockout mouse for the *MBLN* gene (Mbln1 Δ^3/Δ^3) displayed alterations in the alternative splicing of *TNNT2*, *TNNT3*, and *ClCN-1* genes and consequently developed myotonia and cataracts. Comparison of two mouse models for DM1, one expressing the mutant *DMPK* RNA and the other *null* for the *Mbnl1a* gene, revealed that loss of MBNL1a explains only >80% of the splicing pathology due to expanded CUG RNA. Mbnl-independent mis-splicing effects were observed particularly on mRNAs for extracellular matrix proteins (Du et al., 2010).

Finally, the generation and characterization of cellular models for DM1 have additionally contributed to the identification of the molecular mechanism underling this pathology. A study on C2C12 cells, a mouse muscular-cell line, demonstrated that CELF1 sequestration by the mutant *DMPK* RNA impairs the translation of several myogenesis regulators, including MEF2A (myocyte-specific potentiator factor 2A), MyoD (Myogenin 2), and p21 (CdK 1A inhibitor), which ultimately cause impairment in the muscle differentiation program (Ho et al., 2005). Although the brain is considered the second most affected organ in DM1, the molecular basis of this pathology in the nervous system has not yet been elucidated. One of the most distinctive characteristics of brain damage in subjects with DM1 is the presence of hyperphosphorylated Tau aggregates in the neurocortex (Jiang et al., 2004). Tau is expressed abundantly in the peripheral and nervous systems and is especially enriched in the axons of mature and growing neurons, in which it is found associated with microtubules and on which it confers stability. Abnormal phosphorylation of Tau negatively affects its binding to microtubules, and ultimately its function, as has been described in Alzheimer disease. In the human brain, six Tau-protein isoforms are expressed as a result of the alternative splicing of exons 2, 3, and 10. Interestingly, expression of Tau isoforms, with the exclusion of exons 2/3 and 10, is favored in subjects with DM1 (Jiang et al., 2004; Wang et al., 2005). Exon 2 encodes for the N-terminal domain of Tau, which interacts with the axonal membrane, whereas exon 10 encodes for a microtubule-binding domain. Therefore, absence of these domains in the protein product might affect the function of Tau as a microtubule-stabilizer molecule, causing, at least in part, the neuronal damage observed in patients with DM1 (Wang et al., 2005). As mentioned previously, the brain of subjects with DM1 also exhibits alterations in *NMDAR1*-gene transcript maturation (Jiang et al., 2004), specifically in cortical and subcortical neurons. *NMDAR1* regulates synaptic transmission of excitation in the hippocampus, thus participating in the long-term potentiation and learning process (Tsien et al., 1996). Normally, the *NMDAR1* gene produces eight isoforms derived from alternative splicing of its premRNA; nevertheless, patients with DM1 preferentially produce an isoform with the inclusion of exon 5, which affects the affects the receptor's distribution and pharmacological properties. Hence, the presence of this abnormal isoform of NMDAR1 might be related with DM1-associated memory impairment (Cull-Candy et al., 2004; Winblad et al., 2006).

4.3 Leaching of transcription factors from chromatin

It has been recently observed that several transcription factors are sequestered by mutant *DMPK* RNA in muscle cells of subjects with DM1, including Sp1 (Specific protein 1), STAT1, and STAT3 (members of Signal transduction-family proteins and transcription activators), and the gamma subunit of the Retinoic acid receptor (RARγ) (Figure 3). This aberrant event removes the transcription factors from active chromatin, leading to disrupted gene-expression patterns. It is thought that the decreased *ClCN-1* gene expression observed in the muscle cells of patients with DM1 is due to the entrapment of Sp1 in nuclear foci containing mutant *DMPK* RNA, because Sp1 modulates the *ClCN-1* gene promoter positively. Supporting this idea, expression of the *ClCN-1* gene is restored in DM1 muscle cells by over-expression of Sp1 (Ebralidze et al., 2004). Further studies are required to fully understand the influence of mutant DMPK RNA on gene expression.

5. Perspectives of gene therapy

At present, treatment for DM1 is limited to symptomatic intervention and there is no therapeutic approach to prevent or reverse disease progression. However, elucidation of the molecular mechanisms underlying DM1 pathogenesis have allowed for the envisaging and developing of experimental approaches with therapeutic potential that are aimed at reversing DM1 symptomatology. Because the central core of DM1 pathogenesis is the gain-

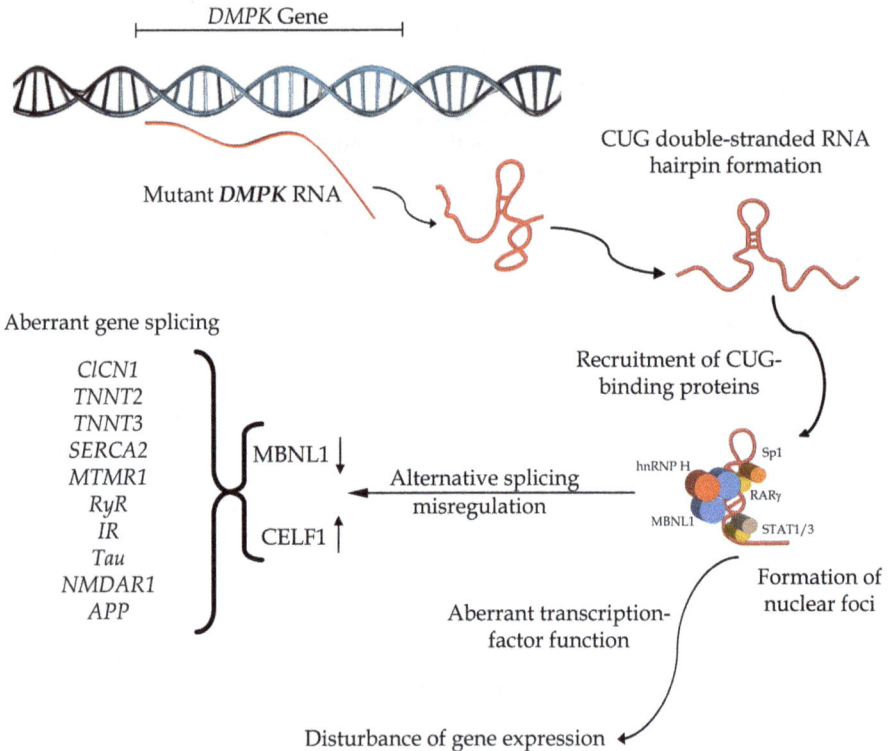

Fig. 3. RNA toxic gain-of-function model for DM1 pathogenesis. Mutant *DMPK* RNA accumulates in the nucleus of muscle and nerve cells, sequestering different regulatory proteins including splicing modulators MBNL1 and hnRNP H and transcription factors Sp1, STAT1, STAT3, and RARγ. Furthermore, expression of expanded CTG repeats causes, by means of an unknown mechanism, an increase in the activity of splicing modulator CELF1. The aberrant behavior of mutant *DMPK* RNA alters the activity of both splicing modulators and transcription factors, giving rise to impairment in the expression and function of a number of genes and ultimately, to the multisystemic DM1 phenotype.

of-function of mutant *DMPK* RNA, the majority of studies have been focused on targeting the mutant transcript to eliminate or ameliorate its toxic effects. However, alternative strategies centered on reversing DM1-associated spliceopathy without targeting the mutant *DMPK* RNA have remerged recently (Magaña & Cisneros, 2011; Mulders et al., 2010).

5.1 Degradation or neutralization of mutant *DMPK* RNA

Different approaches have been applied to target and cleave mutant *DMPK* RNA, including the use of antisense RNA, Antisense oligonucleotides (AONs), small interfering RNA (siRNA), and self-cleaving hammerhead ribozymes (Figure 4A). Antisense RNA complementary to (CUG)13 repeat-sequence AON was employed in human DM1 myoblasts carrying ~750 CTG repeats (Furling et al., 2003), resulting in preferential decay of mutant over wild-type *DMPK* transcripts and consequent normalization of myoblast fusion and glucose uptake via restoration of the expression and binding activity of *CELF1*. Further studies with a 2'-O-Methyl-phosphorothioate-modified AON (2'-MePS-AON) that targets CUG repeats were performed in immortal mouse myoblasts expressing the human *DMPK* gene with 500 CTG repeats (DM500 cell model) (Mulders et al., 2009) and in two following DM1 mouse models: the first carrying the Human skeletal alpha-actin (*HSA*) gene modified by the insertion of 250 CTG repeats in the 3'UTR (*HSA*[LR] mouse model) and the second, bearing the human *DM1* locus with 500 CTG repeats (DM500 mouse model) (Mankodi et al., 2000; Seznec et al., 2000). Promisingly, antisense treatment resulted in decreasing levels of mutant *DMPK*, reduction of ribonuclear foci, and correction of the DM1-associated, aberrant pre-mRNA splicing of several genes. Similar positive effects have been observed in DM1 myoblasts that have ~3,200 CTG repeats with the use of siRNAs (Langlois et al., 2005), and in DM1 myoblasts expressing approximately 750 CTG repeats with the employment of nuclear ribozymes that targeted and cleaved 3'UTR of *DMPK* mRNA (Langlois et al., 2003). However, the main limitation of these strategies lies in that all molecules recognize and cleave both mutant and wild-type *DMPK* mRNA with similar efficacy.

A more recent and attractive strategy against DM1 postulates that disruption of the aberrant RNA-protein interactions exerted by the *DMPK* mutant transcript with the alternative-splicing regulator MBNL1 would correct DM1-associated mis-splicing (Figure 4B). Supporting this hypothesis, a 25-nucleotide morpholino-type AON complementary to CUG-repeated RNA blocks the formation of the CUG-expanded MBNL1 complex in the *HSA*[LR] transgenic mouse model, resulting in several beneficial effects, including decreased number of nuclear foci through MBNL1 protein redistribution in the nucleus, enhanced transport of CUG expanded-containing transcripts to the cytoplasm, alternative-splicing correction of MBNL1-dependent genes, normalization of transmembrane chloride-ion conductance, and reduction of myotonia (Wheeler et al., 2009). In this regard, identification of small molecules or multivalent modular compounds that specifically bind CUG repeats and that could competitively release sequestered MBNL1 would constitute a promising alternative strategy for neutralization of toxic RNA (Warf and Berglund, 2010; Warf et al., 2009).

5.2 Mis-splicing reversal

Sequestration of MBNL1 by mutant *DMPK* transcript in nuclear foci indicates that MBNL1 titration and loss-of-function is linked with the mis-splicing of particular genes. Furthermore, it was recently shown that activation of the PKC signaling pathway by CUG repeats leads to CELF1 hyperphosphorylation and stabilization, implicating this signaling event in DM1-associated mis-splicing (Philips et al., 1998; Savkur et al., 2001; Sergeant et al., 2001). Therefore, it has been hypothesized that modulation of the expression and/or activity of these two splicing factors would reverse DM1-associated spliceopathy (Figure 4C). Consistent with this idea, over-expression of *MBNL1* in a *Drosophila* model of DM1 expressing a non-coding mRNA containing 480 CUG repeats reduced the number of nuclear foci and suppressed the degenerative phenotypes caused by expanded repeats in muscle and eye tissue (de Haro et al., 2006). Moreover, over-expression of *MBNL1* mediated by an adeno-associated viral vector specifically corrected the mis-splicing of MBNL1-dependent genes including *Clcn1*, *Serca1*, and *Tnnt3* and reversed myotonia in the *HSA*[LR] mouse model of DM1 (Kanadia et al., 2006). On the other hand, different mice models have been established to test the role of CELF1 activity in the development of muscle-wasting and cardiac disease in DM1 (Ho et al., 2005; Koshelev et al., 2010). Interestingly, specific blockage of PKC activity in an inducible mouse model for heart-specific expression of 960 CUG RNA repeats that developed cardiac arrhythmias, cardiomyopathy, and CELF1-associated spliceopathy (Wang et al. 2007) resulted in improved cardiac conduction and reduced misregulation of CELF1-mediated splicing events, which correlated with decreased phosphorylation and steady-state levels of CELF1 (Wang et al., 2009). Hence, the use of protein kinase C inhibitors to downregulate or to prevent upregulation of CELF1 activity would be an alternative therapeutic treatment for DM1. Finally, it is important to mention that correction of DM1 mis-splicing by modulation of *CELF1* and *MBNL1* expression should be considered with caution because artificial alteration of MBNL1 and/ CELF1 steady-state levels might alter the splicing pattern of a number of genes regulated by these proteins, with unknown consequences for muscle function.

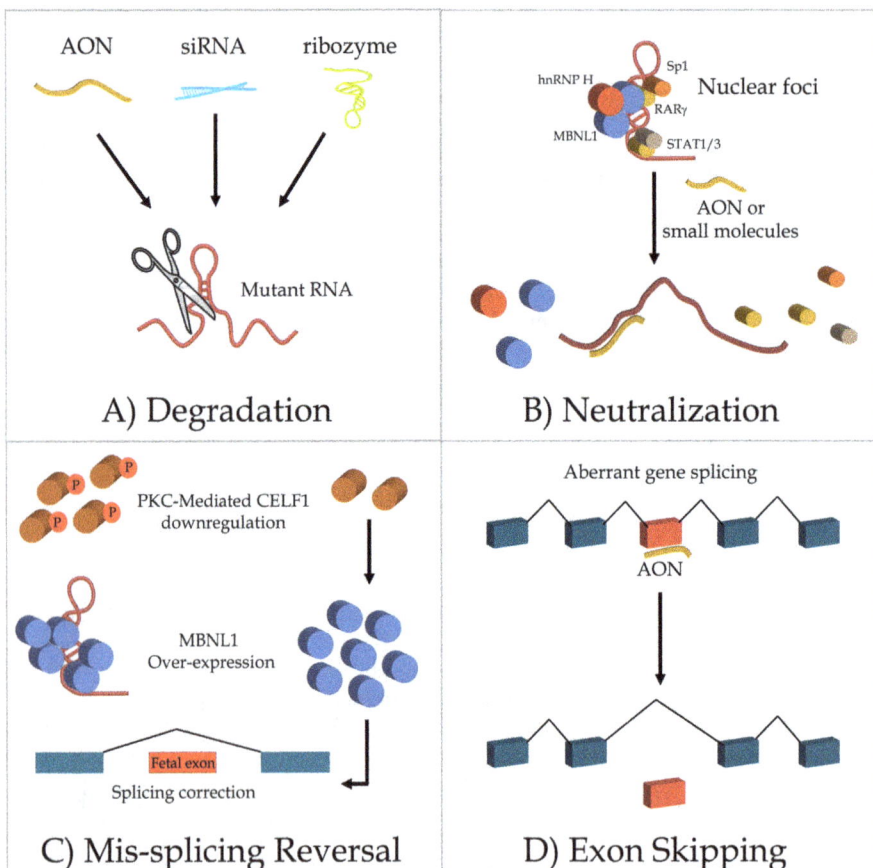

Fig. 4. Strategies for DM1 gene therapy. A) Degradation of mutant RNA by antisense oligonucleotides (AON), ribozyme, or siRNA. B) Neutralization of mutant RNA activity by blocking its interaction with the splicing regulator MBNL1 using AON or small chemical compounds. C) Mis-splicing reversal by ver-expression of MBNL1 or down-regulation of CELF activity. D) Exon skipping of mis-spliced genes (i.e. *CLCN1* gene) by splicing blockage with AON.

5.3 Exon skipping of mis-spliced genes

An alternative strategy to fight DM1 symptomatology is to correct aberrant splicing events by exon skipping of mis-spliced genes. The mechanism of exon skipping is based on the binding of AON to specific-target sense sequences of mis-spliced pre-mRNA genes to block the access of splicing machinery to splice sites, causing the elimination of specific exons(s) and their flanking regions, in order to restore an open-reading frame of the normal isoform (Alter et al., 2006; Lu et al., 2005) (Figure 4D). AON-mediated exon skipping appears to be a potent method for reversing DM1-associated myotonia caused by abnormal inclusion of exon 7a in *ClCN-1* mRNA. Normalization of *ClCN-1* current density, as well as elimination of myotonic discharges, were observed in two murine models (DM1 mouse model HSA^{LR}, and a transgenic mouse homozygous for *MBNL1*-gene disruption) after muscular injection of a morpholino-AON that targeted the 3' splice site of *ClCN-1* mRNA exon 7a and prevented inclusion of this exon in the mature transcript (Wheeler et al., 2007). Future exon-skipping strategies for DM1 should ensure muscle-specific uptake of therapeutic oligos after their systemic delivery, as well as the employment of a multiple AON cocktail designed to correct splicing at two or more transcripts involved in DM1 symptomatology.

6. Conclusions and future outlook

Conventional approaches to treatment of DM1 are supportive and have failed to slow or halt disease progression. Substantial progress has been made in understanding the disease-causing mechanisms of DM1, and now that it is clear that multisystemic phenotype of DM1 results directly from expression of a mutant expanded repeat RNA, the search for novel therapies is underway. Despite the tremendous progress obtained in several cell-based and animal models, in which degradation or neutralization of the mutant *DMPK* RNA results in reversal of mis-splicing and myotonia, there are a number of hurdles to overcome before implementation of RNA-based strategies in clinical trials, such as tissue-specific delivery, sustainability, and effectiveness of the therapeutic molecules.

7. Acknowledgments

This work was supported by the Science and Technology Institute of Mexico City (ICyTDF), Grant PIFUTP08-164.

8. References

Acton, R.T.; Rivers, C.A.; Watson, B.; & Oh S.J. (2007). DMPK-associated myotonic dystrophy and CTG repeats in Alabama African Americans. *Clinical Genetics*, Vol. 72, pp. 448-453, ISSN 0009-9163

Alter, J.; Lou, F.; Rabinowitz, A.; Yin, H.; Rosenfeld, J.; Wilton, S.D.; Partridge, T.A.; & Lu, Q.L. (2006). Systemic delivery of morpholino oligonucleotide restores dystrophin expression bodywide and improves dystrophic pathology. *Nature Medicine*. Vol.12, No.2, pp.175-177., ISSN 1078-8956

Alwazzan, M.; Hamshere, M.G.; Lennon, G.G.; & Brook, J.D. (1998). Six transcripts map within 200 kilobases of the myotonic dystrophy expanded repeat. *Mammalian Genome*. Vol.9, No.6, pp.485-487, ISSN 0938-8990

Alwazzan, M.; Newman, E.; Hamshere, M.G.; & Brook, J.D. (1999). Myotonic dystrophy is associated with a reduced level of RNA from DMWD allele adjacent to the expanded repeat. *Human Molecular Genetics.*Vol.8 pp.1491-1497, ISSN 0964-6906

Ashizawa, T.; & Epstein H.F. (1991). Ethnic distribution of myotonic dystrophy gene. *Lancet.* Vol 338 No. 8767, pp. 642-643. ISSN 0140-6736

Ashizawa, T.; Dunne, C.J.; Dubel, JR.; Perryman, M.B.; Epstein, H.F.; Boerwinkle, E.; & Hejtmancik, J.F.(1992). Anticipation in myotonic dystrophy. I. Statistical verification based on clinical and haplotype findings. *Neurology.* Vol 42, No. 10, pp. 1871-1877, ISSN 0028-3878

Ashizawa, T.; Dunne, P.W.; Ward, P.A.; Seltzer, W.K.; & Richards, CS. (1994). Effects of the sex of myotonic dystrophy patients on the unstable triplet repeat in their affected offspring. *Neurology.* Vol 44 No.1, pp. 120-122 , ISSN 0028-3878

Berul, C.I.; Maguire, C.T.; Gehrmann, J.; & Reddy, S. (2000).Progressive atrioventricular conduction block in a mouse myotonic dystrophy model. *Journal of Interventional Cardiac Electrophysiology.* Vol.4, No.2, pp.351-358 ISSN 1383-875X

Bouchard, G.; Roy, R.; Declos, M.; Mathieu, J.; & Kouladjian, K. (1989). Origin and diffusion of the myotonic dystrophy gene in the Saguenay region (Quebec). *The Canadian Journal of Neurological Sciences.* Vol 16, No.1 ,pp. 119-122 ISSN 0317-1671

Brook, J.D.; McCurrach, M.E.; Harley, H.G.; Buckler, A.J.; Church, D.; Aburatani, H.; Hunter, K.; Stanton, V.P.; Thirion, J.P.; & Hudson, T. (1992). Molecular basis of myotonic dystrophy: expansion of a trinucleotide (CTG) repeat at the 3' end of a transcript encoding a protein kinase family member. *Cell,* Vol 68, No.4, pp.799-808, ISSN 0092-8674.

Charlet, B.N.; Savkur, R.S.; Singh, G.; Philips, A.V.; Grice, E.A.; & Cooper, T.A. (2002). Loss of the muscle-specific chloride channel in type 1 myotonic dystrophy due to misregulated alternative splicing. *Molecular Cell* 2002; Vol. 10, pp.45-53, ISSSN 1097-2765

Cheng, S.; Barceló, J.M.; & Korneluk, RG. (1996). Characterization of large CTG repeat expansions in myotonic dystrophy alleles using PCR. *Human Mutation,* Vol. 7, No.4 , pp. 304-310, ISSN 1059-7794

Cull-Candy, S.G.; & Leszkiewicz, D.N.(2004). Role of distinct NMDA receptor subtypes at central synapses. *Science´s STKE: signal trasduction knowledge environment.* 2004; re16 ISSN 1525-8882

Davis, B.M.; McCurrach, M.E.; Taneja, K.L.; Singer, R.H.; & Housman, D.E. (1997). Expansion of a CUG trinucleotide repeat in the 3' untranslated region of myotonic dystrophy protein kinase transcripts results in nuclear retention of transcripts. *Proceedings National Academy Sciences of United States of America,* Vol.94, No.14, pp.7388-7393, ISSN 0027-8424

Day, J.W. & Ranum, L.P.; (2005). RNA pathogenesis of the myotonic dystrophies. *Neuromuscular Disorders,* Vol. 15, No.1, pp.5-16, ISSN 0960-8966

De Haro, M.; Al-Ramahi, I.; De Gouyon, B.; Ukani, L.; Rosa, A.; Faustino, N.A.; Ashizawa, T.; Cooper, T.A.; & Botas, J. (2006). MBNL1 and CUGBP1 modify expanded CUG-induced toxicity in a Drosophila model of myotonic dystrophy type 1. *Human Molecular Genetics.* Vol.15, No.13, pp.2138-2145, ISSN 0964-6906

De León, M. & Cisneros, B. (2008). Myotonic dystrophy 1 in the nervous system: From the clinic to molecular mechanisms. *Journal Neuroscience Reserch,* Vol. 86, No. 1, pp.18-26, ISSN 0360-4012

De Temmerman, N.; Sermon, K.; Seneca, S.; De Rycke, M.; Hilven, P.; Lissens, W.; Van Steirteghem, A.; & Liebaers, I. (2004). Intergenerational instability of the expanded CTG repeat in the DMPK gene: studies in human gametes and preimplantation embryos. *American Journal of Human Genetics* Vol.75, No.2, pp. 325-329, ISSN 0002-9297

Di Costanzo, A.; Di Salle, F.; Santero, L.; Tessitore, A.; Bonavita, V.; & Tedeschi, G. (2002) Pattern and significance of white matter abnormalities in myotonic dystrophy type 1: an MRI study. *Journal of Neurology.* Vol.249 , No.9, pp. 1175-82, ISSN 0340-5354

Di Costanzo, A.; Santoro, L.; de Cristofaro, M.; Manganelli, F.; Di Salle, F.; & Tedeschi, G. (2008). Familial aggregation of white matter lesions in myotonic dystrophy type 1. *Neuromuscular Disorders.* Vol.18, No.4, pp. 299-305, ISSN 0960-8966

Du, H.; Cline, M.S.; Osborne, R.J.; Tuttle, D.L.; Clark, T.A.; Donohue, J.P.; Hall, M.P.; Shiue, L.; Swanson, M.S.; Thornton, C.A.; & Ares, M. Jr. (2010) Aberrant alternative splicing and extracellular matrix gene expression in mouse models of myotonic dystrophy. *Nature structural & molecular biology.*2010 Feb;17(2):pp.187-93. ISSN 1545-9993

Ebralidze, A.; Wang, Y.; Petkova, V.; Ebralidse, K.; & Junghans, R.P. (2004). RNA leaching of transcription factors disrupts transcription in myotonic dystrophy. *Science*, Vol 303, No.5656, pp.383-387, ISSN 0036-8075.

Ellegren, H. (2000). Heterogeneous mutation processes in human microsatellite DNA sequences. *Nature Genetics*, Vol 24, No. 4, pp. 400-402, ISSN 1061-4036.

Falk, M.; Vojtiskova, M.; Lukas, Z.; Kroupová, I.; & Froster, U. (2006). Simple procedure for automatic detection of unstable alleles in the myotonic dystrophy and Huntington's disease loci. *Genetic Testing,* Vol. 10, No. 2, pp.85-97, ISSN 1090-6576

Fardaei, M.; Rogers, M.T.; Thorpe, H.M.; Larkin, K.; Hamshere, M.G.; Harper, P.S.; & Brook, J.D.(2002). Three proteins, MBNL, MBLL and MBXL, co-localize in vivo with nuclear foci of expanded-repeat transcripts in DM1 and DM2 cells. *Human Moecular Genetics.* Vol.11, No.7, pp.805-814, ISSN 0964-6906

Fortune, M.T.; Vassilopoulos, C.; Coolbaugh, M.I.; Siciliano, M.J.; & Monckton, D.G. (2000). Dramatic, expansion-biased, age-dependent, tissue-specific somatic mosaicism in a transgenic mouse model of triplet repeat instability. *Human Molecular Genetics.* Vol.9, No.3, pp. 439-445, ISSN 0964-6906

Fu, Y.H.; Friedman, D.L.; Richards, S.; Pearlman, J.A.; Gibbs, R.A.; & Pizzuti, A. (1993). Decreased expression of myotonin-protein kinase messenger RNA and protein in adult form of myotonic dystrophy. *Science* 1993; 36: 59-61 ISSN 0964-6906.

Furling, D.; Doucet, G.; Langlois, M.A.; Timchenko, L.; Belanger, E.; Cossette, L.; & Puymirat, J. (2003). Viral vector producing antisense RNA restores myotonic dystrophy myoblast functions. *Gene Therapy.*Vol.10, No.9, pp.795-802, ISSN 0969-7128

García de Andoin, N.; Echeverría, J.; Cobo, A.M.; Rey, A.; Paisán, L.; & López de Munain, A. (2005). A neonatal form of Steinert's myotonic dystrophy in twins after in vitro fertilization. *Fertility and Sterility.* Vol.84, No.3 pp. 756, ISSN 0015-0282

Gennarelli, M.; Pavón, M.; Amicucci, P.; Angelini, C.; Menegazzo, E.; Zelano, G.; Novelli, G.; & Dallapiccola, B. (1999). Reduction of the DM-associated homeo domain protein (DMAHP) mRNA in different brain areas of myotonic dystrophy patients. *Neuromuscular Disorders.* Vol.9, No.4, pp.215-219, ISSN 0960-8966

Goldman, A.; Ramsay, M.; & Jenkins, T. (1994). Absence of myotonic dystrophy in southern African Negroids is associated with a significantly lower number of CTG trinucleotide repeats. *Journal of Medical Genetics* . Vol.31, pp. 37-40, ISSN 002-2593

Gourdon, G.; Radvanyi, F.; Lia, AS.; Duros, C.; Blanche, M.; Abitbol, M.; Junien, C.; & Hofmann-Radvanyi, H. (1997). Moderate intergenerational and somatic instability of a 55-CTG repeat in transgenic mice. *Nature Genetics*. Vol.15, No.2, pp.190- 192, ISSN 1061-4036.

Grover, S.; Fishman, G.A.; & Stone, E.M. (2002). Atypical presentation of pattern dystrophy in two families with peripherin/RDS mutations. *Ophthalmology*. Vol.109, pp. 1110-1117, ISSN 0161-6420

Harley, H.G.; Rundle, S.A.; MacMillan, J.C.; Myring, J.; Brook, J.D.; Crow, S.; Reardon, W.; Fenton, I.; Shaw, DJ.; & Harper, P.S. (1993). Size of the unstable CTG repeat sequence in relation to phenotype and parental transmission in myotonic dystrophy. *American Journal of Human Genetics*. Vol.52, No.6, pp.1164-1174 ISSN 0002-9297

Harper, P.S. (2001). *Myotonic Dystrophy*. WB Saunders (3rd Ed), ISBN 0702021520, London

Harper, P.S.; van Engelen, B.G.; Eymard, B.; Rogers, M.; & Wilcox, D. (2002). 99th ENMC international workshop: myotonic dystrophy: present management, future therapy. 9-11 Naarden, The Netherlands. *Neuromuscular Disorders*, Vol.12, No.6, pp. 596-599, ISSN 0960-8966

Hashem, V.I.; Klysik, E.A.; Rosche, W.A.; & Sinden, R.R.; (2002). Instability of repeated DNAs during transformation in Escherichia coli. *Mutation Reserch*. Vol.502, No 1-2 , pp. 39-46,ISSN 0027-5107

Ho, T.H.; Bundman, D.; Armstrong, D.L.; & Cooper, T.A. (2005). Transgenic mice expressing CUG-BP1 reproduce splicing mis-regulation observed in myotonic dystrophy. *Human Molecular Genetics* Vol.14, No.11, pp.1539-1547, ISSN 0964-6906

Hsiao, K.M.; Chen, S.S.; Li, S.Y.; Chiang, S.Y.; Lin, H.M.; & Pan, H. (2003). Epidemiological and genetic studies of myotonic dystrophy type 1 in Taiwan. *Neuroepidemiology* .Vol.22, pp. 283-289, ISSN 0251-5350

Jakubiczka, S.; Vielhaber, S.; Kress, W.; Küpferling, P.; Reuner, U.; Kunath, B.; & Wieacker, P. (2004). Improvement of the diagnostic procedure in proximal myotonic myopathy/myotonic dystrophy type 2. *Neurogenetics*. Vol.5, No.1, pp. 55-59, ISSN 1364-6745

Jansen, G.; Willems, P.; Coerwinkel, M.; Nillesen, W.; Smeets, H.; Vits, L.; Howeler, C.; Brunner, H.; & Wieringa, B. (1994). Gonosomal mosaicism in myotonic dystrophy patients: involvement of mitotic events in (CTG)n repeat variation and selection against extreme expansion in sperm. *American Journal of Human Genetics* .Vol.54, No.4, pp. 575-585, ISSN 0002-9297

Jiang, H.; Mankodi, A.; Swanson, M.S.; Moxley, R.T.; & Thornton, C.A. (2004). Myotonic dystrophy type 1 is associated with nuclear foci of mutant RNA, sequestration of muscleblind proteins and deregulated alternative splicing in neurons. *Human Molecular Genetics* 2004; Vol,13, No. 24, pp.3079-3088, ISSN 0964-6906

Kakourou, G.; Dhanjal, S.; Mamas, T.; Serhal, P.; Delhanty, J.D.; & SenGupta, S.B. (2010). Modification of the triplet repeat primed polymerase chain reaction method for detection of the CTG repeat expansion in myotonic dystrophy type 1: application in preimplantation genetic diagnosis. *Fertility and Sterility*. Vol.94 , No.5, pp. 1674-1679, ISSN 0015-0282

Kanadia, R.N.; Johnstone, K.A.; Mankodi, A.; Lungu, C.; Thornton, C.A.; Esson, D.; Timmers, A.M.; Hauswirth, W.W.; & Swanson, M.S.(2003). A muscleblind knockout model for myotonic dystrophy. *Science*. Vol.302, No.5652, pp.1978-1980 ISSN 0036-8075

Kanadia, R.N.; Shin, J.; Yuan, Y.; Beattie, S.G.; Wheeler, T.M.; Thornton, C.A.; & Swanson, M.S. (2006). Reversal of RNA missplicing and myotonia after muscleblind overexpression in a mouse poly(CUG) model for myotonic dystrophy. *Proceedings of National Academy of Sciences of United States of America*, Vol.103, No.31, pp.11748-11753, ISSN 0027-8424

Kim, U.S.; Kim, J.S.; & Hwang, J.M. (2009). A Case of Myotonic Dystrophy With Pigmentary Retinal Changes. *Korean Journal of Ophthalmology* ,Vol.23, No.2, pp. 121-123, ISSN 1011-8942

Kimura, T.; Nakamori, M.; Lueck, J.D.; Pouliquin, Aoike F.; Fujimura, H.; Dirksen, R.T.; Takahashi M. P.; Dulhunty, A. F., & Sakoda, S. (2005). Altered mRNA splicing of the skeletal muscle ryanodine receptor and sarcoplasmic/endoplasmic reticulum Ca^{2+} -ATPase in myotonic dystrophy type 1. *Human Molecular Genetics* 2005, Vol.14, No. 15, pp.2189-2200, ISSN 0964-6906

Kirby, R.J.; Hamilton, G.M.; Finnegan, D.J.; Johnson, K.J.; & Jarman, A.P.(2001).Drosophila homolog of the myotonic dystrophy-associated gene, SIX5, is required for muscle and gonad development. *Current Biology*. Vol.10, No.13, pp. 1044-1049, ISSN 0960-9822

Klesert, T.R.; Otten, A.D.; Bird, T.D.; & Tapscott, S.J. (1997). Trinucleotide repeat expansion at the myotonic dystrophy locus reduces expression of DMAHP. *Nature Genetics*. Vol.16, No.4, pp. 402-406, ISSN 1061-4036

Klesert, T.R.; Cho, D.H.; Clark, J.I.; Maylie, J.; Adelman, J.; Snider, L.; Yuen, E.C.; Soriano, P.; & Tapscott S.J. (2000). Mice deficient in Six5 develop cataracts: implications for myotonic dystrophy. *Nature Genetics*. Vol.25, No.1, pp.105-109, ISSN 1061-4036

Koshelev, M.; Sarma, S.; Price, R.E.; Wehrens, X.H.; & Cooper, T.A. (2010). Heart-specific overexpression of CUGBP1 reproduces functional and molecular abnormalities of myotonic dystrophy type 1. *Human Molecular Genetics*. Vol.19, No.6, pp.1066-1075, ISSN 0964-6906

Krahe, R.; Eckhart, M.; Ogunniyi, A.O.; Osuntokun, B.O.; Siciliano, M.J.; & Ashizawa, T. (1995). De novo myotonic dystrophy mutation in a Nigerian kindred. *American Journal of Human Genetics*. Vol.56, No.5, pp.1067-1074, ISSN 0002-9297

Krndija, D.; Savić, D.; Mladenović, J.; Rakocević-Stojanović, V.; Apostolski, S.; Todorović, S.; & Romac, S. (2005). Haplotype analysis of the DM1 locus in the Serbian population. *Acta Neurologica Scandinavica*. Vol.111, No.4 , pp. 274-277, ISSN 0001-6314

krzypczak-Zielinska, M.; Sulek-Piatkowska, A.; Mierzejewski, M.; & Froster, U.G. (2009). New analysis method of myotonic dystrophy 1 based on quantitative fluorescent polymerase chain reaction. *Genetic Testing Molecular Biomarkers*. Vol.13, No.5, pp.651-655. ISSN 1945-0265

Kuyumcu-Martinez, NM; & Cooper, TA.(2006). Misregulation of alternative splicing causes pathogenesis in myotonic dystrophy. *Progress Moecularl Subcellular Biology,* Vol.44, pp. 133-159. ISSN 0079-6484

Laberge, L.; Bégin, P.; Dauvilliers, Y.; Beaudry, M.; Laforte, M.; Jean, S.; & Mathieu, J. (2009). A polysomnographic study of daytime sleepiness in myotonic dystrophy type 1. *Journal of neurology, neurosurgery, and psychiatry,* Vol.80, No.6, pp.642-646, ISSN 0022-3050

Langlois, M.A.; Lee, N.S.; Rossi, J.J.; & Puymirat, J.(2003). Hammerhead ribozyme-mediated destruction of nuclear foci in myotonic dystrophy myoblasts. *Molecular Therapy,* Vo. 7, No.5 Pt 1, pp 670-680, ISSN 1525-0016

Langlois, M.A.; Boniface, C.; Wang, G.; Alluin, J.; Salvaterra, P.M.; Puymirat, J.; Rossi, J.J.; & Lee, N.S. (2005). Cytoplasmic and nuclear retained DMPK mRNAs are targets for

RNA interference in myotonic dystrophy cells. *Journal of Biologial Chemistry* Vol.280, No.17, pp.16949-16954, ISSN 0021-9258

Lavedan, C.; Hofmann-Radvanyi, H.; Rabes, JP.; Roume, J.; & Junien, C. (1993). Different sex-dependent constraints in CTG length variation as explanation for congenital myotonic dystrophy. *Lancet.* Vol.341, No.8839, pp. 237. ISSN 0140-6736

Leifsdóttir, G.; Benedikz, J.E.; Jóhannesson, G.; Jónsson, J.J.; & Sveinbjörnsdóttir, S. (2005). Prevalence of myotonic dystrophy in Iceland. *Laeknabladid.* Vol.91, pp. 829-34, ISSN 0023-7213

Liquori, C.L.; Ricker, K.; Moseley, M.L.; Jacobsen, J.F.; Kress, W.; Naylor, S.L.; Day, J.W.; & Ranum, L.P. (2001). Myotonic dystrophy type 2 caused by a CCTG expansion in intron 1 of ZNF9. *Science*, Vol.293, No.5531, pp.864-867, ISSN 0036-8075.

Llagostera,E; Catalucci, D; Marti, L; Liesa, M; Camps, M; Ciaraldi, TP; Kondo, R; Reddy, S; Dillmann, WH; Palacin, M; Zorzano, A; Ruiz-Lozano, P; Gomis, R; & Kaliman, P. (2007).Role of myotonic dystrophy protein kinase (DMPK) in glucose homeostasis and muscle insulin action. *PLoS One*, Vol. 2, No.11, e1134. ISSN 1932-6203

Llamusi, B; & Artero, R. (2008). Molecular Effects of the CTG Repeats in Mutant Dystrophia Myotonica Protein Kinase Gene. *Current Genomics.* Vol.9, No.8, pp.509-516, ISSN 1389-2029

Louprasong, AC.; Light, DJ.; & Diller, RS. (2010). Spider dystrophy as an ocular manifestation of myotonic dystrophy. *Optometry* . Vol.81, pp. 188-193, ISSN 1529-1839

Lu, Q.L.; Rabinowitz, A.; Chen, Y.C.; Yokota, T.; Yin, H.; Alter, J.; Jadoon, A.; Bou-Gharios, G.; & Partridge, T. (2005). Systemic delivery of antisense oligoribonucleotide restores dystrophin expression in body-wide skeletal muscles. *Proceedings of National Academy of Sciences of United States of America*, Vol.102, No.1, pp.198-203, ISSN 0027-8424

Machuca-Tzili, L; Brook, D; & Hilton-Jones, D. (2005). Clinical and molecular aspects of the myotonic dystrophies: a review. *Muscle & Nerve* , Vol.32, No. 1, pp. 1-18, ISSN 0148-639X

Magaña, J.J.; Leyva-Garcia, N.; & Cisneros, B. (2009). [Pathogenesis of myotonic dystrophy type 1]. *Gaceta Medica de Mexico*, Vol.145, No.4, pp.331-337, ISSN 0016-3813

Magaña, J.J.; Cortés-Reynosa, P.; Escobar-Cedillo, R.; Gómez, R.; Leyva-García, N.; & Cisneros, B. (2011). Distribution of CTG repeats at the DMPK gene in myotonic dystrophy patients and healthy individuals from the Mexican population. *Molecular Biology Reports.* Vol.38, No.2, pp.1341-1346, ISSN 0301-4851

Magaña, J.J. & Cisneros, B. (2011). Perspectives on gene therapy in myotonic dystrophy type 1. *Journal of Neuroscience Research*, Vol.89, No.3, pp.275-285, ISSN 0360-4012

Mankodi, A.; Logigian, E.; Callahan, L.; McClain, C.; White, R.; Henderson, D.; Krym, M.; & Thornton, C.A. (2000). Myotonic dystrophy in transgenic mice expressing an expanded CUG repeat. *Science.* Vol.289, No.5485, pp.1769-1773, ISSN 0036-8075

Mankodi, A.; Urbinati, C.R.; Yuan, Q.P.; Moxley, R.T.; Sansone, V.; Krym, M.; Henderson, D.; Schalling, M.; Swanson M.S.; & Thornton, C. (2001) Muscleblind localizes to nuclear foci of aberrant RNA in myotonic dystrophy types 1 and 2. *Human Molecular Genetics*, Vol.10, No.19, pp. 2165-2170. ISSN 0964-6906

Mankodi, A.; Takahashi, M.P.; Jiang, H.; Beck, C.L.; Bowers, W.J.; Moxley, R.T. Cannon, S. C.; & Thornton C. A. (2002). Expanded CUG repeats trigger aberrant splicing of

ClC-1 chloride channel pre-mRNA and Hyperexcitability of skeletal muscle in myotonic dystrophy. *Molecular Cell*, Vol.10, No.1. pp.35-44, ISSN 1097-2765

Martorell, L.; Monckton, D.G.; Sanchez, A.; Lopez De Munain, A.; & Baiget, M. (2001). Frequency and stability of the myotonic dystrophy type 1 premutation. *Neurology*, Vol.56, No.3, pp. 328-335, ISSN 0028-3878

Martorell, L.; Gámez, J.; Cayuela, M.L.; Gould, F.K.; McAbney, J.P.; Ashizawa, T.; Monckton, D.G.; & Baiget, M. (2004). Germline mutational dynamics in myotonic dystrophy type 1 males: allele length and age effects. *Neurology*. Vol.62, No.2 pp.269-274, ISSN 0028-3878

Mastroyiannopoulos, NP; Feldman, ML; Uney, JB; Mahadevan, MS; & Phylactou, LA.(2005). Woodchuck post-transcriptional element induces nuclear export of myotonic dystrophy 3' untranslated region transcripts. *EMBO Reports,* Vol.6, No.5, pp.458-463, ISSN 1469-21X

Matsumura, T.; Iwahashi, H.; Funahashi, T.; Takahashi, M.P.; Saito, T.; Yasui, K.; Saito, T.; Iyama, A.; Toyooka, K.; Fujimura, H.; & Shinno, S. (2009). A cross-sectional study for glucose intolerance of myotonic dystrophy. *Journal of the Neurological Sciences*. Vol.276, No.1-2, pp. 60-65, INSS 0022-510X

Medica, I.; Logar, N.; Mileta, D.L.; & Peterlin, B. (2004). Genealogical study of myotonic dystrophy in Istria (Croatia). *Annales Genetique*. Vol.47, No.2, pp. 139-146, ISSN 0003-3995

Melacini, P.; Villanova, C.; Menegazzo, E.; Novelli, G.; Danieli, G.; Rizzoli, G.; Fasoli, G.; Angelini, C.; Buja, G.; Miorelli, M. et al. (1995). Correlation between cardiac involvement and CTG trinucleotide repeat length in myotonic dystrophy. *Journal of the American Collage of Cardiology*. Vol.25, No.1, pp.239- 245, ISSN 0735-1097

Michalowski, S.; Miller, J.W.; Urbinati, C.R.; Paliouras, M.; Swanson, M.S.; & Griffith, J.(1999). Visualization of double-stranded RNAs from the myotonic dystrophy protein kinase gene and interactions with CUG-binding protein. *Nucleic Acids Research.*Vol.27, No.17, pp.3534-3542, ISSN 0305-1048

Miller, J.W.; Urbinati, C.R.; Teng-Umnuay, P.; Stenberg, M.G.; Byrne, B.J.; Thornton, C.A.; & Swanson, M.S.(2000). Recruitment of human muscleblind proteins to (CUG)(n) expansions associated with myotonic dystrophy. The *EMBO Journal.*Vol. 19, No.17, pp.4439-4448, ISSN 0261-4189

Mladenovic, J.; Pekmezovic, T.; Todorovic, S.; Rakocevic-Stojanovic, V.; Savi, D. Romac, S; & Apostolski, S. (2006). Epidemiology of myotonic dystrophy type 1 (Steinert disease) in Belgrade (Serbia). *Clinical Neurology Neurosurgery*. Vol. 108, pp.757-760, ISSN 0303-8467

Monckton, D.G.; Coolbaugh, M.I.; Ashizawa, K.T.; Siciliano, M.J.; & Caskey, C.T. (1997) Hypermutable myotonic dystrophy CTG repeats in transgenic mice. *Nature Genetics*. Vol.15, No.2, pp.193-196. ISSN 1061-4036

Mulders, S.A.; Van den Broek, W.J.; Wheeler, T.M.; Croes, H.J.; Van Kuik-Romeijn, P.; De Kimpe, S.J.; Furling, D.; Platenburg, G.J.; Gourdon, G.; Thornton, C.A.; Wieringa, B.; & Wansink, D.G. (2009). Triplet-repeat oligonucleotide-mediated reversal of RNA toxicity in myotonic dystrophy. *Proceedings of National Academy of Sciences of United States of America*, Vol.106, No.33, pp.13915-13920, ISSN 0027-8424

Mulders, S.A.; Van Engelen, B.G.; Wieringa, B.; & Wansink, D.G.(2010). Molecular therapy in myotonic dystrophy: focus on RNA gain-of-function. *Human Molecular Genetics*, Vol.19, No.R1, pp.R90-97, ISSN 0964-6906

Myring, J.; Meredith, AL.; Harley, HG.; Kohn, G.; Norbury, G.; Harper, P.S.; & Shaw, D.J. (1992) Specific molecular prenatal diagnosis for the CTG mutation in myotonic dystrophy. *Journal of Medical Genetics.* Vol.29, No.11 pp. 785-788, ISSN 0022-2593

Ono, S.; Takahashi, K.; Kanda, F.; Jinnai, K.; Fukuoka, Y.; Mitake, S.; Inagaki, T.; Kurisaki, H.; Nagao, K.; & Shimizu, N. (2001). Decrease of neurons in the medullary arcuate nucleus in myotonic dystrophy.*Acta Neuropathologica.* Vol.102, No.1, pp.89-93, ISSN 0001-6322

Otten, A.D.; & Tapscott, S.J.(1995) Triplet repeat expansion in myotonic dystrophy alters the adjacent chromatin structure. *Proceedings of the National Academy of Sciences of the United States of America.*1995 Jun 6; Vol.92, No.12, pp.5465-546, ISSN 0027-8424

Pan, H.; Lin, H.M.; Ku, W.Y.; Li, T.C.; Li, S.Y.; Lin, C.C.; & Hsiao, K.M. (2001). Haplotype analysis of the myotonic dystrophy type 1 (DM1) locus in Taiwan: implications for low prevalence and founder mutations of Taiwanese myotonic dystrophy type 1. *European Journal of Human Genetics.* Vol.9, No.8, pp.638-641. ISSN 1018- 4813

Pearson, C.E; Nichol-Edamura, K.; & Cleary JD. (2005). Repeat instability: mechanisms of dynamic mutations. *Nature Review Genetics,* Vol.6, No10, pp.729-742 ISSN 1471-0056.

Philips, A.V.; Timchenko, L.T.; & Cooper, T.A.(1998). Disruption of splicing regulated by a CUG-binding protein in myotonic dystrophy. *Science.* Vol.280, No.5364, pp.737-741 ISSN 0036-8075

Ranum, LP; & Cooper, TA. (2006).RNA-Mediated Neuromuscular Disorders. *Annual Review of Neuroscience,* Vol. 29, pp. 259-277, ISSN 0147-006X

Reddy, S; Smith, DB; Rich, MM; Leferovich, JM; Reilly, P; Davis, BM; Tran, K; Rayburn, H; Bronson, R; Cros, D; Balice-Gordon, RJ; & Housman, D. (1996). Mice lacking the myotonic dystrophy protein kinase develop a late onset progressive myopathy. *Nature Genetics.* Vol.13, No.3, pp.325-335, ISSN 1061-4036

Rosa, N.; Lanza, M.; Borrelli, M.; De Bernardo, M.; Palladino, A.; Di Gregorio, M.G.; Pascotto, F.; & Politano, L. (2011). Low Intraocular Pressure Resulting from Ciliary Body Detachment in Patients with Myotonic Dystrophy. *Ophthalmology.* Vol.118, pp.260-264, ISSN 0161-6420

Rubinsztein, J.S.; Rubinsztein, D.C.; Goodburn, S.; & Holland, A.J. (1998). Apathy and hypersomnia are common features of myotonic dystrophy. *Journal of Neurology, Neurosurgery and Psychiatry.*Vol.64, No.4, pp.510-515, ISSN 0022-3050

Rubinsztein, J.S.; Rubinsztein, D.C.; McKenna, P.J.; Goodburn, S.; & Holland, A.J. (1997). Mild myotonic dystrophy is associated with memory impairment in the context of normal general intelligence. *Journal of Medical Genetics.* Vol.34, No.3 , pp.229-233, ISSN 0022-2593

Sarkar, P.S.; Appukuttan, B.; Han, J.; Ito, Y.; Ai, C.; Tsai, W.; Chai, Y.; Stout, J.T.; & Reddy, S. (2000). Heterozygous loss of Six5 in mice is sufficient to cause ocular cataracts. *Nature Genetics,* Vol. 25, No. 1, pp.110-114, ISSN 1061-4036

Savkur, R.S.; Philips, A.V.; & Cooper, T.A.(2001).Aberrant regulation of insulin receptor alternative splicing is associated with insulin resistance in myotonic dystrophy. *Nature Genetics* Vol.29, No.1, pp. 40-47, ISSN 1061-4036

Savkur, R.S.; Philips, A.V.; Cooper, T.A.; Dalton, J.C.; Moseley, M.L.; Ranum, L.P.; & Day, J.W.(2004). Insulin receptor splicing alteration in myotonic dystrophy type 2. *American Journal of Human Genetics.*Vol.74, No.6, pp.1309-1313, ISSN 0002-9297

Savouret, C.; Garcia-Cordier, C.; Megret, J.; te Riele, H.; Junien, C.; & Gourdon, G. (2004). MSH2-dependent germinal CTG repeat expansions are produced continuously in spermatogonia from DM1 transgenic mice. *Molecular Cell Biology*. Vol.24, No.2, pp. 629-637.ISSN 0270-7306

Schara, U.; & Schoser, B.G. (2006). Myotonic dystrophies type 1 and 2: a summary on current aspects. *Seminars in Pediatric Neurology*, Vol 13, No.2, pp 71-79, ISSN 1071-9091.

Sergeant, N.; Sablonniere, B.; Schraen-Maschke, S.; Ghestem, A.; Maurage, C.A.; Wattez, A.; Vermersch, P.; & Delacourte, A. (2001). Dysregulation of human brain microtubule-associated tau mRNA maturation in myotonic dystrophy type 1. *Human Molecular Genetics*. Vol.10, No.19, pp.2143-2155, ISSN 0964-6906

Seznec, H.; Lia-Baldini, A.S.; Duros, C.; Fouquet, C.; Lacroix, C.; Hofmann-Radvanyi, H.; Junien, C.; & Gourdon G.(2000). Transgenic mice carrying large human genomic sequences with expanded CTG repeat mimic closely the DM CTG repeat intergenerational and somatic instability. *Human Molecular Genetics* . Vol.9, No.8, pp.1185-1194, ISSN 0964-6906

Seznec, H.; Agbulut, O.; Sergeant, N.; Savouret, C.; Ghestem, A.; Tabti, N.; Willer, J.C.; Ourth, L.; Duros, C.; Brisson, E.; Fouquet, C.; Butler-Browne, G.; Delacourte, A.; Junien, C.; & Gourdon, G. (2002). Mice transgenic for the human myotonic dystrophy region with expanded CTG repeats display muscular and brain abnormalities. *Human Molecular Genetics*. Vol.10, No.23, pp.2717-26, ISSN 0964-6906

Sharma, P.C; Grover, A.; & Kahl, G.(2007). Mining microsatellites in eukaryotic genomes. *Trends in Biotechnology*, Vol.25, No. 11, pp. 490-498, ISSN 0167-7799.

Shimizu, M.; Fujita, R.; Tomita, N.; Shindo, H.; & Wells, R.D. (2001) Chromatin structure of yeast minichromosomes containing triplet repeat sequences associated with human hereditary neurological diseases. *Nucleic Acids Research Supplement*. No.1, pp.71-72, ISSN 0305-1048

Taneja, K.L.; McCurrach, M.; Schalling, M.; Housman, D.; & Singer, R.H. (1995). Foci of trinucleotide repeat transcripts in nuclei of myotonic dystrophy cells and tissues.*The Journal of Cell Biology*. Vol.128, No.6, pp.995-1002, ISSN 0021-9525

The International Myotonic Dystrophy Consortium (IDMC). (2000) New nomenclature and DNA testing guidelines for myotonic dystrophy type 1 (DM1). *Neurology*, Vol.54, No.6, pp.1218-1221, ISSN 0028-3878

Timchenko, N.A.; Cai, Z.J.; Welm, A.L.; Reddy, S.; Ashizawa, T.; & Timchenko, L.T.(2001).RNA CUG repeats sequester CUGBP1 and alter protein levels and activity of CUGBP1. *The Journal of Biological Chemistry*.Vol.276, No.11, pp.7820-7826, ISSN 0021-9258

Tishkoff, S.; Goldman, A.; Calafell, F.; Speed, W.C.; Deinard, A.S.; Bonne-Tamir, B.; Tishkoff, S.; Goldman, A.; Calafell, F.; Speed, W.C.; Deinard, A.S.; Bonne-Tamir, B.; Kidd, J.R,; Pakstis, A.J.; Jenkinns, T.; & Kidd, T.T. (1998). A global haplotype analysis of the myotonic dystrophy locus: implications for the evolution of modern humans and for the origin of myotonic dystrophy mutations. *American Journal of Human Genetics*, Vol.62, pp.1389-1402, ISSN 0002-9297

Tsien, J.Z.; Huerta, P.T.; & Tonegawa, S.(1996).The essential role of hippocampal CA1 NMDA receptor-dependent synaptic plasticity in spatial memory. *Cell* 1996; 87:pp.13271338, ISSN 0092-8674

Van den Broek, W.J.; Nelen, M.R.; Wansink, D.G.; Coerwinkel, M.M.; te Riele, H.; Groenen, P.J.; & Wieringa, B. (2002). Somatic expansion behaviour of the (CTG)n repeat in myotonic dystrophy knock-in mice is differentially affected by Msh3 and Msh6 mismatch-repair proteins. *Human Molecular Genetics.* Vol.11, No.2, pp .191-198, ISSN 0964-6906

Wang, G.S.; Kearney D.L.; De Biasi, M.; Taffet, G.; & Cooper, T.A. (2007). Elevation of RNA-binding protein CUGBP1 is an early event in an inducible heart-specific mouse model of myotonic dystrophy. *The Journal of Clinical Investigation.* Vol.117, No.10, pp.2802-2811, ISSN 0021-9738

Wang, G.S.; Kuyumcu-Martinez, M.N.; Sarma, S.; Mathur, N.; Wehrens, X.H.; & Cooper, T.A. (2009). PKC inhibition ameliorates the cardiac phenotype in a mouse model of myotonic dystrophy type 1. *Journal of Clinical Investigation.* Vol.119, No.12, pp.3797-3806, ISSN 0021-9738

Wang, Y.; Wang, J.; Gao, L.; Lafyatis, R.; Stamm, S.; & Andreadis, A.(2005). Tau exons 2 and 10, which are misregulated in neurodegenerative diseases, are partly regulated by silencers which bind a SRp30c.SRp55 complex that either recruits or antagonizes htra2beta1. *Journal of Biological Chemistry* 2005; 280: pp.14230-14239, ISSN 0021-9258

Wang, Y.H.; Amirhaeri, S.; Kang, S.; Wells, R.D.; & Griffith, J.D.(1994). Preferential nucleosome assembly at DNA triplet repeats from the myotonic dystrophy gene. *Science,* Vol. 265, No. 5172, pp.669-671, ISSN 0036-8075

Warf, M.B.; Nakamori, M.; Matthys, C.M.; Thornton, C.A.; & Berglund, J.A.; (2009). Pentamidine reverses the splicing defects associated with myotonic dystrophy. *Proceedings of National Academy of Sciences of United States of America,* Vol.106, No.44, pp.18551-18556, ISSN 0027-8424

Warf, M.B. & Berglund, J.A. (2010). Role of RNA structure in regulating pre-mRNA splicing. *Trends Biochemical Science.* Vol.35, No.3, pp.169-178, ISSN 0968-0004

Warner, J.P.; Barron, L.H.; Goudie, D.; Kelly, K.; Dow, D.; Fitzpatrick, D.R.; & Brock, D.J. (1996). A general method for the detection of large CAG repeat expansions by fluorescent PCR. *Journal of Medical Genetics,* Vol.33, pp.1022-1026 , ISSN 0022-2593

Wheeler, T.M.; Lueck, J.D., Swanson, M.S.; Dirksen, R.T.; & Thornton, C.A. (2007). Correction of ClC-1 splicing eliminates chloride channelopathy and myotonia in mouse models of myotonic dystrophy. *The Journal Clinical Investigation.* Vol.117, No.12, pp. 3952-3957, ISSN 0021-9738

Wheeler, T.M.; Sobczak K.; Lueck, J.D.; Osborne, R.; Lin, X.; Dirksen, R.T.; & Thornton, C.A. (2009). Reversal of RNA dominance by displacement of protein sequestered on triplet repeat RNA. Science 325(5938):336-339, ISSN 0036-8075

Winblad, S.; Lindberg, C.; & Hansen, S.(2006). Cognitive deficits and CTG repeat expansion size in classical myotonic dystrophy type 1 (DM1). *Behavioral and Brain Functions,* Vol. 2, pp.16. ISSN 1744-9081

Wojciechowska, M.; Bacolla, A.; Larson, J.E.; & Wells, R.D. (2005), The myotonic dystrophy type 1 triplet repeat sequence induces gross deletions and inversions. *Journal of Biological Chemistry.* Vol.280, No.2, pp.941-952, ISSN 0021-9258

Zerylnick, C.A.; Torroni, A.; Sherman, S.L.; & Warren, S.T.(1995). Normal variation at the myotonic dystrophy locus in global human populations. *American Journal of Human Genetics.* Vol.56, pp.123-130, ISSN 0002-9297

Section 2

Pathophysiology and Disease State

5

Duchenne Muscular Dystrophy and Brain Function

J.L. Anderson[1], S.I. Head[2] and J.W. Morley[3]
[1]Childrens Hospital, Westmead, Sydney,
[2]School of Medical Sciences, University of New South Wales, Sydney,
[3]School of Medicine, University of Western Sydney, Sydney,
Australia

1. Introduction

Muscular dystrophies have historically been characterised according to clinical criteria, however in the genomic age the muscular dystrophies are now subdivided into groups according to the primary gene defect. Currently identified are 29 different loci and encoded proteins, giving rise to 34 distinct forms of muscular dystrophy (Dalkilic & Kunkel 2003; Hsu 2004). The majority of these types of muscular dystrophy are caused by perturbations of different components of the dystrophin-glycoprotein complex (DGC) an integral component of the cellular cytoskeleton (see below). Dystrophin is the largest component of the DGC and is absent in Duchenne muscular dystrophy (DMD), and severely truncated with decreased levels in Becker muscular dystrophy (BMD) (Hoffman & Kunkel 1989). DMD and the allelic BMD are the most common forms of muscular dystrophy in humans and together they are termed dystrophinopathies (Kingston et al. 1984; Shaw & Dreifuss 1969). DMD alone accounts for approximately 80% of all the myopathies in the muscular dystrophy group (Culligan et al. 1998).The dystrophin gene is the second largest described to date, totalling 1.5% of the X chromosome, 0.1% of the entire genome. The DMD gene is 99% introns, with a coding sequence of 86 exons (including the promoters) and remains the only known human metagene (Blake et al. 2002; Burmeister et al. 1988; Hamed & Hoffmann 2006; Kenwrick et al. 1987; Koenig et al. 1987; Kunkel et al. 1986; Muntoni et al. 2003; Roberts et al. 1993; Smith et al. 2006; Van Ommen et al. 1987; Wallis et al. 2004). Dystrophin was demonstrated to be localised at the sarcolemma in human skeletal muscle after its' genetic characterisation (Arahata et al. 1988; Sugita et al. 1988; Zubrzycka-Gaarn et al. 1988). This discovery was followed by a report of dystrophin messenger RNA in brain, with the protein being specifically localised at postsynaptic densities (PSD) in the CNS, in particular in the hippocampus, cerebral cortex and in cerebellar Purkinje cells (PC) (Chamberlain et al. 1988; Chelly et al. 1988, 1989; Lidov et al. 1990, Nudel et al. 1988).

From the earliest reports authors have noted a preponderance of cognitive impairment in the Duchenne population and it has been well established that the average IQ of the boys with DMD is 85, one standard deviation below the normal of 100 (Cotton et al. 2005). With a greater understanding of the underlying molecular biology i.e. genotype, the recognised phenotype of dystrophinopathies is expanding (Beggs 1997; Emery 2002, 2002a; Ferlini et al. 1999; Muntoni et al. 1993). More recently investigations into the role of these proteins in the

CNS have commenced. In contrast to skeletal muscle, the function of dystrophin in brain is less well understood in part due to its more recent discovery in the CNS as well as the greater complexity of the dystrophin gene products and DGCs in this location (Culligan et al. 2001). It has been suggested that dystrophin may play a role in anchoring the postsynaptic apparatus, receptor channel clustering and membrane organization (Lidov et al. 1993). This anchoring of molecules, critical for neuronal function, may be achieved by dystrophin/DGC acting as adaptors between the actin cytoskeleton and membrane bound receptors (Yoshihara et al. 2003). It may also play a critical role in the formation and maintenance of macromolecular signalling complexes (Tokarz et al. 1998; Yoshihara et al. 2003). Dystrophin has also been suggested to play a role in stabilizing the postsynaptic apparatus to maintain a certain status of the network after brain maturation and/or episodes of synaptic plasticity (Brunig et al. 2002). Calcium levels have been found to be abnormal in neurons from an animal model of DMD (*mdx* mouse), and in a situation analogous to muscle, this could make these cells more susceptible to necrosis (Culligan et al. 2001). In summary, dystrophin deficiency may significantly alter membrane integrity, ion channel physiology, calcium homeostasis, regional cellular signal integration and structural reorganisation at the synapse (Mehler 2000; Vaillend & Billard 2002; Vaillend et al. 2004). The majority of recent studies support a role for dystrophin in organisation of the mature synapse – particularly GABA-ergic synapses under dynamic conditions. Below is a brief summary of the localisation of dystrophin/DGC in the CNS and a synthesis of the current literature investigating the role of dystrophin in human and murine CNS at the behavioural, morphological, biochemical and electrophysiological level.

1.1 The dystrophin-glycoprotein complex in CNS

Individual members of the DGC show a variety of site-specific specializations leading to many different DGCs (differentiated by binding-partner profile, localization and composition) existing in the CNS. Differences exist between the DGC in muscle and neuromuscular junction and also between both of these DGCs and brain DGCs. Additionally, individual members of the DGC play different roles at different sites. In the brain, unlike in muscle, the association of syntrophin with dystrophin is not crucial for DGC formation (Moukhles & Carbonetto 2001; Waite et al. 2009). Furthermore, Culligan & Ohlendieck (2002) have suggested that the brain DGC consists of four main components, the dystroglycan subcomplex, a dystrophin or utrophin gene product, a dystrobrevin isoform and a syntrophin subcomplex (Fig.1). Complexes including short dystrophin gene products together with syntrophin may also be expressed in both neurons and glia.

A role for the DGC in CNS has been suggested by many investigators, yet unequivocal evidence has yet to emerge. One theory suggests a role for the DGC in cellular communication by acting as a transmembrane signalling complex (Muntoni et al. 2003; Petrof 2002; Rando 2001). Supportive evidence for this theory is seen when mutations of the DGC component genes leads to cell death, thought to be due to a disruption of cell survival pathways and cellular defence mechanisms, both of which are regulated by signalling cascades (Muntoni et al. 2003; Rando 2001). The DGC in CNS may also play a dual function: incorporating both membrane stabilization as well as transmembrane signalling, as has been demonstrated at the neuromuscular junction (Albrecht & Froehner 2002). Additionally, the DGC has been suggested to play a role in the structural/functional organisation and/or stabilization of synapses (Albrecht & Froehner 2002). Dystroglycan and dystrophin, as

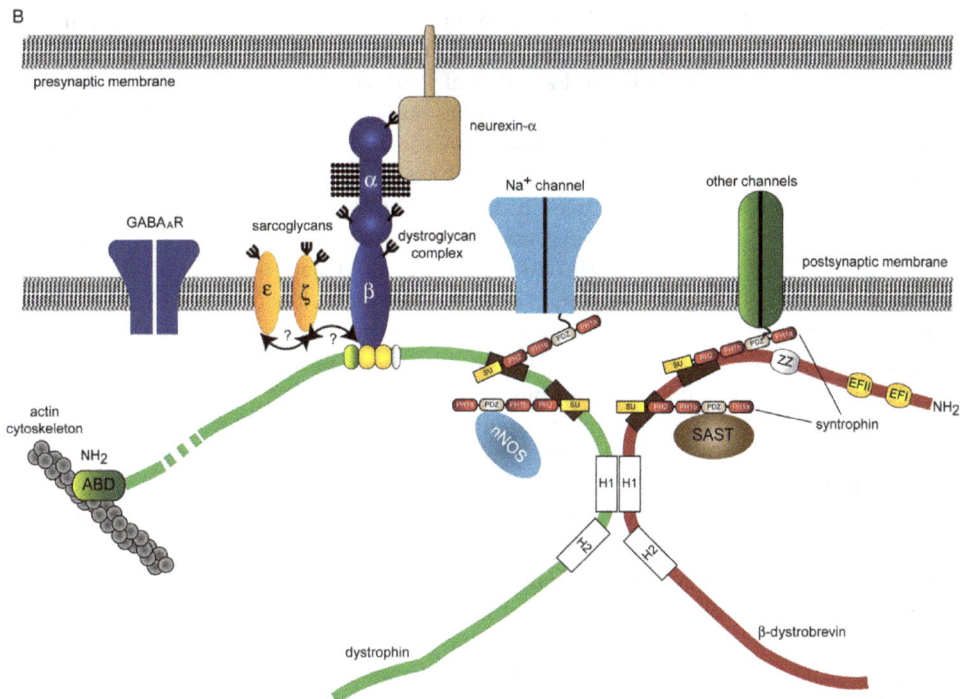

Fig. 1. The molecular organization of the "DGC-like" complexes and associated proteins in neurons (Modified from Waite et al. 2009).

central components of DGCs, have been implicated in the stabilisation of neurotransmitter receptor clusters e.g. GABAergic and cholinergic afferents (Knuesel et al. 1999; Zaccaria et al. 2001). It has been suggested that the DGC may act as a cytoskeletal scaffold on which signalling complexes as well as transmembrane proteins can be assembled and clustered, largely mediated by the syntrophins and dystrobrevins (Albrecht & Froehner 2002; Cavaldesi et al. 1999; Connors et al. 2004; Gee et al. 1998; Hashida-Okumura et al. 1999). Culligan and Ohlendieck (2002) propose that the extracellular component of neuronal DGCs mediates cellular signalling through interactions of specific proteins such as laminin, laminin α2, perlecan, agrin and biglycan. These interactions are believed to play a role in terminal consolidation, integrity and maintenance. Ceccarini et al. (2002) postulate that the DGC may play a role in the neuronal maturation process i.e. in morphological and functional modifications such as neurite outgrowth and synapse formation. Levi et al. (2002) suggest that the DGC may act as a trans-synaptic signal for some aspects of signalling involved in central neuron synaptic differentiation (Levi et al. 2002).

2. Dystrophin and the CNS

2.1 Localization

Dystrophin expression in the CNS is significantly more complicated compared to muscle due to the site specificity, developmental expression and diversity of gene products in this tissue. Levels of dystrophin in the brain are approximately 10% of those found in muscle. However, the CNS has the highest number of different dystrophin gene products of any other organ/tissue in the body (Abdulrazzak et al. 2001; Gorecki et al. 1991, 1992; Gorecki & Barnard 1995; Tokarz et al. 1998). Early studies indicated that in the CNS dystrophin localises primarily to the vascular endothelium, postsynaptic regions, pia and choroid plexus (Kamakura et al. 1994; Lidov et al. 1990; Uchino et al. 1994). Later studies demonstrated that Dp71 a smaller gene product of the dystrophin gene, is present in the wall of blood vessels, but is actually expressed in perivascular astrocyte endfeet (Ueda et al. 2000). Nudel et al. 1998, Chelly et al. (1988 and 1989) and Chamberlain et al. (1988) found dystrophin messenger RNA in brain and suggested that the lack of dystrophin in DMD may be the cause of cognitive impairment known to exist in this population. Lidov et al. (1990) demonstrated that dystrophin was specifically localised at postsynaptic densities (PSD) in the CNS, in particular in the hippocampus, cerebral cortex and in cerebellar Purkinje cells (PC) in rodents. This is in agreement with others who also found Dp427 as well as Dp71 enriched at the PSD (Blake et al. 1999; Jung et al. 1993; Kim et al. 1992; Moukhles & Carbonetto 2001). Uchino et al. (1994) confirmed these findings of PSD localisation in humans in agreement with Kim et al. (1995) and Jancsik & Hajos (1998). This latter group found that dystrophin was in the spines of neurons, with particularly heavy labelling at the PSD (Jancsik & Hajos 1998). There are now known to be three full-length dystrophin gene-products found in the CNS: M-dystrophin has been found in cerebral cortex and hippocampus (CA1, CA2 and CA3), C-dystrophin has also been localised to the cortex (grey matter, parietal layers II-IV, cingulated cortex) and hippocampus (pyramidal layer , layer II of infrahinal cortex, striatum radiatum and striatum oriens). C-dystrophin has also been demonstrated to be present in brainstem (inferior olive and trigeminal complex) and the midbrain (Caudate putamen). The third full-length dystrophin gene product P-dystrophin has been found in foetal cerebral cortex and Purkinje cells from early in the developmental process. Full-length dystrophin gene products are expressed almost exclusively in neurons (Lidov et al. 1990; Waite et al. 2009). The shorter dystrophin-gene products have a nomenclature of 'Dp' followed by their molecular weight: Dp 260 (D'Souza et al. 1995) Dp 140 (Lidov et al. 1995), Dp 116 (Byers et al. 1993; Schofield et al. 1994) and Dp71 (Blake et al. 1992; Iannello et al. 1991; formerly named apo-dystrophin 1 or G-dystrophin). Dp260 is found predominately in the retina (also brain and cardiac tissue) (Cibis et al. 1993; Costa et al. 2007; D'Souza et al. 1995; Pillers et al. 1993). Dp140 is predominately expressed in brain during foetal development and at very low levels in the adult brain, localised to astro-glial processes, vascular endothelium and leptomeningeal surfaces (Bardoni et al. 2000; Lidov et al. 1995). Dp 116 has been localised to adult peripheral nerves, along the Schwann cell membrane and fibroblasts (Byers et al. 1993; Labarque et al. 2008). Dp71 is expressed in a variety of tissues, predominately the CNS (where it is the most abundant dystrophin gene product), it has multiple isoforms each with specific subcellular localisations (Austin et al. 1995, 2000; Bar et al. 1990; Blake & Kroger 2000; Ceccarini et al. 2002; Chamberlain et al. 1988; Greenberg et al. 1996; Holder et al. 1996; Huard et al. 1992; Ilarraza-Lomeli et al. 2007; Lederfein et al. 1992;Miyatake et al. 1991; Rapaport et al. 1992). Dp71 has been localised to hippocampus (CA1 and dentate gyrus), olfactory bulb as well as perivascular astrocyte feet (Daoud et al. 2009). Figure 2 (modified from Blake et al. 2002) is a schematic diagram of the structure of dystrophin gene products. The basic structure consists of four main domains:

i.   the N terminal which shares similarities to α-actin and has an actin-binding domain (Byers 1989; Fabbrizio et al. 1995; Koenig et al. 1988).

ii.   a central rod domain with 24 spectrin-like triple helical repeats conferring an extended rod shape interrupted by four proline-rich spacer domains thought to act as hinges and conferring flexibility (Arahata et al. 1988; Cross et al. 1990; Koenig & Kunkel 1990, Michalak & Opas et al. 2001; O'Brien & Kunkel 2001; Roberts 2001).

iii. Cysteine-rich domain, separated from the rod domain by a WW domain (a protein-binding module found in several signalling and regulatory molecules). The cysteine-rich domain encompasses the EF1, EF2 and ZZ domains which together are termed the dystroglycan-binding domain. Following the ZZ domain is an α-helical domain important in mediating interactions with syntrophin (Bork & Sudol 1994; Huang et al. 2000; Ishikawa-Sakurai et al. 2004; Jung et al. 1995; Ponting et al. 1996; Rentschler et al. 1999; Suzuki et al. 1994; Winder et al. 1995).

iv.   The C-terminal domain which contains binding sites for some dystrophin-associated glycoproteins, as well as putative sites for endogenous protein kinases to act upon (Lederfein et al. 1993; Michalak & Opas et al. 2001; Milner et al. 1993; Zubrzycka-Gaarn et al. 1988).

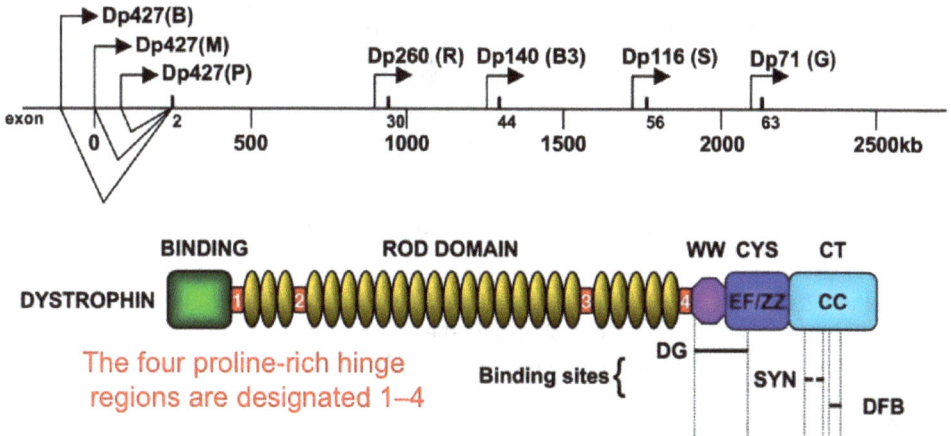

Fig. 2. Schematic showing the organization of the human Duchenne muscular dystrophy (DMD) gene and the dystrophin-related protein family (Modified from Blake et al. 2002).

3. Functional evidence of CNS aberrations in dystrophinopathy

Since the original description of the disease by Duchenne (1868) in which he reported five patients with some degree of cognitive impairment there has been debate as to whether there is a cognitive deficit associated with DMD. A meta-analysis of 32 studies comprising of 1224 patients with DMD with full-scale IQ data available for 1146 DMD patients reported an average IQ of 80.6 (SD 19.3), which was statistically different from the normal population average (Cotton et al. 2001). In this sample 35% of boys had an IQ lower than 70. Of these 79% were characterized as mild, 19% moderate, 1% severe and 0.3% profound (Cotton et al. 2001).

The importance of cognitive impairment in DMD has been demonstrated by a number of reports detailing developmental delay as the first presentation of disease (Essex & Roper 2001;

Kaplan et al. 1986; Mohamed et al. 2000; Smith et al. 1989). Specific subsets in cognitive ability which have been found to be affected in DMD/BMD include: memory/attention/recall (for patterns, numbers and verbal labels, serial position), verbal learning, language/verbal skills/confrontational naming, phonological and graphophonological production, reading, visuospatial organization skills, writing/spelling, comprehension/receptive language, mathematics, locomotor areas, verbal expression/fluency and conceptual ability (Anderson et al. 1988; Billard et al. 1992, 1998; Bresolin et al. 1994; Cotton et al. 1998; D'Angelo & Bresolin 2003; Dorman et al. 1988; Hendriksen & Vles 2006; Hinton et al. 2000, 2001; Karagan et al. 1980; Ogasawara 1989; Palumbo et al. 1996; Savage & Adams 1979; Smith et al. 1989, 1990; Sollee et al. 1985; Whelan 1987). Recent evidence suggests that children with DMD may have a distinct language-based learning deficit, similar to that seen in developmental dysphonetic-dyseidetic dyslexia i.e. problems with phonic analysis and synthesis of words as well as perception of the visual shape of words (Billard et al. 1992, 1998; Cotton et al. 2001). A number of investigators have hypothesized that the cerebellum plays an important role in the manifestation of cognitive deficits in dystrophinopathies (Cyrulnik & Hinton 2008; D'Angelo & Bresolin 2003; Hendriksen & Vles 2006).

Individual studies finding a difference between verbal and performance IQ include Karagan & Zellweger (1976), Karagan & Zellweger (1978), Karagan (1979), Glaub & Mechler (1987), Bresolin et al. (1994), Roccella et al. (2003), and Ogasawara (1989a). In a more recent meta-analysis VIQ and PIQ data was available for >800 children with VIQ = 80.4 +/- 18.8 (SD, n=881) and PIQ 85.4 +/- 16.9 (SD, n=878), both significantly different from the normal population. The discrepancy in VIQ and PIQ was –5.1 +/- 14.4 (SD, n=877). The mean was significantly different from zero but the distribution did not differ significantly from normal and was less than 10, the figure thought to establish clinical significance (Cotton et al. 2001, Wechsler 1997). Although there is a statistical difference between these IQ scores the functional significance is negligible.

Gauld et al. (2005) investigated the influence of IQ on the ability of children with DMD to perform spirometry, as well as assessing the impact of specific interventions for improvement. They found that the mean IQ was 84.7, PIQ 90.6 and VIQ 85.6 in 47 boys tested (mean age 12.6 years). The mean parent reported oppositional behaviour score was 56.3 (range 39 - 87) and mean teacher reported oppositional behaviour score was 56.9 (range 45 - 90) (higher scores on the scale correlate to children more likely to break rules, have problems with authority and who are easily annoyed) (Conners 2000). The oppositional behavioural scores remained stable over a 2.3 year period with a test-retest reliability of r = 0.54 (parent-rated) and r = 0.6 (teacher-rated), P < 0.001 for both (Gauld et al. 2005). They found that the results of spirometry testing were related to the individuals' performance IQ and can be explained by difficulties in understanding or learning to perform the technique required. The use of computer visualised incentives led to an improvement in function of spirometry testing in those shown to have a moderate intellectual or behavioural disturbance (Gauld et al. 2005). Additionally, Uchikawa et al. (2004) found in a group of 7 - 14 year old boys with DMD living in the community, that motor scores were higher in those with good cognitive functioning compared to those with impaired cognitive functioning, even though muscle strength was not significantly different. The authors note that poor cognitive functioning has an adverse effect on activities of daily living in DMD and that this impacts training and performance of these activities. These studies demonstrate the importance of paying attention to the cognitive functioning of individual patients with

DMD, as specific interventions can lead to improved symptom management and quality of life.

The search for a clear genotype-phenotype correlation with the degree of cognitive impairment has been confusing with conflicting reports. A recent study has brought some clarity to this issue. Taylor et al. (2010) have demonstrated that there is a quasi dose-response i.e. the cognitive impairment increases with cumulative loss of dystrophin gene products. A number of studies have suggested a higher incidence of a variety of neuropsychiatric deficits in boys with DMD compared to normal including dysthmic and major depressive disorders, anxiety, attention deficit hyperactivity disorder, obsessive-compulsive disorder and autism spectrum disorder (Fitzpatrick et al. 1986; Hendriksen & Vles 2008; Komoto et al. 1984; Melo et al. 1995; Poysky 2007; Reid & Renwick 2001; Roccella et al. 2003; Sekiguchi 2005; Wu et al. 2005; Young et al. 2008; Zwaigenbaum &Tarnopolsky 2003). As yet Reid & Renwick (2001) have been the only investigators to demonstrate an effect of decreased IQ on mental health in the dystrophinopthies, with no reports to investigate if the converse is true.

3.1 Morphological evidence of a CNS deformity in dystrophinopathy

Morphological studies of the CNS in dystrophinopathy have been inconsistent with some investigators reporting no or minimal changes (Bresolin et al. 1994; Dubowitz and Crome 1969; Rae et al. 1998), cerebral atrophy in later stages of disease (Al-Qudah et al. 1990; Yoshioka et al. 1980), abnormalities in dendritic development and arborisation in visual cortical neurons with extensive Purkinje cell loss (Jagadha & Becker 1988) and pachygyria (Bandoh et al. 1987; Rosman & Kakulas 1966; Wibawa et al. 2000). Some investigators have found a link between morphological abnormalities and impaired cognitive function (Bandoh et al. 1987; Bresolin et al. 1994; Rosman & Kakulas 1966; Septien et al. 1991; Wibawa et al. 2000; Yoshioka et al. 1980), whilst others have not (Al-Qudah et al. 1990).

Sogos et al. (1997) disrupted the expression of dystrophin in human neuronal cultures using *in vitro* techniques. They found a disruption of the morphology of synaptic boutons with alteration of the neuronal cytoskeleton in these cells. This also assessed whether a lack of dystrophin would lead to any perturbations of neuronal NOS (nNOS) using similar techniques (Sogos et al. 2003). They found that nNOS messenger RNA was significantly decreased (~ 35%) in neurones treated with B-dystrophin antisense. These authors postulated that decreased nNOS in neurons deficient for dystrophin may be responsible for alterations in synaptic plasticity (due to known association between nNOS and the NMDA receptor). Alternatively, the involvement of nNOS in CNS development may mean any perturbation could lead to altered neuronal maturation and abnormal synaptogenesis in developing neurons (Sogos et al. 2003).

3.2 Biochemical evidence of a CNS abnormality in dystrophinopathy

The search for the biochemical mechanisms underlying the cognitive deficit associated with lack of dystrophin in humans has been necessarily limited, however, new technologies allowing *in vivo* analysis has enabled some investigations. Not surprisingly oxygen and carbon dioxide levels have been found to be abnormal (especially during sleep), thought to be due to weakened respiratory function secondary to underlying muscle weakness and rib cage deformation (Khan & Heckmatt 1994; Manni et al. 1991; Misuri et al. 2000; Smith et al. 1988). Glucose hypometabolism has been studied by a number of groups as it is a common feature of disorders with associated cognitive deficits, and is generally indicative of lowered synaptic activity (Jueptner & Weiller 1995). Bresolin et al. (1994) found decreased glucose uptake in the cerebellum in DMD boys using PET imaging. Lee et al. (2002) using PET and MRI found four clusters of decreased glucose metabolism in DMD: medial temporal structures and cerebellum bilaterally, the sensorimotor and lateral temporal cortex on the right side (compared to an adult control group). The authors suggest that these findings may reflect local cytoarchitectural changes and abnormalities associated with altered neural development. Tracey et al. (1995), Kato et al. (1997) and Rae et al. (1998) using magnetic resonance spectroscopy and autopsy studies (Kato et al. 1997) focussed on choline-containing compounds which are seen to be elevated in a number of brain disorders and interpreted as symptomatic of increased membrane turnover or decreased membrane stability (Rae et al. 1998). MRI demonstrated significantly increased choline-containing compounds in the cerebellum, but not the cortex of boys < 13 years (Rae et al. 1998). The ratio of choline-containing compounds to N-acetylaspartyl-containing compounds (Cho/NA) was shown to correlate significantly with scores on the Matrix Analogies Test (MAT). The cerebellar and hippocampal focus of the biochemical lesions in DMD are of interest, due to the normally high expression of dystrophin in neurons found in these regions (Bresolin et al. 1994; Lee et al. 2002; Rae et al. 1998). Both Dorman et al. (1988) and Billard et al. (1998) noted that the reading deficits seen in DMD patients are similar to those seen in phonological dyslexia (Castles & Coltheart, 1993). Persons with phonological dyslexia, either developmental (Nicolson et al. 1999; Rae et al. 1998) or acquired (Levisohn et al. 2000), have been shown to have abnormalities in the right cerebellum. Similarly, deficits in verbal working memory, a large component of the DMD cognitive deficit (Hinton et al. 2001) are known to have a cerebellar focus (Desmond et al. 1997).

3.3 Electrophysiological evidence of a CNS abnormality in dystrophinopathy

EEG abnormalities have been reported in DMD although the only large study with appropriate controls (Barwick et al. 1965) found no association between abnormal EEG and dystrophinopathy. To date no studies have examined genotypically confirmed DMD and EEG abnormalities although an increased incidence of epilepsy has been noted in boys with dystrophinopathies compared to the general population (Etemadifar & Molaei 2004; Goodwin et al. 1997). Motor cortex excitability has also been demonstrated to be affected in DMD with reduced excitability thought to be due to aberrant synaptic functioning (Bresolin et al. 1994; Di Lazzaro et al. 1998; Jueptner & Weiller 1995).

4. Evidence from animal models of dystrophinopathy: the *mdx* mouse

The *mdx* mouse (*m*uscular *d*ystrophy *X*-linked) is the most widely studied animal model of dystrophinopathy (Collins & Morgan 2003; Durbeej & Campbell 2002; Partridge 1991). Although its discovery predated the genotyping of this disorder it has since been proven to be an appropriate model with identification of a premature stop codon terminating translation of murine dystrophin resulting in an absence of all full-length dystrophin-gene products (Bulfield et al. 1984; Chamberlain et al. 1987; Hoffman et al. 1987; Sicinski et al. 1989). This mouse model has aided in investigations of the function of dystrophin, particularly in the CNS as invasive functional investigations can be carried out on these animals. The majority of current knowledge of the role of dystrophin in the CNS comes from this animal model.

4.1 Cognitive functioning

Impairments in passive avoidance learning, long-term recognition memory and procedural learning have all been shown to be adversely affected in *mdx* mice compared to controls. Task acquisition, procedural memory spatial discrimination tasks, novelty-seeking behaviour and exploration in an elevated plus maze have all been shown to be unaffected in the *mdx* mouse (Mehler et al. 1992; Muntoni et al. 1991; Perronnet & Vaillend 2010; Sesay et al. 1996; Vaillend et al. 1995, 1998, 1999, 2004). Most recently Sekiguchi et al. (2009) have demonstrated an enhanced defensive freezing response to a brief restraint as well as enhanced unconditioned and conditioned defensive responses to electrical footshock in *mdx* mice compared to wildtype. This abnormal behaviour was ameliorated with intracerebroventricular administration of antisense morpholino oligonucleotide (which induces skipping of the premature stop codon located at exon 23 in the *mdx* mouse and produces a truncated dystrophin with a 71 amino acid deletion in the mid-rod domain) (Alter et al. 2006; Sekiguchi et al. 2009).

4.2 Morphology

No gross abnormalities in brain or spinal cord in the *mdx* mouse have been found (Bulfield et al. 1984; Dunn & Zaim-Wadghiri 1999; Torres & Duchen 1987; Yoshihara et al. 2003). This was most recently confirmed using MRI by Miranda et al. (2009) who found no major alteration of brain anatomy in *mdx* mice, reporting no significant changes in the cortex, hippocampus or cerebellum (normally dystrophin-positive). At the cellular/axonal level dystrophin has been found to localise to the cell membrane, predominately the soma and postsynaptic densities particularly in hippocampus, neocortex, cerebellum and amygdale (Anderson et al. 2002; Lidov 1996; Perronnet & Vaillend 2010). Anatomical alterations have been found in the *mdx* mouse in various brain regions including decreased cell number, altered cell packing density and changes in cell morphology (Carretta et al. 2001; Sbriccoli et al. 1995). It should be noted that these changes were not demonstrated when investigated in the hippocampus. CA1 pyramidal cell packing density, mean nuclear area and circularity has been found to be unaltered in *mdx* mice (Miranda et al. 2009). PSD length of axospinous perforated excitatory synapses has been found to be larger in *mdx* proximal radiatum of the hippocampus (Miranda et al. 2009). These authors note that perforated synapses are the hallmarks of activity dependent synaptic plasticity (Miranda et al. 2009). A more recent report by this group has demonstrated that the presynaptic ultrastructure of excitatory hippocampal synapses is altered in both *mdx* and Dp71-null mice (Miranda et al. 2011). Again examining the proximal radiatum glutaminergic synapses (normally dystrophin-positive) they report an increased number of docked vesicles, with the number and size of vesicles similar in *mdx* mice compared to controls. They also found a decrease in the number of vesicles in the 'reserve pool' i.e. > 300nm away from the synapse) in *mdx* mice compared to controls. In the Dp71-null mice they found that the number and spatial distribution of vesicles was no different from control (Miranda et al. 2011). In contrast to Dp427-null (*mdx*) mice the number of vesicles in the active zone was decreased and the number of vesicles in the reserve pool was increased compared to controls, whilst the number of docked vesicles remained the same. Alterations in parvalbumin-positive and calbindin-positive interneurons (both calcium binding proteins) have been demonstrated to be significantly increased in particular brain regions of *mdx* compared to wildtype (Carretta et al. 2003, 2004). At the receptor level the glucose transporters GLUT1 and GLUT4, $\alpha 1$ and $\alpha 2$ GABA$_A$ receptor subunit and nicotinic ACh receptor gene expression is decreased in specific brain regions of *mdx* mouse (Wallis et al. 2004). Of particular interest is the strong association of dystrophin with the GABA$_A$ receptor. Knuesel et al. (1999) found co-localization of the GABA$_A$ channel with dystrophin in the mouse cerebellum and hippocampus. In these areas of the *mdx* mouse there was a marked reduction of GABA$_A$ clusters. This decrease in clustering was particularly striking around the soma of cerebellar Purkinje cells. In both the cerebellum and hippocampus the number (but not size) of GABA$_A$ clusters was reduced by ~ 50%. Brunig et al. (2002) found that the DGC and GABA$_A$-gephyrin complexes undergo different clustering mechanisms and that the DGC is unchanged by the absence of gephyrin/GABA$_A$. They suggested that selective signalling from presynaptic GABAergic terminals contributes to DGC clustering (Brunig et al. 2002). The authors postulated that the DGC may stabilise GABA$_A$ clusters, in a developmentally regulated manner. They also suggested functions for the DGC at the synapse: i) by stabilizing the postsynaptic apparatus, the DGC may "freeze" GABAergic synapses in order to maintain a certain status of the network once learning processes have been primarily completed or ii) DGC may provide a scaffold enabling changes in clusters of GABA$_A$ receptor without incurring the loss of the postsynaptic apparatus, as may be required in circuits with a high degree of synaptic plasticity.

Grady et al. (2006) generated α-dystrobrevin, β-dystrobrevin (both members of the DGC) and double mutant α – and β-dystrobrevin knockout mice. They examined the localisation of α and β-dystrobrevin, finding both proteins in the hippocampus and cerebral cortex. They found that all larger β-dystrobrevin-positive puncta on the dendrites (but not somata) of PC were colocalised with gephyrin staining (gephyrin is associated with inhibitory synapses in the CNS). When staining for the GABA$_A$ $\alpha 1$ subunit in β-dystrobrevin knockout mice, they found a decrease in the number of GABA$_A$ $\alpha 1$-positive clusters of 33% and reduction in size by approx 50% in cerebellar PC. This finding is comparable with Knuesel et al. (1999) (no such association in the cerebellum of α-dystrobrevin knockout mice was found). They further demonstrated that, in *mdx* mice, a loss of dystrophin led to a loss of dystrobrevin at these sites and in dystrobrevin knockout mice, a loss of dystrobrevin led to a loss of dystrophin at these sites. This interrelationship between dystrobrevin and dystrophin was not demonstrated in the hippocampus. Another member of the DGC – dystroglycan has also been demonstrated to be clustered at GABAergic synapses. Dystroglycan deficient mice have GABAergic clusters lacking dystrophin, however dystrophin-deficient mice (i.e. *mdx*) as well as gephyrin-deficient mice do not lose colocalisation of dystroglycan and GABAergic synapses (Brunig et al. 2002; Levi et al. 2002; Waite et al. 2009). As will be described below Kueh et al. (2011) demonstrated that there is a reduction in the number of functional receptors localised at the GABAergic synapses in the cerebellar PCs of *mdx* mice and an increase in extrasynaptic GABA$_A$ receptors. Vaillend et al. (2010) have demonstrated a re-expression of a truncated dystrophin in the hippocampus after intra-hippocampal injection of adenovirus-associated vector expressing antisense sequences linked to a modified U7 small nuclear RNA that re-directed the splicing of dystrophin pre-mRNA allowing omission of exon 23 of the dystrophin gene in the *mdx* mouse. This allows restoration of the reading frame and a functional dystrophin protein to be expressed. The levels of expression of the truncated dystrophin reached 15-25% of wildtype. They further investigated whether this 'rescue' of dystrophin expression had an impact on GABA$_A$ receptor clustering. They found that the number of clusters and the area of the α2 subunit of the GABA$_A$ receptor was significantly larger in the treated *mdx* mice compared to untreated *mdx* mice, and was actually no longer significantly different from wildtype (Vaillend et al. 2010) suggesting complete recovery of GABA$_A$ receptor clustering after partial dystrophin-rescue. They conclude that although dystrophin is not involved in synpatogenesis it may be important in maintenance and stabilisation of postsynaptic GABA$_A$ receptors. They note that dystrophin is co-localised with α2-containing GABA$_A$ receptors at a relatively low rate and postulate that the remaining dystrophin may be involved in trafficking/targeting processes, expressed in empty synapses transiently devoid of GABA$_A$ receptors (Vaillend et al. 2010).

The overall protein expression levels of GABA$_A$ receptors containing α1 subunits in a whole membrane preparation of murine cerebellum was investigated by our group and found to be no different from littermate controls (Kueh et al. 2008). This finding supports the theory that it is the organisation of the GABA$_A$ receptor (i.e. altered clustering) rather than the expression (i.e. quantity) that is adversely affected by a lack of dystrophin.

4.3 Biochemistry

A number of reports have examined metabolites in *mdx* CNS. Griffin et al. (2001) identified discernable changes in metabolic pathways: glycolysis, β-oxidation, the TCA cycle, phosphocreatine/ATP cycle and lipid metabolism were all altered in *mdx* cerebral cortex and cerebellum. Young *mdx* mice have been found to have normal levels of N-acetylaspartate and total creatinine content, increased whole-brain levels of choline-containing compounds (glycero- and phosphocholine) and *myo*-inositol, and a decrease in the ATP synthase γ subunit in cerebellum and hippocampi (Tracey et al. 1996; Wallis et al. 2004). In older *mdx* mice a decrease in the total creatinine content, increase in inorganic phosphate to phosphocreatine ratio, increased intracellular brain pH, decreased expression of mitochondrial creatine kinase in *mdx* hippocampi, and increased choline containing compounds in cerebellum and hippocampus of *mdx* brain, but not the cortex, have all been reported (Rae et al. 2002; Tracey et al. 1996; Wallis et al. 2004). Together these results indicate that there are significant differences in *mdx* mice CNS metabolism possibly indicating increased membrane turnover or decreased membrane stability. Furthermore, there is a clear exacerbation of these biochemical abnormalities with age, although there is yet no clear explanation of how a lack of dystrophin leads to these changes and why some of these perturbations are increased and others decreased with age.

Other reports have looked at glucose utilisation in CNS of *mdx* mice. Rae et al. (2002) found significantly decreased free glucose in *mdx*, significantly increased fractional enrichment and increased flux of ^{13}C into metabolites such as glutamate and GABA. These authors noted that this may indicate a faster metabolic rate in dystrophin-deficient brain due to abnormal functioning of GABA$_A$ receptors and, therefore, decreased inhibition (as, in general, excitatory stimulation leads to increased glucose metabolism and inhibitory activation leads to decreased glucose metabolism) (Ito et al. 1994; Rae et al. 2000, 2002). In old *mdx* mice there was abnormal metabolism of [1-^{13}C] glucose (Rae et al. 2002). In a follow-on study this group found no significant difference in glucose metabolism in the young *mdx* mice compared to controls, suggesting that changes in glucose metabolism seen in the old *mdx* mice are due to other factors (i.e. not changes in expression of glucose transporters) (Wallis et al. 2004).

AQP4 and osmotic/cellular volume alterations in *mdx* mice has been reported. Increased extracellular and decreased intracellular volume in *mdx* brain as well as altered osmoregulation was reported by Tracey et al. (1996a) and Griffin et al. (2001). Frigeri et al. (2001) found that although AQP4 mRNA staining pattern was unaltered, the level of this protein was decreased in *mdx* CNS. This decrease grew with age (70% decrease at 12 months). Dp71 has been found to be the major dystrophin gene product responsible for anchoring AQP4 and the DGC at the glial endfeet (Amiry-Moghaddam et al. 2004; Neely et al. 2001; Nicchia et al. 2008; Yokota et al. 2000). Nicchia et al. (2004) reported the unpublished observation of Frigeri et al. (2001) that *mdx* mice also demonstrate a resistance to brain oedema. They postulated that the absence and/or mislocalisation of AQP4 at the perivascular endfeet is protective in induced brain oedema. Nico et al. (2003) found a profoundly altered blood-brain-barrier (BBB). Although initial reports suggested no alteration in response to osmotic stress (hypo-osmotic shock) in *mdx* CNS (Rae et al. 2002). Vajda et al. (2002, 2004) found, in osmotic stress experiments, that the *mdx-βgeo* mice had a delayed decompensation and increased survival time (66.5 min compared to 56 min) indicating that Dp71 is necessary for the polarized distribution of AQP4 in brain.

Interestingly, many of these reports propose a link between the biochemical abnormalities and underlying channel dysfunction secondary to a lack of dystrophin. Rae et al.'s (2002) report suggests that the increased glucose use demonstrated in *mdx* brain may be due to decreased inhibitory input from the subset of abnormally clustered GABA$_A$-receptors. Further Griffin et al. (1999) have proposed this elevation is associated with cellular membranes implying a progressive, degenerative or compensatory process (Rae et al. 2002).

Decreased bioenergetic buffering capacity would be expected to influence susceptibility to hypoxia. Mehler and coworkers (Mehler et al. 1992) reported an increase in sensitivity of hippocampal slices from *mdx* mice to loss of synaptic transmission of CA1 hippocampal pyramidal cells during hypoxia. This was partially ameliorated by blocking both sodium-dependent action potentials as well as low-threshold calcium conductances. Yoshihara et al. (2003) suggested that the increased sensitivity to hypoxia found by Mehler et al. (1992) may be due to impaired function of inhibitory synapses at this site. Another group (Godfraind et al. 1998, 2000) has shown increased susceptibility of *mdx* hippocampal tissue slices to irreversible hypoxic failure when kept in 10 mM glucose, but less susceptibility of *mdx* slices when kept in 4 mM glucose, in agreement with Wallis et al. (2004). The latter group suggest that the decrease in GLUT1 and GLUT3 expression they found is most likely related to decreased synaptic integrity, resulting in decreased activity and decreased glucose utilization. These authors noted that dystrophin may be required to maintain synaptic integrity (Knuesel et al. 2001) rather than being directly involved in anchoring/clustering of the GABA$_A$ receptor itself. Additionally, it is known that the expression of components of the GABA$_A$ receptor relate to synaptic activity (Ives et al. 2002). Thus, Wallis et al. (2004) proposed that the lack of dystrophin in the PSD may impede synaptic activity leading to decreased GABA$_A$ receptor components due to decreased GABAergic demand. Wallis et al. (2004) suggested that dystrophin may be involved in the clustering of this complex of proteins (mitochondrial creatine kinase, adenine nucleotide translocase and the gamma subunit of ATP synthase). Furthermore, Rae et al. (2002) suggested that the regulation of oxidative metabolism during hypoxia was impaired, and that this may be another manifestation of calcium overload in the neuronal mitochondria of *mdx* CNS.

4.4 Electrophysiology

The highest levels of dystrophin gene products are in areas in which neurons maintain a high degree of synaptic plasticity: olfactory bulb, hippocampus, neocortex and cerebellum (Gorecki et al. 1997, 1998; Lidov et al. 1990). Synaptic plasticity has been examined in both the hippocampus and cerebellum and found to be altered in the *mdx* mouse in both of these brain regions (Anderson et al. 2004, 2010; Vaillend et al. 1998, 1999, 2004). Vaillend's group examined the CA1 dendritic layer of the hippocampus and found that NMDA-receptor dependent short-term and long-term potentiation, and long-term depression were abnormally enhanced in *mdx* mice (Perronnet & Vaillend 2010; Vaillend et al. 1998, 1999, 2004). Both our and Vaillend's group have investigated the function of the GABA receptor in the *mdx* cerebellum and hippocampus respectively as it is known to colocalise with dystrophin (Knuesel et al. 1999). In *mdx* mice hippocampus and cerebellum there is a marked reduction of GABA$_A$ clusters, with the number (but not size) of GABA$_A$ clusters being reduced by ~ 50% (Knuesel et al. 1999). In both the cerebellum and hippocampus the GABA$_A$ antagonist had a decreased effect (Anderson et al. 2003; Vaillend et al. 2002). When miniature inhibitory postsynaptic potentials were examined in the cerebellum a decrease in frequency and amplitude was found in contrast to the hippocampus where an increase in frequency was demonstrated (Anderson et al. 2003; Kueh et al. 2008; Graciotti et al. 2008). We have noted however that the reduction in amplitude may lead to a falsely lowered frequency due to lowered amplitude IPSCs being below counting threshold. These results have led to the 'dysfunctional inhibition' hypothesis being postulated as the cause of the cognitive impairment seen in DMD (Perronnet & Vaillend 2010). Dallerac et al. (2011) demonstrated that *mdx* mice treated with U7 small nuclear RNAs modified to encode antisense sequences and expressed from recombinant adeno-associated viral vectors to induce skipping of the premature stop codon at exon 23 of the dystrophin gene normalises hippocampal synaptic plasticity. The vector was injected into the hippocampus and months after two months CA1 hippocampal LTP, which is normally enhanced compared to wildtype, was no longer different from wildtype. In studies of seizure induction in mice, dystrophin deficiency has been found to alter the neuronal excitability of AMPA/kainic-type glutamate receptors suggesting a dysfunctional excitatory-inhibitory balance (De Sarro et al. 2004; Perronnet & Vaillend 2010; Yoshihara et al. 2003). Basolateral nucleus of the amygdale pyramidal neurons have also been studied in the *mdx* mouse and have been demonstrated to have decreased inductions of GABA-ergic IPSCs by noradrenalin. These authors note that in the *mdx* there were cells sensitive to noradrenalin (~40%) and a larger subset of cells insensitive to noradrenalin (~60%). Whilst the regular-spiking non-pyramidal basolateral nucleus of the amygdale neurons had similar proportions of noradrenalin-induced depolarisation and AP firing (~50%) in wildtype and *mdx* demonstrating that the mechanism by which noradrenalin depolarises interneurons beyond AP threshold is not impaired in *mdx* mice. Rather it is more likely that a decrease in the number of normal functioning GABAergic synapses between the noradrenalin-responsive interneurons and pyramidal neurons underlies their findings (Sekiguchi et al. 2009).

Work from our laboratory has similarly demonstrated altered GABA-ergic function in the cerebellum of *mdx* mice. We found that evoked excitatory post-synaptic potentials in cerebellar Purkinje cells show a decreased response (approx 50%) to bicuculline (a GABA antagonist) compared to wildtype (Anderson et al. 2003). We also demonstrated that miniature inhibitory postsynaptic currents had a significantly decreased amplitude in *mdx* cerebellar Purkinje cells compared to wildtype. This difference in amplitude was principally due to the absence of large amplitude miniature inhibitory postsynaptic currents in *mdx* mice. We postulate that this decrease is the result of a decrease in the number of postsynaptic GABA-ergic receptors (Nusser et al. 1997). This finding was reproduced in later studies (Fig. 3; Kueh et al. 2008, 2011). We further went on to investigate the number of $GABA_A$ channels located at the GABAergic synapse of cerebellar Purkinje cells. We found a significant reduction in the number of receptors at the PSD in *mdx* compared with littermate controls determined by non-stationary noise analysis of spontaneous miniature inhibitory postsynaptic currents. Single unitary conductance, rise and decay times of the currents were no different from littermate controls demonstrating that although there is a reduction in the number of channels at the postsynaptic membrane in *mdx* cerebellar Purkinje cells, the $GABA_A$ channels that are present are functioning normally. Further, Gaboxadol, an extrasynaptic GABA agonist, was applied inducing an increase in the holding current of the Purkinje cell. In *mdx* mice this increase was significantly greater (~200%) compared to littermate controls (Kueh et al. 2011), indicating that in *mdx* mice the number of extrasynpatic $GABA_A$ receptors is increased.

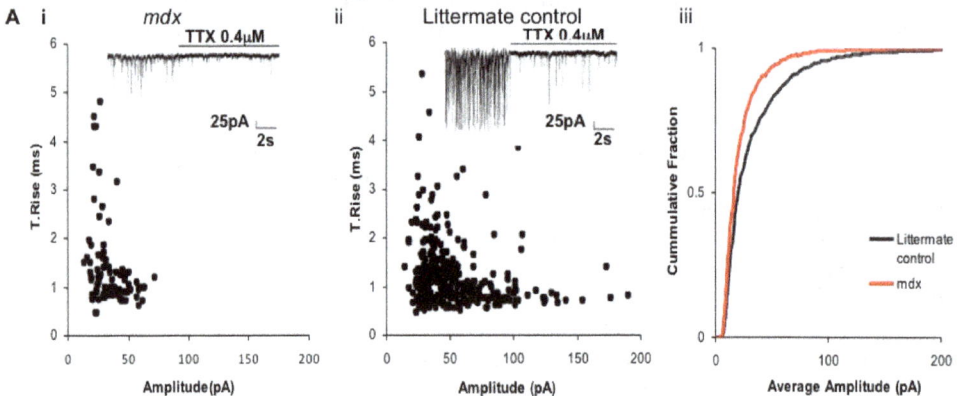

Fig. 3. A scatter plot of rise time versus peak amplitude, showing the distribution of mIPSCs in a (i) *mdx* and a (ii) littermate control mouse. The inserts show a section of the recording in aCSF and when TTX was added to the bath. iii) Cumulative probability of mIPSC amplitudes (average) in *mdx* and littermate control cells. There was a significant difference between mIPSC amplitudes between *mdx* and litermate control cells (Mann Whitney test, p=0.0001) (Modified from Kueh et al. 2011).

Our group has also investigated synaptic plasticity in the *mdx* cerebellum which is uniquely suited to these investigations as the Purkinje cell – the major output neuron of the cerebellum normally expresses a specific full-length dystrophin – P-dystrophin, which is absent in *mdx* mice. The major inputs to the Purkinje cells – parallel fibres and inhibitory interneurons are normally dystrophin negative. Firstly we examined a presynaptic form of synaptic plasticity in the cerebellum – short-term synaptic plasticity mediated at the parallel-fibre to Purkinje cell synapse. We found no difference between wildtype and *mdx* mice in this form of plasticity as expected due to the post-synaptic localisation of

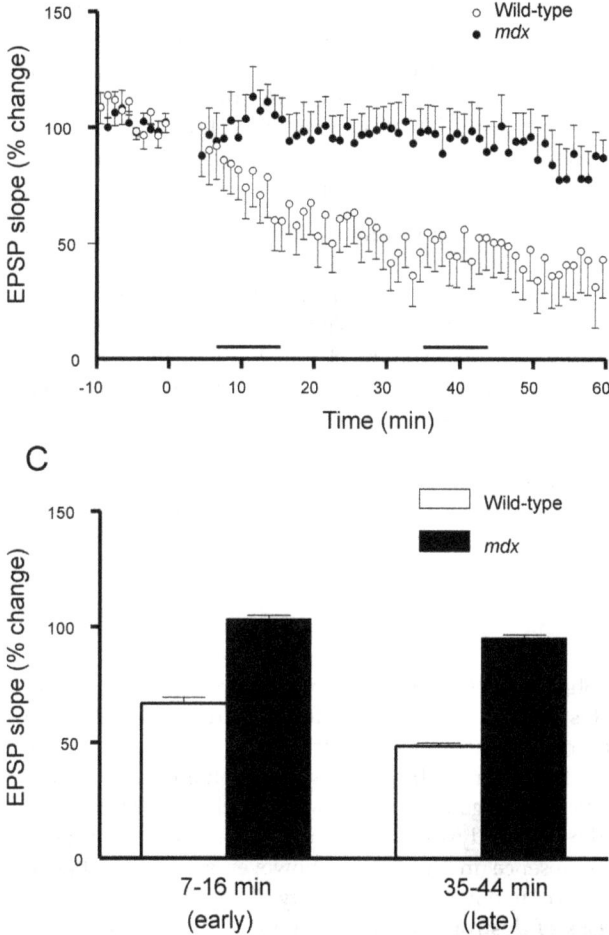

Fig. 4. Long-term depression (LTD) in cerebellar Purkinje cells of wild-type and *mdx* mice. Upper graph shows the average slope of evoked EPSPs in wild-type and *mdx* Purkinje cells before and after LTD induction. Open circles are wildtype Purkinje cells (n=11) and closed circles are *mdx* Purkinje cells (n=12). Slopes are normalised to the average slope for wild-type and *mdx* cells respectively recorded in the 10 minutes preceding LTD induction. Thin horizontal bars above the abscissa represent the two 10 minute time periods during which the EPSP slopes were averaged and represent the magnitude of early and late phases of LTD. Vertical bars are SEM and for clarity are shown on one side of the data points only. Lower bar graph displays the average slope for all wild-type and all *mdx* cells in the early and late phases following LTD induction (Modified from Anderson et al. 2004)

dystrophin. We then went on to examine a post-synaptic mediated form of synaptic plasticity – long-term depression. As postulated the extent of depression was decreased in *mdx* cerebellar Purkinje cells compared to wildtype (Fig, 4; Anderson et al. 2004). We next examined homosynaptic longterm depression at this synapse and found that there was no difference between wildtype and *mdx* cerebellar Purkinje cells in the initial observation period, however the depression was significantly greater in the latter part of the observation period in *mdx* compared to wildtype (Anderson et al. 2010). The three most compelling explanations for the differences demonstrated above are i) an alteration in calcium homeostasis, ii) an indirect effect of altered GABA$_A$ receptor localisation and/or trafficking and iii) an alteration in putative AMPA-receptor localisation/trafficking. The most recent investigations of the multiplicity of effects of the known GABA$_A$ receptor dysfunction on the neurophysiology of the *mdx* mouse is compelling.

Further unpublished data from our laboratory has demonstrated that that short term synaptic plasticity (inhibitory interneuron to Purkinje cell synapse) is no different between *mdx* and wildtype. However rebound potentiation – a form of longterm synaptic plasticity expressed at this synapse is significantly different. Wildtype cerebellar Purkinje cells demonstrated potentiation of the inhibitory postsynaptic potential as previously reported, however the *mdx* cerebellar Purkinje cells depressed. In a pilot study 5/12 wildtype cerebellar Purkinje cells demonstrated rebound potentiation (0 depressed) compared to 0/5 *mdx* cells demonstrating potentiation and 4/5 cells demonstrating depression. Although preliminary, these findings are the first to demonstrate a deficit in GABA-mediated synaptic plasticity. These findings also locate the problem at the post-synaptic (dystrophin-deficient Purkinje cell) locus as the presynaptically-mediated short-term synaptic plasticity of this synapse is preserved. (Anderson 2009).

5. Conclusion

The role of dystrophin in the CNS is complex and incompletely understood. It is clear that the absence of this protein leads to profound functional deficits at the macro-level (behavioural alterations and cognitive impairment) as well as the micro-level (alterations in synaptic plasticity, GABA-ergic functioning). Morphologically there are alterations in cellular architecture and organisation as well as channel localisation. The increase in investigations of the role of dystrophin in the CNS has led to a rapid appreciation of the consequence of its absence in this tissue, however a clear mechanism by which these alterations occur has yet to emerge. The majority of current evidence points convincingly to a link between a lack of dystrophin and alterations in the localisation of GABA$_A$ receptors. Furthermore there is evidence that a lack of dystrophin is associated with abnormal functioning of GABA$_A$ receptor-mediated cellular activity as measured by changes in amplitude of IPSCs. The well-established cognitive-impairment seen in the boys with dystrophinopathies may be due to an underlying abnormality in synaptic plasticity as demonstrated in the *mdx* animal models. However evidence linking the alteration in GABA-ergic localisation and function with alterations in synaptic plasticity is speculative. The postulated dysfunctional excitatory-inhibitory balance – perhaps mediated by chronic alteration of calcium-handling by these neurons, is the most compelling hypothesis to date linking these two major findings (alterations in GABA clustering and function with alterations in synaptic plasticity). Further how a lack of dystrophin leads to the structural alterations seen in found in *mdx* CNS, as well as the plethora of biochemical alterations in seen in both humans and animal models of DMD has yet to emerge. The role of the smaller dystrophin gene products in the brain are now beginning to be appreciated with a recent report demonstrating that a loss of the smallest of these – Dp71, can lead to changes at the behavioural, cell membrane and synaptic levels (Daoud et al. 2009). The role of dystrophin and the dystrophin-glycoprotein complex in the CNS is slowly being elucidated. With a greater understanding of the function of this protein useful therapies may be able to ameliorate the CNS manifestations of Duchenne muscular dystrophy as well as aid in the effort to arrest the devastating muscular degeneration.

6. References

ABDULRAZZAK, H., NORO, N., SIMONS, J. P., GOLDSPINK, G., BARNARD, E. A. & GORECKI, D. C. (2001). Structural diversity despite strong evolutionary conservation in the 5'-untranslated region of the P-type dystrophin transcript. *Molecular & Cellular Neursciences,* 17, 500-13.

ALBRECHT, D. E. & FROEHNER, S. C. (2002). Syntrophins and dystrobrevins: defining the dystrophin scaffold at synapses. *Neurosignals,* 11, 123-9.

AL-QUDAH, A. A., KOBAYASHI, J., CHUANG, S., DENNIS, M. & RAY, P. (1990). Etiology of intellectual impairment in Duchenne muscular dystrophy. *Pediatr Neurol,* 6, 57-9.

ALTER, J., LOU, F., RABINOWITZ, A., YIN, H., ROSENFELD, J., WILTON, S.D., PARTRIDGE, T.A. & LU Q.L. (2006). Systemic delivery of morpholino oligonucleotide restores dystrophin expression bodywide and improves dystrophic pathology. *Nature Medicine* 12, 175-77.

AMIRY-MOGHADDAM, M., XUE, R., FINN-MOGENS, H., NEELY, J.D., BHARDWAJ, A., AGRE, P., ADAMS, M.E., FROEHNER, S.C., MORI, S. & OTTERSEN, O.P. (2004). Alpha-syntrophin deletion removes the perivascular but not the endothelial pool of aquaporin-4 at the blood-brain barrier and delays the development of brain edema in an experimental model of acute hyponatraemia. *The FASEB Journal* 18 542-44.

ANDERSON, J.L. (2009) Cerebellar synaptic plasticity in two animal models of muscular dystrophy. PhD dissertation. University of New South Wales, Sydney Australia.

ANDERSON, J.L., HEAD, S.I., RAE, C. & MORLEY, J.W. (2002). Brain function in Duchenne muscular dystrophy. *Brain* 125: 4-13.

ANDERSON, J.L., HEAD, S.I. & MORLEY, J.W. (2003). Altered inhibitory input to Purkinje cells of dystrophin-deficient mice. *Brain Res* 982: 280-283.

ANDERSON, J.L., HEAD, S.I. & MORLEY, J.W. (2004). Long-term depression is reduced in cerebellar Purkinje cells of dystrophin-deficient mdx mice. *Brain Res* 1019: 289-92.

ANDERSON, J.L., MORLEY, J.W. & HEAD, S.I. (2010). Enhanced homosynaptic LTD in cerebellar Purkinje cells of the dystrophic mdx mouse. *Muscle & Nerve* 41 (3) 329-34.

ANDERSON, S. W., ROUTH, D. K. & IONASESCU, V. V. (1988). Serial position memory of boys with Duchenne muscular dystrophy. *Dev Med Child Neurol,* 30, 328-33.

ARAHATA, K., ISHIURA, S., ISHIGURO, T., TSUKAHARA, T., SUHARA, Y., EGUCHI, C., ISHIHARA, T., NONAKA, I., OZAWA, E. & SUGITA, H. (1988). Immunostaining of skeletal and cardiac muscle surface membrane with antibody against Duchenne muscular dystrophy peptide. *Nature,* 333, 861-3.

AUSTIN, R. C., HOWARD, P. L., D'SOUZA, V. N., KLAMUT, H. J. & RAY, P. N. (1995). Cloning and characterization of alternatively spliced isoforms of Dp71. *Hum Mol Genet*, 4, 1475-83.

AUSTIN, R. C., MORRIS, G. E., HOWARD, P. L., KLAMUT, H. J. & RAY, P. N. (2000). Expression and synthesis of alternatively spliced variants of Dp71 in adult human brain. *Neuromuscul Disord*, 10, 187-93.

BANDOH, T., KAWAI, H., ADACHI, K. & II, K. (1987). [Clinical and pathological studies on intellectual impairment in Duchenne muscular dystrophy, with special reference to patients with severe intellectual impairment]. *Rinsho Shinkeigaku*, 27, 692-701.

BAR, S., BARNEA, E., LEVY, Z., NEUMAN, S., YAFFE, D. & NUDEL, U. (1990). A novel product of the Duchenne muscular dystrophy gene which greatly differs from the known isoforms in its structure and tissue distribution. *Biochem J*, 272, 557-60.

BARDONI, A., FELISARI, G., SIRONI, M., COMI, G., LAI, M., ROBOTTI, M. & BRESOLIN, N. (2000). Loss of Dp140 regulatory sequences is associated with cognitive impairment in the dystrophinopathies. *Neuromuscul Disord* 10(3) 194-199.

BARWICK, D. D., OSSELTON, J. W. & WALTON, J. N. (1965). Electroencephalographic Studies in Hereditary Myopathy. *J Neurol Neurosurg Psychiatry*, 28, 109-14.

BEGGS, A. H. (1997). Dystrophinopathy, the expanding phenotype. Dystrophin abnormalities in X-linked dilated cardiomyopathy. *Circulation*, 95, 2344-7.

BILLARD, C., GILLET, P., SIGNORET, J. L., UICAUT, E., BERTRAND, P., FARDEAU, M., BARTHEZ-CARPENTIER, M. A. & SANTINI, J. J. (1992). Cognitive functions in Duchenne muscular dystrophy: a reappraisal and comparison with spinal muscular atrophy. *Neuromuscul Disord*, 2, 371-8.

BILLARD, C., GILLET, P., BARTHEZ, M., HOMMET, C. & BERTRAND, P. (1998). Reading ability and processing in Duchenne muscular dystrophy and spinal muscular atrophy. *Dev Med Child Neurol*, 40, 12-20.

BLAKE, D. J., LOVE, D. R., TINSLEY, J., MORRIS, G. E., TURLEY, H., GATTER, K., DICKSON, G., EDWARDS, Y. H. & DAVIES, K. E. (1992). Characterization of a 4.8kb transcript from the Duchenne muscular dystrophy locus expressed in Schwannoma cells. *Hum Mol Genet*, 1, 103-9

BLAKE, D. J., HAWKES, R., BENSON, M. A. & BEESLEY, P. W. (1999). Different dystrophin-like complexes are expressed in neurons and glia. *J Cell Biol*, 147, 645-58.

BLAKE, D. J. & KROGER, S. (2000). The neurobiology of duchenne muscular dystrophy: learning lessons from muscle? *Trends Neurosci*, 23, 92-9.

BLAKE, D.J., WEIR, A., NEWEY, S.E. & DAVIES, K.E. (2002). Function and genetics of dystrophin and dystrophin-related proteins in muscle. *Physiol Rev* 82 (2) 291-329.

BORK, P. & SUDOL, M. (1994). The WW domain: a signalling site in dystrophin? *Trends Biochem Sci*, 19, 531-3.

BRESOLIN, N., CASTELLI, E., COMI, G. P., FELISARI, G., BARDONI, A., PERANI, D., GRASSI, F., TURCONI, A., MAZZUCCHELLI, F., GALLOTTI, D. & ET AL. (1994). Cognitive impairment in Duchenne muscular dystrophy. *Neuromuscul Disord*, 4, 359-69.

BRUNIG, I., SUTER, A., KNUESEL, I., LUSCHER, B. & FRITSCHY, J. M. (2002). GABAergic terminals are required for postsynaptic clustering of dystrophin but not of GABA(A) receptors and gephyrin. *J Neurosci*, 22, 4805-13.

BULFIELD, G., SILLER, W. G., WIGHT, P. A. & MOORE, K. J. (1984). X chromosome-linked muscular dystrophy (mdx) in the mouse. *Proc Natl Acad Sci U S A*, 81, 1189-92.

BURMEISTER, M., MONACO, A. P., GILLARD, E. F., VAN OMMEN, G. J., AFFARA, N. A., FERGUSON-SMITH, M. A., KUNKEL, L. M. & LEHRACH, H. (1988). A 10-megabase physical map of human Xp21, including the Duchenne muscular dystrophy gene. *Genomics,* 2, 189-202.

BYERS, T. J., HUSAIN-CHISHTI, A., DUBREUIL, R. R., BRANTON, D. & GOLDSTEIN, L. S. (1989). Sequence similarity of the amino-terminal domain of Drosophila beta spectrin to alpha actinin and dystrophin. *J Cell Biol,* 109, 1633-41.

BYERS, T.J., LIDOV, H.G. & KUNKEL, L.M. (1993). An alternative dystrophin transcript specific to peripheral nerve. *Nat Genet* 4 (1) 77-81.

CARRETTA, D., SANTARELLI, M., VANNI, D., CARRAI, R., SBRICCOLI, A., PINTO, F. & MINCIACCHI, D. (2001). The organisation of spinal projecting brainstem neurons in an animal model of muscular dystrophy. A retrograde tracing study on mdx mutant mice. *Brain Res,* 895, 213-22.

CARRETTA, D., SANTARELLI, M., VANNI, D., CIABATTI, S., SBRICCOLI, A., PINTO, F. & MINCIACCHI, D. (2003). Cortical and brainstem neurons containing calcium-binding proteins in a murine model of Duchenne's muscular dystrophy: selective changes in the sensorimotor cortex. *J Comp Neurol,* 456, 48-59.

CARRETTA, D., SANTARELLI, M., SBRICCOLI, A., PINTO, F., CATINI, C. & MINCIACCHI, D. (2004). Spatial analysis reveals alterations of parvalbumin- and calbindin-positive local circuit neurons in the cerebral cortex of mutant mdx mice. *Brain Res,* 1016, 1-11.

CASTLES, A. & COLTHEART, M. (1993). Varieties of developmental dyslexia. *Cognition,* 47, 149-80.

CAVALDESI, M., MACCHIA, G., BARCA, S., DEFILIPPI, P., TARONE, G. & PETRUCCI, T. C. (1999). Association of the dystroglycan complex isolated from bovine brain synaptosomes with proteins involved in signal transduction. *J Neurochem,* 72, 1648-55.

CECCARINI, M., MACIOCE, P., PANETTA, B. & PETRUCCI, T. C. (2002). Expression of dystrophin-associated proteins during neuronal differentiation of P19 embryonal carcinoma cells. *Neuromuscul Disord,* 12, 36-48.

CHAMBERLAIN, J. S., GRANT, S. G., REEVES, A. A., MULLINS, L. J., STEPHENSON, D. A., HOFFMAN, E. P., MONACO, A. P., KUNKEL, L. M., CASKEY, C. T. & CHAPMAN, V. M. (1987). Regional localization of the murine Duchenne muscular dystrophy gene on the mouse X chromosome. *Somat Cell Mol Genet,* 13, 671-8.

CHAMBERLAIN, J. S., PEARLMAN, J. A., MUZNY, D. M., GIBBS, R. A., RANIER, J. E., CASKEY, C. T. & REEVES, A. A. (1988). Expression of the murine Duchenne muscular dystrophy gene in muscle and brain. *Science,* 239, 1416-8.

CHELLY, J., KAPLAN, J-C., MAIRE, P., GAUTRON, S. & KAHN, A. (1988). Transcription of the dystrophin gene in human muscle and non-muscle tissues. *Nature* 333, 858-60.

CHELLY, J., CONCORDET, J. P., KAPLAN, J. C. & KAHN, A. (1989). Illegitimate transcription: transcription of any gene in any cell type. *Proc Natl Acad Sci U S A,* 86, 2617-21.

CIBIS, G.W., FITZGERALD, K.W., HARRIS, D.J., ROTHBERG, P.G. & RUPANI, M. (1993). The effect of dystrophin gene mutations on the ERG in mice and humans. *Invest Ophthalmol Vis Sci* 34 (13) 3646-52.

COLLINS, C. A. & MORGAN, J. E. (2003). Duchenne's muscular dystrophy: animal models used to investigate pathogenesis and develop therapeutic strategies. *Int J Exp Pathol*, 84, 165-72.

CONNERS, K. (2000). *Technical manual for the Conners rating scales - revised*, North Tonawanda, Multi-Health Systems Inc.

CONNORS, N. C., ADAMS, M. E., FROEHNER, S. C. & KOFUJI, P. (2004). The potassium channel Kir4.1 associates with the dystrophin-glycoprotein complex via alpha-syntrophin in glia. *J Biol Chem*, 279, 28387-92.

COSTA, M.F., OLIVEIRA, A.G., FEITOSA-SANTANA, C., ZATZ, M. & VENTURA, D.F. (2007). Red-green colour vision impairment in Duchenne muscular dystrophy. *Am J Hum Genet* 80 (6) 1064-75.

COTTON, S., CROWE, S. & VOUDOURIS, N. (1998). Neuropsychological Profile of Duchenne Muscular Dystrophy. *Child Neuropsychology*, 4, 110-17.

COTTON, S., VOUDOURIS, N. J. & GREENWOOD, K. M. (2001). Intelligence and Duchenne muscular dystrophy: full-scale, verbal, and performance intelligence quotients. *Dev Med Child Neurol*, 43, 497-501.

COTTON, S. M., VOUDOURIS, N. J. & GREENWOOD, K. M. (2005). Association between intellectual functioning and age in children and young adults with Duchenne muscular dystrophy: further results from a meta-analysis. *Dev Med Child Neurol*, 47, 257-65.

CROSS, R. A., STEWART, M. & KENDRICK-JONES, J. (1990). Structural predictions for the central domain of dystrophin. *FEBS Lett*, 262, 87-92.

CULLIGAN, K. G., MACKEY, A. J., FINN, D. M., MAGUIRE, P. B. & OHLENDIECK, K. (1998). Role of dystrophin isoforms and associated proteins in muscular dystrophy (review). *Int J Mol Med*, 2, 639-48.

CULLIGAN, K., GLOVER, L., DOWLING, P. & OHLENDIECK, K. (2001). Brain dystrophin-glycoprotein complex: persistent expression of beta-dystroglycan, impaired oligomerization of Dp71 and up-regulation of utrophins in animal models of muscular dystrophy. *BMC Cell Biol*, 2, 2.

CULLIGAN, K. & OHLENDIECK, K. (2002). Diversity of the Brain Dystrophin-Glycoprotein Complex. *J Biomed Biotechnol*, 2, 31-36.

CYRULNIK, S. E. & HINTON, V. J. (2008). Duchenne muscular dystrophy: A cerebellar disorder? *Neurosci Biobehav Rev*, 32, 486-96.

D'ANGELO, M. G. & BRESOLIN, N. (2003). Report of the 95th European Neuromuscular Centre (ENMC) sponsored international workshop cognitive impairment in neuromuscular disorders, Naarden, The Netherlands, 13-15 July 2001. *Neuromuscul Disord*, 13, 72-9.

D'SOUZA, V. N., NGUYEN, T. M., MORRIS, G. E., KARGES, W., PILLERS, D. A. & RAY, P. N. (1995). A novel dystrophin isoform is required for normal retinal electrophysiology. *Hum Mol Genet*, 4, 837-42.

DALKILIC, I. & KUNKEL, L. M. (2003). Muscular dystrophies: genes to pathogenesis. *Curr Opin Genet Dev*, 13, 231-8.

DALLERAC, G., PERRONNET, C., CHAGNEAU, C., LEBLANC-VEYRAC, P., SAMSON-DESVIGNES, N., PELTEKIAN, E., DANOS, O., GARCIA LAROCHE, S., BILLARD, J.M. & VAILLEND, C. (2011). Rescue of a dystrophin-like protein by exon skipping normalizes synaptic plasticity in the hippocampus of the mdx mouse. *Neurobiol Dis* 43(3) 635-41.

DAOUD, F., ANGEARD, N., DEMERRE, B., MARTIE, I., BENYAOU, R., LETURCQ, F., COSSÉE, M., DEBURGRAVE, N., SAILLOUR, Y., TUFFERY, S., URTIZBEREA, A., TOUTAIN, A., ECHENNE, B., FRISCHMAN, M., MAYER, M., DESGUERRE, I., ESTOURNET, B., RÉVEILLÈRE, C., PENISSON-BESNIER, CUISSET, J.M., KAPLAN, J.C., HÉRON, D., RIVIER, F. & CHELLY, J. (2009). Analysis of Dp71 contribution in the severity of mental retardation through comparison of Duchenne and Becker patients differing by mutation consequences on Dp71 expression. *Hum Mol Genet* 18 (20) 3779-94.

DE SARRO, G., IBBADU, G. F., MARRA, R., ROTIROTI, D., LOIACONO, A., DONATO DI PAOLA, E. & RUSSO, E. (2004). Seizure susceptibility to various convulsant stimuli in dystrophin-deficient mdx mice. *Neurosci Res*, 50, 37-44.

DESMOND, J. E., GABRIELI, J. D., WAGNER, A. D., GINIER, B. L. & GLOVER, G. H. (1997) Lobular patterns of cerebellar activation in verbal working-memory and finger-tapping tasks as revealed by functional MRI. *J Neurosci*, 17, 9675-85.

DI LAZZARO, V., RESTUCCIA, D., SERVIDEI, S., NARDONE, R., OLIVIERO, A., PROFICE, P., MANGIOLA, F., TONALI, P. & ROTHWELL, J. C. (1998). Functional involvement of cerebral cortex in Duchenne muscular dystrophy. *Muscle Nerve*, 21, 662-4.

DORMAN, C., HURLEY, A. D. & D'AVIGNON, J. (1988). Language and learning disorders of older boys with Duchenne muscular dystrophy. *Dev Med Child Neurol*, 30, 316-27.

DUBOWITZ, V. & CROME, L. (1969). The central nervous system in Duchenne muscular dystrophy. *Brain*, 92, 805-808.

DUCHENNE, G. (1868). Recherche sur la paralysie musculaire pseudo-hypertrophique ou paralysie myosclerosique. *Archives of General Medicine*, 2, 5.

DUNN, J. F. & ZAIM-WADGHIRI, Y. (1999). Quantitative magnetic resonance imaging of the mdx mouse model of Duchenne muscular dystrophy. *Muscle Nerve*, 22, 1367-71.

DURBEEJ, M. & CAMPBELL, K. P. (2002). Muscular dystrophies involving the dystrophin-glycoprotein complex: an overview of current mouse models. *Curr Opin Genet Dev*, 12, 349-61.

EMERY, A. E. (2002). Muscular dystrophy into the new millennium. *Neuromuscul Disord*, 12, 343-9.

EMERY, A. E. (2002a). The muscular dystrophies. *Lancet*, 359, 687-95.

ESSEX, C. & ROPER, H. (2001). Lesson of the week: late diagnosis of Duchenne's muscular dystrophy presenting as global developmental delay. *BMJ*, 323, 37-38.

ETEMADIFAR, M. & MOLAEI, S. (2004). Epilepsy in Boys with Duchenne Muscular Dystrophy. *Journal of Research in Medical Sciences*, 3, 14-17.

FABBRIZIO, E., BONET-KERRACHE, A., LIMAS, F., HUGON, G. & MORNET, D. (1995). Dystrophin, the protein that promotes membrane resistance. *Biochem Biophys Res Commun*, 213, 295-301.

FERLINI, A., SEWRY, C., MELIS, M. A., MATEDDU, A. & MUNTONI, F. (1999). X-linked dilated cardiomyopathy and the dystrophin gene. *Neuromuscul Disord*, 9, 339-46.

FITZPATRICK, C., BARRY, C. & GARVEY, C. (1986). Psychiatric disorder among boys with Duchenne muscular dystrophy. *Dev Med Child Neurol* 28(5):589-95.

FRIGERI, A., NICCHIA, G. P., NICO, B., QUONDAMATTEO, F., HERKEN, R., RONCALI, L. & SVELTO, M. (2001). Aquaporin-4 deficiency in skeletal muscle and brain of dystrophic mdx mice. *Faseb J*, 15, 90-98.

GAULD, L. M., BOYNTON, A., BETTS, G. A. & JOHNSTON, H. (2005). Spirometry is affected by intelligence and behavior in Duchenne muscular dystrophy. *Pediatr Pulmonol*, 40, 408-13.

GEE, S. H., MADHAVAN, R., LEVINSON, S. R., CALDWELL, J. H., SEALOCK, R. & FROEHNER, S. C. (1998). Interaction of muscle and brain sodium channels with multiple members of the syntrophin family of dystrophin-associated proteins. *J Neurosci*, 18, 128-37.

GLAUB, T. & MECHLER, F. (1987). Intellectual function in muscular dystrophies. *Eur Arch Psychiatry Neurol Sci*, 236, 379-82.

GODFRAIND, J.-M., TEKKOK, S. B. & KRNJEVIC, K. (1998). Hypoxia on hippocampal slices from mice deficient in dystrophin (mdx) and dystrophin isoforms (mdx3cv). *Soc Neurosci Abst*

GODFRAIND, J.-M., TEKKOK, S. B. & KRNJEVIC, K. (2000). Hypoxia on Hippocampal Slices From Mice Deficient in Dystrophin (mdx) and Isoforms (mdx3cv). *J Cereb Blood Flow Metab*, 20, 145-152.

GOODWIN, F., MUNTONI, F. & DUBOWITZ, V. (1997). Epilepsy in Duchenne and Becker muscular dystrophies. *Eur J Paediatr Neurol*, 1, 115-9.

GORECKI, D., GENG, Y., THOMAS, K., HUNT, S. P., BARNARD, E. A. & BARNARD, P. J. (1991). Expression of the dystrophin gene in mouse and rat brain. *Neuroreport*, 2, 773-6.

GORECKI, D. C., MONACO, A. P., DERRY, J. M., WALKER, A. P., BARNARD, E. A. & BARNARD, P. J. (1992). Expression of four alternative dystrophin transcripts in brain regions regulated by different promoters. *Hum Mol Genet*, 1, 505-10.

GORECKI, D. C. & BARNARD, E. A. (1995). Specific expression of G-dystrophin (Dp71) in the brain. *Neuroreport*, 6, 893-6.

GORECKI, D. C., ABDULRAZZAK, H., LUKASIUK, K. & BARNARD, E. A. (1997). Differential expression of syntrophins and analysis of alternatively spliced dystrophin transcripts in the mouse brain. *Eur J Neurosci*, 9, 965-76.

GORECKI, D. C., LUKASIUK, K., SZKLARCZYK, A. & KACZMAREK, L. (1998). Kainate-evoked changes in dystrophin messenger RNA levels in the rat hippocampus. *Neuroscience*, 84, 467-77.

GRACIOTTI, L., MINELLI, A., MINCIACCHI, D., PROCOPIO, A. & FULGENZI, G. (2008). GABAergic miniature spontaneous activity is increased in the CA1 hippocampal region of dystrophic mdx mice. *Neuromuscul Disord* 18(3) 220-26.

GRADY, R.M., WOZNIAK, D.F., OHLEMILLER, K.K. & SANES, J.R. (2006). Cerebellar synaptic defects and abnormal motor behavior in mice lacking alpha- and beta-dystrobrevin. *J Neurosci* 26(11) 2841-51.

GREENBERG, D. S., SCHATZ, Y., LEVY, Z., PIZZO, P., YAFFE, D. & NUDEL, U. (1996). Reduced levels of dystrophin associated proteins in the brains of mice deficient for Dp71. *Hum Mol Genet*, 5, 1299-303.

GRIFFIN, J., NICHOLLS, A., MORTSHIRE-SMITH, R., RAE, C. & NICHOLSON, J. (1999). High resolution magic angle spinning ¹H NMR of cerebral tissue as applied to a mouse model of Duchenne muscular dystrophy [abstract]. *International Society Magnetic Resonance Medicine.* British Chapter.

GRIFFIN, J. L., WILLIAMS, H. J., SANG, E., CLARKE, K., RAE, C. & NICHOLSON, J. K. (2001). Metabolic profiling of genetic disorders: a multitissue (1)H nuclear magnetic resonance spectroscopic and pattern recognition study into dystrophic tissue. *Anal Biochem,* 293, 16-21.

HAMED, S. A. & HOFFMAN, E. P. (2006). Automated sequence screening of the entire dystrophin cDNA in Duchenne dystrophy: point mutation detection. *Am J Med Genet B Neuropsychiatr Genet,* 141, 44-50.

HASHIDA-OKUMURA, A., OKUMURA, N., IWAMATSU, A., BUIJS, R. M., ROMIJN, H. J. & NAGAI, K. (1999). Interaction of neuronal nitric-oxide synthase with alpha1-syntrophin in rat brain. *J Biol Chem,* 274, 11736-41.

HENDRIKSEN, J. G. & VLES, J. S. (2006). Are males with Duchenne muscular dystrophy at risk for reading disabilities? *Pediatr Neurol,* 34, 296-300.

HENDRIKSEN, J.G. & VLES, J.S. (2008). Neuropsychiatric disorders in males with duchenne muscular dystrophy: frequency rate of attention-deficit hyperactivity disorder (ADHD), autism spectrum disorder, and obsessive--compulsive disorder. *J Child Neurol* 23(5) 477-81.

HINTON, V. J., DE VIVO, D. C., NEREO, N. E., GOLDSTEIN, E. & STERN, Y. (2000). Poor verbal working memory across intellectual level in boys with Duchenne dystrophy. *Neurology,* 54, 2127-32.

HINTON, V. J., DE VIVO, D. C., NEREO, N. E., GOLDSTEIN, E. & STERN, Y. (2001). Selective deficits in verbal working memory associated with a known genetic etiology: the neuropsychological profile of duchenne muscular dystrophy. *J Int Neuropsychol Soc,* 7, 45-54.

HOFFMAN, E. P., BROWN, R. H., JR. & KUNKEL, L. M. (1987). Dystrophin: the protein product of the Duchenne muscular dystrophy locus. *Cell,* 51, 919-28.

HOFFMAN, E. P. & KUNKEL, L. M. (1989). Dystrophin abnormalities in Duchenne/Becker muscular dystrophy. *Neuron,* 2, 1019-29.

HOLDER, E., MAEDA, M. & BIES, R. D. (1996). Expression and regulation of the dystrophin Purkinje promoter in human skeletal muscle, heart, and brain. *Hum Genet,* 97, 232-9.

HOPF, F. W. & STEINHARDT, R. A. (1992). Regulation of intracellular free calcium in normal and dystrophic mouse cerebellar neurons. *Brain Res,* 578, 49-54.

HSU, Y. D. (2004). Muscular dystrophy: from pathogenesis to strategy. *Acta Neurol Taiwan,* 13, 50-8.

HUANG, X., POY, F., ZHANG, R., JOACHIMIAK, A., SUDOL, M. & ECK, M. J. (2000). Structure of a WW domain containing fragment of dystrophin in complex with beta-dystroglycan. *Nat Struct Biol,* 7, 634-8.

HUARD, J. & TREMBLAY, J. P. (1992) Localization of dystrophin in the Purkinje cells of normal mice. *Neurosci Lett,* 137, 105-8.

IANNELLO, R. C., MAR, J. H. & ORDAHL, C. P. (1991). Characterization of a promoter element required for transcription in myocardial cells. *J Biol Chem,* 266, 3309-16.

ILARRAZA-LOMELI, R., CISNEROS-VEGA, B., CERVANTES-GOMEZ, M.D.E. L., MORNET, D. & MONTAÑEZ, C. (2007). Dp71, utrophin and beta-dystroglycan expression and distribution in PC12/L6 cell cocultures. *NEUROREPORT* 18(16):1657-61.

ISHIKAWA-SAKURAI, M., YOSHIDA, M., IMAMURA, M., DAVIES, K. E. & OZAWA, E. (2004). ZZ domain is essentially required for the physiological binding of dystrophin and utrophin to beta-dystroglycan. *Hum Mol Genet*, 13, 693-702.

ITO, K., SAWADA, Y., SUGIYAMA, Y., SUZUKI, H., HANANO, M. & IGA, T. (1994). Linear relationship between GABAA receptor occupancy of muscimol and glucose metabolic response in the conscious mouse brain. Clinical implication based on comparison with benzodiazepine receptor agonist. *Drug Metab Dispos*, 22, 50-4.

IVES, J. H., DREWERY, D. L. & THOMPSON, C. L. (2002). Neuronal activity and its influence on developmentally regulated GABA(A) receptor expression in cultured mouse cerebellar granule cells. *Neuropharmacology*, 43, 715-25.

JAGADHA, V. & BECKER, L. E. (1988). Brain morphology in Duchenne muscular dystrophy: a Golgi study. *Pediatr Neurol*, 4, 87-92.

JANCSIK, V. & HAJOS, F. (1998). Differential distribution of dystrophin in postsynaptic densities of spine synapses. *Neuroreport*, 9, 2249-51.

JUEPTNER, M. & WEILLER, C. (1995). Review: does measurement of regional cerebral blood flow reflect synaptic activity? Implications for PET and fMRI. *Neuroimage*, 2, 148-56.

JUNG, D., FILLIOL, D., METZ-BOUTIGUE, M. H. & RENDON, A. (1993). Characterization and subcellular localization of the dystrophin-protein 71 (Dp71) from brain. *Neuromuscul Disord*, 3, 515-8.

JUNG, D., YANG, B., MEYER, J., CHAMBERLAIN, J. S. & CAMPBELL, K. P. (1995). Identification and characterization of the dystrophin anchoring site on beta-dystroglycan. *J Biol Chem*, 270, 27305-10.

KAMAKURA, K., TADANO, Y., KAWAI, M., ISHIURA, S., NAKAMURA, R., MIYAMOTO, K., NAGATA, N. & SUGITA, H. (1994). Dystrophin-related protein is found in the central nervous system of mice at various developmental stages, especially at the postsynaptic membrane. *J Neurosci Res*, 37, 728-34.

KAPLAN, L. C., OSBORNE, P. & ELIAS, E. (1986). The diagnosis of muscular dystrophy in patients referred for language delay. *J Child Psychol Psychiatry*, 27, 545-9.

KARAGAN, N. J. & ZELLWEGER, H. U. (1976). IQ studies in Duchenne muscular dystrophy II: test-retest performance. *Developmental Medicine and Child Neurology*, 18, 251.

KARAGAN, N. J. & ZELLWEGER, H. U. (1978). Early verbal disability in children with Duchenne muscular dystrophy. *Dev Med Child Neurol*, 20, 435-41.

KARAGAN, N. J. (1979). Intellectual functioning in Duchenne muscular dystrophy: a review. *Psychol Bull*, 86, 250-9.

KARAGAN, N. J., RICHMAN, L. C. & SORENSEN, J. P. (1980). Analysis of verbal disability in Duchenne muscular dystrophy. *J Nerv Ment Dis*, 168, 419-23.

KATO, T., NISHINA, M., MATSUSHITA, K., HORI, E., AKABOSHI, S. & TAKASHIMA, S. (1997). Increased cerebral choline-compounds in Duchenne muscular dystrophy. *Neuroreport*, 8, 1435-7.

KENWRICK, S., PATTERSON, M., SPEER, A., FISCHBECK, K. & DAVIES, K. (1987). Molecular analysis of the Duchenne muscular dystrophy region using pulsed field gel electrophoresis. *Cell*, 48, 351-7.

KHAN, Y. & HECKMATT, J. Z. (1994). Obstructive apnoeas in Duchenne muscular dystrophy. *Thorax*, 49, 157-61.

KIM, T. W., WU, K., XU, J. L. & BLACK, I. B. (1992). Detection of dystrophin in the postsynaptic density of rat brain and deficiency in a mouse model of Duchenne muscular dystrophy. *Proc Natl Acad Sci U S A*, 89, 11642-4.

KIM, T. W., WU, K. & BLACK, I. B. (1995). Deficiency of brain synaptic dystrophin in human Duchenne muscular dystrophy. *Ann Neurol*, 38, 446-9.

KINGSTON, H. M., SARFARAZI, M., THOMAS, N. S. & HARPER, P. S. (1984). Localisation of the Becker muscular dystrophy gene on the short arm of the X chromosome by linkage to cloned DNA sequences. *Hum Genet*, 67, 6-17.

KNUESEL, I., MASTROCOLA, M., ZUELLIG, R. A., BORNHAUSER, B., SCHAUB, M. C. & FRITSCHY, J. M. (1999). Short communication: altered synaptic clustering of GABAA receptors in mice lacking dystrophin (mdx mice). *Eur J Neurosci*, 11, 4457-62.

KNUESEL, I., ZUELLIG, R. A., SCHAUB, M. C. & FRITSCHY, J. M. (2001). Alterations in dystrophin and utrophin expression parallel the reorganization of GABAergic synapses in a mouse model of temporal lobe epilepsy. *Eur J Neurosci*, 13, 1113-24.

KOENIG, M., HOFFMAN, E. P., BERTELSON, C. J., MONACO, A. P., FEENER, C. & KUNKEL, L. M. (1987). Complete cloning of the Duchenne muscular dystrophy (DMD) cDNA and preliminary genomic organization of the DMD gene in normal and affected individuals. *Cell*, 50, 509-17.

KOENIG, M., MONACO, A. P. & KUNKEL, L. M. (1988). The complete sequence of dystrophin predicts a rod-shaped cytoskeletal protein. *Cell*, 53, 219-26

KOENIG, M. & KUNKEL, L. M. (1990). Detailed analysis of the repeat domain of dystrophin reveals four potential hinge segments that may confer flexibility. *J Biol Chem*, 265, 4560-6.

KOMOTO, J., USUI, S., OTSUKI, S. & TERAO, A. (1984). Infantile autism and Duchenne muscular dystrophy. *J Autism Dev Disord*, 14, 191-5.

KUEH, S.L., HEAD, S.I. & MORLEY, J.W. (2008). GABA(A) receptor expression and inhibitory post-synaptic currents in cerebellar Purkinje cells in dystrophin-deficient mdx mice. *Clin Exp Pharmacol Physiol* 35(2):207-10.

KUEH, S.L., DEMPSTER, J., HEAD, S.I. & MORLEY, J.W. (2011). Reduced postsynaptic GABAA receptor number and enhanced gaboxadol induced change in holding currents in Purkinje cells of the dystrophin-deficient mdx mouse. *Neurobiol Dis* 43(3):558-64.

KUNKEL, L. M., MONACO, A. P., BERTELSON, C. J. & COLLETTI, C. A. (1986). Molecular genetics of Duchenne muscular dystrophy. *Cold Spring Harb Symp Quant Biol*, 51 Pt 1, 349-51.

LABARQUE, V., FRESON, K., THYS, C., WITTEVRONGEL, C., HOYLAERTS, M.F., DE VOS, R., GOEMANS, N. & VAN GEET, C. (2008). Increased Gs signalling in platelets and impaired collagen activation, due to a defect in the dystrophin gene, result in increased blood loss during spinal surgery. *Hum Mol Genet* 17(3):357-66.

LEDERFEIN, D., LEVY, Z., AUGIER, N., MORNET, D., MORRIS, G., FUCHS, O., YAFFE, D. & NUDEL, U. (1992). A 71-kilodalton protein is a major product of the Duchenne muscular dystrophy gene in brain and other nonmuscle tissues. *Proc Natl Acad Sci U S A,* 89, 5346-50.

LEDERFEIN, D., YAFFE, D. & NUDEL, U. (1993). A housekeeping type promoter, located in the 3' region of the Duchenne muscular dystrophy gene, controls the expression of Dp71, a major product of the gene. *Hum Mol Genet,* 2, 1883-8.

LEE, J. S., PFUND, Z., JUHASZ, C., BEHEN, M. E., MUZIK, O., CHUGANI, D. C., NIGRO, M. A. & CHUGANI, H. T. (2002). Altered regional brain glucose metabolism in Duchenne muscular dystrophy: a pet study. *Muscle Nerve,* 26, 506-12.

LEVI, S., GRADY, R. M., HENRY, M. D., CAMPBELL, K. P., SANES, J. R. & CRAIG, A. M. (2002). Dystroglycan is selectively associated with inhibitory GABAergic synapses but is dispensable for their differentiation. *J Neurosci,* 22, 4274-85.

LEVISOHN, L., CRONIN-GOLOMB, A. & SCHMAHMANN, J. D. (2000). Neuropsychological consequences of cerebellar tumour resection in children: cerebellar cognitive affective syndrome in a paediatric population. *Brain,* 123 (Pt 5), 1041-50.

LIDOV, H. G., BYERS, T. J., WATKINS, S. C. & KUNKEL, L. M. (1990). Localization of dystrophin to postsynaptic regions of central nervous system cortical neurons. *Nature,* 348, 725-8.

LIDOV, H. G., BYERS, T. J. & KUNKEL, L. M. (1993). The distribution of dystrophin in the murine central nervous system: an immunocytochemical study. *Neuroscience,* 54, 167-87.

LIDOV, H. G., SELIG, S. & KUNKEL, L. M. (1995). Dp140: a novel 140 kDa CNS transcript from the dystrophin locus. *Hum Mol Genet,* 4, 329-35.

LIDOV, H. G. (1996). Dystrophin in the nervous system. *Brain Pathol,* 6, 63-77.

MANNI, R., ZUCCA, C., GALIMBERTI, C. A., OTTOLINI, A., CERVERI, I., BRUSCHI, C., ZOIA, M. C., LANZI, G. & TARTARA, A. (1991). Nocturnal sleep and oxygen balance in Duchenne muscular dystrophy. A clinical and polygraphic 2-year follow-up study. *Eur Arch Psychiatry Clin Neurosci,* 240, 255-7.

MEHLER, M. F., HAAS, K. Z., KESSLER, J. A. & STANTON, P. K. (1992). Enhanced sensitivity of hippocampal pyramidal neurons from mdx mice to hypoxia-induced loss of synaptic transmission. *Proc Natl Acad Sci U S A,* 89, 2461-5.

MEHLER, M. F. (2000). Brain dystrophin, neurogenetics and mental retardation. *Brain Res Brain Res Rev,* 32, 277-307.

MELO, M., LAURIANO, V., GENTIL, V., EGGERS, S., DEL BIANCO, S. S., GIMENEZ, P. R., AKIYAMA, J., OKABAIASHI, H., FROTA-PESSOA, O., PASSOS-BUENO, M. R. & ET AL. (1995). Becker and limb-girdle muscular dystrophies: a psychiatric and intellectual level comparative study. *Am J Med Genet,* 60, 33-8.

MICHALAK, M. & OPAS, M. (2001). *Duchenne muscular dystrophy,* Chichester, John Wiley & Sons LTD.

MILNER, R. E., BUSAAN, J. L., HOLMES, C. F., WANG, J. H. & MICHALAK, M. (1993). Phosphorylation of dystrophin. The carboxyl-terminal region of dystrophin is a substrate for in vitro phosphorylation by p34cdc2 protein kinase. *J Biol Chem,* 268, 21901-5.

MIRANDA, R., SÉBRIÉ, C., DEGROUARD, J., GILLET, B., JAILLARD, D., LAROCHE, S., VAILLEND, C. (2009). Reorganization of inhibitory synapses and increased PSD length of perforated excitatory synapses in hippocampal area CA1 of dystrophin-deficient mdx mice. *Cereb Cortex* 19(4):876-88.

MIRANDA, R., NUDEL, U., LAROCHE, S. & VAILLEND, C. (2011). Altered presynaptic ultrastructure in excitatory hippocampal synapses of mice lacking dystrophins Dp427 or Dp71. *Neurobiol Dis* 43(1):134-41,

MISURI, G., LANINI, B., GIGLIOTTI, F., IANDELLI, I., PIZZI, A., BERTOLINI, M. G. & SCANO, G. (2000). Mechanism of CO_2 retention in patients with neuromuscular disease. *Chest*, 117, 447-53.

MIYATAKE, M., MIIKE, T., ZHAO, J. E., YOSHIOKA, K., UCHINO, M. & USUKU, G. (1991). Dystrophin: localization and presumed function. *Muscle Nerve*, 14, 113-9.

MOHAMED, K., APPLETON, R. & NICOLAIDES, P. (2000). Delayed diagnosis of Duchenne muscular dystrophy. *Eur J Paediatr Neurol*, 4, 219-23.

MOUKHLES, H. & CARBONETTO, S. (2001). Dystroglycan contributes to the formation of multiple dystrophin-like complexes in brain. *J Neurochem*, 78, 824-34.

MUNTONI, F., MATEDDU, A. & SERRA, G. (1991). Passive avoidance behaviour deficit in the mdx mouse. *Neuromuscul Disord*, 1, 121-3.

MUNTONI, F., CAU, M., GANAU, A., CONGIU, R., ARVEDI, G., MATEDDU, A., MARROSU, M. G., CIANCHETTI, C., REALDI, G., CAO, A. & ET AL. (1993). Brief report: deletion of the dystrophin muscle-promoter region associated with X-linked dilated cardiomyopathy. *N Engl J Med*, 329, 921-5.

MUNTONI, F., TORELLI, S. & FERLINI, A. (2003). Dystrophin and mutations: one gene, several proteins, multiple phenotypes. *Lancet Neurol*, 2, 731-40.

NEELY, J. D., AMIRY-MOGHADDAM, M., OTTERSEN, O. P., FROEHNER, S. C., AGRE, P. & ADAMS, M. E. (2001). Syntrophin-dependent expression and localization of Aquaporin-4 water channel protein. *Proc Natl Acad Sci U S A*, 98, 14108-13.

NICCHIA, G.P., NICO, B., CAMASSA, L.M., MOLA, M.G., LOH, N., DERMIETZEL, R., SPRAY, D.C., SVELTO, M. & FRIGERI, A. (2004). The role of aquaporin-4 in the blood-brain barrier development and integrity: studies in animal and cell culture models. *Neuroscience* 129(4):935-45.

NICCHIA, G.P., ROSSI, A., NUDEL, U., SVELTO, M. & FRIGERI, A. (2008). Dystrophin-dependent and -independent AQP4 pools are expressed in the mouse brain. *Glia* 56(8):869-76.

NICO, B., FRIGERI, A., NICCHIA, G. P., CORSI, P., RIBATTI, D., QUONDAMATTEO, F., HERKEN, R., GIROLAMO, F., MARZULLO, A., SVELTO, M. & RONCALI, L. (2003). Severe alterations of endothelial and glial cells in the blood-brain barrier of dystrophic mdx mice. *Glia*, 42, 235-51.

NICOLSON, R. I., FAWCETT, A. J., BERRY, E. L., JENKINS, I. H., DEAN, P. & BROOKS, D. J. (1999). Association of abnormal cerebellar activation with motor learning difficulties in dyslexic adults. *Lancet*, 353, 1662-7.

NUDEL, U., ROBZYK, K. & YAFFE, D. (1988). Expression of the putative Duchenne muscular dystrophy gene in differentiated myogenic cell cultures and in the brain. *Nature*, 331, 635-8.

NUSSER, Z., CULL-CANDY, S. & FARRANT, M. (1997) Differences in synaptic GABA(A) receptor number underlie variation in GABA mini amplitude. *Neuron*, 19, 697-709.

O'BRIEN, K. F. & KUNKEL, L. M. (2001). Dystrophin and muscular dystrophy: past, present, and future. *Mol Genet Metab*, 74, 75-88.

OGASAWARA, A. (1989). Similarity of IQs of siblings with Duchenne progressive muscular dystrophy. *Am J Ment Retard*, 93, 548-50.

OGASAWARA, A. (1989a). Downward shift in IQ in persons with Duchenne muscular dystrophy compared to those with spinal muscular atrophy. *Am J Ment Retard*, 93, 544-7.

PALUMBO, D., PANDYA, S., MOXLEY, R. & SILVERSTEIN, S. (1996). Cognitive Dysfunction in Boys with Duchenne Muscular Dystrophy. *Archives of Clinical Neuropsychology*, 11, 431.

PARTRIDGE, T. (1991). Animal models of muscular dystrophy--what can they teach us? *Neuropathol Appl Neurobiol*, 17, 353-63.

PERRONNET, C. & VAILLEND, C. (2010). Dystrophins, utrophins, and associated scaffolding complexes: role in mammalian brain and implications for therapeutic strategies. *J Biomed Biotechnol* 2010:849426.

PETROF, B. J. (2002). Molecular pathophysiology of myofiber injury in deficiencies of the dystrophin-glycoprotein complex. *Am J Phys Med Rehabil*, 81, S162-74.

PILLERS, D.A., BULMAN, D.E., WELEBER, R.G., SIGESMUND, D.A., MUSARELLA, M.A., POWELL, B.R., MURPHEY, W.H., WESTALL, C., PANTON, C., BECKER, L.E., WORTON, R.G. & RAY, P.N. (1993). Dystrophin expression in the human retina is required for normal function as defined by electroretinography. *Nat Genet* 4(1):82-6.

PONTING, C. P., BLAKE, D. J., DAVIES, K. E., KENDRICK-JONES, J. & WINDER, S. J. (1996). ZZ and TAZ: new putative zinc fingers in dystrophin and other proteins. *Trends Biochem Sci*, 21, 11-13.

POYSKY J. (2007). Behavior patterns in Duchenne muscular dystrophy: report on the Parent Project Muscular Dystrophy behavior workshop 8-9 of December 2006, Philadelphia, USA. *Neuromuscul Disord.* 17(11-12):986-94.

RAE, C., LEE, M. A., DIXON, R. M., BLAMIRE, A. M., THOMPSON, C. H., STYLES, P., TALCOTT, J., RICHARDSON, A. J. & STEIN, J. F. (1998). Metabolic abnormalities in developmental dyslexia detected by 1H magnetic resonance spectroscopy. *Lancet*, 351, 1849-52.

RAE, C., SCOTT, R. B., THOMPSON, C. H., DIXON, R. M., DUMUGHN, I., KEMP, G. J., MALE, A., PIKE, M., STYLES, P. & RADDA, G. K. (1998). Brain biochemistry in Duchenne muscular dystrophy: a 1H magnetic resonance and neuropsychological study. *J Neurol Sci*, 160, 148-57.

RAE, C., LAWRANCE, M. L., DIAS, L. S., PROVIS, T., BUBB, W. A. & BALCAR, V. J. (2000). Strategies for studies of neurotoxic mechanisms involving deficient transport of L-glutamate: antisense knockout in rat brain in vivo and changes in the neurotransmitter metabolism following inhibition of glutamate transport in guinea pig brain slices. *Brain Res Bull*, 53, 373-81.

RAE, C., GRIFFIN, J. L., BLAIR, D. H., BOTHWELL, J. H., BUBB, W. A., MAITLAND, A. & HEAD, S. (2002). Abnormalities in brain biochemistry associated with lack of dystrophin: studies of the mdx mouse. *Neuromuscul Disord*, 12, 121-9.

RANDO, T. A. (2001). The dystrophin-glycoprotein complex, cellular signaling, and the regulation of cell survival in the muscular dystrophies. *Muscle Nerve*, 24, 1575-94.

RAPAPORT, D., LEDERFEIN, D., DEN DUNNEN, J. T., GROOTSCHOLTEN, P. M., VAN OMMEN, G. J., FUCHS, O., NUDEL, U. & YAFFE, D. (1992). Characterization and cell type distribution of a novel, major transcript of the Duchenne muscular dystrophy gene. *Differentiation*, 49, 187-93.

REID, D. T. & RENWICK, R. M. (2001). Relating familial stress to the psychosocial adjustment of adolescents with Duchenne muscular dystrophy. *Int J Rehabil Res*, 24, 83-93.

RENTSCHLER, S., LINN, H., DEININGER, K., BEDFORD, M. T., ESPANEL, X. & SUDOL, M. (1999). The WW domain of dystrophin requires EF-hands region to interact with beta-dystroglycan. *Biol Chem*, 380, 431-42.

ROBERTS, R. G., COFFEY, A. J., BOBROW, M. & BENTLEY, D. R. (1993). Exon structure of the human dystrophin gene. *Genomics*, 16, 536-8.

ROBERTS, R. G. (2001). Dystrophins and dystrobrevins. *Genome Biol*, 2, REVIEWS3006.

ROCCELLA, M., PACE, R. & DE GREGORIO, M. T. (2003). Psychopathological assessment in children affected by Duchenne de Boulogne muscular dystrophy. *Minerva Pediatr*, 55, 267-73, 273-6.

ROSMAN, N. P. & KAKULAS, B. A. (1966). Mental deficiency associated with muscular dystrophy. A neuropathological study. *Brain*, 89, 769-88.

SAVAGE, R. & ADAMS, M. (1979). Cognitive Functioning and Neurological Deficit: Duchenne Muscular Dystrophy and Cerebral Palsy. *Australian Psychologist* 14, 59-75.

SBRICCOLI, A., SANTARELLI, M., CARRETTA, D., PINTO, F., GRANATO, A. & MINCIACCHI, D. (1995). Architectural changes of the cortico-spinal system in the dystrophin defective mdx mouse. *Neurosci Lett*, 200, 53-6.

SCHOFIELD, J. N., BLAKE, D. J., SIMMONS, C., MORRIS, G. E., TINSLEY, J. M., DAVIES, K. E. & EDWARDS, Y. H. (1994). Apo-dystrophin-1 and apo-dystrophin-2, products of the Duchenne muscular dystrophy locus: expression during mouse embryogenesis and in cultured cell lines. *Hum Mol Genet*, 3, 1309-16.

SEKIGUCHI, M. (2005). The role of dystrophin in the central nervous system: a mini review. *Acta Myol*, 24, 93-7.

SEKIGUCHI, M., ZUSHIDA, K., YOSHIDA, M., MAEKAWA, M., KAMICHI, S., YOSHIDA, M., SAHARA, Y., YUASA, S., TAKEDA, S. & WADA, K. (2009). A deficit of brain dystrophin impairs specific amygdala GABAergic transmission and enhances defensive behaviour in mice. *Brain* 132(Pt 1):124-35.

SEPTIEN, L., GRAS, P., BORSOTTI, J. P., GIROUD, M., NIVELON, J. L. & DUMAS, R. (1991). [Mental development in Duchenne muscular dystrophy. Correlation of data of the brain scanner]. *Pediatrie*, 46, 817-9.

SESAY, A. K., ERRINGTON, M. L., LEVITA, L. & BLISS, T. V. (1996). Spatial learning and hippocampal long-term potentiation are not impaired in mdx mice. *Neurosci Lett*, 211, 207-10.

SHAW, R. F. & DREIFUSS, F. E. (1969). Mild and severe forms of X-linked muscular dystrophy. *Arch Neurol*, 20, 451-60.

SICINSKI, P., GENG, Y., RYDER-COOK, A. S., BARNARD, E. A., DARLISON, M. G. & BARNARD, P. J. (1989). The molecular basis of muscular dystrophy in the mdx mouse: a point mutation. *Science*, 244, 1578-80.

SMITH, D. I., ZHU, Y., MCAVOY, S. & KUHN, R. (2006). Common fragile sites, extremely large genes, neural development and cancer. *Cancer Lett*, 232, 48-57.

SMITH, P. E., CALVERLEY, P. M. & EDWARDS, R. H. (1988). Hypoxemia during sleep in Duchenne muscular dystrophy. *Am Rev Respir Dis*, 137, 884-8.

SMITH, R. A., SIBERT, J. R., WALLACE, S. J. & HARPER, P. S. (1989). Early diagnosis and secondary prevention of Duchenne muscular dystrophy. *Arch Dis Child*, 64, 787-90.

SMITH, R. A., SIBERT, J. R. & HARPER, P. S. (1990). Early development of boys with Duchenne muscular dystrophy. *Dev Med Child Neurol*, 32, 519-27.

SOGOS, V., ENNAS, M. G., MUSSINI, I. & GREMO, F. (1997). Effect of dystrophin antisense oligonucleotides on cultured human neurons. *Neurochem Int*, 31, 447-57.

SOGOS, V., REALI, C., FANNI, V., CURTO, M. & GREMO, F. (2003). Dystrophin antisense oligonucleotides decrease expression of nNOS in human neurons. *Brain Res Mol Brain Res*, 118, 52-9.

SOLLEE, N. D., LATHAM, E. E., KINDLON, D. J. & BRESNAN, M. J. (1985). Neuropsychological impairment in Duchenne muscular dystrophy. *J Clin Exp Neuropsychol*, 7, 486-96.

SUGITA, H., ARAHATA, K. & ISHIGURO, T. (1988). Negative immunostaining of Duchenne muscular dystrophy (DMD) and mdx muscle surface membrane with antibody against synthetic peptide fragment predicted from DMD cDNA. *Proc Jap Acad*, 64, 37-39.

SUZUKI, A., YOSHIDA, M., HAYASHI, K., MIZUNO, Y., HAGIWARA, Y. & OZAWA, E. (1994). Molecular organization at the glycoprotein-complex-binding site of dystrophin. Three dystrophin-associated proteins bind directly to the carboxy-terminal portion of dystrophin. *Eur J Biochem*, 220, 283-92.

TAYLOR, P.J., BETTS, G.A., MAROULIS, S., GILISSEN, C., PEDERSEN, R.L., MOWAT, D.R., JOHNSTON, H.M. & BUCKLEY, M.F. (2010). Dystrophin gene mutation location and the risk of cognitive impairment in Duchenne muscular dystrophy. *PLOS ONE* 20;5(1):e8803.

TOKARZ, S. A., DUNCAN, N. M., RASH, S. M., SADEGHI, A., DEWAN, A. K. & PILLERS, D. A. (1998). Redefinition of dystrophin isoform distribution in mouse tissue by RT-PCR implies role in nonmuscle manifestations of duchenne muscular dystrophy. *Mol Genet Metab*, 65, 272-81.

TORRES, L. F. & DUCHEN, L. W. (1987). The mutant mdx: inherited myopathy in the mouse. Morphological studies of nerves, muscles and end-plates. *Brain*, 110 (Pt 2), 269-99.

TRACEY, I., SCOTT, R. B., THOMPSON, C. H., DUNN, J. F., BARNES, P. R., STYLES, P., KEMP, G. J., RAE, C. D., PIKE, M. & RADDA, G. K. (1995). Brain abnormalities in Duchenne muscular dystrophy: phosphorus-31 magnetic resonance spectroscopy and neuropsychological study. *Lancet*, 345, 1260-4.

TRACEY, I., DUNN, J. F. & RADDA, G. K. (1996). Brain metabolism is abnormal in the mdx model of Duchenne muscular dystrophy. *Brain*, 119 (Pt 3), 1039-44.

TRACEY, I., DUNN, J. F., PARKES, H. G. & RADDA, G. K. (1996a). An in vivo and in vitro H-magnetic resonance spectroscopy study of mdx mouse brain: abnormal development or neural necrosis? *J Neurol Sci*, 141, 13-8.

UCHIKAWA, K., LIU, M., HANAYAMA, K., TSUJI, T., FUJIWARA, T. & CHINO, N. (2004). Functional staus and muscle strength in people with Duchenne muscular dystrophy living in the community. *Journal of Rehabilitation Medicine*, 36, 124-129.

UCHINO, M., YOSHIOKA, K., MIIKE, T., TOKUNAGA, M., UYAMA, E., TERAMOTO, H., NAOE, H. & ANDO, M. (1994). Dystrophin and dystrophin-related protein in the brains of normal and mdx mice. *Muscle Nerve*, 17, 533-8.

UEDA, H., BABA, T., KASHIWAGI, K., IIJIMA, H. & OHNO, S. (2000) Dystrobrevin localization in photoreceptor axon terminals and at blood-ocular barrier sites. *Invest Ophthalmol Vis Sci*, 41, 3908-14.

VAILLEND, C., RENDON, A., MISSLIN, R. & UNGERER, A. (1995). Influence of dystrophin-gene mutation on mdx mouse behavior. I. Retention deficits at long delays in spontaneous alternation and bar-pressing tasks. *Behav Genet*, 25, 569-79.

VAILLEND, C., BILLARD, J. M., CLAUDEPIERRE, T., RENDON, A., DUTAR, P. & UNGERER, A. (1998). Spatial discrimination learning and CA1 hippocampal synaptic plasticity in mdx and mdx3cv mice lacking dystrophin gene products. *Neuroscience*, 86, 53-66.

VAILLEND, C., UNGERER, A. & BILLARD, J.M. (1999). Facilitated NMDA receptor-mediated synaptic plasticity in the hippocampal CA1 area of dystrophin-deficient mice. *Synapse* 33(1):59-70.

VAILLEND, C. & BILLARD, J. M. (2002). Facilitated CA1 hippocampal synaptic plasticity in dystrophin-deficient mice: role for GABAA receptors? *Hippocampus*, 12, 713-7.

VAILLEND, C., BILLARD, J. M. & LAROCHE, S. (2004). Impaired long-term spatial and recognition memory and enhanced CA1 hippocampal LTP in the dystrophin-deficient Dmd(mdx) mouse. *Neurobiol Dis*, 17, 10-20.

VAILLEND, C., PERRONNET, C., ROS, C., GRUSZCZYNSKI, C., GOYENVALLE, A., LAROCHE, S., DANOS, O., GARCIA, L. & PELTEKIAN, E. (2010). Rescue of a dystrophin-like protein by exon skipping in vivo restores GABAA-receptor clustering in the hippocampus of the mdx mouse. *Mol Ther* 8(9):1683-8.

VAJDA, Z., PEDERSEN, M., FUCHTBAUER, E. M., WERTZ, K., STODKILDE-JORGENSEN, H., SULYOK, E., DOCZI, T., NEELY, J. D., AGRE, P., FROKIAER, J. & NIELSEN, S. (2002). Delayed onset of brain edema and mislocalization of aquaporin-4 in dystrophin-null transgenic mice. *Proc Natl Acad Sci U S A*, 99, 13131-6.

VAJDA, Z., PEDERSEN, M., DOCZI, T., SULYOK, E. & NIELSEN, S. (2004). Studies of mdx mice. *Neuroscience*, 129, 993-8.

VAN OMMEN, G. J., BERTELSON, C., GINJAAR, H. B., DEN DUNNEN, J. T., BAKKER, E., CHELLY, J., MATTON, M., VAN ESSEN, A. J., BARTLEY, J., KUNKEL, L. M. & ET AL. (1987). Long-range genomic map of the Duchenne muscular dystrophy (DMD) gene: isolation and use of J66 (DXS268), a distal intragenic marker. *Genomics*, 1, 329-36.

WAITE, A., TINSLEY, C.L., LOCKE, M. & BLAKE DJ. (2009). The neurobiology of the dystrophin-associated glycoprotein complex. *Ann Med* 1(5):344-59.

WALLIS, T., BUBB, W. A., MCQUILLAN, J. A., BALCAR, V. J. & RAE, C. (2004). For want of a nail. ramifications of a single gene deletion, dystrophin, in the brain of the mouse. *Front Biosci*, 9, 74-84.

WECHSLER, D. (1997). *WAIS-III/WMS-III Technical Manual*, San Antonio TX, Psychological Corporation.

WHELAN, T. B. (1987) Neuropsychological performance of children with Duchenne muscular dystrophy and spinal muscle atrophy. *Dev Med Child Neurol*, 29, 212-20.

WIBAWA, T., TAKESHIMA, Y., MITSUYOSHI, I., WADA, H., SURONO, A., NAKAMURA, H. & MATSUO, M. (2000). Complete skipping of exon 66 due to novel mutations of the dystrophin gene was identified in two Japanese families of Duchenne muscular dystrophy with severe mental retardation. *Brain Dev*, 22, 107-12.

WINDER, S. J., GIBSON, T. J. & KENDRICK-JONES, J. (1995). Dystrophin and utrophin: the missing links! *FEBS Lett*, 369, 27-33.

WU, J. W., KUBAN, K. C. K., ALLRED, E., SHAPIRO, F. & DARRAS, B. T. (2005). Association of Duchenne Muscular Dystrophy With Autism Spectrum Disorder. *Journal of Child Neurology*, 20, 790-795.

YOKOTA, T., MIYAGOE, Y., HOSAKA, Y., TSUKITA, K., KAMEYA, S., SHIBUYA, S., MATSUDA, R., WAKAYAMA, Y. & TAKEDA, S. (2000). Aquaporin-4 is absent at the sarcolemma and at perivascular astrocyte endfeet in .ALPHA.1-syntrophin knockout mice. *Proceedings of the Japanese Academy Series B*, 76B, 22-27.

YOSHIHARA, Y., ONODERA, H., IINUMA, K. & ITOYAMA, Y. (2003). Abnormal kainic acid receptor density and reduced seizure susceptibility in dystrophin-deficient mdx mice. *Neuroscience*, 117, 391-5.

YOSHIOKA, M., OKUNO, T., HONDA, Y. & NAKANO, Y. (1980). Central nervous system involvement in progressive muscular dystrophy. *Arch Dis Child*, 55, 589-94.

YOUNG, H.K., BARTON, B.A., WAISBREN, S., PORTALES DALE, L., RYAN, M.M., WEBSTER, R.I. & NORTH, K.N. (2008). Cognitive and psychological profile in males with Becker muscular dystrophy. *J Child Neurol* 23(2):155-62.

ZACCARIA, M. L., PERRONE-CAPANO, C., MELUCCI-VIGO, G., GAETA, L., PETRUCCI, T. C. & PAGGI, P. (2001). Differential regulation of transcripts for dystrophin Isoforms, dystroglycan, and alpha3AChR subunit in mouse sympathetic ganglia following postganglionic nerve crush. *Neurobiol Dis*, 8, 513-24.

ZUBRZYCKA-GAARN, E. E., BULMAN, D. E., KARPATI, G., BURGHES, A. H., BELFALL, B., KLAMUT, H. J., TALBOT, J., HODGES, R. S., RAY, P. N. & WORTON, R. G. (1988). The Duchenne muscular dystrophy gene product is localized in sarcolemma of human skeletal muscle. *Nature*, 333, 466-9.

ZWAIGENBAUM, L. & TARNOPOLSKY, M. (2003). Two children with muscular dystrophies ascertained due to referral for diagnosis of autism. *J Autism Dev Disord*, 33, 193-9.

6

Abnormal Ion Homeostasis and Cell Damage in Muscular Dystrophy

Yuko Iwata and Shigeo Wakabayashi
National Cerebral and Cardiovascular Center Research Institute
Japan

1. Introduction

Disruption of cytoskeletal organization caused by genetic defects in the components of the dystrophin-glycoprotein complex (DGC) results in muscular dystrophy and/or cardiomyopathy in human patients and animal models. Accumulating evidence obtained from studies by using skeletal muscle fibers, cultured myotubes, and cardiac muscle preparations from dystrophic animals suggest that defects in DGC components cause altered membrane properties in the sarcolemma of myocytes. For example, disruption of the DGC can cause increased susceptibility to mechanical stress or increased permeability to ions such as Ca^{2+} and Na^+, leading to a chronic increase in the concentrations of intracellular Ca^{2+} ($[Ca^{2+}]_i$) and Na^+ ($[Na^+]_i$). Abnormal ion homeostasis, especially under conditions of mechanical stress, is thought to be a key molecular event in the pathology of muscular dysgenesis. In this chapter, we will review the stretch-induced cell damage pathways that result in abnormal Ca^{2+} and Na^+ concentrations. In particular, we will focus on stretch-activated channels, transient receptor potential cation channels, and Na^+-dependent ion transporters, which have been reported to be of critical pathological significance. We will also discuss the therapeutic potential of these ion handling membrane proteins for the treatment of muscular dystrophy.

2. Sarcolemmal weakness and abnormal ion homeostasis in muscular dystrophy

Table 1 shows the genes and their products, which are involved in muscular dystrophy. Disruption of some genes (highlighted in pink) lead to heart failure, most often caused by dilated cardiomyopathy, as well as muscular dystrophy. In Duchenne muscular dystrophy (DMD), in which the protein dystrophin is defective, expression of dystrophin-associated proteins is also greatly reduced (Ervasti and Campbell, 1991). In addition, other types of muscular dystrophy are caused by mutations in genes encoding the components of the DGC (Campbell, 1995; Duclos et al., 1998; Nigro et al., 1997). The DGC is a multi-subunit complex (Campbell, 1995; Campbell & Kahl, 1989; Tinsley et al., 1994) that spans the sarcolemma to structurally link extracellular matrix proteins such as laminin to the actin cytoskeleton (Ervasti & Campbell, 1993), providing mechanical strength to the muscle cell membranes. Therefore, disruption of the DGC could significantly destroy membrane integrity or stability during contraction/relaxation, and cause cell damage. Importantly, defects in different genes cause similar end-stage symptoms, i.e., muscle dysgenesis. Understanding the pathway that leads to cell damage is important for the development of common therapeutic strategies, not only for muscular dystrophy, but also for inherited and non-inherited cases of dilated cardiomyopathy. Two animal models are commonly used for the study of muscular dystrophy: the dystrophin-deficient mouse (*mdx*), which is representative of human DMD, and the delta-sarcoglycan-deficient hamster (BIO14.6), which is a model for human delta-sarcoglycanopathy.

inheritance	disease	gene	gene product	locus	OMIM number
X-linked	Duchenne Muscular Dystrophy	DMD	dystrophin	Xp21.2	300377
	Becker Muscular Dystrophy	BMD	dystrophin	Xp21.2	300376
	Emery-Dreifus Muscular Dystrophy	EMD,FHL1	emerin, FHL1	Xq28, Xq27.2	310300
Autosomal Recessive	Fukuyama-type	FCMD	fukutin	9q31-q33	607440
	Merosin-deficient	LAMA2	laminin α-2 chain	6q22-q23	156225
	Integrin-deficient	ITGA7	integrin α-7	12q13	600536
	Ullrich	COL6A1,2,3	collagenVI	2q37, 21q22.3	254090
	Muscle-eye-brain (MEB)	POMGNT1	POMGNT1	1p34-p33	606822
	Walker-Warburg syndrome(WWS)	POMT1,2	POMT1,2	9q34.1, 14q24.3	236670
	Limb-girdle				
	Calpainopathy	CAPN3	calpain-3	15q15.1-q21.1	114240
	Dysferlinopathy, Miyoshi distal	DYSF	dysferlin	2p13	603009
	Gamma-sarcoglycanopathy	SGCG	γ-sarcoglycan	13q12	253700
	Alpha-sarcoglycanopathy	SGCA	α-sarcoglycan	17q21	600119
	Beta-sarcoglycanopathy	SGCB	β-sarcoglycan	4q12	600900
	Delta-sarcoglycanopathy	SGCD	δ-sarcoglycan	5q33	601411
	Telethoninopathy	TCAP	telethonin	17q12	604488
	LGMD2H	TRIM32	E3 ubiquitin-protein ligase	9q31-q34.1	254110
	LGMD2I	FKRP	fukutin-related protein	19q13.32	606596
	LGMD2J	TTN	titin	2q31	608807
	LGMD2K	POMT1	POMT1	9q34.1	609308
	LGMD2L	ANO5	Ca^{2+} activated Cl^- channel	11p12-p13	611307
	LGMD2M	FKTN	fukutin	9q31	607440
	LGMD2N	POMT2	POMT2	14q24.3	607439
	LGMD2O	POMGNT1	POMGNT1	1p34-p33	606822
Autosomal Dominant	Limb-girdle				
	Myotilinopathy(LGMD1A)	MYOT	myotilin	5q31	604103
	LGMD1B	LMNA	lamin A/C	1q21.2	150330
	Caveolinopathy(LGMD1C)	CAV3	caveolin-3	3p25	601253
	LGMD1D	unknown	unknown	6q23	603511
	Facioscapulohumeral (FSHD)	DUX4	DUX4	4q35	158900
	Myotonic dystrophy	DMPK	myotonica protein kinase	19q13.2-q13.3	605377
	Myoclonus dystonia	SGCE	ε-sarcoglycan	7q21.3	604149

OMIM number: National Center for Biotechnology Information (http://www.ncbi.nlm.nih.gov/)

Common gene and gene product of cardiomyopathy

POMGNT;protein O-mannose beta 1,2-N-acetylglucosaminyltransferase
POMT ; protein O-mannosyltransferase

Table 1. Genes and their products responsible for muscular dystrophy

In an initial investigation, we found that sarcolemma from BIO14.6 hamster cardiomyopathic hearts has a fragile nature and is highly susceptible to mechanical stress, as evidenced by the ease of extraction of sarcolemma and T-tubules by relatively weak mechanical homogenization in low strength homogenization buffer (Tawada-Iwata et al., 1993). As a result, the amount of dystrophin extracted from BIO14.6 hamsters was 5 times more than that extracted from control hamsters, despite similar or lower dystrophin expression levels in BIO14.6 hamsters (Iwata et al., 1993a). The physical association between dystrophin and dystroglycan in BIO14.6 hearts was very weak (Iwata et al., 1993b). Mechanical membrane weakness was also observed in the skeletal muscle myotubes from BIO14.6 hamsters. Under hypo-osmotic stress (70% osmolarity), extensive cell bleb formation was seen in cultured BIO14.6 myotubes; however, this was not observed in control myotubes (Fig.1 A). Similarly, bleb formation was also seen in *mdx* mouse fibers, but not in control fibers (Fig.1 B). Upon cyclic stretching of up to 20% elongation for 1 h, creatine phosphokinase (CK) efflux (a marker of cell damage) was elevated with increasing strength of stretch in BIO14.6 myotubes, but not in controls (Fig.1 C). Such cell damage in *mdx* myotubes has also been reported by other groups (Menke & Jockusch, 1991; Petrof et al., 1993). These data suggest that skeletal and cardiac muscle is highly sensitive to mechanical stretch in animal models of DGC deficiency.

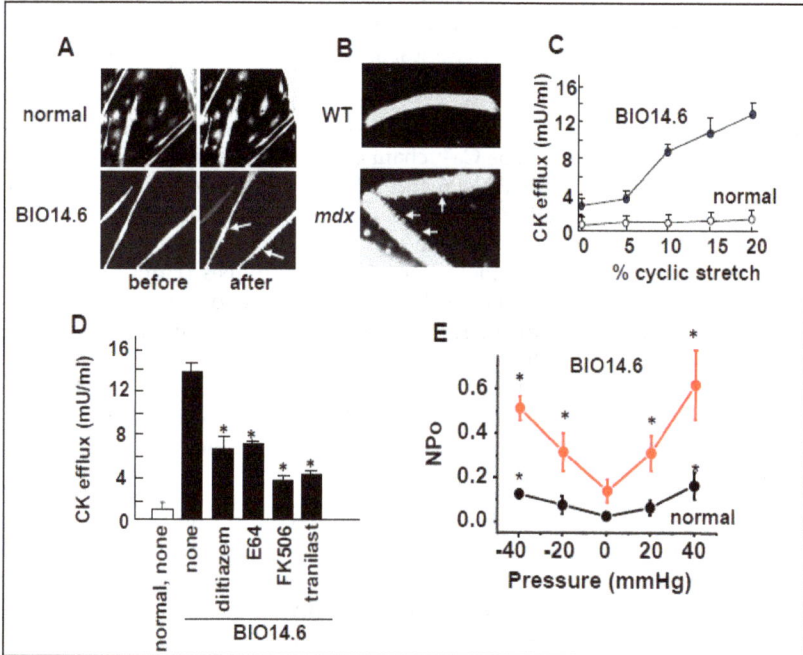

(A) Hypo-osmotic stress-induced cell damage in cultured dystrophic myotubes. Normal and BIO14.6 myotubes were preloaded with 5 mM calcein-AM and exposed to hypo-osmotic medium (70% osmolarity) for 17 min. Extensive bleb formation was observed in BIO14.6 myotubes (arrow). (B) Hypo-osmotic stress-induced cell damage in the single skeletal muscle fibers from WT and *mdx* muscle. Note the extensive bleb formation in *mdx* fibers. (C) Cyclic stretch of up to 20% for 1 h induced CK efflux from BIO14.6 myotubes, indicating the high susceptibility of dystrophic myotubes to mechanical stress. (D) Effect of various agents on stretch-induced CK efflux. The TRPV2 inhibitor tranilast effectively blocked CK efflux. The Ca^{2+} channel blocker diltiazem, the Ca^{2+}-dependent protease calpain inhibitor E64, and the Ca^{2+}-dependent phosphatase calcineurin inhibitor FK506 also blocked CK efflux, suggesting that these Ca^{2+} handling and Ca^{2+} effector proteins are involved in stretch-induced membrane damage. (E) A stretch-induced Ca^{2+}-permeable channel is activated in BIO14.6 myotubes. Positive or negative pressures were applied to the pipette using cell-attached patches that were held at -60 mV. $BaCl_2$ (110 mM) was used as the charge carrier. Note the higher open probability (NP_o) in BIO14.6 myotubes.

Fig. 1. Mechanical membrane weakness in the DGC-defective myotubes

It has been reported that myocyte degeneration may be caused by increased membrane permeability to Ca^{2+}, which is probably linked with membrane weakness. Many studies have reported chronic elevations in $[Ca^{2+}]_i$ underneath the sarcolemma, or within other intracellular compartments, in the skeletal muscle fibers or myotubes from DMD patients and *mdx* mice

(Brown, 1997; Mallouk et al., 2000; Robert et al., 2001). Elevated $[Ca^{2+}]_i$ has been causally linked to a greater rate of protein degradation, catalyzed by the Ca^{2+}-dependent protease calpain (Alderton & Steinhardt, 2000a; MacLennan et al., 1991; Spencer et al., 1995; Turner et al., 1988). Concurrently, myocyte contractile activity would cause physical damage to the sarcolemma, leading to leakage of cytosolic enzymes such as CK. The $[Ca^{2+}]_i$ in the muscle tissue is regulated by numerous ion channels, Ca^{2+} pumps, and transporters in the sarcolemma and sarcoplasmic reticulum (SR). Of these, the sarcolemmal Ca^{2+}-permeable channels (Ca^{2+}-specific leak channels) or the mechanosensitive non-selective cation channels, which contribute to abnormal Ca^{2+} handling in dystrophic myocytes, have been the focus of attention.

In 1990, the Steinhardt group (Fong et al., 1990) reported the existence of Ca^{2+} leak channels with a higher open probability in myotubes from *mdx* mice or DMD patients. These channels were activated by the L-type Ca^{2+} channel blocker nifedipine, but inhibited by the other dihydropyridine compounds AN406 and AN1043 (Alderton et al., 2000a). Treatment with the calpain inhibitor leupeptin decreased opening probabilities of the leak channels and prevented elevation in resting $[Ca^{2+}]_i$ in *mdx* myotubes (Turner et al., 1993). The leak channels were activated by store depletion in control myotubes (Hopf et al., 1996). From these data, Steinhardt et al. proposed a mechanism of myocyte degeneration caused by leak channel activation; contraction-induced sarcolemmal tears in dystrophin-deficient myotubes lead to localized Ca^{2+} entry, which initiates the repair of the defect. Activation of proteolysis is thought to be essential for the activation of leak channels, which accelerate Ca^{2+} entry and further increase Ca^{2+}-dependent proteolysis, the final common pathway of cell damage (Alderton & Steinhardt, 2000b). However, molecular identification and characterization of Ca^{2+} leak channels has not been carried out.

Mechanosensitive stretch-activated channels (SACs) have been described to contribute to increased Ca^{2+} permeability in dystrophic myotubes. The open probability of these channels increases when negative pressure is applied to a patch pipette. This is observed in both control and *mdx* muscle, but to a greater extent in *mdx* myotubes and fibers (Franco-Obregon & Lansman, 1994). SACs are non-selective cation channels permeable to Na^+, K^+, Ca^{2+}, and Ba^{2+}, and have a conductance of 13 pS when a patch pipette is filled with 110 mM Ca^{2+} (Franco & Lansman, 1990). In addition, a stretch-inactivated channel has been reported to exist only in *mdx* muscle cells (Franco et al., 1990), which was later reported to have identical conductance properties to SACs (Franco-Obregon & Lansman, 2002). These channels are blocked by Gd^{3+}, streptomycin (Hamill & McBride, 1996), and the spider venom toxin GsMtx4 (Suchyna et al., 2000). Abnormalities in SACs have been detected in the recordings from the muscle biopsy samples of DMD patients (Vandebrouck et al., 2001; Vandebrouck et al., 2002a). These results suggest that SACs are important for pathological Ca^{2+} entry into the dystrophin-deficient muscle, at early stages of the pathogenesis.

Research has shown that store-operated Ca^{2+} channels (SOCs) may also be involved in the pathogenesis of muscular dystrophy. SOCs have voltage-independent properties and a unitary conductance between 7 and 8 pS (with 110 mM Ca^{2+} in a patch pipette). Their open probability increases when luminal Ca^{2+} in the SR is depleted by the Ca^{2+} pump inhibitor thapsigargin. SOC activity was reported to be about twice as high in *mdx* compared to wild-type mice, and contributes to increased $[Ca^{2+}]_i$ in DMD (Vandebrouck et al., 2002b). Recently, Ca^{2+}-independent phospholipase A2 was found to be localized in the sarcolemma of *mdx* muscle, and its enzymatic product, lysophosphatidylcholine, was found to trigger Ca^{2+} entry through SOCs (Boittin et al., 2006). SACs and SOCs share several biophysical and pharmacological properties in adult muscle fibers; they have the same unitary conductance, and a similar sensitivity to Gd^{3+}, SKF-96365, 2-aminoethoxydiphenyl borate (2-APB), GsMTx4 toxin, and IGF-1 stimulation (Ducret et al., 2006). These observations suggest that SACs and SOCs may share common constituents, although molecular identification of these components is still required.

3. Therapeutic targets for muscular dystrophy

3.1 TRPV channels

Since a large body of evidence indicates the pathological significance of increased $[Ca^{2+}]_i$ in muscular dystrophy, much effort has been made to identify the genes responsible for abnormal Ca^{2+} handling in this disease. Our group has shown that stretch-sensitive cation-selective channels, similar to those recorded in *mdx* skeletal muscle, are active in cultured myotubes prepared from BIO14.6 hamsters (Nakamura et al., 2001). Positive or negative pressure increases the open probability of this channel in BIO14.6 myotubes (Fig.1 E). To identify the Ca^{2+} entry pathway responsible for myocyte degeneration, we searched for mammalian homologs of the *Drosophila* stretch sensor *NompA*, which were expressed in the striated muscle. We were successful in identifying a candidate that belongs to the transient receptor potential (TRP) channel family, which is similar to *NompA*. Many members of this family are Ca^{2+}-permeable cation channels sensitive to physical stimuli such as osmotic stress or heat (Montell et al., 2002). The candidate channel was previously reported as growth factor responsive channel (GRC) (Kanzaki et al., 1999), and later renamed TRP vanilloid type 2 (TRPV2) channel. We showed that TRPV2 is activated by mechanical stimuli and plays a critical role in the pathogenesis of muscular dystrophy and cardiomyopathy (Iwata et al., 2003; Muraki et al., 2003). TRPV2 is normally localized in the intracellular membrane compartment, but translocates to the plasma membrane in response to stretch or growth factor stimulation. Importantly, TRPV2 was observed to accumulate in the sarcolemma of the skeletal muscle from human patients with muscular dystrophy, BIO14.6 hamsters, and *mdx* mice (Fig.2) (Iwata et al., 2003), thus contributing to a sustained increase in $[Ca^{2+}]_i$ in diseased myocytes.

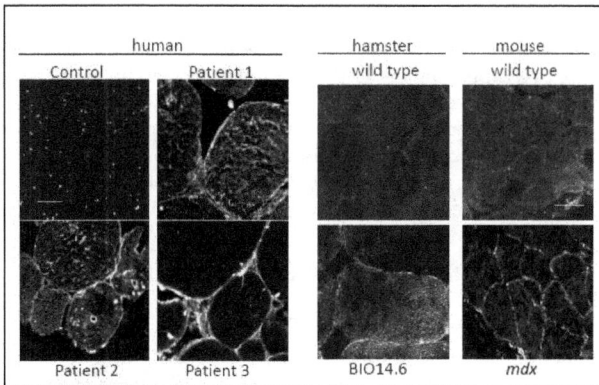

TRPV2 was immunolocalized in the frozen sections of the skeletal muscle from dystrophic patients and a non-dystrophic control, or from wild-type and dystrophic animals (Iwata et al., 2003). Note extensive sarcolemmal localization of TRPV2 in dystrophic patients and animal models. Bars, 50 μm.

Fig. 2. Immunohistochemical localization of TRPV2

In order to determine whether TRPV2 contributes to Ca^{2+}-induced muscle damage, we used a dominant-negative mutant strategy. We produced loss-of-function TRPV2 mutants in the pore region of the protein, which have a dominant-negative effect on the channel function by forming a non-functional oligomer, thereby abrogating the activity of endogenous TRPV2 (Fig.3 A). This dominant-negative TRPV2 mutant was incorporated into *mdx* mice by using a transgenic strategy or into BIO14.6 hamsters by adenoviral transfer. We found that these approaches significantly reduced resting $[Ca^{2+}]_i$ as well as the increase in $[Ca^{2+}]_i$ induced by high Ca^{2+} and the TRPV2 agonist 2-APB observed in dystrophic muscles (Fig.3 B).

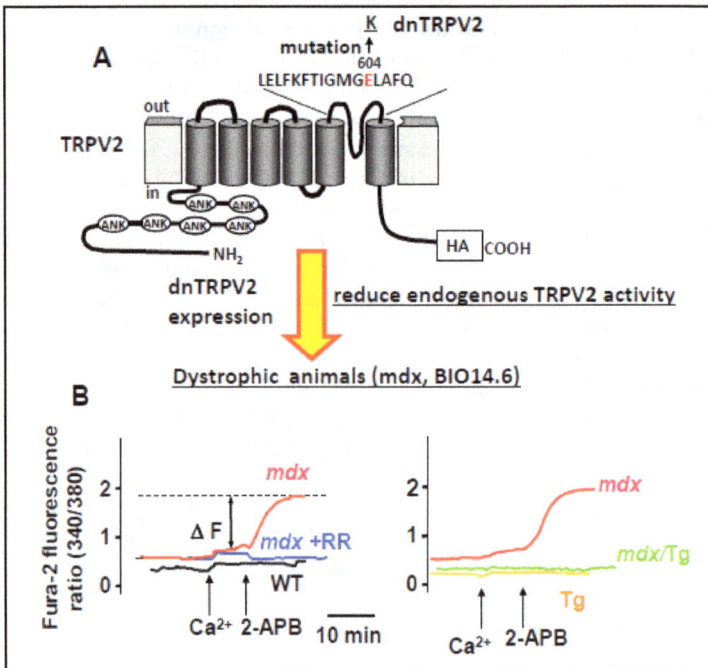

(A) Transgenic (Tg) mice overexpressing the TRPV2 mutant with a mutation in the putative pore region (Glu604) were produced, and crossed with *mdx* mice to introduce dnTRPV2 and inhibit endogenous TRPV2 activity. ANK, ankyrin repeat domain. HA, epitope tag. (B) Agonist (2-APB)-induced $[Ca^{2+}]_i$ increase in the isolated flexor digitorum brevis fibers of *mdx* mice, which is inhibited by ruthenium red (RR) (left). Note that no large $[Ca^{2+}]_i$ increase was detected in the fibers from wild-type mice. Such $[Ca^{2+}]_i$ increases in the *mdx* fibers were markedly reduced by expression of dnTRPV2 (*mdx*/Tg) (right) (Iwata et al., 2009).

Fig. 3. Production of a dominant-negative (dn) TRPV2 mutant

Transgenic or adenoviral expression of dnTRPV2 resulted in a 40%–70% reduction of impaired muscle function, as determined by an increased number of central nuclei and improvements in fiber size variability, fibrosis, apoptosis, elevated serum creatine kinase levels, and reduced muscle performance in dystrophic animals (Fig.4 A) (Iwata et al., 2009). Furthermore, *mdx* muscles were largely protected from eccentric work-induced force drop by the same transgenic strategy (Zanou et al., 2009). These results suggest that the entry of Ca^{2+} through TRPV2 channels precedes and is involved in membrane damage. Interestingly, expression of dnTRPV2 also promoted the removal of endogenous TRPV2 from the sarcolemma (Fig.4 B), suggesting that Ca^{2+} entering the cell via TRPV2 is required for the sarcolemmal retention of TRPV2 expression in dystrophic muscles. The pathological importance of TRPV2 was also verified using a pharmacological approach. A non-selective cation channel blocker tranilast was shown to be an effective inhibitor of TRPV2 (Iwata et al., 2005). Oral administration of tranilast reduced various symptoms of muscular dystrophy, such as elevated serum CK levels, progressive muscle degeneration, and increased infiltration of immune cells (Fig.5 A) (Iwata et al., 2005). Therefore, specific inhibitors of TRPV2 could be potentially useful and effective treatments for various muscle degenerative diseases, including hereditary diseases.

Although the relationship between muscular dystrophy and other types of TRPV channel has not yet been investigated, TRPV4 was recently identified as a responsive gene in inherited neurodegenerative disease, which indirectly causes muscle atrophy (Deng et al., 2010; Landoure et al., 2010).

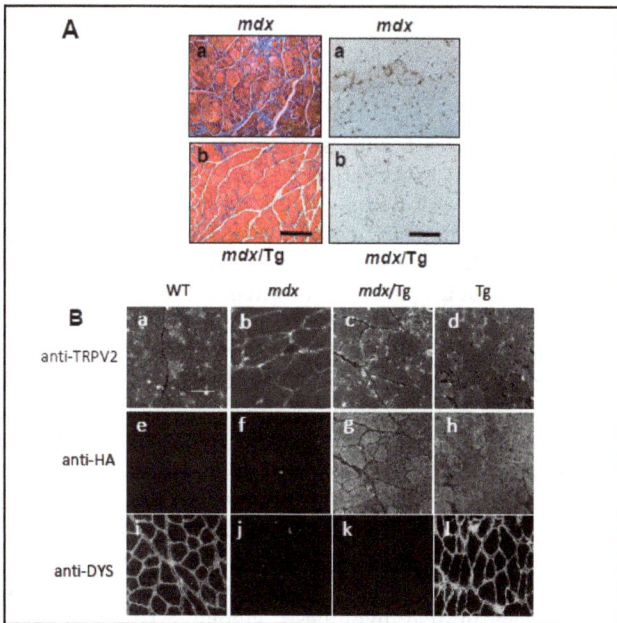

(A) Masson's trichrome staining (left) or TUNEL labeling (right) of the gastrocnemius muscle sections from *mdx* (a) or *mdx*/Tg (b) mice. Note the beneficial effect of dnTRPV2 (*mdx*/Tg). Scale bar, 100 μm. (B) Immunohistochemical analysis of TRPV2 (a-d) and dystrophin (i-l) in frozen cross sections of skeletal muscle. Dominant negative TRPV2 was immunolocalized with rat anti-HA (e-h). Note the removal of TRPV2 from the sarcolemma promoted by dnTRPV2 (*mdx*/Tg). Scale bar, 50 μm.

Fig. 4. Dominant-negative TRPV2 prevents muscle degeneration in *mdx* mice

3.2 TRPC channels

TRPC channels represent another important candidate for a therapeutic target in the treatment of muscular dystrophy. TRPC1, 4, and 6 are expressed in the sarcolemma of the skeletal muscle (Vandebrouck et al., 2002b). Knockdown of TRPC1 and TRPC4, but not TRPC6, was reported to reduce abnormal Ca^{2+} influx in dystrophic fibers (Vandebrouck et al., 2002b). TRPC1 has been shown to form the stretch-activated channel (Maroto et al., 2005), although contrary data also exists (Gottlieb et al., 2008). TRPC1, together with its binding partner caveolin-3, accumulates at higher levels in the sarcolemma of the dystrophin-deficient muscle and contributes to abnormal Ca^{2+} influx, which is activated by reactive oxygen species and Src kinase (Allen & Whitehead, 2011; Gervasio et al., 2008). Furthermore, mice lacking the scaffolding protein Homer-1, which interacts with TRPC1, exhibit myopathy associated with increased spontaneous cation influx (Stiber et al., 2008b). A recent study (Millay et al., 2009) also showed that overexpression of TRPC3 resulted in a phenotype of muscular dystrophy nearly identical to that observed in dystrophic animal models with abnormal DGC. Transgene-mediated inhibition of TRPC channels dramatically reduced the dystrophic phenotype in this animal model. These results suggest that Ca^{2+} entry through TRPC channels is sufficient to induce muscular dystrophy *in vivo*, and that TRPC channels are also promising therapeutic targets for muscular dysgenesis.

3.3 STIM1 and Orai1

Recently, the molecules involved in store-operated Ca^{2+} entry (SOCE) were identified. Stromal interaction molecules (STIM) were identified as the endoplasmic reticulum (ER) Ca^{2+} sensor, and found to interact with sarcolemmal Orai1 channels after Ca^{2+} store depletion to trigger SOCE. STIM1 and Orai1 are highly expressed in skeletal muscle: STIM1 is pre-localized at junctions of the SR with the T-tubule system, which contains pre-localized Orai1 (Stiber et al., 2008a). STIM1/Orai1 couples with TRPC channels (Dirksen, 2009) and the resulting STIM1/Orai1/TRPC1 ternary complexes have been shown to assemble during store depletion, thereby contributing to SOCE (Yuan et al., 2007; Zeng et al., 2008). Recently, the amount of STIM1/Orai1 proteins was reported to be upregulated in *mdx* muscle fibers, and the thresholds for the activation and deactivation of SOCE shifted to higher SR Ca^{2+} concentrations. This contributes to increased Ca^{2+} influx during long stimulation periods in *mdx* muscles (Edwards et al., 2010). In contrast, knockdown or inhibition of STIM1/Orai1 function was reported to cause myopathy resulting from impaired muscle development, which is different to muscular dystrophy caused by DGC defects. For example, mice lacking either STIM1 or Orai1 display skeletal muscle myopathy (Stiber et al., 2008a), and severe combined immunodeficiency patients characterized by loss-of-function mutations in STIM1/Orai1 signaling display similar skeletal muscle myopathy (Feske et al., 2006). Knockdown of STIM1 or expression of the Orai1 dominant negative E106Q caused a marked decrease in SOCE in skeletal muscle myotubes (Lyfenko & Dirksen, 2008). These findings suggest that STIM1/Orai1 proteins are involved in the fine-tuning of Ca^{2+} regulation, and physiological levels are required for normal skeletal muscle function.

3.4 Na⁺-dependent ion transporters

In addition to $[Ca^{2+}]_i$, $[Na^+]_i$ is also reported to be elevated in skeletal muscle of *mdx* mice (Dunn et al., 1993). The increase in $[Na^+]_i$ is accompanied by a compensatory increase in membrane-bound Na^+/K^+ ATPase contents (Dunn et al., 1995). A possible cause of increased $[Na^+]_i$ in the *mdx* skeletal muscle may be enhanced activity of stretch-activated channels, since it was inhibited by Gd^{3+} and streptomycin, which are known to be broad inhibitors of this channel type (Yeung et al., 2003a; Yeung et al., 2003b). It has also been shown that increases in $[Na^+]_i$ under the sarcolemma in *mdx* mice may be due to alterations in localization and gating properties of Nav1.4; the skeletal muscle isoform of the voltage-gated sodium channel may be correlated with increased cell death because $[Na^+]_i$ overload is reversed by tetrodotoxin, a specific Nav1.4 blocker (Hirn et al., 2008).

Recently, we have shown that the sarcolemmal Na^+/H^+ exchanger (NHE), which is known to be stimulated in response to various stimuli, including growth factors and osmotic stress, is significantly activated in dystrophic myocytes (from BIO14.6 hamsters). This is evidenced by an alkaline shift in the intracellular pH (pH_i) dependent on NHE activity, enhanced $^{22}Na^+$ influx, and elevated $[Na^+]_i$ (Iwata et al., 2007). In dystrophic myotubes, NHE was found to be a major Na^+ influx pathway, since the specific NHE inhibitor cariporide markedly (65%) inhibited it. Interestingly, NHE inhibition also significantly reduced the increase in intracellular Ca^{2+} and stretch-induced CK release in dystrophic myotubes, and ameliorated myopathic damage *in vivo* (Fig.5 B) (Iwata et al., 2007), indicating that the inhibition of NHE protects muscle cells against injury. Elevation in $[Na^+]_i$ may contribute to abnormal Ca^{2+} homeostasis by influencing the activity of the Na^+/Ca^{2+} exchanger.

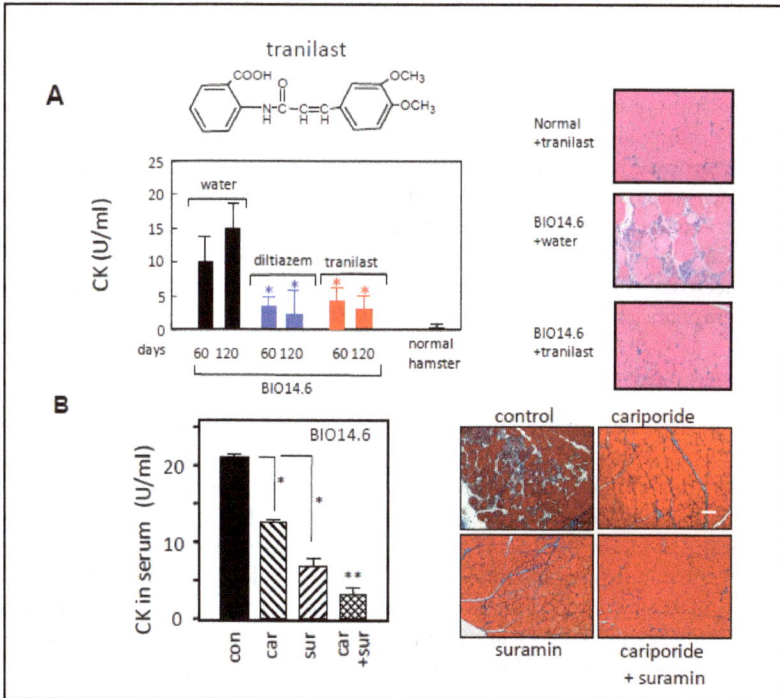

(A) Beneficial effect of the Ca^{2+}-handling drugs diltiazem and tranilast. Chemicals were administered orally to 30-day-old BIO14.6 hamsters for 60 or 120 days. The TRPV2 inhibitor tranilast effectively reduces CK release (left) and prevents muscle degeneration (H&E staining, right) (Iwata et al., 2005). (B) Beneficial effect of the P2 receptor antagonist suramin (sur) and the NHE inhibitor cariporide (car). In particular, note an excellent amelioration of muscle degeneration by combined administration of the two chemicals (Masson's trichrome staining of the quadriceps muscle sections, right) (Iwata et al., 2007). Scale bar, 100 μm.

Fig. 5. Effects of pharmacological agents on muscle degeneration in BIO14.6 hamsters

Furthermore, ATP was released more easily from the dystrophic myotubes in response to mechanical stretch. Thus, it is likely that P2 receptor stimulation with ATP activates the NHE, thereby leading to $[Ca^{2+}]_i$ overload (Iwata et al., 2007). These molecules also represent good targets for muscular dystrophy therapy. In fact, combined treatment with the P2 receptor antagonist suramin and the NHE1-specific inhibitor cariporide resulted in efficient amelioration of muscular dystrophy in BIO14.6 hamsters (Fig.5 B).

3.5 SR proteins

Recently, the occurrence of increased Ca^{2+} sparks, an indication of abnormalities in the SR Ca^{2+} release channel ryanodine receptor (RyR1), was reported in dystrophic fibers (Bellinger et al., 2009; Wang et al., 2005). RyR1 from *mdx* mice were shown to be excessively cystein-nitrosylated, which was coupled with depletion of calstabin-1 (calcium channel-stabilizing binding protein-1, also known as FKBP12) from RyR1. As a consequence, this led to increased spontaneous RyR1 openings (Ca^{2+} sparks), and reduced specific muscle force. Prevention of calstabin-1 depletion from RyR1 inhibited SR Ca^{2+} leak, reduced muscle damage, improved muscle function, and increased exercise performance in *mdx* mice (Bellinger et al., 2009).

One strategy to reduce the effects associated with chronic Ca^{2+} leak from activated channels and membrane rupture is to increase the rate of Ca^{2+} reuptake into the SR, by overexpression of the SR Ca^{2+} pump SERCA1. Indeed, transgenic overexpression of SERCA1 dramatically rescued the dystrophic phenotype of delta-sarcoglycan-null mice (Goonasekera et al., 2011). Furthermore, Ca^{2+} removal by adenovirus-mediated overexpression of SERCA1a reduced susceptibility to contraction-induced damage in *mdx* mice (Morine et al., 2010). These results suggest that Ca^{2+} is a common risk factor in the transmission of most genetic defects to downstream necrosis pathways in muscular dystrophy. Thus, control of $[Ca^{2+}]_i$ would provide a universal therapeutic strategy that reduces the dystrophic phenotype.

3.6 Other candidates

Dystrophic muscles are always exposed to oxidative and immune stress, as well as mechanical stress. Although not discussed in detail in this chapter, there are many important stress-dependent factors leading to muscle injury in muscular dystrophy (Lawler, 2011; Tidball & Wehling-Henricks, 2007). For example, NADPH oxidase in the muscles was recently reported to be an important source of oxidative stress, which stimulates stretch-activated Ca^{2+} entry in dystrophic muscles (Whitehead et al., 2010). Futhermore, nitric oxide (NO) synthase in macrophages may be another risk factor that promotes membrane injury in dystrophic muscles (Villalta et al., 2009). Therapeutic interventions that regulate stress pathways may be useful in protecting against dystrophic phenotypes.

4. Conclusion

As described above, disruption of the DGC results in increased mechanical stress and abnormal ion homeostasis. Sustained increases in $[Ca^{2+}]_i$ are the key pathological event leading to muscle degeneration (Fig.6). Many key players contribute to abnormal Ca^{2+} handling. Among these molecules, we consider TRPV2 to have high therapeutic potential for the treatment of muscular dystrophy, because most TRPV2 localizes to the intracellular

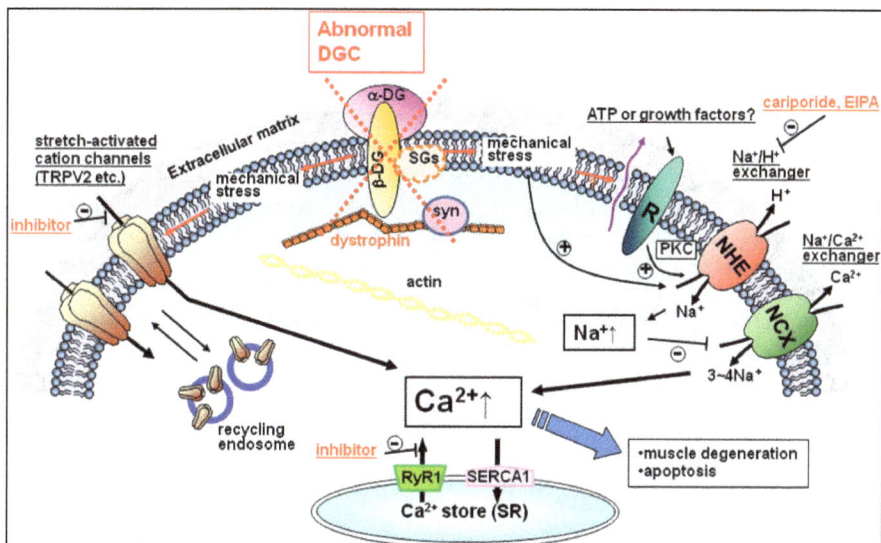

Fig. 6. Schematic drawing showing a possible pathway leading to abnormal Ca^{2+} handling and subsequent muscle degeneration in DGC-defective dystrophic muscles, according to our recent studies (Iwata et al., 2003; 2009; 2007; 2005) Increased mechanical stress caused by DGC defects induces sarcolemmal translocation and TRPV2 activation, leading to sustained [Ca^{2+}]$_i$ increase. On the other hand, mechanical stress also induces release of bioactive substances such as ATP and growth factors, which, in turn, activates NHE, increases [Na$^+$]$_i$, and results in further increase in [Ca^{2+}]$_i$ via inhibition of the NCX forward mode. Ca^{2+} handling proteins in the SR may also contribute to cytosolic Ca^{2+} overload. Therapeutic intervention at the level of Ca^{2+}-handling proteins would be useful for reducing the dystrophic phenotype.

membranes in the healthy skeletal muscles, while it translocates to the surface membrane upon muscle degeneration. Hence, specific inhibitors against TRPV2 are expected to act only on degenerative muscles. Given the lack of a definitive strategy to cure muscular dystrophy, identifying new therapeutic targets appears to be extremely important. We hope that this chapter might help to provide an opportunity to promote such studies.

5. Acknowledgments

We thank all the members of our laboratory who participated in the studies described in this chapter for their contribution and advice. We also thank the staff in the National Cerebral and Cardiovascular Center and the National Center of Neurology and Psychiatry for financial support and helpful suggestions.

6. References

Alderton, J. M. & Steinhardt, R. A. 2000a. Calcium influx through calcium leak channels is responsible for the elevated levels of calcium-dependent proteolysis in dystrophic myotubes. *Journal of Biological Chemistry*, 275(13): 9452-9460.

Alderton, J. M. & Steinhardt, R. A. 2000b. How calcium influx through calcium leak channels is responsible for the elevated levels of calcium-dependent proteolysis in dystrophic myotubes. *Trends in Cardiovascular Medicine*, 10(6): 268-272.

Allen, D. G. & Whitehead, N. P. 2011. Duchenne muscular dystrophy--what causes the increased membrane permeability in skeletal muscle? *International Journal of Biochemistry and Cell Biology*, 43(3): 290-294.

Bellinger, A. M.; Reiken, S.; Carlson, C.; Mongillo, M.; Liu, X.; Rothman, L.; Matecki, S.; Lacampagne, A. & Marks, A. R. 2009. Hypernitrosylated ryanodine receptor calcium release channels are leaky in dystrophic muscle. *Nature Medicine*, 15(3): 325-330.

Boittin, F. X.; Petermann, O.; Hirn, C.; Mittaud, P.; Dorchies, O. M.; Roulet, E. & Ruegg, U. T. 2006. Ca^{2+}-independent phospholipase A2 enhances store-operated Ca^{2+} entry in dystrophic skeletal muscle fibers. *Journal of Cell Science*, 119(Pt 18): 3733-3742.

Brown, R. H., Jr. 1997. Dystrophin-associated proteins and the muscular dystrophies. *Annual Review of Medicine*, 48: 457-466.

Campbell, K. P. 1995. Three muscular dystrophies: loss of cytoskeleton-extracellular matrix linkage. *Cell*, 80(5): 675-679.

Campbell, K. P. & Kahl, S. D. 1989. Association of dystrophin and an integral membrane glycoprotein. *Nature*, 338(6212): 259-262.

Deng, H. X.; Klein, C. J.; Yan, J.; Shi, Y.; Wu, Y.; Fecto, F.; Yau, H. J.; Yang, Y.; Zhai, H.; Siddique, N.; Hedley-Whyte, E. T.; Delong, R.; Martina, M.; Dyck, P. J. & Siddique, T. 2010. Scapuloperoneal spinal muscular atrophy and CMT2C are allelic disorders caused by alterations in TRPV4. *Nature Genetics*, 42(2): 165-169.

Dirksen, R. T. 2009. Checking your SOCCs and feet: the molecular mechanisms of Ca^{2+} entry in skeletal muscle. *J Physiol*, 587(Pt 13): 3139-3147.

Duclos, F.; Straub, V.; Moore, S. A.; Venzke, D. P.; Hrstka, R. F.; Crosbie, R. H.; Durbeej, M.; Lebakken, C. S.; Ettinger, A. J.; van der Meulen, J.; Holt, K. H.; Lim, L. E.; Sanes, J. R.; Davidson, B. L.; Faulkner, J. A.; Williamson, R. & Campbell, K. P. 1998. Progressive muscular dystrophy in alpha-sarcoglycan-deficient mice. *Journal of Cell Biology*, 142(6): 1461-1471.

Ducret, T.; Vandebrouck, C.; Cao, M. L.; Lebacq, J. & Gailly, P. 2006. Functional role of store-operated and stretch-activated channels in murine adult skeletal muscle fibres. *J Physiol*, 575(Pt 3): 913-924.

Dunn, J. F.; Bannister, N.; Kemp, G. J. & Publicover, S. J. 1993. Sodium is elevated in mdx muscles: ionic interactions in dystrophic cells. *Journal of the Neurological Sciences*, 114(1): 76-80.

Dunn, J. F.; Burton, K. A. & Dauncey, M. J. 1995. Ouabain sensitive Na^+/K^+-ATPase content is elevated in mdx mice: implications for the regulation of ions in dystrophic muscle. *Journal of the Neurological Sciences*, 133(1-2): 11-15.

Edwards, J. N.; Friedrich, O.; Cully, T. R.; von Wegner, F.; Murphy, R. M. & Launikonis, B. S. 2010. Upregulation of store-operated Ca^{2+} entry in dystrophic mdx mouse muscle. *Am J Physiol Cell Physiol*, 299(1): C42-50.

Ervasti, J. M. & Campbell, K. P. 1993. A role for the dystrophin-glycoprotein complex as a transmembrane linker between laminin and actin. *Journal of Cell Biology*, 122(4): 809-823.

Feske, S.; Gwack, Y.; Prakriya, M.; Srikanth, S.; Puppel, S. H.; Tanasa, B.; Hogan, P. G.; Lewis, R. S.; Daly, M. & Rao, A. 2006. A mutation in Orai1 causes immune deficiency by abrogating CRAC channel function. *Nature*, 441(7090): 179-185.

Fong, P. Y.; Turner, P. R.; Denetclaw, W. F. & Steinhardt, R. A. 1990. Increased activity of calcium leak channels in myotubes of Duchenne human and mdx mouse origin. *Science*, 250(4981): 673-676.

Franco-Obregon, A., Jr. & Lansman, J. B. 1994. Mechanosensitive ion channels in skeletal muscle from normal and dystrophic mice. *J Physiol*, 481 (Pt 2): 299-309.

Franco-Obregon, A. & Lansman, J. B. 2002. Changes in mechanosensitive channel gating following mechanical stimulation in skeletal muscle myotubes from the mdx mouse. *J Physiol*, 539(Pt 2): 391-407.

Franco, A., Jr. & Lansman, J. B. 1990. Calcium entry through stretch-inactivated ion channels in mdx myotubes. *Nature*, 344(6267): 670-673.

Gervasio, O. L.; Whitehead, N. P.; Yeung, E. W.; Phillips, W. D. & Allen, D. G. 2008. TRPC1 binds to caveolin-3 and is regulated by Src kinase - role in Duchenne muscular dystrophy. *Journal of Cell Science*, 121(Pt 13): 2246-2255.

Goonasekera, S. A.; Lam, C. K.; Millay, D. P.; Sargent, M. A.; Hajjar, R. J.; Kranias, E. G. & Molkentin, J. D. 2011. Mitigation of muscular dystrophy in mice by SERCA overexpression in skeletal muscle. *Journal of Clinical Investigation*, 121(3): 1044-1052.

Gottlieb, P.; Folgering, J.; Maroto, R.; Raso, A.; Wood, T. G.; Kurosky, A.; Bowman, C.; Bichet, D.; Patel, A.; Sachs, F.; Martinac, B.; Hamill, O. P. & Honore, E. 2008. Revisiting TRPC1 and TRPC6 mechanosensitivity. *Pflugers Archiv. European Journal of Physiology*, 455(6): 1097-1103.

Hamill, O. P. & McBride, D. W., Jr. 1996. The pharmacology of mechanogated membrane ion channels. *Pharmacological Reviews*, 48(2): 231-252.

Hirn, C.; Shapovalov, G.; Petermann, O.; Roulet, E. & Ruegg, U. T. 2008. Nav1.4 deregulation in dystrophic skeletal muscle leads to Na^+ overload and enhanced cell death. *Journal of General Physiology*, 132(2): 199-208.

Hopf, F. W.; Turner, P. R.; Denetclaw, W. F., Jr.; Reddy, P. & Steinhardt, R. A. 1996. A critical evaluation of resting intracellular free calcium regulation in dystrophic mdx muscle. *American Journal of Physiology*, 271(4 Pt 1): C1325-1339.

Iwata, Y.; Katanosaka, Y.; Arai, Y.; Komamura, K.; Miyatake, K. & Shigekawa, M. 2003. A novel mechanism of myocyte degeneration involving the Ca^{2+}-permeable growth factor-regulated channel. *Journal of Cell Biology*, 161(5): 957-967.

Iwata, Y.; Katanosaka, Y.; Arai, Y.; Shigekawa, M. & Wakabayashi, S. 2009. Dominant-negative inhibition of Ca^{2+} influx via TRPV2 ameliorates muscular dystrophy in animal models. *Human Molecular Genetics*, 18(5): 824-834.

Iwata, Y.; Katanosaka, Y.; Hisamitsu, T. & Wakabayashi, S. 2007. Enhanced Na^+/H^+ Exchange Activity Contributes to the Pathogenesis of Muscular Dystrophy via Involvement of P2 Receptors. *American Journal of Pathology*, 171(5):1576-1587.

Iwata, Y.; Katanosaka, Y.; Shijun, Z.; Kobayashi, Y.; Hanada, H.; Shigekawa, M. & Wakabayashi, S. 2005. Protective effects of Ca^{2+} handling drugs against abnormal Ca^{2+} homeostasis and cell damage in myopathic skeletal muscle cells. *Biochemical Pharmacology*, 70(5): 740-751.

Iwata, Y.; Nakamura, H.; Fujiwara, K. & Shigekawa, M. 1993a. Altered membrane-dystrophin association in the cardiomyopathic hamster heart muscle. *Biochemical and Biophysical Research Communications*, 190(2): 589-595.

Iwata, Y.; Nakamura, H.; Mizuno, Y.; Yoshida, M.; Ozawa, E. & Shigekawa, M. 1993b. Defective association of dystrophin with sarcolemmal glycoproteins in the cardiomyopathic hamster heart. *FEBS Letters*, 329(1-2): 227-231.

Kanzaki, M.; Zhang, Y. Q.; Mashima, H.; Li, L.; Shibata, H. & Kojima, I. 1999. Translocation of a calcium-permeable cation channel induced by insulin-like growth factor-I. *Nat Cell Biol*, 1(3): 165-170.

Landoure, G.; Zdebik, A. A.; Martinez, T. L.; Burnett, B. G.; Stanescu, H. C.; Inada, H.; Shi, Y.; Taye, A. A.; Kong, L.; Munns, C. H.; Choo, S. S.; Phelps, C. B.; Paudel, R.; Houlden, H.; Ludlow, C. L.; Caterina, M. J.; Gaudet, R.; Kleta, R.; Fischbeck, K. H. & Sumner, C. J. 2010. Mutations in TRPV4 cause Charcot-Marie-Tooth disease type 2C. *Nature Genetics*, 42(2): 170-174.

Lawler, J. M. 2011. Exacerbation of pathology by oxidative stress in respiratory and locomotor muscles with Duchenne muscular dystrophy. *J Physiol*, 589(Pt 9): 2161-2170.

Lyfenko, A. D. & Dirksen, R. T. 2008. Differential dependence of store-operated and excitation-coupled Ca^{2+} entry in skeletal muscle on STIM1 and Orai1. *J Physiol*, 586(Pt 20): 4815-4824.

MacLennan, P. A.; McArdle, A. & Edwards, R. H. 1991. Effects of calcium on protein turnover of incubated muscles from mdx mice. *American Journal of Physiology*, 260(4 Pt 1): E594-598.

Mallouk, N.; Jacquemond, V. & Allard, B. 2000. Elevated subsarcolemmal Ca^{2+} in mdx mouse skeletal muscle fibers detected with Ca^{2+}-activated K^+ channels. *Proceedings of the National Academy of Sciences of the United States of America*, 97(9): 4950-4955.

Maroto, R.; Raso, A.; Wood, T. G.; Kurosky, A.; Martinac, B. & Hamill, O. P. 2005. TRPC1 forms the stretch-activated cation channel in vertebrate cells. *Nat Cell Biol*, 7(2): 179-185.

Menke, A. & Jockusch, H. 1991. Decreased osmotic stability of dystrophin-less muscle cells from the *mdx* mouse. *Nature*, 349(6304): 69-71.

Millay, D. P.; Goonasekera, S. A.; Sargent, M. A.; Maillet, M.; Aronow, B. J. & Molkentin, J. D. 2009. Calcium influx is sufficient to induce muscular dystrophy through a TRPC-dependent mechanism. *Proceedings of the National Academy of Sciences of the United States of America*, 106(45): 19023-19028.

Montell, C.; Birnbaumer, L. & Flockerzi, V. 2002. The TRP channels, a remarkably functional family. *Cell*, 108(5): 595-598.

Morine, K. J.; Sleeper, M. M.; Barton, E. R. & Sweeney, H. L. 2010. Overexpression of SERCA1a in the *mdx* diaphragm reduces susceptibility to contraction-induced damage. *Human Gene Therapy*, 21(12): 1735-1739.

Muraki, K.; Iwata, Y.; Katanosaka, Y.; Ito, T.; Ohya, S.; Shigekawa, M. & Imaizumi, Y. 2003. TRPV2 is a component of osmotically sensitive cation channels in murine aortic myocytes. *Circulation Research*, 93(9): 829-838.

Nakamura, T. Y.; Iwata, Y.; Sampaolesi, M.; Hanada, H.; Saito, N.; Artman, M.; Coetzee, W. A. & Shigekawa, M. 2001. Stretch-activated cation channels in skeletal muscle myotubes from sarcoglycan-deficient hamsters. *Am J Physiol Cell Physiol*, 281(2): C690-699.

Nigro, V.; Okazaki, Y.; Belsito, A.; Piluso, G.; Matsuda, Y.; Politano, L.; Nigro, G.; Ventura, C.; Abbondanza, C.; Molinari, A. M.; Acampora, D.; Nishimura, M.; Hayashizaki, Y. & Puca, G. A. 1997. Identification of the Syrian hamster cardiomyopathy gene. *Human Molecular Genetics*, 6(4): 601-607.

Petrof, B. J.; Shrager, J. B.; Stedman, H. H.; Kelly, A. M. & Sweeney, H. L. 1993. Dystrophin protects the sarcolemma from stresses developed during muscle contraction. *Proceedings of the National Academy of Sciences of the United States of America*, 90(8): 3710-3714.

Robert, V.; Massimino, M. L.; Tosello, V.; Marsault, R.; Cantini, M.; Sorrentino, V. & Pozzan, T. 2001. Alteration in calcium handling at the subcellular level in *mdx* myotubes. *Journal of Biological Chemistry*, 276(7): 4647-4651.

Spencer, M. J.; Croall, D. E. & Tidball, J. G. 1995. Calpains are activated in necrotic fibers from *mdx* dystrophic mice. *Journal of Biological Chemistry*, 270(18): 10909-10914.

Stiber, J.; Hawkins, A.; Zhang, Z. S.; Wang, S.; Burch, J.; Graham, V.; Ward, C. C.; Seth, M.; Finch, E.; Malouf, N.; Williams, R. S.; Eu, J. P. & Rosenberg, P. 2008a. STIM1 signalling controls store-operated calcium entry required for development and contractile function in skeletal muscle. *Nat Cell Biol*, 10(6): 688-697.

Stiber, J. A.; Zhang, Z. S.; Burch, J.; Eu, J. P.; Zhang, S.; Truskey, G. A.; Seth, M.; Yamaguchi, N.; Meissner, G.; Shah, R.; Worley, P. F.; Williams, R. S. & Rosenberg, P. B. 2008b. Mice lacking Homer 1 exhibit a skeletal myopathy characterized by abnormal transient receptor potential channel activity. *Molecular and Cellular Biology*, 28(8): 2637-2647.

Suchyna, T. M.; Johnson, J. H.; Hamer, K.; Leykam, J. F.; Gage, D. A.; Clemo, H. F.; Baumgarten, C. M. & Sachs, F. 2000. Identification of a peptide toxin from Grammostola spatulata spider venom that blocks cation-selective stretch-activated channels. *Journal of General Physiology*, 115(5): 583-598.

Tawada-Iwata, Y.; Imagawa, T.; Yoshida, A.; Takahashi, M.; Nakamura, H. & Shigekawa, M. 1993. Increased mechanical extraction of T-tubule/junctional SR from cardiomyopathic hamster heart. *American Journal of Physiology*, 264(5 Pt 2): H1447-1453.

Tidball, J. G. & Wehling-Henricks, M. 2007. The role of free radicals in the pathophysiology of muscular dystrophy. *Journal of Applied Physiology*, 102(4): 1677-1686.

Tinsley, J. M.; Blake, D. J.; Zuellig, R. A. & Davies, K. E. 1994. Increasing complexity of the dystrophin-associated protein complex. *Proceedings of the National Academy of Sciences of the United States of America*, 91(18): 8307-8313.

Turner, P. R.; Schultz, R.; Ganguly, B. & Steinhardt, R. A. 1993. Proteolysis results in altered leak channel kinetics and elevated free calcium in *mdx* muscle. *Journal of Membrane Biology*, 133(3): 243-251.

Turner, P. R.; Westwood, T.; Regen, C. M. & Steinhardt, R. A. 1988. Increased protein degradation results from elevated free calcium levels found in muscle from *mdx* mice. *Nature*, 335(6192): 735-738.

Vandebrouck, C.; Duport, G.; Cognard, C. & Raymond, G. 2001. Cationic channels in normal and dystrophic human myotubes. *Neuromuscular Disorders*, 11(1): 72-79.

Vandebrouck, C.; Duport, G.; Raymond, G. & Cognard, C. 2002a. Hypotonic medium increases calcium permeant channels activity in human normal and dystrophic myotubes. *Neuroscience Letters*, 323(3): 239-243.

Vandebrouck, C.; Martin, D.; Colson-Van Schoor, M.; Debaix, H. & Gailly, P. 2002b. Involvement of TRPC in the abnormal calcium influx observed in dystrophic (*mdx*) mouse skeletal muscle fibers. *Journal of Cell Biology*, 158(6): 1089-1096.

Villalta, S. A.; Nguyen, H. X.; Deng, B.; Gotoh, T. & Tidball, J. G. 2009. Shifts in macrophage phenotypes and macrophage competition for arginine metabolism affect the severity of muscle pathology in muscular dystrophy. *Human Molecular Genetics*, 18(3): 482-496.

Wang, X.; Weisleder, N.; Collet, C.; Zhou, J.; Chu, Y.; Hirata, Y.; Zhao, X.; Pan, Z.; Brotto, M.; Cheng, H. & Ma, J. 2005. Uncontrolled calcium sparks act as a dystrophic signal for mammalian skeletal muscle. *Nat Cell Biol*, 7(5): 525-530.

Whitehead, N. P.; Yeung, E. W.; Froehner, S. C. & Allen, D. G. 2010. Skeletal muscle NADPH oxidase is increased and triggers stretch-induced damage in the *mdx* mouse. *PLoS One*, 5(12): e15354.

Yeung, E. W.; Ballard, H. J.; Bourreau, J. P. & Allen, D. G. 2003a. Intracellular sodium in mammalian muscle fibers after eccentric contractions. *Journal of Applied Physiology*, 94(6): 2475-2482.

Yeung, E. W.; Head, S. I. & Allen, D. G. 2003b. Gadolinium reduces short-term stretch-induced muscle damage in isolated *mdx* mouse muscle fibres. *J Physiol*, 552(Pt 2): 449-458.

Yuan, J. P.; Zeng, W.; Huang, G. N.; Worley, P. F. & Muallem, S. 2007. STIM1 heteromultimerizes TRPC channels to determine their function as store-operated channels. *Nat Cell Biol*, 9(6): 636-645.

Zanou, N.; Iwata, Y.; Schakman, O.; Lebacq, J.; Wakabayashi, S. & Gailly, P. 2009. Essential role of TRPV2 ion channel in the sensitivity of dystrophic muscle to eccentric contractions. *FEBS Letters*, 583(22): 3600-3604.

Zeng, W.; Yuan, J. P.; Kim, M. S.; Choi, Y. J.; Huang, G. N.; Worley, P. F. & Muallem, S. 2008. STIM1 gates TRPC channels, but not Orai1, by electrostatic interaction. *Molecular Cell*, 32(3): 439-448.

7

Proteomic Analysis of Signalling Pathway Deregulation in Dystrophic Dog Muscle

Marie Féron[1], Karl Rouger[2] and Laetitia Guével[1,2]
[1]University of Nantes CNRS UMR6204,
[2]ONIRIS/INRA UMR 703,
France

1. Introduction

During recent years, considerable effort has been made to develop proteomics technologies, with the aim of providing a complementary approach to the genomics tools already used in biomedical settings. This development has been extremely fast, and a number of emerging methodological proteomics tools now allow scientists to study the variable aspects of proteins in particular cell types, tissues or disease states. These tools include antibody arrays, two-dimensional-gel electrophoresis (2D-GE) and mass spectrometry (MS), the latter knowing an increasing use. In particular, candidate or non-candidate-based analyses of cell signalling represent powerful approaches for the investigation of the answers developed by cells in response to genetic modifications. Signalling molecules are key players in the regulation of the numerous and various biological processes occurring in a cell, and the alteration of signalling pathways has been associated with multiple diseases. Alterations in individual signalling pathways have been described in neuromuscular disorders, however, little information is available regarding their putative implication in Duchenne Muscular Dystrophy (DMD).

DMD is an X-linked neuromuscular disorder that affects 1 newborn in 3500. This recessive disease represents the most common and severe form of muscular dystrophy. Although the genetic basis of the disease is well resolved, the cellular mechanisms associated with the physiopathology remain largely unknown. Increasing evidence suggests that mechanisms secondary to the dystrophin deficiency at the basis of the disease, such as alterations in key signalling pathways, may play an important role. Proteomic profiling of dystrophic *vs* healthy skeletal muscle can help to generate a DMD-specific proteomic signature. Understanding which particular signal transduction pathways are involved in muscular dystrophy might provide a basis for new target and therapeutic agents discovery. This chapter examines signalling pathways status in skeletal muscles from the Golden Retriever Muscular Dystrophy (GRMD) dog, the only clinically relevant animal model for DMD (Valentine et al., 1988; Cooper et al., 1988). More specifically, we will describe how proteomic studies were successfully used to identify reliable biomarkers of the disease in animal models.

2. Signalling pathways and DMD

In dystrophic muscles, the absence of dystrophin, and the consequent destabilization of the dystrophin-glycoprotein associated complex DGC (a multiprotein transmembrane complex), lead to the loss of sarcolemma integrity, calcium overload, calpains activation and finally, necrosis of the myofibers (Muntoni et al., 2003). Besides providing mechanical stability, the DGC interacts with several proteins, including growth factor receptor-bound protein 2 (Grb2) (Yang et al., 1995), neuronal nitric oxide synthase (nNOS) (Brenman et al., 1995), calmodulin (Madhavan et al., 1992), focal adhesion kinase (FAK) (Cavaldesi et al., 1999) and caveolin-3 (Crosbie et al., 1998), that play a role in cell signalling. Grb2 has been identified as a component of the Ras/ mitogen-activated protein kinases (MAPK) signalling pathway and both FAK and Grb2 function as mediators of survival signalling in various cell types, often working through the phosphatidyl inositol 3-kinase (PI3K)/Akt pathway (Langenbach&Rando, 2002). Even if this mechanism can, in part, account for the degenerative phenotype observed in DMD, it seems increasingly obvious that the deregulation of intracellular signalling pathways also plays a role. These pathways, which are implicated in the regulation of crucial processes such as the balance between apoptosis and cell survival or the equilibrium between atrophy and hypertrophy, involve cascades of phosphorylation/dephosphorylation events. Protein kinases represent key enzymes responsible for the phosphorylation of specific targets. Moreover, altered cell signalling is thought to increase the susceptibility of muscle fibers to secondary triggers, such as functional ischemia and oxidative stress, and free-radical scavengers can have a direct impact on the activity/phosphorylation of some components of the MAPK cascades (Hnia et al., 2007). In progressive muscular dystrophy, muscles are characterized by hypertrophy in the early phase, while atrophic changes are observed with aging (Noguchi, 2005).

Studies of the X chromosome-linked muscular dystrophy (*mdx*) mouse model of DMD (Bulfield et al., 1984) revealed modulations in MAPK signalling cascades, as dystrophic animals exhibited increased phosphorylation of extracellular signal-regulated kinases 1 and 2 (ERK1/2) (Kumar et al., 2004; Lang et al., 2004) and c-jun N-terminal kinases 1 and 2 (JNK1/2) (Kolodziejczyk et al., 2001; Nakamura et al., 2005; St-Pierre et al., 2004), and decreased phosphorylation of p38 (Lang et al., 2004). The PI3K/Akt signalling pathway has also been shown to be affected in the *mdx* mouse, with an increased synthesis and phosphorylation of Akt observed (Dogra et al., 2006; Peter&Crosbie, 2006). Studies finally demonstrated that directly modulating signalling pathways activity could improve *mdx* muscle function (Kim et al., 2010; Tang et al., 2010). More specifically, increasing Akt activity by transgenic overexpression of the activated kinase itself has been shown to be able to reverse the dystrophic phenotype (Blaauw et al., 2009; Peter et al., 2009).

Moreover, the phosphorylation status of Akt was shown to be altered in human and canine dystrophic biopsies (Peter&Crosbie, 2006; Feron et al., 2009). Enhanced expression and activity of the phosphatidylinositol-3,4,5-trisphosphate 3-phosphatase (PTEN) has been observed in dystrophin-deficient dog muscle, and proposed to be at the origin of Akt inactivation (Feron et al., 2009). Indeed, PTEN opposes PI3K action by dephosphorylating phosphatidylinositol (3,4,5)-triphosphate (PtdIns(3,4,5)P_3) (Maehama&Dixon, 1998) and the increased activity detected in GRMD muscle would presumably lead to a decreased level of the phosphoinositide, which should limit the recruitment and activation of Akt (see Figure 1 for a schematic representation of the signalling pathway deregulation in dystrophic dog muscle).

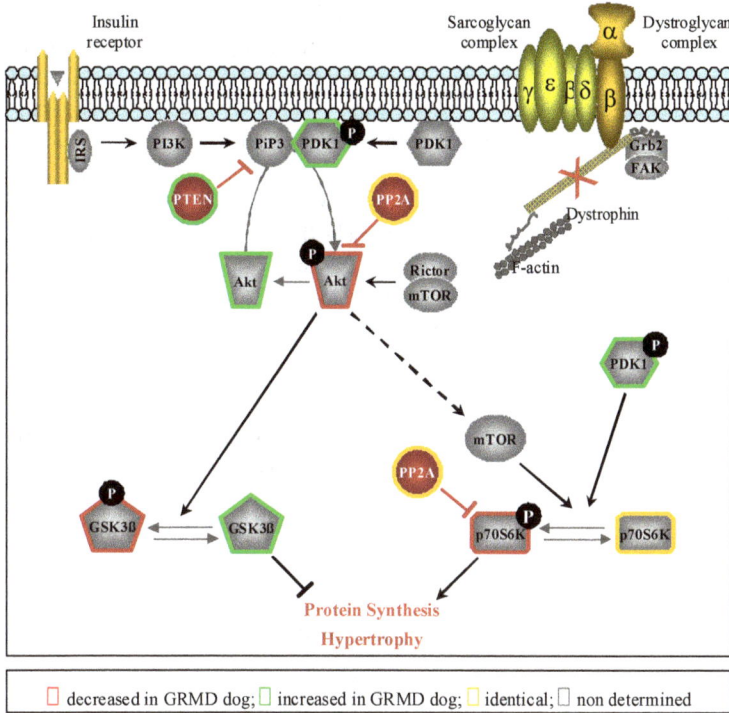

Fig. 1. Schematic diagram of signalling in the PI3K/Akt pathway and deregulations detected in GRMD skeletal muscle. Proteins shown in red, green and yellow indicate decreased, increased and unchanged level of expression or activity of these enzymes in GRMD vs. healthy muscle, respectively. As protein phosphatase 2A (PP2A) activity was not statistically modulated in GRMD muscle, the protein is shown in yellow. The deregulations detected in GRMD skeletal muscle could lead to decreased protein synthesis and block compensatory hypertrophy.

Akt directly phosphorylates glycogen synthase kinase-3 (GSK3β) at Ser9, thereby repressing its activity (Cross et al., 1995), and catalyses, via the mammalian target of rapamycin (mTOR), 70-kDa ribosomal protein S6 kinase (p70S6K) phosphorylation and activation (Chung et al., 1992; Glass, 2005; Inoki et al., 2002; Inoki et al., 2005; Price et al., 1992) (Figure 1). The PI3K/Akt/GSK3β and PI3K/Akt/mTOR/p70S6K pathways have been implicated in the regulation of skeletal muscle mass. Akt/mTOR signals were found to be upregulated during hypertrophy and downregulated during atrophy and the activation of Akt or p70S6K (or inactivation of GSK3β) appeared to be sufficient to induce hypertrophy. Moreover, in addition to acting as an inductive cue for hypertrophy, activation of the Akt/mTOR pathway could also prevent muscle atrophy in vivo (Bodine et al., 2001; Rommel et al., 2001). Furthermore, it has been shown in vitro that the overexpression of Src homology 2 (SH2) domain-containing inositol-5'-phosphatase 2 (SHIP-2), which, like PTEN, decreases PIP3 level, led to atrophy whereas the overexpression of a dominant negative mutant, which increases PIP3 level, induced hypertrophy (Rommel et al., 2001). The overexpression of

SHIP-2 in healthy mice muscle had no effect on fiber size but the overexpression of the phosphatase in a model of compensatory hypertrophy completely blocked the hypertrophy response (Bodine et al., 2001). It is thereby likely that the overexpression and increased activity of PTEN detected in GRMD muscle (by decreasing Akt activity and p70S6K phosphorylation, and by activating GSK3β) could prevent compensatory muscle hypertrophy. More recently, the peroxisome proliferator-activated receptor-gamma co-activator 1 alpha (PGC-1α) and PTEN inhibitor DJ-1/Parkinson disease (autosomal recessive early-onset) 7 (PARK7) appeared substantially reduced in GRMD *vs* healthy muscle (Feron et al., 2009; Guevel et al., 2011). Given the role of DJ-1 in the regulation of PTEN, this suggests that PTEN activation in GRMD dog muscle may originate from the under-expression of DJ-1. Noteworthy, in addition to its role in PTEN's regulation, DJ-1 also promotes the activity of PGC-1α (Zhong&Xu, 2008). As such, DJ-1 sensitive signalling pathways may provide high priority targets for the development of novel drug therapies for DMD.

Thus, compelling evidence suggest that alterations in signal transduction pathways may represent significant contributing factors to the progression of DMD. Proteomic profiling performed on the *mdx* mouse (Doran et al., 2006; Lewis et al., 2009; Ohlendieck, 2011) and GRMD dog models (Feron et al., 2009; Guevel et al., 2011) identified signalling proteins and reliable biomarkers of the secondary changes taking place in dystrophic muscles.

3. Proteomic analysis of dystrophic dog muscle

Proteomic approaches have been developed in order to try to identify putative biomarkers of DMD. The proteome-wide investigation of proteins requires technological efforts in three essential steps: the separation, the identification and the quantification of multiple proteins. Reversible protein phosphorylation is arguably the most common and significant mechanism for the dynamic control of biological processes. Phosphorylation can dramatically alter a protein's biological location and/or activity and recent studies clearly highlighted the involvement of phosphoproteins and kinases in DMD (Kolodziejczyk et al., 2001; Kumar et al., 2004; Lang et al., 2004; Peter&Crosbie, 2006; Feron et al., 2009). Although up to one-third of the total proteome might be phosphorylated, the absolute levels of any single protein specie might be very low. In contrast to the traditional biochemical study of single proteins or isolated pathways in the context of muscular dystrophy, technical advances in the high-throughput screening by MS and array-based technology have established new ways of identifying entire cellular proteins populations in one shift analytical approach.

Global identification of signalling proteins can be done by a dedicated approach using antibody arrays. Antibody arrays also serve as an attractive option to carry out phosphoproteomic profiling in disease (Feron et al., 2009; Gembitsky et al., 2004; Kingsmore, 2006). Phospho-specific antibody arrays commercially available facilitate the investigation of specific activated pathways in muscular disorders. On the other hand, a considerable number of proteomic studies have employed unbiased technology such as 2D-GE and stable isotope-labelling techniques combined with MS. To construct an accurate model of the proteome variations occurring in dystrophic dog muscle, complementary proteomic screenings have been done (Figure 2).

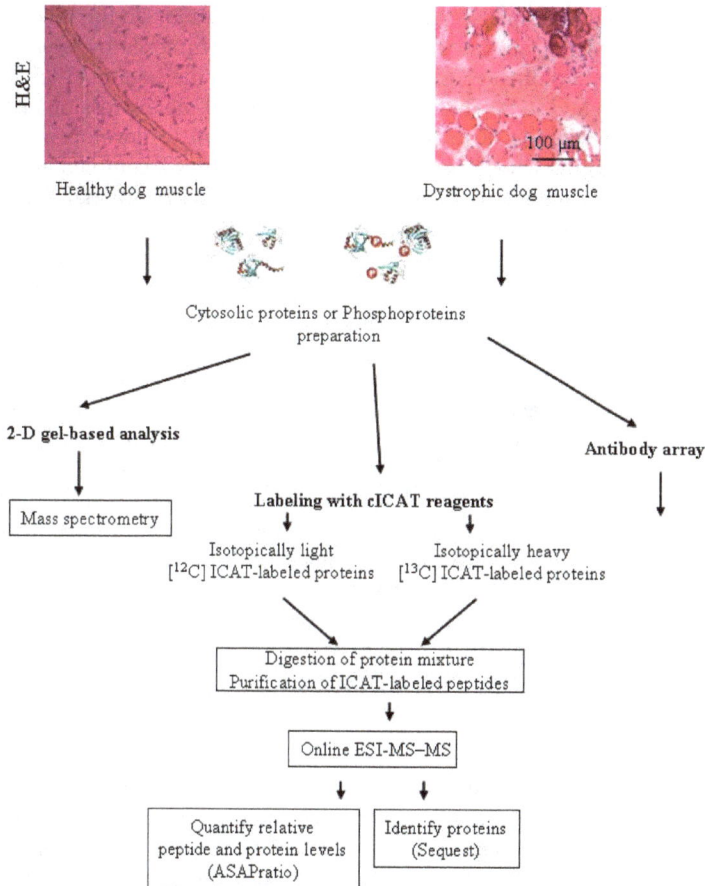

Fig. 2. Schematic diagram of the proteomic analysis of dystrophic dog muscle. H&E (hematoxylin and eosin) staining showing classical pathological changes of DMD, including fiber size variation, fiber splitting, and central nucleation in skeletal muscle. 2D-GE, isotope-coded affinity tag (ICAT) quantitative proteomic analysis and antibody array of proteins purified from 4-month-old healthy and GRMD dog muscle.

3.1 Protein array profiling

Biomedical research of the 21st century will largely be based on the results of studies focusing on the evaluation of gene expression and performed in order to develop molecular tools for the diagnosis and treatment of human diseases. Currently, DNA arrays represent the most commonly used means to follow gene expression in health and disease, and in muscular dystrophies in particular (Chen et al., 2000; Rouger et al., 2002). However, gene expression studies are limited by several aspects: i) gene expression levels do not necessarily reflect the level of proteins (that can also be regulated by degradation), ii) the activity of some proteins is regulated by posttranslational modifications (PTM) such as phosphorylation, glycosylation, carbonylation, acetylation and ubiquitylation, or by allosteric modifications and iii) localization changes can also play roles in this regulation. On the other hand, a lot of studies have been focusing on single proteins, protein complexes or isolated pathways, limiting the understanding of the pathogenesis of DMD at the organism level. In order to obtain this information and to be able to measure in parallel the expression and the state of activation of several hundreds of proteins, it was important to develop new approaches. Protein array-based approaches can provide not only data complementary to DNA microarrays but also provide unique information about the functional state of proteins under normal and pathological conditions (Hanash, 2003; MacBeath, 2002). Miniaturized protein array technology has opened a new chapter in biotechnology due to its ability to compare, characterize and quantify simultaneously a large number of proteins in the form of spots, thus replacing numerous individual protein by protein tests.It also allows parallel evaluation of several parameters in complex biological solutions. Moreover, a minute spot with immobilized protein sample on an array slide provides greater sensitivity for the detection of molecular interactions compared to other binding assays (Ekins&Chu, 1999). For the first time, antibody arrays were used by Anderson group to look for protein expression changes in spinal muscular atrophy (Anderson&Davison, 1999). A relatively small number of differences were found within a group of proteins that function as both RNA binding proteins and transcription factors. A second group used microarrays to profile the level of proteins associated with calcium regulation in sarcoplasmic reticulum isolated from muscle (Schulz et al., 2006). They used a reverse-phase protein array printed with proteins from genotyped animals and probed with seven target proteins important in calcium regulation. Reverse-phase arrays have been used for profiling phosphorylated proteins in various cancers (Grubb et al., 2003; Sheehan et al., 2005), and it was hoped that these arrays would become a powerful clinical tool for diagnosis and therapy guidance in different diseases.

More recently, the antibody array technology was used to assess the phosphorylation status of key proteins of the MAPK and PI3K/Akt signalling pathways in the *Vastus lateralis* muscle from 4-month old GRMD *vs* healthy dogs. The antibody array technology represents a powerful tool for the semi-quantitative comparison of the expression and/or phosphorylation level of a high number of proteins in a limited number of samples (Sakanyan, 2005; Yeretssian et al., 2005). The main advantage resides in the gain of time that it provides, as a high number of proteins can be studied in just one experiment. Moreover (and in contrary to the ICAT technology for example), antibody arrays give access to information about PTM, such as phosphorylation, which is of course crucial in the context of cell signalling. Though it represents a biased technique (data is obtained only for the antibodies initially spotted on the membrane) but, as hundreds of different antibodies can be spotted onto the same membrane, it can easily be used for screening purposes such asfor disease diagnosis using disease biomarkers. This study indicated that Akt1, GSK3β and p70S6K, as well as ERK1/2 and the p38δ and γ kinases all displayed a decreased phosphorylation level in canine dytrophic muscle (Figure 3). Antibody arrays allow the detection of the presence of specific proteins, and the level of expression of phospho-proteins in disease tissue (Cahill, 2001), thus having a potential for biomedical and diagnostic applications. However, it had not been possible to address the systematic analysis of proteins using this dedicated approach.

A lot of evidence now indicates that various signalling and metabolic pathways are altered in DMD, and a global, unbiased, proteomics study was necessary to identify these perturbations. In order to characterize the complete dystrophic proteome, the use the recent 2D-GE technology coupled to MS became favorable.

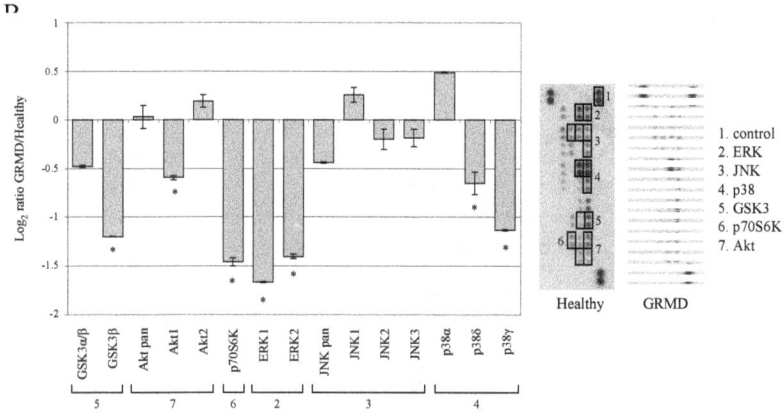

Fig. 3. Antibody array analysis revealed PI3K/Akt and MAPK signalling pathway modulation in GRMD skeletal muscle. Healthy and GRMD muscle extracts from 4-month-old dogs were incubated with two antibody arrays. A ratio of signal intensity (GRMD/healthy) was calculated, and log transformed (base2). A cutoff value was determined by ANOVA analysis at 95% confidence level (p<0.05). * - significantly different from healthy muscle.

3.2 Mass spectrometry-based proteomic analyses

MS-based proteomics represents an unbiased approach allowing the comprehensive cataloging of the whole protein alterations associated with a specific disease. This chapter outlines the findings from recent applications of MS-based proteomics for studying alterations in dystrophic dog muscle, and examines novel strategies to establish DMD-specific biomarkers.

3.2.1 Separation of muscle proteins by two-dimensional gel electrophoresis

2D-GE represents a highly reproducible and discriminatory technique that allows the analysis of the accessible (meaning soluble and abundant) muscle proteins. The proteins that appear differentially expressed between the different samples analyzed are then identified by high-throughput MS (matrix-assisted laser desorption/ionization time-of-flight - MALDI-ToF or electrospary ionization - ESI). Proteomics dataset are finally interlinked with international web-based gel electrophoretic and protein sequence databanks for comparative analysis. Modern mass spectrometers produce and separate ions according to their mass-to-charge ratio (m/z) with an extraordinary resolving power. MS-based analysis of the skeletal muscle proteome has already been successfully used in the context of muscle development, fiber type specification, fast-to-slow transformation, muscle growth and aging, and in the context of denervation-induced fiber damage, atrophy, obesity, diabetes and muscular dystrophies (Ohlendieck, 2010). Detailed 2D maps of the major soluble muscle proteome, including proteins involved in actomyosin apparatus, regulation of contraction, ion homeostasis, signalling, cytosolic and mitochondrial metabolism and stress response, have been established for various mammals (Doran et al., 2009a). The results obtained by this high-throughput technology should then be confirmed by more classical techniques such as western immunoblotting and immunohistochemistry. For example, the *mdx* mouse model was employed in recent proteomics profiling studies which revealed new disease markers in dystrophin-deficient fibres (Doran et al., 2004; Doran et al., 2006a, 2006b; Gardan-Salmon et al., 2011). A differential in-gel analysis (DIGE) analysis of *mdx vs* normal diaphragm muscle revealed a drastic differential expression pattern of 35 proteins, with 21 proteins being decreased (including the F-box only protein 11 - Fbxo11, adenylate kinase 1 – AK1, and the calcium-binding protein regucalcin) and 14 proteins being increased, including the small cardiovascular heat shock protein cvHSP and muscle proteins such as vimentin, desmin and myosin heavy chain (MHC) (Doran et al., 2006a).

More recently, the GRMD dog model was used to profile changes in protein abundance associated with DMD using 2D-GE. To eliminate the structural and contractile proteins that are over-abundant in crude protein extracts prepared from skeletal muscle, and to enrich the samples in signalling proteins, the study restricted the analysis to the cytosolic and phospho-enriched proteins of the *Vastus lateralis* muscle removed from 4-month-old healthy and dystrophic dogs. Among the differentially expressed proteins , 8 were chosen, according to their high level of dysregulation, for further identification by MS. This led to the identification of skeletal muscle markers involved in the contractile function and mitochondrial proteins involved in energy metabolism (Guevel et al., 2011). Although 2D-GE analysis represents an efficient technique to identify relative changes in protein expression, it is not well suited for studying low-abundant proteins, which are often important regulators of cell signalling. The high abundance of cytoskeletal, contractile and chaperone proteins identified in the phospho-enriched sample combined with dynamic range issues associated with the 2D-GE approach hampered studies on skeletal muscle analysis. Recently, Hojlund and colleague used 1D-GE and high-performance liquid chromatography (HPLC)-ESI-MS/MS to characterize the proteome of human skeletal muscle (Hojlund et al., 2008). The proteins identified in this study provide a representation of the major biological function of healthy human skeletal muscle. To elucidate changes in the proteome associated with DMD, and to overcome disadvantages of 2D-GE, peptide-centric approach can be used, which allows quantitative comparison of two samples. Numerous stable isotope-labelling techniques have been employed in quantitative shotgun proteomics, including isobaric tag for relative and absolute quantification (iTRAQ); isotope-coded affinity tag (ICAT); and stable isotope labelling by amino-acids in cell culture (SILAC) (Ohlendieck, 2011). In dystrophic skeletal muscle, the ICAT labelling approach has been used for the quantitative proteomic profiling of healthy and GRMD dog muscles.

3.2.2 Quantitative proteomic analysis

ICAT labelling followed by LC-MS/MS was used to analyze the quantitative variations of the proteome in both a cytoplasmic and a phospho-enriched fraction prepared from the *Vastus lateralis* muscle of 4-month old healthy and GRMD dogs (Guevel et al., 2011). A total of 84 proteins appeared significantly altered (61 proteins from the cytosolic fraction and 36 proteins from the phospho-enriched fraction, with an overlap of 13 proteins). These proteins were classified into 7 major categories including: i) muscle development and contraction, ii) glycolytic metabolism, iii) oxidative metabolism, iv) calcium ion homeostasis, v) intracellular signalling, vi) regulation of apoptosis, and vii) other functions. Gene Ontology

(GO) annotation of the altered proteome led to several key findings which might reflect the ongoing muscle regeneration taking place in dystrophic muscle. Among the proteins altered in the intracellular signalling category in the dystrophic muscle, protein phosphatase 1 (PP1) and DJ-1 appear particularly interesting. PP1, which is present in skeletal muscle, is known to regulate both glycogen and fatty metabolism, while promoting the dephosphorylation of myosin. The protein DJ-1 (also called PARK7) was recently described as a negative regulator of PTEN (Kim et al., 2005; Villa-Moruzzi et al., 1996). Interestingly, the under-expressed proteins primarily composed of metabolic proteins, many of which have been shown to be regulated by PGC-1α. Interestingly, among the several PGC-1α targets identified to be under-expressed in dystrophic dog muscle, 5 (namely 6-phosphofructokinase, phosphoglucomutase-1, aconitase 2, cytochrome c1 and fatty acid binding protein 3) have already been identified in a different transcriptomic study as under-expressing in DMD compared to healthy human biopsies (Pescatori et al., 2007). PGC-1α has been described as a potent regulator of mitochondrial biogenesis and oxidative metabolism in skeletal muscle (Wu et al., 1999; Lin et al., 2002). In addition, activation of the peroxysome proliferator-activated receptor (PPAR)/PGC-1α pathway has been shown, by preventing the bioenergetic deficit observed, to efficiently improve a mitochondrial myopathy phenotype (Wenz et al., 2008), suggesting that PGC-1α mediated improvement of dystrophic muscle may rely (in part) on the restoration of PGC-1α mitochondrial targets (Handschin et al., 2007). Interestingly, a recent study has shown that pharmacologic activation of PPARβ/δ also leads to an upregulation in the expression of utrophin A, which was concurrent with a partial correction of the dystrophic phenotype (Miura et al., 2009). Taken together, these results provide compelling new evidence that defects in PTEN and PGC-1α contribute to profound signalling pathway deregulation in the canine model of DMD as well as to the disease progression. In addition, they demonstrate that proteomics tools are of particular interest for the study of muscular disorders. Recently, the combination of proteomics, metabolomics and fluoximics has confirmed the existence in the *mdx* mouse of perturbations that reflect mitochondrial energetic alterations (Griffin&Des Rosiers, 2009). The broad aim of these studies has been two-fold, first the identification of co-founding factors that promote or limit the disease progression and second, the identification of new biomarkers that could be used to more accurately define the disease status.

4. Reliable biomarkers of DMD, with a special focus on signalling proteins

As previously mentioned, the absence of a single protein (dystrophin) in muscle has devastating consequences. Despite the tremendous efforts that have been made for more than 20 years in order to try to understand how this initial genetic defect could lead to the progressive and irreversible muscle wasting observed, the pathogenesis of DMD has not been fully characterized. Furthermore, no curative treatment is yet available and DMD patients are still dying during early adulthood. The identification, at the proteome level, of the alterations associated with DMD is important for at least five reasons. By providing a better understanding of the pathogenesis of DMD, they should i) improve diagnosis, ii) enable a better monitoring of disease progression, iii) lead to the proposal of new therapeutic targets (in the perspective of a pharmacological treatment – alone or in combination with a gene or cell therapy approach), iv) enable the fast and efficient evaluation of the benefits provided by the treatments currently under study (are they able to reverse the secondary changes associated with the absence of dystrophin?) and v) in some cases, they could even enable the improvement of a given therapy. Ideally, serum biomarkers should be identified (Cacchiarelli et al., 2011) allowing an easy and non invasive analysis, but a muscle muscular biopsy could always be used if necessary.

Skeletal muscle proteomics represents a new and powerful analytical tool for the swift separation and identification of new biomarkers and, in the recent years, several reviews written mainly by Doran, Ohlendieck and their colleagues focused on the proteomics analysis, by 2D-GE and high-throughput MS, of skeletal muscle during aging or disease (Lewis et al., 2009; Griffin&Des Rosiers, 2009; Doran et al., 2009a; Doran et al., 2007a, 2007b). Although being extremely powerful for the identification of new biomarkers, the proteomics analysis of skeletal muscle encounters some limitations. In the particular case of DMD, some complications are also due to the increase in endomysial fat and connective tissue, changes in the interstitial volume, infiltration by immune cells, residual blood components or drastic transformations in contractile fiber types. However, MS is so sensitive that it can differentiate these effects in heterogeneous cell mixtures. On the other hand, it is not always easy to distinguish between a DMD-specific biomarker and a biomarker that is more linked to muscle degeneration in general. The detailed analysis of the overlapping results obtained in the studies of DMD *vs* dysferlinopathies *vs* age-induced muscle wasting may help to distinguish between common and more specific biomarkers. In parallel to 2D-GE, we successfully used the antibody array technology to compare cell signalling in dystrophic *vs* healthy dog skeletal muscle (Feron et al., 2009). Finally, metabolomics and fluxomics (metabolic flux anlysis) studies have been successfully performed on skeletal muscle (Griffin&Des Rosiers, 2009).

In 2003, Ge and colleagues published the results of a proteomic analysis, using 2D-GE/MS, of *mdx* hindlimb skeletal muscle (Ge et al., 2003). Among the 60 proteins identified as differentially expressed in dystrophic *vs* healthy muscle (40 in the cytosolic fraction and 20 in the microsomal one), AK1 (cytosolic fraction) appeared to be of particular interest, because of its dramatic decrease (> four-fold) and because of its role, along with creatine kinase (CK), in the regulation of nucleotide ratios and energy metabolism. The expression and activity of AK1 was reduced in *mdx* muscle at different stages (one, three and six months), suggesting a direct link with the deficiency in dystrophin. Decreased AK1 activity in *mdx* muscle could contribute to the energetic defect, the decreased force and the increased fatigability exhibited. At the same time, the redistribution of energy flow through the alternative and compensatory CK phosphotransfer system could limit cellular energy failure. In DMD patients, lower ATP levels and impaired energy metabolism had been reported very early, and several studies suggest that defects in energy metabolism could contribute to DMD pathogenesis.

Ge and colleagues, in 2004, also published a study in which they compared by 2D-GE the proteome of *mdx* vs control hindlimb muscles at different stages of the disease (Ge et al., 2004). Among the 46 differentially expressed cytosolic proteins detected at three months (10 down- and 36 up-regulated proteins), 24 could be identified by MS. These proteins belong to five different functional categories, and illustrate the increase in protein turnover caused by the cycles of degeneration/regeneration characteristic of *mdx* muscles. Concerning metabolism and energy production (i), the reduction in AK1 was confirmed and an increase in the expression level of the CK, ATP synthase, ATP succinyl-CoA synthetase and pyrophosphatase enzymes was detected, highlighting the general mitochondrial dysfunction and metabolism crisis taking place in dystrophic muscles. Concerning the serine protease inhibitor family (ii), an up-regulation was detected for protease inhibitor member 1a and serine protease inhibitors 3, 6 and 1-5, suggesting a partial inhibition of proteolysis in *mdx* muscles. Concerning growth and differentiation (iii), an increase was detected in the expression level of PP1, cofilin 2 (CFL2) and ε 14-3-3, indicating active proliferation and differentiation. Of interest, an increase in CFL2 had also been observed in human DMD biopsies. As far as calcium homeostasis is concerned (iv), the up-regulation of PP1 can also be cited, as the phosphatase binds to the ryanodine-sensitive calcium release channel protein to regulate calcium flux. The calcium-binding protein annexin V was also increased. Finally, and concerning cytoskeleton reorganization and biogenesis (v), RhoGDI-1, γ-actin and tropomyosin 1 were found to be up-regulated in *mdx* muscles, indicating cytoskeleton remodeling. At one and six months, 62 and 48 differentially expressed proteins were detected, respectively. At one month, most of the proteins detected were down-regulated whereas at six months (as it was the case at three months), most of them were up-regulated. These results confirmed the specificity of the one month stage ("DMD-like" crisis) in the evolution of the disease in the *mdx* mouse. Six proteins were detected as differentially expressed in *mdx vs* healthy muscles at the three stages tested: AK1 (down-regulated), CK (up-regulated), myosin light chain 2 (MLC2, up-regulated), annexin V, tropomyosin and ε 14-3-3 (all down-regulated at one month and up-regulated at three and six months). Some of these changes thus appear directly linked to the absence of dystrophin whereas some others appear more dependent of the phenotype on the muscle. The elevation detected in MLC2 levels could reflect the proliferation/differentiation processes occurring in *mdx* muscles, as the protein is involved in muscle differentiation, and its consistent elevation during the progression of the disease suggests that *mdx* muscles may assume a chronic or abnormal differentiation state.

In another study, Doran and colleagues performed a 2D-GE/MS-based subproteomics analysis of calcium-binding proteins by using the cationic carbocyanine dye 'Stains-All' (Doran et al., 2004). Among the 8 dye-positive proteins identified as greatly reduced in *mdx vs* healthy skeletal muscle, calsequestrin was present. Calsequestrin represents the main luminal sarcoplasmic reticulum calcium reservoir protein. It is a terminal cisternae constituent with high-capacity and medium-affinity, and acts as a mediator of the excitation-contraction-relaxation cycle, both as a luminal ion trap and an endogenous regulator of the ryanodine receptor. The authors could also confirm the reduction in sarcalumenin, a calcium-shuttle element of the longitudinal tubules. These results of course confirm the calcium hypothesis of DMD. The reduction in calsequestrin could explain the impaired calcium buffering capacity of dystrophic sarcoplasmic reticulum, which is known to cause an increase in free cytosolic calcium level and thus in proteolysis. Previous microsomal study had not detected any change in the expression level of calsequestrin, highlighting the power of the technique used here.

More recently, Doran and colleagues could also show, using 2D-GE/MS again, that another protein involved in calcium homeostasis, regucalcin, was reduced in young and aged *mdx vs* healthy diaphragm, limb and heart muscles (Doran et al., 2006a). Regucalcin represented the most interesting hit in respect to the calcium hypothesis of DMD as its reduced level could render *mdx* fibers more susceptible to necrosis. Regucalcin is a cytosolic calcium-handling protein involved in signalling. By enhancing the calcium-pumping activity in the plasma membrane, endoplasmic reticulum and mitochondria, regucalcin appears as an important regulator that maintains low cytosolic calcium levels. Its reduced expression level could be confirmed by immunoblotting in the diaphragm muscle from 3-week-, 9-week-, 11-month- and 20-month-old *mdx* mice. At 9 weeks, a reduced level of the protein could also be observed in hindlimb and heart muscles. Doran and colleagues finally used the powerful DIGE technique and identified 2398 proteins among which 35 exhibited a differential expression level in *mdx* vs healthy diaphragm muscle (Doran et al., 2006b). These proteins are involved in muscle contraction, cytoskeleton formation, mitochondrial function, metabolism, ion homeostasis and chaperone function. The most interesting finding concerned the dramatic increase in the expression level of the small heat shock protein cvHSP (highest fold change). This drastic increase could be observed in 9-week- and 11-month-old *mdx* diaphragm muscles (it increases with the age – in correlation with the severity of the phenotype). Whereas the protein was concentrated in subsarcolemmal regions in healthy muscle, it was shown to be present throughout the cytoplasm of *mdx* fibers, with a typical striated appearance suggesting an association with contractile elements and/or cytoskeletal components and a role in the stress response developed by *mdx* damaged fibers. This increase in cvHSP was associated with the differential expression of others key heat shock proteins (HSP20, GRP75, HSP90 and HSP110), emphasizing stress response as an important mechanism in DMD pathogenesis, and suggesting that it could be targeted by new pharmacological treatments. Heat shock chaperon proteins can be activated, besides by heat shock *per se*, by other stress factors such as inflammation, ischemia, oxidative stress, exposure to heavy metals or certain amino acids analogs. They prevent the aggregation of misfolded proteins as well as they influence the transport of mature proteins. The up-regulation of cvHSP observed in *mdx* diaphragm indicates an attempt of damaged muscle fibers to repair their cytoskeletal network. The change observed in the localization of the protein also suggests a protective role in muscle fiber degeneration. The up-regulation of chaperones probably represents an autoprotective mechanism, whereby the stress response can be considered as a reaction to the pathological increase in abnormally folded muscle proteins.

More recently, a magnetic bead fractionation and MS-based serum protein profiling was performed in the *mdx* mouse and described coagulation Factor XIIIa, previously identified in human serum, as a potential biomarker of muscular dystrophy (Alagaratnam et al., 2008). Factor XIIIa plays roles in coagulation and cardiovascular biology, possibly through macrophage activation, and macrophages are known to infiltrate dystrophic muscles. Because blood serum analysis is fast, economical and non invasive, this type of study is of high interest, and a study with serum from DMD patients should be performed. However, this factor alone may not be sufficient to distinguish between DMD and other inflammatory context.

Finally, our lab identified two signalling molecules (PTEN and PGC1-α) as biomarkers in GRMD dog model, strongly reinforcing the hypothesis that signalling pathways alteration could play a role in DMD pathogenesis. In a first study (Feron et al., 2009), we were able to show that an increase in the activity of PTEN, a phosphatase that counteracts Akt activation by dephosphorylating the PIP3 generated by PI3K (Maehama&Dixon, 1998), in dystrophin-deficient dog muscle leads to a profound and long-term deregulation of the PI3K/Akt signalling pathway. All the GSK3β+ fibers observed in dystrophic muscle appeared to exhibit a strong accumulation of PTEN, whereas the fibers with weak PTEN labelling were systematically GSK3β-. In order to see if the alterations initially detected at 4-months were specific of this age, the double labelling experiment was repeated at 3 months (when the morphological features of muscular dystrophy are yet very few) and 36 months (which corresponds to a very advanced stage). PTEN+/GSK3β+ fibers could be observed at all stages, and we demonstrated that the alteration of the pathway could not be attributed only to a feature or regeneration or to a consequence of inflammatory changes. In conclusion, increased PTEN activity revealed to be a signature of muscular dystrophy pathogenesis in dog, leading to long-term and deep PI3K/Akt signalling pathway alteration. This dysregulation probably limits compensatory hypertrophy, thus exacerbating muscle degeneration, and these results could open the door to new potential therapeutic targets for the treatment of DMD.

In a second analysis, a quantitative proteomic analysis of dystrophic *vs* healthy dog muscle was performed using the ICAT technology coupled to LC/MS/MS (Guevel et al., 2011). This study, performed on both a cytoplasmic and a phospho-enriched fractions, identified 84 proteins as being differentially represented in GRMD *vs* healthy dog muscle. Interestingly, many of the under-expressed proteins detected have been previously shown to be regulated by PGC-1α, and we were able to show that PGC1-α expression was indeed dramatically reduced in GRMD *vs* healthy muscle. These results confirmed that defective energy metabolism is a central hallmark of the disease in the canine model, and reinforced once more the hypothesis that secondary changes may play an active role in DMD pathogenesis.

In conclusion, proteomics studies performed in the recent years on dystrophic *vs* healthy muscles led to the identification of new biomarkers of DMD, such as AK1 (nucleotide metabolism), calsequestrin, regucalcin (calcium homeostais) and cvHSP (cellular stress response) in the *mdx* mouse and PTEN and PGC-1α (cell signalling: atrophy/hypertrophy and energy metabolism) in the GRMD dog. Other putative biomarkers were also identified in the following processes: nucleotide metabolism (CK, Atp5b), calcium homeostasis (sarcalumenin), cellular stress response (αBC, chaperonins), muscle contraction (MHC and MLC, troponin, actin), intermediate filament formation (vimentin, desmin), glycolysis (glyceraldehyde-3-phosphate dehydrogenase, aldolase), polyol pathway of glucose metabolism (sorbitol dehydrogenase), citric acid cycle (isocitrate dehydrogenase), fatty acid oxidation (electron transferring flavoprotein), aldehyde metabolism (aldehyde reductase, aldehyde dehydrogenase), formation of acetyl-coenzyme A (dihydrolipoamide dehydrogenase), remethylation pathway of homocysteine homeostasis (betaine-homocysteine methyltransferase), acid-base balance (carbonic anhydrase), oxygen transport (β-haemoglobin, α-globin), protein ubiquitination (Fbxo11) and transcriptional control (Jmjd1a). Taken together, these results indicate a drastic reduction in key metabolic regulators and a compensatory up-regulation of structural elements.

5. Proteomic profiling of experimental therapy

As previously mentioned, no curative treatment is yet available for DMD patients that can benefit only from palliative care and generally die during early adulthood. Two therapeutic strategies can be envisaged to treat, or at least to alleviate the symptoms of DMD: try to restore dystrophin expression in dystrophic muscle fibers (through gene or cell therapy approaches), or target the molecular pathways lying downstream of dystrophin (through pharmacological treatments). Several strategies have been recently set up in order to rescue dystrophin synthesis in animal models of DMD and some of them have now entered clinical trials (Kinali et al., 2009; van Deutekom et al., 2007). One of the major problems in comparing the benefit of different therapeutic treatments is to find common outcome measurements. This paragraph does not aim at describing in details the therapies currently under study [for a review, please see (Sugita&Takeda, 2010; Guglieri&Bushby, 2010; Zhang et al., 2007)], but rather to show how proteomic profiling could be used to evaluate the efficiency of therapeutic treatments. Recently, Doran and colleagues (Doran et al., 2009b) used DIGE analysis to evaluate the efficiency of an exon skipping-based strategy in the *mdx* mouse.

The idea behind the study is that, as secondary mechanisms such as abnormal signalling, energy metabolism defects, alterations in ion homeostasis or in excitation-contraction coupling, probably play a crucial role in DMD pathogenesis, any novel therapeutic strategy should be evaluated on several aspects: re-expression of dystrophin (except for therapeutic treatments targeting downstream events), muscle function tests, but also correction of the secondary changes previously detected in the above mentioned processes.

Proteomic profiling of exon skipping-treated *mdx* muscles showed that the re-expression of dystrophin led to the correction of the previously detected alterations in calcium handling, nucleotide metabolism, bioenergetic pathways, acid-base balance and cellular stress response. More precisely, the re-expression of dystrophin was associated with the restoration of β-dystroglycan and nNOS (two proteins associated with the DGC at the sarcolemma), and a normal expression level of some biomarkers previously identified (namely calsequestrin, adenylate kinase, aldolase, mitochondrial creatine kinase and cvHsp).

Both the primary and secondary abnormalities provoked by the absence of dystrophin were reversed, reinforcing the interest of the exon skipping strategy for the treatment of DMD. This study reinforced the role ofsecondary mechanisms in DMD pathogenesis, and it demonstrated for the first time the utility of evaluation of the effect of any novel therapeutic approach on both the re-expression of dystrophin and the indirect alterations associated with its absence. AK1, that had previously been reported as down-regulated in *mdx* diaphragm muscle (Ge et al., 2003), was restored after the antisense-induced exon skipping. Also, the down-regulation of the mitochondrial isozyme of CK was partially reversed. Accordingly, the known down-regulation of two others metabolic enzymes, namely aldolase and isocitrate dehydrogenase (Doran et al., 2006b) was also partially reversed. Conversely, the major increase previously reported in the level of cvHSP in *mdx* diaphragm was significantly reduced after treatment. As far as the acid-base balance is concerned, the expression level of carbonic anhydrase was also restored after treatment. For calsequestrin, an immunoblotting experiment (as DIGE is not well suited for the analysis of membrane proteins) was performed that revealed that exon skipping treatment was again able to restore its expression (Doran et al., 2004), suggesting a partial abolishment of the secondary changes in calcium homeostasis associated with DMD. The exon skipping strategy presented here effectively reverses both the metabolic crisis and the compensatory up-regulation of different chaperones and enzymes associated with muscular dystrophy in the mouse.

Lastly, miRNAs specifically expressed in muscle cells and known to be released in the blood of DMD patients in a way proportional to the extent of muscle degeneration, could be used as biomarkers in the evaluation of therapeutic strategies (Cacchiarelli et al., 2011).

To sum up, even though many different DMD therapeutic approaches are now entering clinical trials, a unifying method for assessing the benefit of different treatments is still lacking.

6. Conclusion

In conclusion, proteomics analysis plays a significant role in our ability to understand molecular mechanisms associated with DMD. Various technological platforms are now available for proteomic studies enabling us to address different aspects of dystrophic muscle governed by signalling pathways. We foresee proteomics emerging as a vital technique in clinical research to assist us in understanding which particular signal transduction pathways are involved in muscular dystrophy and to evaluate the benefit of clinical trials.

7. Acknowledgment

Research in the author's laboratory on proteomics handling in Duchenne muscular dystrophy was supported by projects grants from the AFM (Association Française contre les Myopathies).

8. References

Alagaratnam, S.;Mertens, B. J.;Dalebout, J. C.;Deelder, A. M.;Van Ommen, G. J.;Den Dunnen, J. T. & T Hoen, P. A. (2008) Serum protein profiling in mice: identification of Factor XIIIa as a potential biomarker for muscular dystrophy. *Proteomics*, 8, 8, pp. 1552-63, ISSN 1615-9861

Anderson, L. V. & Davison, K. (1999) Multiplex Western blotting system for the analysis of muscular dystrophy proteins. *Am J Pathol*, 154, 4, pp. 1017-22

Blaauw, B.;Canato, M.;Agatea, L.;Toniolo, L.;Mammucari, C.;Masiero, E.;Abraham, R.;Sandri, M.;Schiaffino, S. & Reggiani, C. (2009) Inducible activation of Akt increases skeletal muscle mass and force without satellite cell activation. *FASEB J*, ISSN 1530-6860

Bodine, S. C.;Stitt, T. N.;Gonzalez, M.;Kline, W. O.;Stover, G. L.;Bauerlein, R.;Zlotchenko, E.;Scrimgeour, A.;Lawrence, J. C.;Glass, D. J. & Yancopoulos, G. D. (2001) Akt/mTOR pathway is a crucial regulator of skeletal muscle hypertrophy and can prevent muscle atrophy in vivo. *Nat Cell Biol*, 3, 11, pp. 1014-9

Brenman, J. E.;Chao, D. S.;Xia, H.;Aldape, K. & Bredt, D. S. (1995) Nitric oxide synthase complexed with dystrophin and absent from skeletal muscle sarcolemma in Duchenne muscular dystrophy. *Cell*, 82, 5, pp. 743-52

Bulfield, G;Siller, W.G;Wight , P.A.G. & Moore, K.J (1984) X chromosome-linked muscular dystrophy (mdx) in the mouse. *Proc Natl Acad Sci U S A*, 81, pp. 1189-1192

Cacchiarelli, D.;Legnini, I.;Martone, J.;Cazzella, V.;D'amico, A.;Bertini, E. & Bozzoni, I. (2011) miRNAs as serum biomarkers for Duchenne muscular dystrophy. *EMBO Mol Med*, 3, 5, pp. 258-65, ISSN 1757-4684

Cahill, D. J. (2001) Protein and antibody arrays and their medical applications. *J Immunol Methods*, 250, 1-2, pp. 81-91, ISSN 0022-1759

Cavaldesi, M.;Macchia, G.;Barca, S.;Defilippi, P.;Tarone, G. & Petrucci, T. C. (1999) Association of the dystroglycan complex isolated from bovine brain synaptosomes with proteins involved in signal transduction. *J Neurochem*, 72, 4, pp. 1648-55

Chen, Y. W.;Zhao, P.;Borup, R. & Hoffman, E. P. (2000) Expression profiling in the muscular dystrophies: identification of novel aspects of molecular pathophysiology. *J Cell Biol*, 151, 6, pp. 1321-36

Chung, J.;Kuo, C. J.;Crabtree, G. R. & Blenis, J. (1992) Rapamycin-FKBP specifically blocks growth-dependent activation of and signaling by the 70 kd S6 protein kinases. *Cell*, 69, 7, pp. 1227-36, ISSN 0092-8674

Cooper, B. J.;Winand, N. J.;Stedman, H.;Valentine, B. A.;Hoffman, E. P.;Kunkel, L. M.;Scott, M. O.;Fischbeck, K. H.;Kornegay, J. N.;Avery, R. J. & Et Al. (1988) The homologue of the Duchenne locus is defective in X-linked muscular dystrophy of dogs. *Nature*, 334, 6178, pp. 154-6

Crosbie, R. H.;Yamada, H.;Venzke, D. P.;Lisanti, M. P. & Campbell, K. P. (1998) Caveolin-3 is not an integral component of the dystrophin glycoprotein complex. *FEBS Lett*, 427, 2, pp. 279-82, ISSN 0014-5793

Cross, D. A.;Alessi, D. R.;Cohen, P.;Andjelkovich, M. & Hemmings, B. A. (1995) Inhibition of glycogen synthase kinase-3 by insulin mediated by protein kinase B. *Nature*, 378, 6559, pp. 785-9

Dogra, C.;Changotra, H.;Wergedal, J. E. & Kumar, A. (2006) Regulation of phosphatidylinositol 3-kinase (PI3K)/Akt and nuclear factor-kappa B signaling pathways in dystrophin-deficient skeletal muscle in response to mechanical stretch. *J Cell Physiol*, 208, 3, pp. 575-85

Doran, P.;Donoghue, P.;O'connell, K.;Gannon, J. & Ohlendieck, K. (2007a) Proteomic profiling of pathological and aged skeletal muscle fibres by peptide mass fingerprinting (Review). *Int J Mol Med*, 19, 4, pp. 547-64, ISSN 1107-3756

Doran, P.;Donoghue, P.;O'connell, K.;Gannon, J. & Ohlendieck, K. (2009a) Proteomics of skeletal muscle aging. *Proteomics*, 9, 4, pp. 989-1003, ISSN 1615-9861

Doran, P.;Dowling, P.;Donoghue, P.;Buffini, M. & Ohlendieck, K. (2006a) Reduced expression of regucalcin in young and aged mdx diaphragm indicates abnormal cytosolic calcium handling in dystrophin-deficient muscle. *Biochim Biophys Acta*, 1764, 4, pp. 773-85

Doran, P.;Dowling, P.;Lohan, J.;Mcdonnell, K.;Poetsch, S. & Ohlendieck, K. (2004) Subproteomics analysis of Ca+-binding proteins demonstrates decreased calsequestrin expression in dystrophic mouse skeletal muscle. *Eur J Biochem*, 271, 19, pp. 3943-52, ISSN 0014-2956

Doran, P.;Gannon, J.;O'connell, K. & Ohlendieck, K. (2007b) Proteomic profiling of animal models mimicking skeletal muscle disorders. *Proteomics Clin Appl*, 1, 9, pp. 1169-84, ISSN 1862-8346

Doran, P.;Martin, G.;Dowling, P.;Jockusch, H. & Ohlendieck, K. (2006b) Proteome analysis of the dystrophin-deficient MDX diaphragm reveals a drastic increase in the heat shock protein cvHSP. *Proteomics*, 6, 16, pp. 4610-21

Doran, P.;Wilton, S. D.;Fletcher, S. & Ohlendieck, K. (2009b) Proteomic profiling of antisense-induced exon skipping reveals reversal of pathobiochemical abnormalities in dystrophic mdx diaphragm. *Proteomics*, 9, 3, pp. 671-85, ISSN 1615-9861

Ekins, R. & Chu, F. W. (1999) Microarrays: their origins and applications. *Trends Biotechnol*, 17, 6, pp. 217-8

Feron, M.;Guevel, L.;Rouger, K.;Dubreil, L.;Arnaud, M. C.;Ledevin, M.;Megeney, L. A.;Cherel, Y. & Sakanyan, V. (2009) PTEN contributes to profound PI3K/Akt signaling pathway deregulation in dystrophin-deficient dog muscle. *Am J Pathol*, 174, 4, pp. 1459-70, ISSN 1525-2191

Gardan-Salmon, D.;Dixon, J. M.;Lonergan, S. M. & Selsby, J. T. (2011) Proteomic assessment of the acute phase of dystrophin deficiency in mdx mice. *Eur J Appl Physiol*, ISSN 1439-6327

Ge, Y.;Molloy, M. P.;Chamberlain, J. S. & Andrews, P. C. (2003) Proteomic analysis of mdx skeletal muscle: Great reduction of adenylate kinase 1 expression and enzymatic activity. *Proteomics*, 3, 10, pp. 1895-903, ISSN 1615-9853

Ge, Y.;Molloy, M. P.;Chamberlain, J. S. & Andrews, P. C. (2004) Differential expression of the skeletal muscle proteome in mdx mice at different ages. *Electrophoresis*, 25, 15, pp. 2576-85, ISSN 0173-0835

Gembitsky, D. S.;Lawlor, K.;Jacovina, A.;Yaneva, M. & Tempst, P. (2004) A prototype antibody microarray platform to monitor changes in protein tyrosine phosphorylation. *Mol Cell Proteomics*, 3, 11, pp. 1102-18

Glass, D. J. (2005) Skeletal muscle hypertrophy and atrophy signaling pathways. *Int J Biochem Cell Biol*, 37, 10, pp. 1974-84, ISSN 1357-2725

Griffin, J. L. & Des Rosiers, C. (2009) Applications of metabolomics and proteomics to the mdx mouse model of Duchenne muscular dystrophy: lessons from downstream of the transcriptome. *Genome Med*, 1, 3, pp. 32, ISSN 1756-994X

Grubb, R. L.;Calvert, V. S.;Wulkuhle, J. D.;Paweletz, C. P.;Linehan, W. M.;Phillips, J. L.;Chuaqui, R.;Valasco, A.;Gillespie, J.;Emmert-Buck, M.;Liotta, L. A. & Petricoin, E. F. (2003) Signal pathway profiling of prostate cancer using reverse phase protein arrays. *Proteomics*, 3, 11, pp. 2142-6

Guevel, L. ;Lavoie, Jr.;Perez-Iratxeta, C. ;Rouger, K. ;Dubreil, L. ;Feron, M. ;Talon, S. ;Brand, M. & Megeney, L. (2011) Quantitative proteomic analysis of dystrophic dog muscle. *J Proteome Res.*, 10, 5, pp. 2465-78, ISSN 1535-3907

Guglieri, M. & Bushby, K. (2010) Molecular treatments in Duchenne muscular dystrophy. *Curr Opin Pharmacol*, 10, 3, pp. 331-7, ISSN 1471-4973

Hanash, S. (2003) Disease proteomics. *Nature*, 422, 6928, pp. 226-32

Handschin, C.;Kobayashi, Y. M.;Chin, S.;Seale, P.;Campbell, K. P. & Spiegelman, B. M. (2007) PGC-1alpha regulates the neuromuscular junction program and ameliorates Duchenne muscular dystrophy. *Genes Dev*, 21, 7, pp. 770-83, ISSN 0890-9369

Hnia, K.;Hugon, G.;Rivier, F.;Masmoudi, A.;Mercier, J. & Mornet, D. (2007) Modulation of p38 Mitogen-Activated Protein Kinase Cascade and Metalloproteinase Activity in Diaphragm Muscle in Response to Free Radical Scavenger Administration in Dystrophin-Deficient Mdx Mice. *Am J Pathol*, 170, 2, pp. 633-43

Hojlund, K.;Yi, Z.;Hwang, H.;Bowen, B.;Lefort, N.;Flynn, C. R.;Langlais, P.;Weintraub, S. T. & Mandarino, L. J. (2008) Characterization of the human skeletal muscle proteome by one-dimensional gel electrophoresis and HPLC-ESI-MS/MS. *Mol Cell Proteomics*, 7, 2, pp. 257-67, ISSN 1535-9484

Inoki, K.;Li, Y.;Zhu, T.;Wu, J. & Guan, K. L. (2002) TSC2 is phosphorylated and inhibited by Akt and suppresses mTOR signalling. *Nat Cell Biol*, 4, 9, pp. 648-57, 1465-7392

Inoki, K.;Ouyang, H.;Li, Y. & Guan, K. L. (2005) Signaling by target of rapamycin proteins in cell growth control. *Microbiol Mol Biol Rev*, 69, 1, pp. 79-100, ISSN 1092-2172

Kim, M. H.;Kino-Oka, M.;Saito, A.;Sawa, Y. & Taya, M. (2010) Myogenic induction of human mesenchymal stem cells by culture on dendrimer-immobilized surface with d-glucose display. *J Biosci Bioeng*, 109, 1, pp. 55-61, ISSN 1347-4421

Kim, R. H.;Peters, M.;Jang, Y.;Shi, W.;Pintilie, M.;Fletcher, G. C.;Deluca, C.;Liepa, J.;Zhou, L.;Snow, B.;Binari, R. C.;Manoukian, A. S.;Bray, M. R.;Liu, F. F.;Tsao, M. S. & Mak, T. W. (2005) DJ-1, a novel regulator of the tumor suppressor PTEN. *Cancer Cell*, 7, 3, pp. 263-73

Kinali, M.;Arechavala-Gomeza, V.;Feng, L.;Cirak, S.;Hunt, D.;Adkin, C.;Guglieri, M.;Ashton, E.;Abbs, S.;Nihoyannopoulos, P.;Garralda, M. E.;Rutherford, M.;Mcculley, C.;Popplewell, L.;Graham, I. R.;Dickson, G.;Wood, M. J.;Wells, D. J.;Wilton, S. D.;Kole, R.;Straub, V.;Bushby, K.;Sewry, C.;Morgan, J. E. & Muntoni, F. (2009) Local restoration of dystrophin expression with the morpholino oligomer AVI-4658 in Duchenne muscular dystrophy: a single-blind, placebo-controlled, dose-escalation, proof-of-concept study. *Lancet Neurol*, 8, 10, pp. 918-28, ISSN 1474-4465

Kingsmore, S. F. (2006) Multiplexed protein measurement: technologies and applications of protein and antibody arrays. *Nat Rev Drug Discov*, 5, 4, pp. 310-20, ISSN 1474-1776

Kolodziejczyk, S. M.;Walsh, G. S.;Balazsi, K.;Seale, P.;Sandoz, J.;Hierlihy, A. M.;Rudnicki, M. A.;Chamberlain, J. S.;Miller, F. D. & Megeney, L. A. (2001) Activation of JNK1 contributes to dystrophic muscle pathogenesis. *Curr Biol*, 11, 16, pp. 1278-82

Kumar, A.;Khandelwal, N.;Malya, R.;Reid, M. B. & Boriek, A. M. (2004) Loss of dystrophin causes aberrant mechanotransduction in skeletal muscle fibers. *FASEB J*, 18, 1, pp. 102-13

Lang, J. M.;Esser, K. A. & Dupont-Versteegden, E. E. (2004) Altered activity of signaling pathways in diaphragm and tibialis anterior muscle of dystrophic mice. *Exp Biol Med (Maywood)*, 229, 6, pp. 503-11

Langenbach, K. J. & Rando, T. A. (2002) Inhibition of dystroglycan binding to laminin disrupts the PI3K/AKT pathway and survival signaling in muscle cells. *Muscle Nerve*, 26, 5, pp. 644-53

Lewis, C.;Carberry, S. & Ohlendieck, K. (2009) Proteomic profiling of x-linked muscular dystrophy. *J Muscle Res Cell Motil*, 30, 7-8, pp. 267-9, ISSN 1573-2657

Lin, J.;Wu, H.;Tarr, P. T.;Zhang, C. Y.;Wu, Z.;Boss, O.;Michael, L. F.;Puigserver, P.;Isotani, E.;Olson, E. N.;Lowell, B. B.;Bassel-Duby, R. & Spiegelman, B. M. (2002) Transcriptional co-activator PGC-1 alpha drives the formation of slow-twitch muscle fibres. *Nature*, 418, 6899, pp. 797-801, ISSN 0028-0836

Macbeath, G. (2002) Protein microarrays and proteomics. *Nat Genet*, 32 Suppl, pp. 526-32

Madhavan, R.;Massom, L. R. & Jarrett, H. W. (1992) Calmodulin specifically binds three proteins of the dystrophin-glycoprotein complex. *Biochem Biophys Res Commun*, 185, 2, pp. 753-9

Maehama, T. & Dixon, J. E. (1998) The tumor suppressor, PTEN/MMAC1, dephosphorylates the lipid second messenger, phosphatidylinositol 3,4,5-trisphosphate. *J Biol Chem*, 273, 22, pp. 13375-8, ISSN 0021-9258

Miura, P.;Chakkalakal, J. V.;Boudreault, L.;Belanger, G.;Hebert, R. L.;Renaud, J. M. & Jasmin, B. J. (2009) Pharmacological activation of PPAR{beta}/{delta} stimulates utrophin A expression in skeletal muscle fibers and restores sarcolemmal integrity in mature mdx mice. *Hum Mol Genet*, ISSN 1460-2083

Muntoni, F.;Torelli, S. & Ferlini, A. (2003) Dystrophin and mutations: one gene, several proteins, multiple phenotypes. *Lancet Neurol*, 2, 12, pp. 731-40

Nakamura, A.;Yoshida, K.;Ueda, H.;Takeda, S. & Ikeda, S. (2005) Up-regulation of mitogen activated protein kinases in mdx skeletal muscle following chronic treadmill exercise. *Biochim Biophys Acta*, 1740, 3, pp. 326-31, ISSN 0006-3002

Noguchi, S. (2005) The biological function of insulin-like growth factor-I in myogenesis and its therapeutic effect on muscular dystrophy. *Acta Myol*, 24, 2, pp. 115-8,

Ohlendieck, K. (2010) Proteomics of skeletal muscle differentiation, neuromuscular disorders and fiber aging. *Expert Rev Proteomics*, 7, 2, pp. 283-96

Ohlendieck, K. (2011) Skeletal muscle proteomics: current approaches, technical challenges and emerging techniques. *Skeletal muscle*, 1, 6, pp. 1-15

Pescatori, M.;Broccolini, A.;Minetti, C.;Bertini, E.;Bruno, C.;D'amico, A.;Bernardini, C.;Mirabella, M.;Silvestri, G.;Giglio, V.;Modoni, A.;Pedemonte, M.;Tasca, G.;Galluzzi, G.;Mercuri, E.;Tonali, P. A. & Ricci, E. (2007) Gene expression profiling in the early phases of DMD: a constant molecular signature characterizes DMD muscle from early postnatal life throughout disease progression. *FASEB J*, 21, 4, pp. 1210-26, ISSN 1530-6860

Peter, A. K. & Crosbie, R. H. (2006) Hypertrophic response of Duchenne and limb-girdle muscular dystrophies is associated with activation of Akt pathway. *Exp Cell Res*, 312, 13, pp. 2580-91

Peter, A. K.;Ko, C. Y.;Kim, M. H.;Hsu, N.;Ouchi, N.;Rhie, S.;Izumiya, Y.;Zeng, L.;Walsh, K. & Crosbie, R. H. (2009) Myogenic Akt signaling upregulates the utrophin-glycoprotein complex and promotes sarcolemma stability in muscular dystrophy. *Hum Mol Genet*, 18, 2, pp. 318-27, ISSN 1460-2083

Price, D. J.;Grove, J. R.;Calvo, V.;Avruch, J. & Bierer, B. E. (1992) Rapamycin-induced inhibition of the 70-kilodalton S6 protein kinase. *Science*, 257, 5072, pp. 973-7, ISSN 0036-8075

Rommel, C.;Bodine, S. C.;Clarke, B. A.;Rossman, R.;Nunez, L.;Stitt, T. N.;Yancopoulos, G. D. & Glass, D. J. (2001) Mediation of IGF-1-induced skeletal myotube hypertrophy by PI(3)K/Akt/mTOR and PI(3)K/Akt/GSK3 pathways. *Nat Cell Biol*, 3, 11, pp. 1009-13

Rouger, K.;Le Cunff, M.;Steenman, M.;Potier, M. C.;Gibelin, N.;Dechesne, C. A. & Leger, J. J. (2002) Global/temporal gene expression in diaphragm and hindlimb muscles of dystrophin-deficient (mdx) mice. *Am J Physiol Cell Physiol*, 283, 3, pp. C773-84

Sakanyan, V. (2005) High-throughput and multiplexed protein array technology: protein-DNA and protein-protein interactions. *J Chromatogr B Analyt Technol Biomed Life Sci*, 815, 1-2, pp. 77-95, ISSN 1570-0232

Schulz, J. S.;Palmer, N.;Steckelberg, J.;Jones, S. J. & Zeece, M. G. (2006) Microarray profiling of skeletal muscle sarcoplasmic reticulum proteins. *Biochim Biophys Acta*, 1764, 9, pp. 1429-35

Sheehan, K. M.;Calvert, V. S.;Kay, E. W.;Lu, Y.;Fishman, D.;Espina, V.;Aquino, J.;Speer, R.;Araujo, R.;Mills, G. B.;Liotta, L. A.;Petricoin, E. F., 3rd & Wulfkuhle, J. D. (2005)

Use of reverse phase protein microarrays and reference standard development for molecular network analysis of metastatic ovarian carcinoma. *Mol Cell Proteomics*, 4, 4, pp. 346-55

St-Pierre, S. J.;Chakkalakal, J. V.;Kolodziejczyk, S. M.;Knudson, J. C.;Jasmin, B. J. & Megeney, L. A. (2004) Glucocorticoid treatment alleviates dystrophic myofiber pathology by activation of the calcineurin/NF-AT pathway. *Faseb J*, 18, 15, pp. 1937-9

Sugita, H. & Takeda, S. (2010) Progress in muscular dystrophy research with special emphasis on gene therapy. *Proc Jpn Acad Ser B Phys Biol Sci*, 86, 7, pp. 748-56, ISSN 1349-2896

Tang, Y.;Reay, D. P.;Salay, M. N.;Mi, M. Y.;Clemens, P. R.;Guttridge, D. C.;Robbins, P. D.;Huard, J. & Wang, B. (2010) Inhibition of the IKK/NF-kappaB pathway by AAV gene transfer improves muscle regeneration in older mdx mice. *Gene Ther*, 17, 12, pp. 1476-83, ISSN 1476-5462

Valentine, B. A.;Cooper, B. J.;De Lahunta, A.;O'quinn, R. & Blue, J. T. (1988) Canine X-linked muscular dystrophy. An animal model of Duchenne muscular dystrophy: clinical studies. *J Neurol Sci*, 88, 1-3, pp. 69-81, ISSN 0022-510X

Van Deutekom, J. C.;Janson, A. A.;Ginjaar, I. B.;Frankhuizen, W. S.;Aartsma-Rus, A.;Bremmer-Bout, M.;Den Dunnen, J. T.;Koop, K.;Van Der Kooi, A. J.;Goemans, N. M.;De Kimpe, S. J.;Ekhart, P. F.;Venneker, E. H.;Platenburg, G. J.;Verschuuren, J. J. & Van Ommen, G. J. (2007) Local dystrophin restoration with antisense oligonucleotide PRO051. *N Engl J Med*, 357, 26, pp. 2677-86, ISSN 1533-4406

Villa-Moruzzi, E.;Puntoni, F. & Marin, O. (1996) Activation of protein phosphatase-1 isoforms and glycogen synthase kinase-3 beta in muscle from mdx mice. *Int J Biochem Cell Biol*, 28, 1, pp. 13-22, ISSN 1357-2725

Wenz, T.;Diaz, F.;Spiegelman, B. M. & Moraes, C. T. (2008) Activation of the PPAR/PGC-1alpha pathway prevents a bioenergetic deficit and effectively improves a mitochondrial myopathy phenotype. *Cell Metab*, 8, 3, pp. 249-56, ISSN 1932-7420

Wu, Z.;Puigserver, P.;Andersson, U.;Zhang, C.;Adelmant, G.;Mootha, V.;Troy, A.;Cinti, S.;Lowell, B.;Scarpulla, R. C. & Spiegelman, B. M. (1999) Mechanisms controlling mitochondrial biogenesis and respiration through the thermogenic coactivator PGC-1. *Cell*, 98, 1, pp. 115-24, ISSN 0092-8674

Yang, B.;Jung, D.;Motto, D.;Meyer, J.;Koretzky, G. & Campbell, K. P. (1995) SH3 domain-mediated interaction of dystroglycan and Grb2. *J Biol Chem*, 270, 20, pp. 11711-4

Yeretssian, G.;Lecocq, M.;Lebon, G.;Hurst, H. C. & Sakanyan, V. (2005) Competition on nitrocellulose-immobilized antibody arrays: from bacterial protein binding assay to protein profiling in breast cancer cells. *Mol Cell Proteomics*, 4, 5, pp. 605-17, ISSN 1535-9476

Zhang, S.;Xie, H.;Zhou, G. & Yang, Z. (2007) Development of therapy for Duchenne muscular dystrophy. *Zhongguo Xiu Fu Chong Jian Wai Ke Za Zhi*, 21, 2, pp. 194-203, ISSN 1002-1892

Zhong, N. & Xu, J. (2008) Synergistic activation of the human MnSOD promoter by DJ-1 and PGC-1alpha: regulation by SUMOylation and oxidation. *Hum Mol Genet*, 17, 21, pp. 3357-67, ISSN 1460-2083

8

Mitogen-Activated Protein Kinases and Mitogen-Activated Protein Kinase Phosphatases in Regenerative Myogenesis and Muscular Dystrophy

Hao Shi[1] and Anton M. Bennett[1,2]
[1]Department of Pharmacology
[2]Program in Integrative Cell Signaling and Neurobiology of Metabolism,
Yale University School of Medicine,
United States

1. Introduction

The mitogen-activated protein kinase (MAPK) signal transduction pathway is required to promote skeletal myogenesis and maintain skeletal muscle function. Although it has been long appreciated that the MAPK pathway plays a critical role in skeletal myogenesis it is still unclear as to whether the MAPKs are involved in the development of skeletal muscle diseases such as muscular dystrophies. Much evidence has demonstrated that MAPK activation is important for skeletal myogenesis. The cessation of MAPK activity is also an important part of the process of skeletal myogenesis. The MAPK phosphatases (MKPs) are responsible for inactivating the MAPKs. The role of the MKPs in physiological and pathophysiological functions of skeletal muscle remains to be fully understood. In this review, we will summarize the current state of understanding of the functional roles of the MAPKs, and the emerging role of the MKPs in the regulation of physiological skeletal muscle function, and their potential involvement in skeletal muscle diseases.

2. Mitogen-activated Protein Kinase signaling and myogenesis

The mitogen-activated protein kinase (MAPK) cascade plays an essential role in conveying extracellular signals from growth factors, stress, and cytokines into biological responses that include differentiation, proliferation, apoptosis and cell motility (Cuevas et al., 2007; Pearson et al., 2001). Up until now, at least 4 MAPK signaling pathways have been identified: 1) extracellular signal-regulated kinase 1 and 2 (ERK1/2), 2) p38α/β/γ/δ MAPK, 3) c-Jun NH_2-terminal kinases 1, 2, and 3 (JNK1/2/3) and 4) ERK5 (Bogoyevitch, 2006; Bogoyevitch and Court, 2004; Whitmarsh, 2006; Zarubin and Han, 2005). MAPKs when phosphorylated on their regulatory threonine and tyrosine residues by their upstream MAPK kinases become activated. Once activated, these MAPKs phosphorylate substrates that include transcription factors, phospholipases, protein kinases and cytoskeletal proteins (Johnson and Lapadat, 2002; Turjanski et al., 2007).

A large body of data suggests that the p38 MAPK pathway is pro-myogenic. p38 MAPK promotes myogenesis through 1) interaction with transcription factors. At the early stage of differentiation, p38 MAPK phosphorylates E-protein E47, which dimerizes with the transcription factor MyoD to activate muscle-specific gene expression (Lluis et al., 2005). Whereas, at later stages of differentiation, p38 MAPK phosphorylates the transcription factor MRF4 thereby repressing its transcriptional activity (Suelves et al., 2004). 2) phosphorylation of the SWI/SNF chromatin-remodeling complex, recruiting this complex to myogenic loci (Simone et al., 2004); 3) phosphorylation of the transcription factor myocyte enhancer factor-2 (MEF2) thereby enhancing its transcriptional activity (Black and Olson, 1998; Zetser et al., 1999); 4) stabilization of myogenic mRNA by directly phosphorylating KSRP, an important factor for decaying AU-rich element mRNA, and compromising its function to promote mRNA decay (Briata et al., 2005). These observations provide strong mechanistic insight into how p38 MAPK couples to the myogenic machinery.

Evidence derived from mouse models also supports the functional role of p38 MAPK in muscle differentiation (Perdiguero et al., 2007). In an effort to dissect the role of different p38 MAPK isoforms in myogenesis, Perdiguero *et al* used p38α, p38β, p38γ, and p38δ-deficient mice and analyzed the function of each. p38α rather than p38β and p38γ-deficient myoblasts failed to form multinucleated myotubes, whereas p38δ-deficient myoblasts exhibited attenuated differentiation (Perdiguero et al., 2007). Although a wide body of evidence supports the pro-myogenic role of p38 MAPK, several reports also imply the involvement of p38 MAPK in muscle cell proliferation. The concomitant activation of p38 MAPKα/β and satellite cells imply that p38 MAPK may also be involved in satellite cell activation, since blockade of p38 MAPK by pharmacological inhibitors of p38 MAPK prevents both satellite cell proliferation and differentiation (Jones et al., 2005; Shi et al., 2010). A recent study using p38γ-deficient mice revealed that muscles lacking this isoform of p38 MAPK contain 50% less satellite cells, and these cells exhibit reduced proliferation (Gillespie et al., 2009) implying that this p38 MAPK isoform may also be an important regulator of satellite cell deposition and proliferation.

Although a critical role for ERK1/2 in satellite cell proliferation is established, surprisingly the role of ERK1/2 in myogenesis has not been well defined. Conflicting data from various groups suggest that this pathway may be tailored to respond to distinct cellular and extracellular conditions. Using 10T1/2 fibroblasts, Gredinger el showed that MEK1 and/or Raf1 positively regulates myogenesis by enhancing MyoD transcriptional activity, addition of the MEK inhibitor PD098059 represses MyoD-responsive genes (Gredinger et al., 1998). PD098059 also partially inhibits the formation of multinucleated myotubes in C2 myoblasts (Gredinger et al., 1998). In contrast, others have reported a negative effect of ERK1/2 in the regulation of myogenesis (Dorman and Johnson, 1999; Weyman and Wolfman, 1998). In 23A2 and C2C12 myoblasts, IGF-1 and FGF-2 inhibit myoblast differentiation through ERK1/2 signaling as PD098059 blocked this effect (Kontaridis et al., 2002; Weyman and Wolfman, 1998). Persistent activation of Raf/MEK/ERK1/2 by overexpression of a constitutively active Raf inhibits the fusion of embryonic chick myoblasts into multinucleated myotubes. This inhibition can be rescued by addition of PD098059 (Dorman and Johnson, 1999). Yet there is another layer of regulation of Ras/Raf/ERK1/2 on myogenesis. A novel regulator of the Ras-Raf interaction, named DA-Raf, lacks the Raf kinase domain and interferes with the binding of Ras to other targets. It was found that DA-

Raf serves as a positive regulator of myogenic differentiation (Yokoyama et al., 2007). A recent study revealed that Grb2-associated binder 1 (Gab1) interacts with the protein tyrosine phosphatase SHP-2 to activate downstream ERK signaling, thereby inhibiting IGF-1-mediated myogenic differentiation (Koyama et al., 2008). These results are consistent with other data in which conditional deletion of SHP-2 in skeletal muscle impairs skeletal muscle growth (Fornaro et al., 2006). Taken together, these findings tend to support the notion that ERK1/2 signaling promotes myoblast proliferation and inhibits myogenic differentiation. However, further genetic data using ERK-deficient mice needs to be provided to fully conclude the relevance of ERK1/2 in myoblast proliferation and differentiation.

ERK5 is a novel member of the MAPK family and its physiological function in myogenesis remains to be fully defined. ERK5 is enriched in skeletal muscle, it is activated upon myogenic differentiation, and anti-sense RNA to ERK5 blocks entry into myogenesis (Dinev et al., 2001). A recent study revealed an essential role of ERK5 in muscle cell fusion through the transcription factors Sp1 and Klf2/4 (Sunadome et al., 2011). ERK5 has also been shown to be responsible for muscle cell fusion without interference with other differentiation processes (Sunadome et al., 2011).

Although the JNK pathway has been implicated in myoblast proliferation (Perdiguero et al., 2007) its role in myogenic differentiation remains controversial. JNK has been demonstrated to be either dispensable or negative for myogenesis (Gallo et al., 1999; Khurana and Dey, 2004; Meriane et al., 2002). It would be extremely informative if myoblasts derived from mice lacking either of the JNK isoforms were analyzed for their effects on cell proliferation and differentiation to resolve these issues.

3. Duchenne muscular dystrophy

The most common form of muscular dystrophy is Duchenne muscular dystrophy (DMD) which affects up to 1:3,500 males in the United States (Porter, 2000). The regenerative capacity of skeletal muscle in DMD-stricken patients is impaired due to the loss of dystrophin (Davies and Nowak, 2006). DMD patients lose muscle strength and mobility and the disease often results in death. There is neither a cure, nor an effective treatment for DMD, or similar skeletal muscle degenerative diseases (Bhatnagar and Kumar, 2010; Tedesco et al., 2010). DMD is caused by the loss or partial deficiency in the dystrophin protein, which serves as a critical component of the dystrophin glycoprotein complex (DGC) linking the cytoskeleton of the muscle fibers to that of the extracellular matrix. The loss of dystrophin cripples the functionality of the DGC rendering the muscle fiber more susceptible to stress-induced injury. Although the primary defect of DMD is the loss of dystrophin, there are multiple secondary events that contribute to the progression of the disease. These include profound inflammatory responses, extracellular matrix degradation and fibrosis. Strategies therefore that curtail some of these secondary responses have been considered as potential therapeutic avenues to treating the progression of the disease in DMD patients.

Although the DGC and its components such as dystrophin appear to primarily serve structural roles to couple the muscle fiber to the extracellular matrix, there is clearly an important intracellular role played by providing a platform from which signaling pathways are launched. These links to downstream pathways suggest that the DGC engages active signaling in order to regulate muscle fiber function. Hence, DGC dysregulation may lead to alterations in intracellular signaling cascades, which may contribute to the pathogenesis of the muscular dystrophies. In this regard, understanding the signaling pathways such as the MAPKs in skeletal muscle function and muscular dystrophy may provide important insight into new avenues of therapies for these diseases.

4. MAPKs and Muscular dystrophy

A link between the MAPKs and muscular dystrophy has been indirectly suggested by the fact that the DGC not only functions as a mechanical infrastructure to stabilize skeletal muscle cell membranes, but it also serves as a bridge between stimuli from the extracellular matrix and intracellular signaling through physically interacting with distinct proteins (Rando, 2001). For example, Grb2, an adapter protein involved in MAPK signal transduction and cytoskeletal organization, interacts with β-dystroglycan at the C-terminal proline-rich domains (Yang et al., 1995). Furthermore, β-dystroglycan can physically interact with MAPK kinase 2 (MEK2) and its downstream kinase ERK1/2 in a yeast two-hybrid screen (Spence et al., 2004). These findings imply that MAPK signaling may play an important role in the mechano- and signal transduction of extracellular stimuli to intracellular biological responses that control muscle fiber viability. However, the reports regarding the activity of the MAPKs in the pathogenesis of muscular dystrophy remain inconclusive and vary in different experimental settings. For example, it has been reported that JNK1 is highly activated in a mouse model of DMD (*mdx* mouse) and compound intercrosses between an *mdx* mouse and a MyoD-deficient mouse (*mdx/MyoD-/-*) contributes to the progressive dystrophinopathy without appreciable changes in either ERK1/2 or p38 MAPK activities (Kolodziejczyk et al., 2001). In contrast, stable over-expression of the JNK1-specific upstream kinase MKK7 disrupts the formation of myotubes in C2C12 skeletal myoblasts and H9C2 cardiac myoblasts (Kolodziejczyk et al., 2001). Adenoviral infection of the JNK1 specific inhibitor JIP1 (JNK interacting protein) increased the diameter of myofibers (Kolodziejczyk et al., 2001), suggesting that the MAPKs can affect the structural integrity of the myofiber. In an attempt to test whether loss of dystrophin causes aberrant mechanotransduction, Kumar et al measured the activity of the MAPKs following stretching of *mdx* and wild type diaphragm muscles. ERK1/2, but not JNK or p38 MAPKs were significantly activated in the muscles derived from *mdx* mice (Kumar et al., 2004). In addition, the downstream effector of ERK1/2, AP-1 was highly up-regulated (Kumar et al., 2004). In another exercise model, *mdx* mice were subjected to treadmill exercise, p38 MAPK and ERK1/2, but not JNK1 were highly elevated in *mdx* cardiac muscles in comparison with wild type muscles (Nakamura et al., 2002). Elevated p38 MAPK was also observed in utrophin-dystrophin double knock-out cardiac muscles (Nakamura et al., 2001). Together, these findings suggest that MAPK signaling is likely involved in the pathogenesis of muscular dystrophy, but to what extent and how exactly MAPK contributes at the molecular level to the pathogenesis of DMD remains to be established.

5. MAPK phosphatases in skeletal muscle function and muscular dystrophy

Equally important as the activation of the MAPKs is their inactivation, which is catalyzed by the MKPs. The MKPs belong to a sub-class of protein tyrosine phosphatases known as the dual-specificity protein phosphatases (DUSP) (Boutros et al., 2008; Soulsby and Bennett,

2009; Tonks, 2006). The DUSPs are characterized by a consensus signature motif represented by $HC(X)_5R$ which defines the active site of these enzymes (Soulsby and Bennett, 2009; Tonks, 2006). MKPs inactivate the MAPKs by directly dephosphorylating the MAPKs on its regulatory threonine and tyrosine residues. The MKPs share largely the same structure comprising of a cdc25 homology domain and a MAPK binding domain in the NH_2 terminus and a COOH-terminus PTP catalytic domain. The NH_2 terminus of the MKPs controls MAPK binding and sub-cellular targeting (Wu et al., 2005), both of these attributes contribute to MAPK signaling specificity. In this regard, although the MKPs dephosphorylate the MAPKs they do so with varying degrees of potency that depends upon both their MAPK binding affinity and sub-cellular localization. There are 10 catalytically active members in this group and they exhibit distinct sub-cellular localization, responses to extracellular stimuli, tissue distribution and affinity to their substrates (Boutros et al., 2008; Groom et al., 1996; Ishibashi et al., 1994; Misra-Press et al., 1995; Muda et al., 1997; Noguchi et al., 1993; Rohan et al., 1993).

Binding of MKPs to their MAPK substrates increases phosphatase activity (Camps et al., 1998a; Hutter et al., 2000; Slack et al., 2001) and this is due to stabilization of the active enzyme-substrate complex (Field et al., 2000). MKP-3 exhibits high fidelity to its substrate ERK1/2 and upon binding its catalytic activity is enhanced (Camps et al., 1998b). Despite the fact that the MKPs dephosphorylate a common pool of MAPKs these enzymes exhibit remarkably unique physiological effects (Chi et al., 2006; Christie et al., 2005; Wu et al., 2006). Studies from MKP knock-out mice provide convincing genetic evidence to support the notion that these MKPs function in distinct ways (Nunes-Xavier et al., 2011). The complexity of the signaling pathways and biological responses that the MKPs are involved with strongly suggest that these enzymes serve as central players in the regulation of the MAPKs. Therefore, the MKPs, which have the capacity to regulate multiple MAPKs simultaneously, represent a critical signaling node of MAPK convergence. Molecules that act as signalling (before nodes) in signal transduction can be defined as those which represent a point of convergence of multiple pathways, and one that is represented by several isoforms that are both positively and negatively involved in divergent signaling. We propose that the MKPs satisfy these criteria and constitute a critical signaling node in the MAPK pathway. Given the established role of the MAPKs in skeletal myogenesis, the actions of the MKPs as critical signaling nodes of the MAPKs is likely to make them important players in this system.

MKPs in skeletal myogenesis and skeletal muscle function. Studies of the MKPs in myogenesis and skeletal muscle function remain mainly an uncharted area. Much of the work on the MKPs in skeletal muscle function has focused on the role of MKP-1. The first MKP to be implicated in skeletal muscle function was MKP-1 (Bennett and Tonks, 1997). MKP-1 is a ubiquitously expressed, nuclear localized dual-specificity phosphatase, whose substrates include predominantly p38 MAPK, JNK and to a lesser extent, ERK1/2 (Boutros et al., 2008; Owens and Keyse, 2007). MKP-1 is an immediate-early gene and is induced by numerous stresses (Owens and Keyse, 2007). Initial reports demonstrated that MKP-1-deficient mice exhibit an unremarkable phenotype, suggesting that the MKPs largely serve redundant physiological roles (Dorfman et al., 1996). However, we have shown that mice lacking MKP-1 exhibit enhanced ERK1/2, JNK and p38 MAPK activities in skeletal muscle, as well as in other tissues, demonstrating that MKP-1 plays an essential physiological role as a negative regulator of the MAPKs (Wu et al., 2006). The earliest suggestion that MKP-1, and hence the MAPKs, participate in myogenic regulation emerged from studies in which conditional overexpression of MKP-1 was shown to stimulate precocious myogenesis in the context of the inhibitory actions of growth factors (Bennett and Tonks, 1997). MKP-1 expression levels in proliferating myoblasts are initially high, at levels presumably sufficient to allow cell proliferation but not differentiation, and declines upon the onset of myogenesis, suggesting that extinguishing the expression of MKP-1 might be a prerequisite for myogenic entry and/or progression (Bennett and Tonks, 1997; Kondoh et al., 2007; Perdiguero et al., 2007). Consistent with this, overexpression of MKP-1 when myoblasts have become irrevocably committed to myogenesis inhibits multinucleated myotube formation (Bennett and Tonks, 1997; Kondoh et al., 2007). Hence, MKP-1 plays both positive and negative roles in myogenesis in a temporal manner by selectively regulating one or more MAPKs (**Figure 1**). MKP-1 appears to be directly coupled to the myogenic transcriptional machinery as studies have shown that MKP-1 is a target for upregulation by MyoD (Shi et al., 2010). Within the proximal promoter of MKP-1 there resides an E-box binding site that serves to mediate MKP-1 activation by MyoD (Shi et al., 2010). Hence, upon the initiation of myogenesis the activation of MyoD leads to an initial upregulation of MKP-1, which may be required to inactivate ERK1/2 and thus facilitate cell cycle exit in the transition towards myogenic entry. Later on during myogenesis MyoD was shown to uncouple from the MKP-1 promoter and hence downregulate MKP-1 expression (**Figure 1**). Downregulation of MKP-1 during the later stages of myogenesis may facilitate the increased p38 MAPK activation, which is important for multinucleated myotube formation. As such, the complexity of the outcome through which MKP-1 integrates multiple MAPK activities cannot be simply inferred by the implied actions of a single MAPK family member. These results using cultured myoblast cell lines are supported by *in vivo* data where it has been shown that regenerative myogenesis in response to cardiotoxin-induced injury is impaired in MKP-1-deficient mice (Shi et al., 2010). These results support the notion that MKP-1 is an important regulator of myogenesis.

MKP-1 is also implicated in adult skeletal muscle fiber specialization (Shi et al., 2008). Overexpression of MKP-1 in adult type IIb (glycolytic) myofibers converts these fibers to slower-twitch type IIa or type I (oxidative) fibers, suggesting that MKP-1-mediated dephosphorylation of MAPK signaling is required to maintain the glycolytic fiber phenotype through the repression of slow myofibers (Shi et al., 2008). Consistent with these data, it has been shown that MKP-1-deficient mice are protected from the loss of oxidative myofibers during high fat diet-induced obesity (Roth et al., 2009). Hence, decreased MKP-1 expression results in enhanced MAPK signaling, which protects from the loss of glycolytic myofibers by driving oxidative myofiber conversion. The mechanistic basis for these data is based upon the observation that MKP-1 mediates p38 MAPK phosphorylation of the peroxisome proliferator-activated receptor γ co-activator 1α (PGC-1α) (Roth et al., 2009), which is required to promote oxidative myofiber conversion. Collectively, these results suggest that MKP-1 plays an essential role in the maintenance of glycolytic/oxidative myofiber composition. MKP-1 is also suggested to be involved in the maintenance of muscle mass (Shi et al., 2009). Overexpression of MKP-1 in slow-twitch soleus muscles and in fast-twitch gastrocnemius muscles reduces muscle fiber size, though this reduction in fiber size may go through distinct molecular mechanisms (Shi et al., 2009).

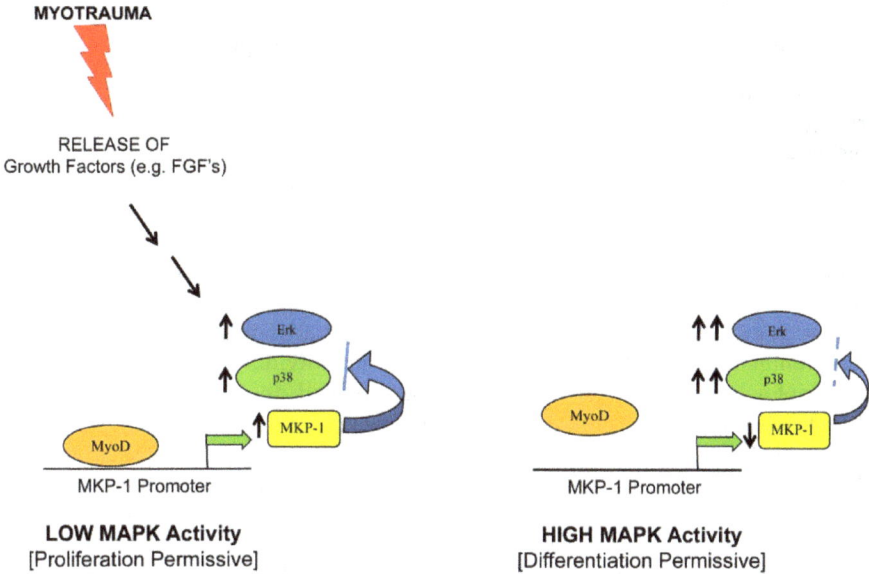

Fig. 1. MAPK/MKP signaling coordinates myogenesis. Following myotrauma the MAPKs become activated to drive cell proliferation. MKP-1 is upregulated by these MAPKs and MyoD. MKP-1 sets the threshold of MAPK activity that permits myoblast proliferation [Proliferation Permissive] but not differentiation. Upon the initiation of differentiation, MyoD uncouples from the MKP-1 promoter causing its expression levels to fall, thereby removing the inhibitory actions of MKP-1 on the MAPKs. This allows for higher levels of MAPK activity to be achieved, in particular p38 MAPK, which promotes differentiation [Differentiation Permissive].

MKP-1 also plays a regulatory role in estrogen-related receptor α (ERRα) and PGC-1α mediated myogenic differentiation. Direct up-regulation of MKP-1 by ERRα and PGC-1α at the early stage of myogenesis inactivate ERK1/2 signaling and facilitate the progression of myogensis as MEK inhibition rescues the myogenic defect in ERRα-/- myoblasts (Murray and Huss, 2011). Recent work from this laboratory suggests that other MKPs, in addition to MKP-1, also contribute to the regulation of skeletal muscle function. Mice lacking MKP-5, which interestingly also dephosphorylates predominately p38 MAPK and JNK, exhibit enhanced skeletal muscle regeneration distinct from that observed with MKP-1-deficient mice (H.S. and A.M.B., *unpublished observations*). These results suggest that the MKPs might play distinct roles in not only coordinating myogenic activation and progression but they may do so through specific and non-overlapping mechanisms.

A role for MKP-1 in muscular dystrophy. The generation, maintenance, and repair of adult skeletal muscle is critically dependent upon the activation and self-renewal of satellite cells (Wagers and Conboy, 2005). In response to skeletal muscle injury, myofiber-released growth factors and cytokines stimulate satellite cell proliferation, migration and differentiation by activating signaling cascades including the MAPK pathway. It is thought that the depletion of satellite cells during the progression of DMD is a major factor that precipitates the ultimate failure of muscle function. Therefore, by modulating satellite cell activation, differentiation and/or self-renewal DMD can theoretically be improved.

Several reports have addressed the role of the MAPKs in *mdx* mice, however there is no underlying consensus as to whether the MAPKs are definitively involved in the pathogenesis of the dystrophic phenotype. Some reports show upregulation of ERK1/2, JNK2 and p38 MAPK (Nakamura et al., 2005), whereas others have shown a downregulation of p38 MAPK and an upregulation of ERK1/2 (Lang et al., 2004), yet others find no consistent differences in p38 MAPK (Nakamura et al., 2001). To study the pathophysiological role of MKP-1 in Duchenne muscular dystrophy, we inter-crossed MKP-1 knockout mice into the *mdx* background in order to determine whether loss of MKP-1 ameliorates or exacerbates the dystrophic phenotype. The advantage of generating an MKP-1-deficient animal model is that instead of studying an individual MAPK, we examined the integration of several MAPKs that become hyperactivated due to the lack of MKP-1. We found that *mdx/mkp-1-/-* mice have reduced body weight and muscle mass in comparison with *mdx/mkp-1+/+* mice (Shi et al., 2010). The reduction of body weight may be attributed to the chronic elevated levels of inflammation or it is also likely that this is due to an underlying metabolic defect that we have observed in mice lacking MKP-1 that is related to increased energy expenditure (Roth et al., 2009; Wu et al., 2006). Histological analysis of muscle sections from *mdx/mkp-1-/-* mice revealed that MKP-1 deficiency exacerbates the pathogenesis of muscular dystrophy (Shi et al., 2010). This exacerbation may be accounted for by a combination of two factors that are cell autonomous and/or directly related to defects in satellite cell function as well as a contribution from a hyperactivated immune response. Satellite cells from MKP-1-deficient muscles exhibit reduced proliferative capacity whereas precocious differentiation was evident even under high serum conditions (Shi et al., 2010). Additionally, increased levels of macrophage and neutrophil infiltrates into damaged myofibers in *mdx/mkp-1-/-* mice compared to MKP-1 wild type *mdx* mice, this was observed along with serum and skeletal muscle cytokine levels that are significantly increased in *mdx/mkp-1-/-* mice (Shi et al., 2010). Collectively, these findings suggest that MKP-1 is critical for the regulation of muscle regeneration in DMD by modulating both immune responses and satellite cell proliferation and differentiation (**Figure 2**). Further studies employing conditional deletion of MKP-1 in the satellite cell and hematopoietic compartments will be required in order to determine the contribution of MKP-1 in these tissues to the overall skeletal muscle regenerative defect.

6. Therapeutic targeting of MAPK/MKPs in muscular dystrophy

Research on MKP-1 and its involvement in regenerative myogenesis and muscular dystrophy suggests that MKP-1 may play an important role in the progression of muscular dystrophy and possibly other degenerative skeletal muscle diseases. Therefore, targeting the MAPK/MKP signaling pathway in order to ameliorate skeletal muscle disease and specifically, muscular dystrophy, merits further investigation. However, definitive validation that the MAPK/MKP module is a valid therapeutic target for muscular dystrophy is still lacking. There has been some suggestion that interference with the MAPK/MKP signaling module may have therapeutic value. It has been shown that adenoviral delivery of the JNK1 inhibitory protein, JIP1, can attenuate the pathogenesis of dystrophic fibers (Kolodziejczyk et al., 2001), implying that inhibition of JNK1 may serve as

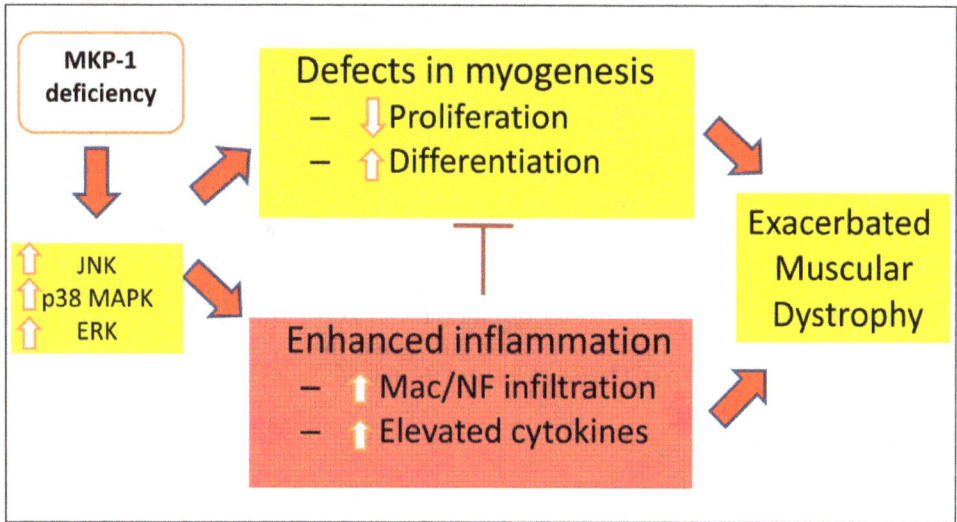

Fig. 2. MKP-1 and Duchenne Muscular Dystrophy. MKP-1 regulates both myoblast
proliferation and differentiation (see Figure 1). Loss of MKP-1 in a mouse model of
Duchennes' muscular dystrophy exacerbates the dystrophic phenotype due to enhanced
MAPK activity, which inhibits myoblast proliferation, and ectopically enhances
differentiation. In conjunction, MKP-1 has a profound effect in macrophages (Mac) and
neutrophils (NF), which as a result of enhanced MAPK activity, in the absence of MKP-1
become hyper-responsive leading to increased inflammatory responses. Together, both the
increased inflammatory response and dysfunctional myoblast proliferation and
differentiation exacerbates the dystrophic phenotype.

a potential therapeutic target for the treatment of certain dystrophies. However, given the
uncertain role played by JNK in skeletal muscle regeneration this target should be
approached cautiously. A recent study shows that treating dystrophic mice with the free
radical scavenger α-lipoic acid and L-carnitine improved muscular dystrophy with a
concomitant repression of ERK1/2, JNK and p38 MAPK activation (Hnia et al., 2007). This is
quite a provocative result since reactive oxygen species have been shown to inhibit the
actions of certain protein tyrosine phosphatases through modification of the catalytic
cysteine residue (Tonks, 2005). Therefore, treatment of dystrophic muscle with free radical
scavengers would be predicted to ameliorate the loss of PTP activity, including MKP
activity, resulting in increased inactivation of MAPKs. However, it is not yet clear whether
the improved myopathy is caused by the decreased activation of a particular MAPK and/or
a combination thereof. In an Emery-Dreyfuss muscular dystrophy mouse model, which
lacks the inner nuclear membrane protein A-type lamins (LMNA), JNK and ERK1/2 are
highly activated in heart tissue and cardiomycytes (Muchir et al., 2007). Inhibition of the
ERK1/2 upstream kinase MEK by PD098059 improves cardiomyopathy in *Lmna* mutant
knock-in mice (Muchir et al., 2009), implying that molecules in the ERK1/2 pathway have
therapeutic potential for the treatment of human Emery-Dreyfuss muscular dystrophy and
potentially related disorders.

Although the MAPK/MKP pathway represents a potentially attractive therapeutic target to treat muscular dystrophy, it is a challenging one given the fact that the MAPK/MKP module is a universal pathway serving a number of common control points in the regulation of cell proliferation, differentiation, migration, and survival. The challenge will be to identify MAPK/MKP family members that exhibit signaling preferences to skeletal muscle with those functions further selectively controlling the appropriate physiological response in dystrophic skeletal muscle tissue. Given the importance of p38 MAPK in promoting regenerative myogenesis an attractive strategy could involve enhancing p38 MAPK activity so as to promote either satellite cell activation, proliferation and/or differentiation in dystrophic tissue. This could conceivably be achieved either through activation of p38 MAPK itself or through inhibition of the MKP that opposes the physiologically relevant pool of p38 MAPK in these cells. Clearly, significant gaps in our knowledge need to be filled in this area, nevertheless it is an important goal given the devastating nature of these skeletal muscle diseases that still lack a successful treatment.

7. Acknowledgements

A.M.B. is supported by the National Institutes of Health and H.S. by a grant from the Muscular Dystrophy Association.

8. References

Bennett, A.M., and N.K. Tonks. 1997. Regulation of distinct stages of skeletal muscle differentiation by mitogen-activated protein kinases. *Science*. 278:1288-1291.

Bhatnagar, S., and A. Kumar. 2010. Therapeutic targeting of signaling pathways in muscular dystrophy. *J Mol Med (Berl)*. 88:155-166.

Black, B.L., and E.N. Olson. 1998. Transcriptional control of muscle development by myocyte enhancer factor-2 (MEF2) proteins. Annu Rev Cell Dev Biol. 14:167-196.

Bogoyevitch, M.A. 2006. The isoform-specific functions of the c-Jun N-terminal Kinases (JNKs): differences revealed by gene targeting. *Bioessays*. 28:923-934.

Bogoyevitch, M.A., and N.W. Court. 2004. Counting on mitogen-activated protein kinases-- ERKs 3, 4, 5, 6, 7 and 8. *Cell Signal*. 16:1345-1354.

Boutros, T., E. Chevet, and P. Metrakos. 2008. Mitogen-activated protein (MAP) kinase/MAP kinase phosphatase regulation: roles in cell growth, death, and cancer. *Pharmacol Rev*. 60:261-310.

Briata, P., S.V. Forcales, M. Ponassi, G. Corte, C.Y. Chen, M. Karin, P.L. Puri, and R. Gherzi. 2005. p38-dependent phosphorylation of the mRNA decay-promoting factor KSRP controls the stability of select myogenic transcripts. *Mol Cell*. 20:891-903.

Camps, M., C. Chabert, M. Muda, U. Boschert, C. Gillieron, and S. Arkinstall. 1998a. Induction of the mitogen-activated protein kinase phosphatase MKP3 by nerve growth factor in differentiating PC12. *FEBS Lett*. 425:271-276.

Camps, M., A. Nichols, C. Gillieron, B. Antonsson, M. Muda, C. Chabert, U. Boschert, and S. Arkinstall. 1998b. Catalytic activation of the phosphatase MKP-3 by ERK2 mitogen-activated protein kinase. *Science*. 280:1262-1265.

Chi, H., S.P. Barry, R.J. Roth, J.J. Wu, E.A. Jones, A.M. Bennett, and R.A. Flavell. 2006. Dynamic regulation of pro- and anti-inflammatory cytokines by MAPK phosphatase 1 (MKP-1) in innate immune responses. *Proc Natl Acad Sci U S A*. 103:2274-2279.

Christie, G.R., D.J. Williams, F. Macisaac, R.J. Dickinson, I. Rosewell, and S.M. Keyse. 2005. The dual-specificity protein phosphatase DUSP9/MKP-4 is essential for placental function but is not required for normal embryonic development. *Mol Cell Biol.* 25:8323-8333.

Cuevas, B.D., A.N. Abell, and G.L. Johnson. 2007. Role of mitogen-activated protein kinase kinase kinases in signal integration. *Oncogene.* 26:3159-3171.

Davies, K.E., and K.J. Nowak. 2006. Molecular mechanisms of muscular dystrophies: old and new players. *Nat Rev Mol Cell Biol.* 7:762-773.

Deconinck, N., and B. Dan. 2007. Pathophysiology of duchenne muscular dystrophy: current hypotheses. *Pediatr Neurol.* 36:1-7.

Dorfman, K., D. Carrasco, M. Gruda, C. Ryan, S.A. Lira, and R. Bravo. 1996. Disruption of the erp/mkp-1 gene does not affect mouse development: normal MAP kinase activity in ERP/MKP-1-deficient fibroblasts. *Oncogene.* 13:925-931.

Dorman, C.M., and S.E. Johnson. 1999. Activated Raf inhibits avian myogenesis through a MAPK-dependent mechanism. *Oncogene.* 18:5167-5176.

Field, C.J., C.A. Thomson, J.E. Van Aerde, A. Parrott, A. Euler, E. Lien, and M.T. Clandinin. 2000. Lower proportion of CD45R0+ cells and deficient interleukin-10 production by formula-fed infants, compared with human-fed, is corrected with supplementation of long-chain polyunsaturated fatty acids. *J Pediatr Gastroenterol Nutr.* 31:291-299.

Fornaro, M., P.M. Burch, W. Yang, L. Zhang, C.E. Hamilton, J.H. Kim, B.G. Neel, and A.M. Bennett. 2006. SHP-2 activates signaling of the nuclear factor of activated T cells to promote skeletal muscle growth. *J Cell Biol.* 175:87-97.

Gallo, R., M. Serafini, L. Castellani, G. Falcone, and S. Alema. 1999. Distinct effects of Rac1 on differentiation of primary avian myoblasts. *Mol Biol Cell.* 10:3137-3150.

Gillespie, M.A., F. Le Grand, A. Scime, S. Kuang, J. von Maltzahn, V. Seale, A. Cuenda, J.A. Ranish, and M.A. Rudnicki. 2009. p38-{gamma}-dependent gene silencing restricts entry into the myogenic differentiation program. *J Cell Biol.* 187:991-1005.

Gredinger, E., A.N. Gerber, Y. Tamir, S.J. Tapscott, and E. Bengal. 1998. Mitogen-activated protein kinase pathway is involved in the differentiation of muscle cells. *J Biol Chem.* 273:10436-10444.

Groom, L.A., A.A. Sneddon, D.R. Alessi, S. Dowd, and S.M. Keyse. 1996. Differential regulation of the MAP, SAP and RK/p38 kinases by Pyst1, a novel cytosolic dual-specificity phosphatase. *Embo J.* 15:3621-3632.

Hammer, M., J. Mages, H. Dietrich, A. Servatius, N. Howells, A.C. Cato, and R. Lang. 2006. Dual specificity phosphatase 1 (DUSP1) regulates a subset of LPS-induced genes and protects mice from lethal endotoxin shock. *J Exp Med.* 203:15-20.

Hnia, K., G. Hugon, F. Rivier, A. Masmoudi, J. Mercier, and D. Mornet. 2007. Modulation of p38 mitogen-activated protein kinase cascade and metalloproteinase activity in diaphragm muscle in response to free radical scavenger administration in dystrophin-deficient Mdx mice. *Am J Pathol.* 170:633-643.

Hutter, D., P. Chen, J. Barnes, and Y. Liu. 2000. Catalytic activation of mitogen-activated protein (MAP) kinase phosphatase-1 by binding to p38 MAP kinase: critical role of the p38 C-terminal domain in its negative regulation. *Biochem J.* 352 Pt 1:155-163.

Ishibashi, T., D.P. Bottaro, P. Michieli, C.A. Kelley, and S.A. Aaronson. 1994. A novel dual specificity phosphatase induced by serum stimulation and heat shock. *J Biol Chem.* 269:29897-29902.

Johnson, G.L., and R. Lapadat. 2002. Mitogen-activated protein kinase pathways mediated by ERK, JNK, and p38 protein kinases. *Science.* 298:1911-1912.

Jones, N.C., K.J. Tyner, L. Nibarger, H.M. Stanley, D.D. Cornelison, Y.V. Fedorov, and B.B. Olwin. 2005. The p38alpha/beta MAPK functions as a molecular switch to activate the quiescent satellite cell. *J Cell Biol.* 169:105-116.

Khurana, A., and C.S. Dey. 2004. Involvement of c-Jun N-terminal kinase activities in skeletal muscle differentiation. *J Muscle Res Cell Motil.* 25:645-655.

Kolodziejczyk, S.M., G.S. Walsh, K. Balazsi, P. Seale, J. Sandoz, A.M. Hierlihy, M.A. Rudnicki, J.S. Chamberlain, F.D. Miller, and L.A. Megeney. 2001. Activation of JNK1 contributes to dystrophic muscle pathogenesis. *Curr Biol.* 11:1278-1282.

Kondoh, K., K. Sunadome, and E. Nishida. 2007. Notch signaling suppresses p38 MAPK activity via induction of MKP-1 in myogenesis. *J Biol Chem.* 282:3058-3065.

Kontaridis, M.I., X. Liu, L. Zhang, and A.M. Bennett. 2002. Role of SHP-2 in fibroblast growth factor receptor-mediated suppression of myogenesis in C2C12 myoblasts. *Mol Cell Biol.* 22:3875-3891.

Koyama, T., Y. Nakaoka, Y. Fujio, H. Hirota, K. Nishida, S. Sugiyama, K. Okamoto, K. Yamauchi-Takihara, M. Yoshimura, S. Mochizuki, M. Hori, T. Hirano, and N. Mochizuki. 2008. Interaction of scaffolding adaptor protein Gab1 with tyrosine phosphatase SHP2 negatively regulates IGF-I-dependent myogenic differentiation via the ERK1/2 signaling pathway. *J Biol Chem.* 283:24234-24244.

Kumar, A., N. Khandelwal, R. Malya, M.B. Reid, and A.M. Boriek. 2004. Loss of dystrophin causes aberrant mechanotransduction in skeletal muscle fibers. *Faseb J.* 18:102-113.

Lang, J.M., K.A. Esser, and E.E. Dupont-Versteegden. 2004. Altered activity of signaling pathways in diaphragm and tibialis anterior muscle of dystrophic mice. *Exp Biol Med (Maywood).* 229:503-511.

Lluis, F., E. Ballestar, M. Suelves, M. Esteller, and P. Munoz-Canoves. 2005. E47 phosphorylation by p38 MAPK promotes MyoD/E47 association and muscle-specific gene transcription. *Embo J.* 24:974-984.

Meriane, M., S. Charrasse, F. Comunale, and C. Gauthier-Rouviere. 2002. Transforming growth factor beta activates Rac1 and Cdc42Hs GTPases and the JNK pathway in skeletal muscle cells. *Biol Cell.* 94:535-543.

Misra-Press, A., C.S. Rim, H. Yao, M.S. Roberson, and P.J. Stork. 1995. A novel mitogen-activated protein kinase phosphatase. Structure, expression, and regulation. *J Biol Chem.* 270:14587-14596.

Muchir, A., P. Pavlidis, V. Decostre, A.J. Herron, T. Arimura, G. Bonne, and H.J. Worman. 2007. Activation of MAPK pathways links LMNA mutations to cardiomyopathy in Emery-Dreifuss muscular dystrophy. *J Clin Invest.* 117:1282-1293.

Muchir, A., J. Shan, G. Bonne, S.E. Lehnart, and H.J. Worman. 2009. Inhibition of extracellular signal-regulated kinase signaling to prevent cardiomyopathy caused by mutation in the gene encoding A-type lamins. *Hum Mol Genet.* 18:241-247.

Muda, M., U. Boschert, A. Smith, B. Antonsson, C. Gillieron, C. Chabert, M. Camps, I. Martinou, A. Ashworth, and S. Arkinstall. 1997. Molecular cloning and functional characterization of a novel mitogen-activated protein kinase phosphatase, MKP-4. *J Biol Chem.* 272:5141-5151.

Murray, J., and J.M. Huss. 2011. Estrogen-related receptor {alpha} regulates skeletal myocyte differentiation via modulation of the ERK MAP kinase pathway. *Am J Physiol Cell Physiol.* 301:C630-645.

Nakamura, A., G.V. Harrod, and K.E. Davies. 2001. Activation of calcineurin and stress activated protein kinase/p38-mitogen activated protein kinase in hearts of utrophin-dystrophin knockout mice. *Neuromuscul Disord.* 11:251-259.

Nakamura, A., K. Yoshida, S. Takeda, N. Dohi, and S. Ikeda. 2002. Progression of dystrophic features and activation of mitogen-activated protein kinases and calcineurin by physical exercise, in hearts of mdx mice. *FEBS Lett.* 520:18-24.

Nakamura, A., K. Yoshida, H. Ueda, S. Takeda, and S. Ikeda. 2005. Up-regulation of mitogen activated protein kinases in mdx skeletal muscle following chronic treadmill exercise. *Biochim Biophys Acta.* 1740:326-331.

Noguchi, T., R. Metz, L. Chen, M.G. Mattei, D. Carrasco, and R. Bravo. 1993. Structure, mapping, and expression of erp, a growth factor-inducible gene encoding a nontransmembrane protein tyrosine phosphatase, and effect of ERP on cell growth. *Mol Cell Biol.* 13:5195-5205.

Nunes-Xavier, C., C. Roma-Mateo, P. Rios, C. Tarrega, R. Cejudo-Marin, L. Tabernero, and R. Pulido. 2011. Dual-specificity MAP kinase phosphatases as targets of cancer treatment. *In* Anticancer Agents Med Chem. Vol. 11. 109-132.

Owens, D.M., and S.M. Keyse. 2007. Differential regulation of MAP kinase signalling by dual-specificity protein phosphatases. *Oncogene.* 26:3203-3213.

Pearson, G., F. Robinson, T. Beers Gibson, B.E. Xu, M. Karandikar, K. Berman, and M.H. Cobb. 2001. Mitogen-activated protein (MAP) kinase pathways: regulation and physiological functions. *Endocr Rev.* 22:153-183.

Perdiguero, E., V. Ruiz-Bonilla, L. Gresh, L. Hui, E. Ballestar, P. Sousa-Victor, B. Baeza-Raja, M. Jardi, A. Bosch-Comas, M. Esteller, C. Caelles, A.L. Serrano, E.F. Wagner, and P. Munoz-Canoves. 2007. Genetic analysis of p38 MAP kinases in myogenesis: fundamental role of p38alpha in abrogating myoblast proliferation. *Embo J.* 26:1245-1256.

Porter, J.D. 2000. Introduction to muscular dystrophy. *Microsc Res Tech.* 48:127-130.

Rando, T.A. 2001. The dystrophin-glycoprotein complex, cellular signaling, and the regulation of cell survival in the muscular dystrophies. *Muscle Nerve.* 24:1575-1594.

Rohan, P.J., P. Davis, C.A. Moskaluk, M. Kearns, H. Krutzsch, U. Siebenlist, and K. Kelly. 1993. PAC-1: a mitogen-induced nuclear protein tyrosine phosphatase. *Science.* 259:1763-1766.

Roth, R.J., A.M. Le, L. Zhang, M. Kahn, V.T. Samuel, G.I. Shulman, and A.M. Bennett. 2009. MAPK phosphatase-1 facilitates the loss of oxidative myofibers associated with obesity in mice. *J Clin Invest.* 119:3817-3829.

Salojin, K.V., I.B. Owusu, K.A. Millerchip, M. Potter, K.A. Platt, and T. Oravecz. 2006. Essential role of MAPK phosphatase-1 in the negative control of innate immune responses. *J Immunol.* 176:1899-1907.

Shi, H., E. Boadu, F. Mercan, A.M. Le, R.J. Flach, L. Zhang, K.J. Tyner, B.B. Olwin, and A.M. Bennett. 2010. MAP kinase phosphatase-1 deficiency impairs skeletal muscle regeneration and exacerbates muscular dystrophy. *Faseb J.* 24:2985-2997.

Shi, H., J.M. Scheffler, J.M. Pleitner, C. Zeng, S. Park, K.M. Hannon, A.L. Grant, and D.E. Gerrard. 2008. Modulation of skeletal muscle fiber type by mitogen-activated protein kinase signaling. *Faseb J.* 22:2990-3000.

Shi, H., J.M. Scheffler, C. Zeng, J.M. Pleitner, K.M. Hannon, A.L. Grant, and D.E. Gerrard. 2009. Mitogen-activated protein kinase signaling is necessary for the maintenance of skeletal muscle mass. *Am J Physiol Cell Physiol.* 296:C1040-1048.

Simone, C., S.V. Forcales, D.A. Hill, A.N. Imbalzano, L. Latella, and P.L. Puri. 2004. p38 pathway targets SWI-SNF chromatin-remodeling complex to muscle-specific loci. *Nat Genet.* 36:738-743.

Slack, D.N., O.M. Seternes, M. Gabrielsen, and S.M. Keyse. 2001. Distinct binding determinants for ERK2/p38alpha and JNK map kinases mediate catalytic activation and substrate selectivity of map kinase phosphatase-1. *J Biol Chem.* 276:16491-16500.

Soulsby, M., and A.M. Bennett. 2009. Physiological signaling specificity by protein tyrosine phosphatases. *Physiology (Bethesda).* 24:281-289.

Spence, H.J., A.S. Dhillon, M. James, and S.J. Winder. 2004. Dystroglycan, a scaffold for the ERK-MAP kinase cascade. *EMBO Rep.* 5:484-489.

Suelves, M., F. Lluis, V. Ruiz, A.R. Nebreda, and P. Munoz-Canoves. 2004. Phosphorylation of MRF4 transactivation domain by p38 mediates repression of specific myogenic genes. *Embo J.* 23:365-375.

Sunadome, K., T. Yamamoto, M. Ebisuya, K. Kondoh, A. Sehara-Fujisawa, and E. Nishida. 2011. ERK5 regulates muscle cell fusion through Klf transcription factors. *Dev Cell.* 20:192-205.

Tedesco, F.S., A. Dellavalle, J. Diaz-Manera, G. Messina, and G. Cossu. 2010. Repairing skeletal muscle: regenerative potential of skeletal muscle stem cells. *J Clin Invest.* 120:11-19.

Tonks, N.K. 2005. Redox redux: revisiting PTPs and the control of cell signaling. *Cell.* 121:667-670.

Tonks, N.K. 2006. Protein tyrosine phosphatases: from genes, to function, to disease. *Nat Rev Mol Cell Biol.* 7:833-846.

Turjanski, A.G., J.P. Vaque, and J.S. Gutkind. 2007. MAP kinases and the control of nuclear events. *Oncogene.* 26:3240-3253.

Wagers, A.J., and I.M. Conboy. 2005. Cellular and molecular signatures of muscle regeneration: current concepts and controversies in adult myogenesis. *Cell.* 122:659-667.

Weyman, C.M., and A. Wolfman. 1998. Mitogen-activated protein kinase kinase (MEK) activity is required for inhibition of skeletal muscle differentiation by insulin-like growth factor 1 or fibroblast growth factor 2. *Endocrinology.* 139:1794-1800.

Whitmarsh, A.J. 2006. The JIP family of MAPK scaffold proteins. *Biochem Soc Trans.* 34:828-832.

Wu, J.J., R.J. Roth, E.J. Anderson, E.-G. Hong, M.-K. Lee, C.S. Choi, P.D. Neufer, G.I. Shulman, J.K. Kim, and A.M. Bennett. 2006. Mice lacking MAP kinase phosphatase-1 have enhanced MAP kinase activity and resistance to diet-induced obesity. *Cell Metab.* 4:61-73.

Wu, J.J., L. Zhang, and A.M. Bennett. 2005. The noncatalytic amino terminus of mitogen-activated protein kinase phosphatase 1 directs nuclear targeting and serum response element transcriptional regulation. *Mol Cell Biol.* 25:4792-4803.

Yang, B., D. Jung, D. Motto, J. Meyer, G. Koretzky, and K.P. Campbell. 1995. SH3 domain-mediated interaction of dystroglycan and Grb2. *J Biol Chem.* 270:11711-11714.

Yokoyama, T., K. Takano, A. Yoshida, F. Katada, P. Sun, T. Takenawa, T. Andoh, and T. Endo. 2007. DA-Raf1, a competent intrinsic dominant-negative antagonist of the Ras-ERK pathway, is required for myogenic differentiation. *J Cell Biol.* 177:781-793.

Zarubin, T., and J. Han. 2005. Activation and signaling of the p38 MAP kinase pathway. *Cell Res.* 15:11-18.

Zetser, A., E. Gredinger, and E. Bengal. 1999. p38 mitogen-activated protein kinase pathway promotes skeletal muscle differentiation. Participation of the Mef2c transcription factor. *J Biol Chem.* 274:5193-5200.

Zhao, Q., X. Wang, L.D. Nelin, Y. Yao, R. Matta, M.E. Manson, R.S. Baliga, X. Meng, C.V. Smith, J.A. Bauer, C.H. Chang, and Y. Liu. 2006. MAP kinase phosphatase 1 controls innate immune responses and suppresses endotoxic shock. *J Exp Med.* 203:131-140.

9

Altered Gene Expression Pathways in Duchenne Muscular Dystrophy

Nevenka Juretić, Francisco Altamirano,
Denisse Valladares and Enrique Jaimovich
Centro de Estudios Moleculares de la Célula, Facultad de Medicina,
Universidad de Chile, Santiago,
Chile

1. Introduction

Duchenne muscular dystrophy (DMD) is caused by the absence of functional dystrophin (Blake et al. 2002). Dystrophin is a cytoskeleton protein normally expressed in the inner face of the plasma membrane (Ahn and Kunkel 1993). In normal skeletal muscle, dystrophin is associated with a complex of glycoproteins known as dystrophin-associated proteins (DAPs), providing a linkage between the extracellular matrix (ECM) and cytoskeleton (Batchelor and Winder 2006). Lack of dystrophin in dystrophic muscle results in loss of the complex integrity and allegedly impairs the stability of the plasma membrane causing mechanical stress fragility, and an increase in Ca^{2+} permeability (Alderton and Steinhardt 2000). But the pathophysiology of muscular dystrophy is not only explained by this increased mechanical fragility and a role for dystrophin and DAPs has been suggested as being part of a protein signaling complex involved in cell survival (Rando 2001). In this chapter we discuss evidence of such a role, which may evidence possible interactions between dystrophin and proteins other than those involved in DAP and possible cell location of dystrophin in regions other than the sarcolemma cytoskeleton.

2. Calcium homeostasis

Ca^{2+} is a highly versatile second messenger that can regulate several cellular functions. Skeletal muscles use Ca^{2+} for contraction process and as regulatory signaling molecule. Subsequently, muscle plasticity is closely related with calcium signals (Berchtold et al. 2000).

Under resting conditions, wild type *(wt)* skeletal muscle cells maintain the cytosolic calcium concentration ($[Ca^{2+}]_i$) around 100-120 nM (Lopez et al. 1987; Eltit et al. 2010). Since the chemical gradient between $[Ca^{2+}]_i$ and extracellular medium or sarcoplasmic reticulum (SR) is about 10,000 fold, to constantly keep the $[Ca^{2+}]_i$ in the nM range, skeletal muscle cells uses a complex machinery to finely regulate calcium concentration. Plasma membrane Ca^{2+}-ATPase (PMCA), Na^+/Ca^{2+} exchanger (NCX) in the plasma membrane and the SR Ca^{2+}-ATPase (SERCA) extrudes the Ca^{2+} to extracellular space or to SR, respectively. These functions are opposed, under resting conditions, for the SR Ca^{2+} leak type-1 ryanodine receptor (RyR1) channels and the basal sarcolemma Ca^{2+} influx (Eltit et al. 2010).

2.1 Altered resting calcium in DMD

Several reports demonstrate that the $[Ca^{2+}]_i$ is elevated in *mdx* mice and DMD human fibers (Lopez et al. 1987; Yeung et al. 2005; Allen et al. 2010). Lopez et al. (1987) have shown that the $[Ca^{2+}]_i$ in DMD muscle fibers is 370 nM, while in normal muscle fibers was around 100 nM (Lopez et al. 1987). Similar results were obtained in *mdx* adult fibers compared with the *wt* counterpart (Yeung et al. 2005; Allen et al. 2010). The authors demonstrated that $[Ca^{2+}]_i$ was elevated under resting conditions in *mdx* fibers and when the fibers were exposed to stretch-induced damage, $[Ca^{2+}]_i$ increased to higher levels, around 700 nM (Yeung et al. 2005; Allen et al. 2010).

Increased $[Ca^{2+}]_i$ has been related with necrosis through calpain activation and mitochondrial permeability transition pore (MPTP) (Turner et al. 1988; Spencer et al. 1995; Millay et al. 2008).

The mechanism that has been proposed for dystrophin function involves a role in sarcolemma stabilization, so in muscle fibers that lack this protein, membrane damage would be recurrent (Petrof et al. 1993; Mokri and Engel 1998). These evidences suggested the hypothesis of Ca^{2+} leak into the cell through damaged membrane. There are several evidences in *mdx* muscle fibers that relate the calcium entry with the transient receptor potential channels (TRPC1) and the store-operated calcium entry (SOCE) mechanism. TRPC1-dependent calcium entry is increased in *mdx* muscle fibers (Vandebrouck et al. 2002; Yeung et al. 2005; Gervasio et al. 2008). The blockage of these cationic channels with streptomycin or spider venom toxin (GsMTx4) reduced $[Ca^{2+}]_i$ and prevented the rise of the $[Ca^{2+}]_i$ following stretch (eccentric) contractions. This maneuver, partially reduced the decline in both the tetanic Ca^{2+} increase and force (Yeung et al. 2005; Allen et al. 2010). Gervasio et al. 2008 showed that TRPC1, caveolin-3 and Src-kinase protein levels are increased in *mdx* muscle (Gervasio et al. 2008). The authors propose that the stretch-induced muscle damage and the increase in the $[Ca^{2+}]_i$ is produced by the ROS production, activation of Src-kinase and TRPC-induced Ca^{2+} entry. Furthermore, administration of streptomycin reduced muscle damage and increased myofiber regeneration (Yeung et al. 2005).

More recently, store-operated calcium entry has been implicated in the exacerbated resting Ca^{2+} entry observed in *mdx* fibers (Boittin et al. 2006; Vandebrouck et al. 2006; Edwards et al. 2010). These Ca^{2+} entries are modulated by a Ca^{2+}-independent phospholipase A_2, which is overexpressed in dystrophic fibers (Boittin et al. 2006). Vandebrouck et al. (2005) demonstrate that the high store-operated Ca^{2+} transients observed in dystrophin-deficient myotubes were associated with sustained cytosolic Ca^{2+} transients and high intra-mitochondrial entries, that can be reduced by mini-dystrophin expression or FCCP (uncoupler of oxidative phosphorylation) (Vandebrouck et al. 2006). In addition, the thresholds for SOCE activation and deactivation occur at higher $[Ca^{2+}]_{SR}$ and the proteins levels of STIM1 and Orai1 was 3-fold increased in *extensor digitorum longus* (EDL) muscles from *mdx* mice (Edwards et al. 2010).

2.2 SR Ca^{2+} loading capacity

There is a controversy about the loading capacity of the SR $[Ca^{2+}]_{SR}$ in dystrophic skeletal muscle cells compared with normal skeletal muscle cells. Roberts et al. (2001), using a Ca^{2+}-sensitive photoprotein aequorin chimera with SR destination sequence, show that after SR

Ca^{2+} depletion, the re-addition of Ca^{2+} to the media increases the $[Ca^{2+}]_{SR}$ rapidly up to a steady state that is 50% higher that the *wt* myotubes (Robert et al. 2001). In contrast, Culligan et al. (2002) shows a reduction in Ca^{2+} binding in the SR microsomes from *mdx* mice, associated with a drastic reduction in the calsequestrin-like proteins and normal SERCA1 expression and activity (Culligan et al. 2002). However, a reduction in SERCA activity has been observed in dystrophic muscle (Kargacin and Kargacin 1996; Divet et al. 2005), which could account for the increased $[Ca^{2+}]_i$. SERCA1a overexpression in *mdx* diaphragm muscle by adeno-associated virus gene transfer, resulted in a reduction of centrally located nuclei and reduced susceptibility to eccentric contraction-induced damage (Morine et al. 2010). More recently, δ-sarcoglycan-null and *mdx* mice transgenic animals that overexpress SERCA1, show a reduction in myofiber central nucleation, tissue fibrosis and serum creatine kinase levels. In addition SERCA1 overexpression enhances excitation-contraction (E-C) coupling and restore the $[Ca^{2+}]_i$ and $[Ca^{2+}]_{SR}$ in both dystrophic models (Goonasekera et al. 2011).

2.3 Excitation-Contraction (E-C) coupling

The proteins involved in E-C coupling are normally expressed in dystrophic muscle. The expression of α1-, α2- and β-subunits of the dihydropyridine receptor (DHPR) are similar in microsomes from control and *mdx* mice (Culligan et al. 2002). RyR1 and SERCA1 are also found in comparable amounts in control and dystrophin-deficient muscles (Culligan et al. 2002).

In skeletal muscle cells, membrane depolarization induces a conformational change in Cav1.1 DHPRs that is transmitted to the ryanodine receptor (RyR1), causing it to release Ca^{2+} from the SR, that it is necessary for the contraction process.

Several evidences indicate that the dystrophic skeletal muscle cells have an unpaired E-C coupling. Comparisons of the cytosolic calcium transients evoked by single action potential have shown that the calcium transients are reduced in *mdx* fibers compared with *wt* fibers (Woods et al. 2004; Hollingworth et al. 2008). Recently, similar results have been found in fibers from *utr -/- mdx* mice (Capote et al. 2010). Muscle weakness observed in isolated fibers from *mdx* mice and DMD patients has not been fully explained. The reduction in the Ca^{2+} transient evoked by single action potential, reduction in $[Ca^{2+}]_{SR}$ and increased $[Ca^{2+}]_i$ could provide a mechanism for contractile dysfunction and impaired force production in DMD patients.

3. Excitation-Transcription (E-T) coupling

We have previously described that membrane depolarization of skeletal myotubes evokes a fast Ca^{2+} transient during the stimuli, that promotes a contractile response through "E-C coupling", and a slow Ca^{2+} transient peaking 60-100 seconds later, mostly associated to cell nuclei (Jaimovich et al. 2000; Estrada et al. 2001; Powell et al. 2001; Araya et al. 2003; Cardenas et al. 2005). Slow Ca^{2+} transients are involved in the "E-T coupling" mechanism, which relates membrane depolarization with gene expression (Powell et al. 2001; Araya et al. 2003; Carrasco et al. 2003; Juretic et al. 2006; Juretic et al. 2007). The signaling pathway begins at the DHPR, which by a mechanism involving G protein (Eltit et al. 2006), activates

PI3 kinase and PLC to produce inositol 1,4,5-trisphosphate (IP$_3$) that diffuses in the cytosol and reaches IP$_3$ receptors (IP$_3$Rs) located both at the SR membrane and at the nuclear envelope, promoting Ca^{2+} release (Araya et al. 2003). IP$_3$ mediated Ca^{2+} signals induce both a transient activation of ERK$\frac{1}{2}$ and transcription factor CREB, and an increase in early genes (*c-fos, c-jun* and *egr-1*) and in late genes (troponin I, interleukin-6, hmox and hsp70) mRNA levels after depolarization of normal skeletal muscle cells (Carrasco et al. 2003; Juretic et al. 2006; Juretic et al. 2007; Jorquera et al. 2009). Moreover, in electrically stimulated adult muscle fibers, slow Ca^{2+} signals mediate the frequency-dependent activation of slow-phenotype muscle fiber genes (slow troponin I, TnIs) and repression of fast-phenotype ones (TnIf) (Casas et al. 2010). These evidences link slow Ca^{2+} transients with muscular effects of nerve activity and with the process of muscle cell plasticity.

Recently we described a new role for ATP signaling in skeletal muscle in a process called "E-T" coupling (Buvinic et al. 2009, see Fig.1). We were able to show that the main ATP efflux pathway is through pannexin 1 hemichannels. We know that DHPR receptors and pannexin 1 interact with each other but it is not clear whether it is a direct interaction. The ATP released will locally activate the purinergic receptors P2X and P2Y localized in the membrane. This activation induces a transient increase in intracellular Ca^{2+} with specific kinetics. We demonstrated that ATP participates in the fast calcium transient related to contraction because apyrase (catalyses the hydrolysis of ATP) reduced the depolarization-evoked Ca^{2+} transient by about 20%. We can speculate that activation of P2X receptors may contribute to improve the skeletal muscle cells Ca^{2+} availability needed to sustain contractions. Moreover, we could also show that ATP participates in "E-T" coupling due to the total inhibition by apyrase of the second Ca^{2+} transient induced by depolarization. Additionally, the use of apyrase during the electrical stimulation completely abolished the increase in gene expression related with muscle plasticity (unpublished data). We can conclude that gene expression is regulated through activation of P2Y receptors mediated by the ATP released during depolarization.

3.1 Extracellular ATP: a major mediator for signal transduction

ATP for a long time was considering as a molecule that was involved with energy and metabolism of many cells. Nevertheless in the last few years ATP has been considered as an extracellular messenger for autocrine and paracrine signaling (Corriden and Insel 2010). It has been described as a regulator of inflammation, in embryonic and stem cell development, ischemia, among others (Bours et al. 2006; Burnstock and Ulrich 2011). In skeletal muscle ATP has been implicated in the regulation of proliferation, differentiation and regeneration (Ryten et al. 2002; Ryten et al. 2004) and also promoting the stabilization of the neuromuscular junction (Jia et al. 2007).

ATP release is induced in response to several kinds of stress in many cells type, including hypoxia, ischemia, osmotic swelling and mechanical stimulation (Corriden and Insel 2010). ATP can exit cells using several different purinergic signal efflux pathways (Fitz 2007). The main source of extracellular ATP is cell lysis, which occurs when massive cell death takes place during trauma, injury or inflammation. A non-lytic source of ATP is the release of secretory granules during stimulated exocytosis, which occurs in secretory cell types like epithelial cells of the liver, lung, kidney, neurons and astrocytes (Volonte and D'Ambrosi

2009). A non-lytic, and also non-exocytotic release of ATP can occur by channel- or transporter-mediated mechanisms, such as: (a) hemichannels, such as connexins and pannexin (Dubyak 2009); (b) anion channels, such as plasmalemma voltage dependent anion channel, voltage-dependent maxi-anion channel, volume sensitive Cl- channel and P2X7 receptor (Sabirov and Okada 2005; Suadicani et al. 2006; Liu et al. 2008); (c) ATP-binding cassette transporters, such as cystic fibrosis transmembrane conductance regulator Cl- channel and P-glycoprotein (Campbell et al. 2003; Sabirov and Okada 2005); and (d) exchange carriers such as ADP/ATP exchange carrier (Sabirov and Okada 2005; Volonte and D'Ambrosi 2009). Several studies have recently demonstrated that ATP can be released by pannexin hemichannels in a variety of cells types that include myotubes (D'Hondt et al. 2011). Pannexin is widely distributed among tissues with cell communication via calcium waves (Shestopalov and Panchin 2008). The channel formed by this protein can be opened by mechanical perturbation at the resting membrane potential. The channel is permeable for ATP and it can be opened at physiological calcium concentration (Barbe et al. 2006). These properties make pannexin 1 (Panx1) a very attractive candidate for an ATP-releasing channel. The widespread distribution of Panx1 has been confirmed in a variety of human tissues, with the highest levels being found in skeletal muscle (Baranova et al. 2004). Results of our laboratory indicate that this hemichannel is expressed in myotubes and adult fibers of rat and mouse.

Once released, ATP acts as an extracellular signal trough the binding to purinergic receptors expressed in most cell types. Purinergic receptors comprise both ionotropic P2X receptor subtypes and G-protein-coupled P2Y receptor subtypes (Burnstock 2004). Between the purinergic receptors and the purine-generating reactions, there exist purino-converting enzymes. These enzymes named ectonucleotidases, consist of several different families with well-characterized molecular and functional features (Yegutkin 2008). They operate to metabolize nucleotides down to the respective nucleoside analogues, thus having the potential to decrease the extracellular concentrations of nucleotides. Consequently these enzymes modulate ligand availability at both nucleotide and nucleoside receptors (Yegutkin 2008). The contribution of the diverse ectonucleotidases to the modulation of purinergic signaling depends on their availability of different ectonucleotidases and their selectivity for substrates, but also on their abundance and cell distribution (Volonte and D'Ambrosi 2009).

ATP signaling has been implicated in many cell functions ranging from proliferation, differentiation, toxic actions, neurotransmission, smooth and cardiac muscle contraction, vasodilation, chemosensory signaling and secretion, to complex phenomena such as immune responses, male reproduction, fertilization, embryonic development, and so on (Burnstock 2004). This vast heterogeneity of their biological responses is influenced by different parameters such as the presence of endogenous ligands at receptor sites and the time and distance from the source of release; the concentration gradient of a ligand that simultaneously can activate more than one receptor subtype; the different composition of purinergic receptors in a given cell, or even more the composition in the diverse sub membrane compartments in which each ligand operates (Volonte and D'Ambrosi 2009).

3.2 Purinergic receptors

Purinergic receptors are subdivided into two major groups: eight G-protein-coupled seven-transmembrane P2Y subunits (P2Y$_{1, 2, 4, 6, 11-14}$), and seven P2X ligand-gated ion channels

(P2X$_{1-7}$). These two types of receptor have larger differences in their aminoacid sequences, molecular/physiological properties and relative sensitivities to ATP, with ranges of nanomolar for P2Y, low micromolar for most P2X, to high micromolar for P2X7. Moreover the complexity of these receptors is augmented because both subtypes can form homomers and heteromers and these different combinations can change the agonist and antagonist selectivity, transmission signaling, channel and desensitization properties (Nakata et al. 2004).

P2X receptors are ATP-gated ion channels that mediate sodium influx, potassium efflux and, to varying extents, calcium influx, leading to depolarization of the cell membrane. Membrane depolarization subsequently activates voltage-gated calcium channels, thus causing accumulation of calcium ions in the cytoplasm. The predicted structure of the P2X subunits is a transmembrane protein with two membrane spanning domains that are involved in gating the ion channel and lining the ion pore (Surprenant and North 2009). Functional P2X receptor ion channels are now thought to consist of three subunits that could be homomers and heteromers (North 2002). The different combinations present different desensitization and permeability properties, as well as agonist and antagonist specificities. P2X receptors are widely distributed, and in neurons, glial cells, bone, muscle, endothelium, epithelium, and hematopoietic cells, they have functional roles. Moreover, several studies have implicated these receptors in the pathophysiology of Parkinson's disease, Alzheimer's disease, and multiple sclerosis (Jarvis and Khakh 2009).

P2Y receptors are G-protein-coupled receptors (GPCRs) that are activated by purine and/or pyrimidine nucleotides. Like other members of the GPCR superfamily, they are composed of seven transmembrane spanning regions that assist in forming the ligand binding pocket and also the purinergic receptor (Abbracchio et al. 2006). Stimulation leads to activation of heterotrimeric G proteins and their dissociation into α and $\beta\gamma$ subunits that can then interact with a variety of effector proteins. Some of P2Y receptors are activated mainly by nucleoside diphosphates (P2Y$_{1,6,12}$), while others are activated mainly by nucleoside triphosphates (P2Y$_{2,4}$). Otherwise, some P2Y receptors are activated by both purine and pyrimidine nucleotides (P2Y$_{2,4,6}$), and others only by purine nucleotides (P2Y$_{1,\,11,\,12}$) (Jacobson et al. 2009). Each individual P2Y receptor subtypes can couple to distinct G proteins that are specific for each cell type or tissue. The abilities to activate different G proteins were inferred from their capability to induce increases in inositol tris-phosphate, cytoplasmic Ca^{2+}, or cyclic AMP levels, and determination of sensitivity to the Gi/o protein inhibitors pertussis toxin (PTX) (Abbracchio et al. 2006). P2Y receptors can also be coupled to the activation of monomeric G proteins like Rac and RhoA. Even more, in the last few years many studies have revealed that a cross-talk exist between different GPCRs and their downstream effectors as well as between GPCRs and other signaling proteins, such as ion channels, integrins, and receptor and non-receptor tyrosine kinases (von Kugelgen 2006). These properties explain how the activation of particular P2Y receptors can lead to the induction of more than one signaling pathway in the same cell type. These receptors are able to regulate many different functions in a variety of cell types, and for that reason an intense effort has been developed to design selective agonist and antagonist ligands, both as pharmacological tools and as potential therapeutic agents (Abbracchio et al. 2003; Brunschweiger and Muller 2006). For cystic fibrosis, dry eye disease, and thrombosis the application of P2Y receptor ligands has been tested as drug candidates. The development of new chemical compounds will provide new opportunities for therapeutics of several diseases, including cardiovascular diseases, inflammatory diseases, and neurodegeneration (Jacobson and Boeynaems 2010).

Between the many functions that P2 receptors can regulate is ion channel activity. The studies have been performed mainly in neurons, in which specific P2 subtype can regulate the N-type Ca^{2+} channel and the M-current K^+ channel. Nevertheless, recent studies have demonstrated that P2 receptors can induce fast inhibitory junction potential in rat colon (Grasa et al. 2009), membrane hyperpolarization in vascular endothelial cells (Raqeeb et al. 2011), Ca^{2+} influx mediated contraction in intestinal myofibroblasts (Nakamura et al. 2011), and contraction induced by electrical field stimulation in smooth muscle (Cho et al. 2010). These data suggest that ATP signaling is important in excitable cells for their normal function. In skeletal muscle there are many evidences of the importance of ATP signaling. The activation of P2 receptors has been associated with modulation of Ca^{2+} influx and signaling (Sandona et al. 2005; May et al. 2006), activation of the $ERK\frac{1}{2}$ (May et al. 2006), muscle contractility (Sandona et al. 2005; Grishin et al. 2006), and regulation of excitability of muscle fibers (Voss 2009; Broch-Lips et al. 2010). Also extracellular nucleotides play important functions during skeletal muscle development and regeneration (Ryten et al. 2002; Ryten et al. 2004). Importantly, it has been shown that ATP promotes differentiation of rat skeletal muscle satellite cells (Araya et al. 2004; Banachewicz et al. 2005).

4. Alterations in both IP_3Rs and E-T coupling in DMD models

We have described that the amount of IP_3Rs, as well as the total mass of IP_3, are largely increased in both an *mdx* mice derived cell line and in a human DMD derived cell line compared to normal cells (Liberona et al. 1998). In dystrophic skeletal muscle, it has been suggested that an alteration of Ca^{2+} homeostasis occurs and might be responsible for muscle degeneration (Turner et al. 1988; Turner et al. 1991). Several studies indicate that IP_3 pathways could be involved in the DMD pathophysiology (Liberona et al. 1998; Balghi et al. 2006a; Balghi et al. 2006b). We recently found that both expression and localization of IP_3Rs are different in normal and dystrophic human skeletal muscle and cell lines (Cárdenas et al. 2010). On the other hand, experiments performed using two types of myotubes originated from the same Sol8 cell line – dystrophin deficient myotubes, SolC1(-), and myotubes transfected to express the minidystrophin, SolD(+) - show that Ca^{2+} rise evoked by potassium depolarization was higher in SolC1(-) than in SolD(+) myotubes (Balghi et al. 2006a). Analysis of the kinetics of the Ca^{2+} rise, reveals that the slow IP_3-dependent release may be increased in the SolC1(-) as compared to the SolD(+), suggesting an inhibitory effect of mini-dystrophin on IP_3R-dependent K^+-evoked Ca^{2+} release (Balghi et al. 2006a). Moreover, it has been described that IP_3 production after membrane depolarization is significantly elevated in dystrophin-deficient myotubes and that the presence of mini-dystrophin under the membrane leads to reduced IP_3 production (Balghi et al. 2006a). In fact, we have recently demonstrated, using normal (RCMH) and dystrophic (RCDMD) human skeletal muscle cell lines, that IP_3 dependent, slow Ca^{2+} transients evoked by electrical stimulation are faster in dystrophic cells, compared to normal myotubes (Cárdenas et al. 2010). Electrical stimulation induced an important phosphorylation of $ERK\frac{1}{2}$ in normal but not in dystrophic cells, and a differential pattern of gene expression between cell lines.

In normal adult mice skeletal muscle, we observed that IP_3R immuno-labeling follows distinctive patters resembling the SR (types 1, 2 and 3 IP_3Rs), sarcolemmal (types 1 and 3 IP_3Rs) or nuclear localizations (types 1 and 3 IP_3Rs) (Casas et al. 2010). The labeling for both type 1 and type 2 IP_3Rs subtypes showed a fiber type-specific distribution with much higher expression in fast (type II) muscle fibers, whereas type 3 IP_3R showed a uniform distribution in both fiber types, as shown by co-labeling with slow myosin heavy chain antibody. Likewise, mice muscle fibers show a characteristic mosaic pattern for type 1 IP_3R (Casas et al. 2010). When human muscle was studied, type II muscle fibers showed a much more intense labeling for the IP_3R subtype 1 compared to type I (slow) fibers. In biopsies from DMD patients, we found that $24 \pm 7\%$ of type II fibers have totally lost type 1 IP_3R labeling, compared to age-matched control biopsies (Cárdenas et al. 2010). On the other hand, RCDMD cells show a five-fold over expression of type 2 IP_3Rs and down regulation of type 3 IP_3Rs compared to normal RCMH cells (Cárdenas et al. 2010). Unlike normal muscle cells, type 2 IP_3R locate in the nucleus in RCDMD cells, while type 1 and type 3 IP_3Rs also display a particular subcellular location for each line (Cárdenas et al. 2010). These results showed that IP_3Rs expression and localization are different in muscle affected by DMD.

5. Signaling by extracellular nucleotides in dystrophic skeletal muscle

A number of skeletal muscle pathologies have been associated with alterations in the metabolism of extracellular ATP, changes in the sensitivity towards ATP and altered expression of purinergic receptors; among these pathologies we have DMD. In recent works, ATP signaling has been implicated in abnormal calcium homeostasis in dystrophic muscle and proposed to have implications in the pathogenesis of muscular dystrophies. Moreover, in myoblasts of a dystrophin negative muscle cell line, exposure to extracellular ATP elicited a strong increase in cytoplasmic Ca^{2+} concentrations. This increased susceptibility to ATP was due to changes in expression and function of P2X receptors and proposed to be a significant contributor to pathogenic Ca^{2+} entry in dystrophic mouse muscle (Yeung et al. 2006). The plasma membrane Na^+/H^+ exchanger (NHE) has been proposed to be involved in the pathogenesis of muscular dystrophy, most probably through the sustained increase in intracellular Ca^{2+}. The mechanism by which NHE is constitutive activated appears to be through stimulation of P2 receptors with ATP being continuously released in response to stretching (Iwata et al. 2007).

Nevertheless, these works failed to explain the mechanism by which ATP is released from skeletal muscle. ATP in skeletal muscle was proposed to be co-released with acetylcholine from motor nerve terminals during nerve activation (Smith 1991; Silinsky and Redman 1996) and released from muscle fibers during contraction (Cunha and Sebastiao 1993; Hellsten et al. 1998). Dystrophic muscle would be expected to contain high levels of extracellular ATP due mainly to fiber injury.

We propose now that in skeletal muscle, ATP is released upon contraction or electrical stimulation mainly through activation of pannexin 1 hemichannels. Any disturbance in either pannexin 1 channels or changes in P2 receptors expression or activity will have implications in skeletal muscle normal function. The possibility that this system is altered in muscular dystrophies raises new possibilities of therapeutic strategies in the treatment of diseases like DMD.

In addition to the structural role for dystrophin and its known associated proteins, there is clear evidence for signal transduction roles. The best studied signaling protein linked is the nNOS pathway. In DMD nNOS appears to be either drastically reduced or even absent (Niebroj-Dobosz and Hausmanowa-Petrusewicz 2005). It has been propose that part of muscle degeneration in DMD may result from the reduction in the production of nNOS/NO (Niebrój-Dobosz, 2005). Lately many additional signaling pathways have been demonstrated to be altered in dystrophy, such as: nuclear factor kappa-B (NF-kB), tumor necrosis factor (TNF)-alpha and interleukin (IL)-6 (Messina et al. 2011). The precise role of these signaling pathways remains mysterious, it is interesting to investigate whether the abnormal regulation of one (or more) of these pathways contributes to skeletal muscle pathogenesis in dystrophy.

To address the different pathways that could be altered in muscular dystrophy, many studies have compared gene expression profile between normal and dystrophic muscle based on microarray analysis. These analysis have been done in patients with DMD and in *mdx* mice. These studies include different types of muscle and in different times of the human disease (Chen et al. 2000) or in different life periods of *mdx* mice (Porter et al. 2003b; Lang et al. 2004; Porter et al. 2004; Dogra et al. 2008). In DMD patients biopsies that were individually analyzed, the upregulated genes are related with ECM and cytoskeleton, muscle structure and regeneration, immune response, signal transduction and cell-cell communication (Chen et al. 2000). In the mouse model there are many gene expression studies. The main muscles studied are diaphragm, extraocular muscles and leg muscle groups (Porter et al. 2003b; Lang et al. 2004; Dogra et al. 2008). Among the results, it is worth mentioning that the response to the lack of dystrophin varies in different muscle groups of human and *mdx* mice, and it was proposed that changes in gene expression could be related with the progression of the disease (Porter et al. 2003b; Lang et al. 2004; Porter et al. 2004; Dogra et al. 2008). Moreover, some groups studied the profile of gene expression in skeletal muscle implicated in specific pathways such as regeneration (Turk et al. 2005), inflammation (Evans et al. 2009a), immune system (Evans et al. 2009b) and specific transcription factors (Dogra et al. 2008). Also there are some studies that propose that expression of utrophin in the *mdx* mouse muscle results in a gene expression profile that is similar to that seen for the *wt* mouse (Baban and Davies 2008).

The analysis performed by Porter et al. (2002) established that numerous pathogenic pathways in *mdx* skeletal muscles are closely related and share features with DMD (Porter et al. 2002). Among the genes that were increased in *mdx* muscle is purinergic receptor P2X. The $P2X_4$ up regulation in dystrophic muscle has been attributed to vascular permeability changes and to inflammatory responses (Porter et al. 2002). Later, Yeung et al. (2004) demonstrated that P2X4 were expressed in infiltrating macrophages in dystrophic human and mouse muscle, and could be related with the inflammatory process (Yeung et al. 2004). Jiang et al. 2005 demonstrated that there is a differential expression of P2X receptors that change during the progression of the disease in both human and mouse dystrophic muscle (Jiang et al. 2005). They found that the $P2X_1$ and $P2X_6$ receptors are expressed during the process of regeneration in mouse muscular dystrophy, and the expression of $P2X_2$ is associated with type 1 fibers. Nevertheless, the work of Yeung et al. (2006) demonstrated that increase in P2X receptors increased the susceptibility of dystrophic myoblasts to extracellular ATP (Yeung et al. 2006). They proposed that changes in P2X will significant contribute to pathogenic Ca^{2+} entry.

Moreover, studies of Ryten et al. (2002, 2004) identified a role for ATP in the regulation of skeletal muscle formation, through inhibiting the proliferation and increase the rate of differentiation of satellite cells (Ryten et al. 2002; Ryten et al. 2004) Later, they show that the P2X$_2$, P2X$_5$ and P2Y$_1$ receptors were strongly expressed in *mdx* skeletal muscle and in the cells known to be important for muscle regeneration.

As previously described, P2 receptors have been implicated in the alteration on intracellular calcium. This could also be releated with some of the signaling pathways that are dependent on calcium homeostasis, like the activation of proteases. It has been demonstrated that changes in intracellular calcium can activate calpain and proteolytic damage to sarcomer proteins, like titin (Goll et al. 2003; Zhang et al. 2008).

The original sarcoglycan (SG) complex has four subunits and comprises a subcomplex of the dystrophin-associated protein complex (Hack et al. 2000). Gene defects in α-sarcoglycan also lead to a severe muscular dystrophy, type 2D limb-girdle muscular dystrophy (Roberds et al. 1994). The role of sarcoglycans in dystrophin complex function is not entirely understood. The α-sarcoglycan was described as an ecto-ATPase with distinctive enzymatic properties *in vitro* (Betto et al. 1999). Later on, α-sarcoglycan was demonstrated to significantly contribute to total ecto-nucleotidase activity of C2C12 myotubes and during the differentiation of this cell type (Sandona et al. 2004). As a result, mutations of the α-sarcoglycan gene causing the loss of its enzymatic function could represent an important mechanism to explain the pathogenesis mechanisms leading to dystrophy.

Taken these studies together, we can conclude that modifications in ATP signaling, due to changes in ATP release mechanism or receptors expression and availability, could be implicated in several mechanisms potentially involved in diseases. For these reasons ATP signaling has been considered as a good candidate for therapeutic targets for the treatment of muscle diseases

6. Gene expression in DMD

Microarrays analysis has been the basis of a number of publications in which dystrophic muscle is compared with unaffected muscle. Gene expression comparison of human biopsies from DMD and normal skeletal muscle has shown that many of the differentially expressed genes reflect in histo-pathology changes. For example, immune response signals and ECM genes are overexpressed in DMD muscle, an indication of the infiltration of inflammatory cells and connective tissue (Haslett et al. 2002). cDNA analysis of individual DMD patients have shown that genes related to immune response, sarcomere, ECM and signaling/cell growth were increased. Up-regulation of these genes accompanies dystrophic changes in DMD muscles such as myofiber necrosis, inflammation and muscle regeneration (Noguchi et al. 2003). Up-regulated inflammatory gene expression and activated immune cells are present in dystrophic muscle and play a critical role in muscle wasting (Evans et al. 2009b). The pro-inflammatory cytokines TNF-alpha, IL-1beta and IL-6 are up-regulated in Duchenne patients and *mdx* mice (Porreca et al. 1999; Porter et al. 2002; Kumar and Boriek 2003; Acharyya et al. 2007; Hnia et al. 2008). The fact that a number of chemokines are expressed directly by the muscle cell suggests that muscle tissue may contribute to chemotaxis process (Porter et al. 2003a). Using microarray technology we have shown that membrane depolarization induces expression and repression of a number of genes in both normal (RCMH) and DMD (RCDMD) human skeletal muscle cell lines. Importantly, modulated genes are mostly different for these two cell lines (Cárdenas et al. 2010). Nevertheless, the expression of only 44 of them is modified in both cell lines. The pattern of expression (up- or down-regulation) of these common genes is strikingly different between cell lines, and they appear to be regulated in opposite ways (Cárdenas et al. 2010).

Within these 44 genes we identified genes related to the immune response (HLA-DQB1), cytoskeleton/ECM proteins (ADD1, KRT1, and FBLN1), and signaling (NRG and POU2F2), among others. We found that 18 of these 44 genes are related to processes associated with Ca^{2+}, and 10 of them have been related in some way to dystrophy (Cárdenas et al. 2010).

Within the genes whose expression increases in RCDMD cells, particularly interesting in relation to muscle function and development, are those coding for the two isoforms of neuregulin (NGR1-β2 and NRG1-γ) and the POU2F2 gene (Cárdenas et al. 2010). NRG1 is a growth factor that potentiates myogenesis and may play an important role in differentiation of satellite cells in muscle regeneration (Hirata et al. 2007). Moreover, NRG stimulates Ca^{2+}-induced glucose transport during contraction (Canto et al. 2006) and is implicated in the metabolic and proliferative response of muscle to exercise (Lebrasseur et al. 2003). POU2F2 has been described as a transcription factor expressed in developing mouse skeletal muscle (Dominov and Miller 1996).

In addition, we found variations in the expression of ICEBERG, HLA-DQB1, ADD1, FBLN1 and TRIO genes that also have been associated with Ca^{2+} and dystrophy (Cárdenas et al. 2010). Considering that changes observed in DMD muscle biopsies have been related to elevation of intracellular Ca^{2+} concentration, which could activate Ca^{2+}-dependent degradation pathways, resulting in myofibril disruption and muscle necrosis (Turner et al. 1993). It will be interesting to analyze the roles described for the above mentioned genes. To our knowledge, there are no studies describing the role of membrane depolarization on the expression of these genes, and further studies are needed to explore the involvement of IP_3-mediated slow Ca^{2+} signals in the expression of some of these particular genes in skeletal muscle cells (Cárdenas et al. 2010).

Gene expression profiling at different stages in *mdx* models have also evidenced the highly dynamic process of the disease onset. These works, show that dystrophy in *mdx* models have an onset at 3 weeks of age, with a peak in pathology around 8 weeks. Interestingly, at this stage, there is a marked upregulation of almost 9 fold of the puringeric receptor $P2X_4$ (Porter et al. 2003b).

Although no therapy described to date can effectively slow or halt muscle degeneration in dystrophic patients (Kapsa et al. 2003), a promising pharmacological treatment for DMD aims to increase levels of utrophin and to identify molecules that modulate utrophin expression (regulatory pathways) by activation of its promoter (Dennis et al. 1996), in muscle fibers of affected patients to compensate for the absence of dystrophin (Miura and Jasmin 2006).

Indeed, utrophin is considered the autosomal homolog of dystrophin because it shares structural and functional motifs throughout the length of the molecule (Love et al. 1989; Khurana et al. 1990; Nguyen et al. 1991; Ohlendieck et al. 1991; Tinsley et al. 1992). It is capable of associating with members of the DAPs with similar affinity to dystrophin as well (Matsumura et al. 1992; Winder et al. 1995). Studies in the dystrophin-deficient *mdx* mice have established that the elevation of utrophin levels in dystrophic muscle fibers can restore sarcolemmal expression of DAPs members and alleviate the dystrophic pathology (Miura and Jasmin 2006). Direct evidence for the ability of utrophin to functionally substitute for dystrophin comes from experiments demonstrating that transgene-driven utrophin overexpression can effectively rescue dystrophin-deficient muscle in *mdx* mice (Tinsley et al. 1996; Deconinck et al. 1997; Tinsley et al. 1998).

6.1 Electrical stimulation induces calcium-dependent up-regulation of neuregulin-1β in dystrophic skeletal muscle cell lines

Neuregulin (NRG) is one of many factors that increase utrophin expression (Miura and Jasmin 2006). It belongs to a family of proteins structurally related to the epidermal growth factor (EGF) that are synthesized in and secreted from motoneurons and muscle (Falls 2003). Four members of NRG proteins, NRG-1 to NRG-4, have been identified. The best-studied and most characterized products are those encoded by NRG-1 gene.

Neuregulin-1 (NRG-1) was initially described as a neurotrophic factor involved in neuromuscular junction formation in skeletal muscle, but recently it has emerged as a myokine, with relevant effects on myogenesis, muscle metabolism and regeneration, and has been considered as a strong candidate to transduce muscle adaptation to chronic exercise (Lebrasseur et al. 2003; Guma et al. 2010).

Interestingly, NRG-1 treatment increases utrophin mRNA levels and transcriptional activity in mouse and human myotubes (Gramolini et al. 1999; Khurana et al. 1999). Moreover, Krag et al. (2004) described that intraperitoneal injection of a small peptide region of NRG-1 ectodomain increases utrophin expression in *mdx* mice (Krag et al. 2004). Observed increase was accompanied by a reduction in muscle degeneration and inflammation, and by decreased susceptibility to the damage induced by lengthening contractions. Improvement in muscle function was deemed to result specifically from the up-regulation of utrophin because NRG-1 administration has no beneficial effect in dystrophin/utrophin double-knockout animals (Krag et al. 2004).

However, regardless the evidences supporting such important roles for NRG-1 in skeletal muscle, the molecular mechanisms involved in its expression are still unclear.

When we investigated the effect of membrane depolarization on global gene expression in dystrophic RCDMD cells using microarrays technology, our data revealed that membrane potential changes, induced by electrical stimulation, resulted in significant up or down regulation of 150 genes after 4 h. Interestingly, two NRG-1 isoforms (β and γ) appear within the ten highest up-regulated genes (Cárdenas et al. 2010).

Taking into account the important biological effects of NRG-1 in the muscle and its potential clinical implication in DMD, we focused our study on the regulation of muscle NRG-1 expression, specifically on NRG-1β isoform, that displays a higher affinity for NRG receptor (Juretić et al. n.d.). NRG-1β increased expression was confirmed by quantitative PCR. We observed that electrical stimulation induces a significant increase of NRG-1β mRNA level in RCDMD cells, with a maximun at 4 h post-stimuli, but has no effect on NRG-1β expression in RCMH cells treated with the same procedure, suggesting that activation of molecular pathways involved in the regulation of NRG-1β gene expression are different in normal and dystrophic cells. Western blot analysis of stimulated RCDMD cells demonstrates that observed increase in NRG-1β mRNA levels was followed by actual enhancement of the corresponding protein (Juretić et al. n.d.).

Accumulating evidence suggests that integral dystrophin-DAPs complex components are also implicated in signaling in DMD, and that mutations in non-DAP protein encoding genes may lead to the muscular dystrophy phenotype, supporting the idea that more than one molecular pathway is implicated in the disease (Haslett et al. 2002). Thus, it is likely that the lack of DAP proteins in the cell membrane will somehow affect the regulation of Ca^{2+} transients and gene expression in dystrophic cells after electrical stimulation. In fact, Balghi et al. (2006) have demonstrated that IP_3 production after depolarization is significantly elevated in SolC1(-) dystrophin deficient myotubes and that the presence of mini-dystrophin under the membrane leads to reduced IP_3 production (Balghi et al. 2006b).

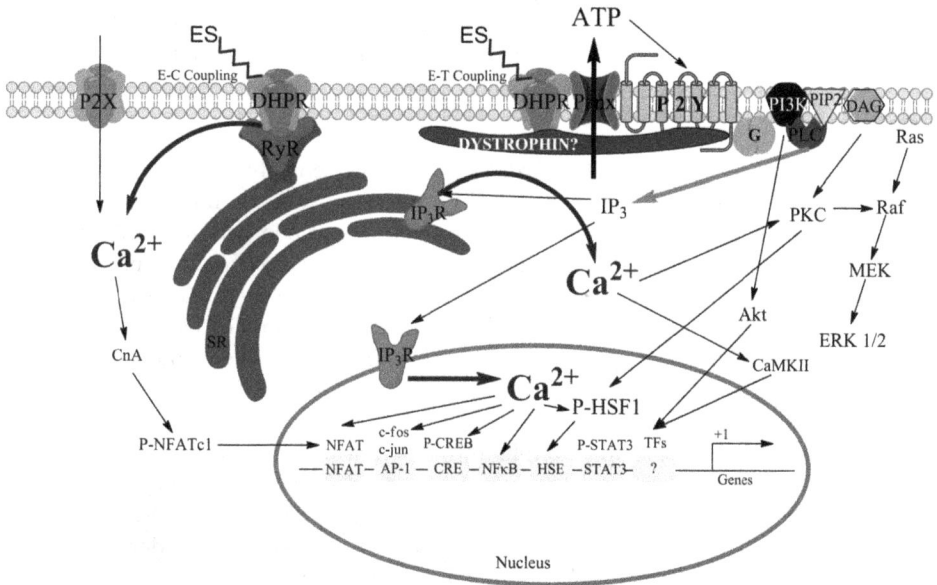

Fig. 1. **Diagram for the model for excitation-transcription coupling in skeletal muscle.**
Two protein complexes are proposed to be present in the transverse tubule (T-T) membrane. The first one is the excitation-contraction (E-C) complex, comprising the voltage sensing dihydropyridine receptor (DHPR, Cav1.1) and the ryanodine receptor (RyR). We propose that purinergic P2X receptors also contribute to the fast calcium transient associated to E-C coupling. The excitation-transcription (E-T) coupling complex comprises also the DHPR, pannexin1 (Panx), the purinergic receptor P2Y linked to a G protein and possibly the phosphatidyl inositol 3 kinase (PI3K) and phospholipase C (PLC). It is likely that dystrophin is playing a role stabilizing this complex in the membrane. Upon electrical stimulation (ES), membrane depolarization will trigger a conformational change in DHPR which somehow will induce opening of Panx channel and ATP will be released. ATP acting on P2Y receptors will activate PI3K via G protein and in turn PLC will be recruited to the membrane producing inositol (1,4,5) trisphosphate (IP_3) and diacyl glycerol (DAG). IP_3R- mediated calcium signals will be responsible for activation of kinases (PKC, CaMK II, ERK½) and transcription factors leading finally to gene expression.

7. Final remarks

Results discussed here point out to the important role of slow Ca^{2+} transients evoked by electrical stimulation in the activation of the pathways that couple excitation to gene expression in dystrophin-deficient muscle cells (a putative role for dystrophin is schematized in Fig. 1). If we find ways to intervene such pathways in a manner that can compensate dystrophin dysfunction, the understanding of this new role of dystrophin will give new insights to the design of a therapeutic strategy in order to potentiate muscle survival and regeneration in DMD.

8. Acknowledgements

We thank Sonja Buvinic, Mariana Casas and Nora Riveros, whose work and ideas provided input to this chapter. This work was supported by FONDECYT 1110467, 11100267, FONDAP 15010006, and CONICYT AT-24100066 (FA) and AT-24110211 (DV).

9. References

Abbracchio, MP, Boeynaems, JM, Barnard, EA, Boyer, JL, Kennedy, C, Miras-Portugal, MT, King, BF, Gachet, C, Jacobson, KA, Weisman, GA & Burnstock, G (2003). Characterization of the UDP-glucose receptor (re-named here the P2Y14 receptor) adds diversity to the P2Y receptor family. *Trends Pharmacol Sci*, 24, 2, pp. 52-55.

Abbracchio, MP, Burnstock, G, Boeynaems, JM, Barnard, EA, Boyer, JL, Kennedy, C, Knight, GE, Fumagalli, M, Gachet, C, Jacobson, KA & Weisman, GA (2006). International Union of Pharmacology LVIII: update on the P2Y G protein-coupled nucleotide receptors: from molecular mechanisms and pathophysiology to therapy. *Pharmacol Rev*, 58, 3, pp. 281-341.

Acharyya, S, Villalta, SA, Bakkar, N, Bupha-Intr, T, Janssen, PM, Carathers, M, Li, ZW, Beg, AA, Ghosh, S, Sahenk, Z, Weinstein, M, Gardner, KL, Rafael-Fortney, JA, Karin, M, Tidball, JG, Baldwin, AS & Guttridge, DC (2007). Interplay of IKK/NF-kappaB signaling in macrophages and myofibers promotes muscle degeneration in Duchenne muscular dystrophy. *J Clin Invest*, 117, 4, pp. 889-901.

Ahn, AH & Kunkel, LM (1993). The structural and functional diversity of dystrophin. *Nat Genet*, 3, 4, pp. 283-291.

Alderton, JM & Steinhardt, RA (2000). How calcium influx through calcium leak channels is responsible for the elevated levels of calcium-dependent proteolysis in dystrophic myotubes. *Trends Cardiovasc Med*, 10, 6, pp. 268-272.

Allen, DG, Gervasio, OL, Yeung, EW & Whitehead, NP (2010). Calcium and the damage pathways in muscular dystrophy. *Can J Physiol Pharmacol*, 88, 2, pp. 83-91.

Araya, R, Liberona, JL, Cardenas, JC, Riveros, N, Estrada, M, Powell, JA, Carrasco, MA & Jaimovich, E (2003). Dihydropyridine receptors as voltage sensors for a depolarization-evoked, IP3R-mediated, slow calcium signal in skeletal muscle cells. *J Gen Physiol*, 121, 1, pp. 3-16.

Araya, R, Riquelme, MA, Brandan, E & Saez, JC (2004). The formation of skeletal muscle myotubes requires functional membrane receptors activated by extracellular ATP. *Brain Res Brain Res Rev*, 47, 1-3, pp. 174-188.

Baban, D & Davies, KE (2008). Microarray analysis of mdx mice expressing high levels of utrophin: therapeutic implications for dystrophin deficiency. *Neuromuscul Disord*, 18, 3, pp. 239-247.

Balghi, H, Sebille, S, Constantin, B, Patri, S, Thoreau, V, Mondin, L, Mok, E, Kitzis, A, Raymond, G & Cognard, C (2006a). Mini-dystrophin expression down-regulates overactivation of G protein-mediated IP3 signaling pathway in dystrophin-deficient muscle cells. *J Gen Physiol*, 127, 2, pp. 171-182.

Balghi, H, Sebille, S, Mondin, L, Cantereau, A, Constantin, B, Raymond, G & Cognard, C (2006b). Mini-dystrophin expression down-regulates IP3-mediated calcium release events in resting dystrophin-deficient muscle cells. *J Gen Physiol*, 128, 2, pp. 219-230.

Banachewicz, W, Suplat, D, Krzeminski, P, Pomorski, P & Baranska, J (2005). P2 nucleotide receptors on C2C12 satellite cells. *Purinergic Signal*, 1, 3, pp. 249-257.

Baranova, A, Ivanov, D, Petrash, N, Pestova, A, Skoblov, M, Kelmanson, I, Shagin, D, Nazarenko, S, Geraymovych, E, Litvin, O, Tiunova, A, Born, TL, Usman, N, Staroverov, D, Lukyanov, S & Panchin, Y (2004). The mammalian pannexin family is homologous to the invertebrate innexin gap junction proteins. *Genomics*, 83, 4, pp. 706-716.

Barbe, MT, Monyer, H & Bruzzone, R (2006). Cell-cell communication beyond connexins: the pannexin channels. *Physiology (Bethesda)*, 21, pp. 103-114.

Batchelor, CL & Winder, SJ (2006). Sparks, signals and shock absorbers: how dystrophin loss causes muscular dystrophy. *Trends Cell Biol*, 16, 4, pp. 198-205.

Berchtold, MW, Brinkmeier, H & Muntener, M (2000). Calcium ion in skeletal muscle: its crucial role for muscle function, plasticity, and disease. *Physiol Rev*, 80, 3, pp. 1215-1265.

Betto, R, Senter, L, Ceoldo, S, Tarricone, E, Biral, D & Salviati, G (1999). Ecto-ATPase activity of alpha-sarcoglycan (adhalin). *J Biol Chem*, 274, 12, pp. 7907-7912.

Blake, DJ, Weir, A, Newey, SE & Davies, KE (2002). Function and genetics of dystrophin and dystrophin-related proteins in muscle. *Physiol Rev*, 82, 2, pp. 291-329.

Boittin, FX, Petermann, O, Hirn, C, Mittaud, P, Dorchies, OM, Roulet, E & Ruegg, UT (2006). Ca2+-independent phospholipase A2 enhances store-operated Ca2+ entry in dystrophic skeletal muscle fibers. *J Cell Sci*, 119, Pt 18, pp. 3733-3742.

Bours, MJ, Swennen, EL, Di Virgilio, F, Cronstein, BN & Dagnelie, PC (2006). Adenosine 5'-triphosphate and adenosine as endogenous signaling molecules in immunity and inflammation. *Pharmacol Ther*, 112, 2, pp. 358-404.

Broch-Lips, M, Pedersen, TH & Nielsen, OB (2010). Effect of purinergic receptor activation on Na+-K+ pump activity, excitability, and function in depolarized skeletal muscle. *Am J Physiol Cell Physiol*, 298, 6, pp. C1438-1444.

Brunschweiger, A & Muller, CE (2006). P2 receptors activated by uracil nucleotides--an update. *Curr Med Chem*, 13, 3, pp. 289-312.

Burnstock, G (2004). Introduction: P2 receptors. *Curr Top Med Chem*, 4, 8, pp. 793-803.

Burnstock, G & Ulrich, H (2011). Purinergic signaling in embryonic and stem cell development. *Cell Mol Life Sci*, 68, 8, pp. 1369-1394.

Buvinic, S, Almarza, G, Bustamante, M, Casas, M, Lopez, J, Riquelme, M, Saez, JC, Huidobro-Toro, JP & Jaimovich, E (2009). ATP released by electrical stimuli elicits calcium transients and gene expression in skeletal muscle. *J Biol Chem*, 284, 50, pp. 34490-34505.

Campbell, L, Abulrob, AN, Kandalaft, LE, Plummer, S, Hollins, AJ, Gibbs, A & Gumbleton, M (2003). Constitutive expression of p-glycoprotein in normal lung alveolar epithelium and functionality in primary alveolar epithelial cultures. *J Pharmacol Exp Ther*, 304, 1, pp. 441-452.

Canto, C, Chibalin, AV, Barnes, BR, Glund, S, Suarez, E, Ryder, JW, Palacin, M, Zierath, JR, Zorzano, A & Guma, A (2006). Neuregulins mediate calcium-induced glucose transport during muscle contraction. *J Biol Chem*, 281, 31, pp. 21690-21697.

Capote, J, DiFranco, M & Vergara, JL (2010). Excitation-contraction coupling alterations in mdx and utrophin/dystrophin double knockout mice: a comparative study. *Am J Physiol Cell Physiol*, 298, 5, pp. C1077-1086.

Cárdenas, C, Juretic, N, Bevilacqua, J, García, N, Figueroa, R, Hartley, R, Taratuto, AL, Gejman, L, Riveros, N, Molgó, J & Jaimovich, E (2010). Abnormal distribution of inositol 1,4,5-trisphosphate receptors in human muscle can be related to altered calcium signals and gene expression in Duchenne dystrophy derived cells. *FASEB J*. 24, 9, pp. 3210-3221

Cardenas, C, Liberona, JL, Molgo, J, Colasante, C, Mignery, GA & Jaimovich, E (2005). Nuclear inositol 1,4,5-trisphosphate receptors regulate local Ca2+ transients and modulate cAMP response element binding protein phosphorylation. *J Cell Sci*, 118, Pt 14, pp. 3131-3140.

Carrasco, MA, Riveros, N, Rios, J, Muller, M, Torres, F, Pineda, J, Lantadilla, S & Jaimovich, E (2003). Depolarization-induced slow calcium transients activate early genes in skeletal muscle cells. *Am J Physiol Cell Physiol*, 284, 6, pp. C1438-1447.

Casas, M, Figueroa, R, Jorquera, G, Escobar, M, Molgo, J & Jaimovich, E (2010). IP(3)-dependent, post-tetanic calcium transients induced by electrostimulation of adult skeletal muscle fibers. *J Gen Physiol*, 136, 4, pp. 455-467.

Chen, YW, Zhao, P, Borup, R & Hoffman, EP (2000). Expression profiling in the muscular dystrophies: identification of novel aspects of molecular pathophysiology. *J Cell Biol*, 151, 6, pp. 1321-1336.

Cho, YR, Jang, HS, Kim, W, Park, SY & Sohn, UD (2010). P2X and P2Y Receptors Mediate Contraction Induced by Electrical Field Stimulation in Feline Esophageal Smooth Muscle. *Korean J Physiol Pharmacol*, 14, 5, pp. 311-316.

Corriden, R & Insel, PA (2010). Basal release of ATP: an autocrine-paracrine mechanism for cell regulation. *Sci Signal*, 3, 104, pp. re1.

Culligan, K, Banville, N, Dowling, P & Ohlendieck, K (2002). Drastic reduction of calsequestrin-like proteins and impaired calcium binding in dystrophic mdx muscle. *J Appl Physiol*, 92, 2, pp. 435-445.

Cunha, RA & Sebastiao, AM (1993). Adenosine and adenine nucleotides are independently released from both the nerve terminals and the muscle fibres upon electrical stimulation of the innervated skeletal muscle of the frog. *Pflugers Arch*, 424, 5-6, pp. 503-510.

D'Hondt, C, Ponsaerts, R, De Smedt, H, Vinken, M, De Vuyst, E, De Bock, M, Wang, N, Rogiers, V, Leybaert, L, Himpens, B & Bultynck, G (2011). Pannexin channels in

ATP release and beyond: an unexpected rendezvous at the endoplasmic reticulum. *Cell Signal*, 23, 2, pp. 305-316.

Deconinck, N, Tinsley, J, De Backer, F, Fisher, R, Kahn, D, Phelps, S, Davies, K & Gillis, JM (1997). Expression of truncated utrophin leads to major functional improvements in dystrophin-deficient muscles of mice. *Nat Med*, 3, 11, pp. 1216-1221.

Dennis, CL, Tinsley, JM, Deconinck, AE & Davies, KE (1996). Molecular and functional analysis of the utrophin promoter. *Nucleic Acids Res*, 24, 9, pp. 1646-1652.

Divet, A, Lompre, AM & Huchet-Cadiou, C (2005). Effect of cyclopiazonic acid, an inhibitor of the sarcoplasmic reticulum Ca-ATPase, on skeletal muscles from normal and mdx mice. *Acta Physiol Scand*, 184, 3, pp. 173-186.

Dogra, C, Srivastava, DS & Kumar, A (2008). Protein-DNA array-based identification of transcription factor activities differentially regulated in skeletal muscle of normal and dystrophin-deficient mdx mice. *Mol Cell Biochem*, 312, 1-2, pp. 17-24.

Dominov, JA & Miller, JB (1996). POU homeodomain genes and myogenesis. *Dev Genet*, 19, 2, pp. 108-118.

Dubyak, GR (2009). Both sides now: multiple interactions of ATP with pannexin-1 hemichannels. Focus on "A permeant regulating its permeation pore: inhibition of pannexin 1 channels by ATP". *Am J Physiol Cell Physiol*, 296, 2, pp. C235-241.

Edwards, JN, Friedrich, O, Cully, TR, von Wegner, F, Murphy, RM & Launikonis, BS (2010). Upregulation of store-operated Ca2+ entry in dystrophic mdx mouse muscle. *Am J Physiol Cell Physiol*, 299, 1, pp. C42-50.

Eltit, JM, Garcia, AA, Hidalgo, J, Liberona, JL, Chiong, M, Lavandero, S, Maldonado, E & Jaimovich, E (2006). Membrane electrical activity elicits inositol 1,4,5-trisphosphate-dependent slow Ca2+ signals through a Gbetagamma/phosphatidylinositol 3-kinase gamma pathway in skeletal myotubes. *J Biol Chem*, 281, 17, pp. 12143-12154.

Eltit, JM, Yang, T, Li, H, Molinski, TF, Pessah, IN, Allen, PD & Lopez, JR (2010). RyR1-mediated Ca2+ leak and Ca2+ entry determine resting intracellular Ca2+ in skeletal myotubes. *J Biol Chem*, 285, 18, pp. 13781-13787.

Estrada, M, Cardenas, C, Liberona, JL, Carrasco, MA, Mignery, GA, Allen, PD & Jaimovich, E (2001). Calcium transients in 1B5 myotubes lacking ryanodine receptors are related to inositol trisphosphate receptors. *J Biol Chem*, 276, 25, pp. 22868-22874.

Evans, NP, Misyak, SA, Robertson, JL, Bassaganya-Riera, J & Grange, RW (2009a). Dysregulated intracellular signaling and inflammatory gene expression during initial disease onset in Duchenne muscular dystrophy. *Am J Phys Med Rehabil*, 88, 6, pp. 502-522.

Evans, NP, Misyak, SA, Robertson, JL, Bassaganya-Riera, J & Grange, RW (2009b). Immune-mediated mechanisms potentially regulate the disease time-course of duchenne muscular dystrophy and provide targets for therapeutic intervention. *PM R*, 1, 8, pp. 755-768.

Falls, DL (2003). Neuregulins: functions, forms, and signaling strategies. *Exp Cell Res*, 284, 1, pp. 14-30.

Fitz, JG (2007). Regulation of cellular ATP release. *Trans Am Clin Climatol Assoc*, 118, pp. 199-208.

Gervasio, OL, Whitehead, NP, Yeung, EW, Phillips, WD & Allen, DG (2008). TRPC1 binds to caveolin-3 and is regulated by Src kinase - role in Duchenne muscular dystrophy. *J Cell Sci*, 121, Pt 13, pp. 2246-2255.

Goll, DE, Thompson, VF, Li, H, Wei, W & Cong, J (2003). The calpain system. *Physiol Rev*, 83, 3, pp. 731-801.

Goonasekera, SA, Lam, CK, Millay, DP, Sargent, MA, Hajjar, RJ, Kranias, EG & Molkentin, JD (2011). Mitigation of muscular dystrophy in mice by SERCA overexpression in skeletal muscle. *J Clin Invest*, 121, 3, pp. 1044-1052.

Gramolini, AO, Angus, LM, Schaeffer, L, Burton, EA, Tinsley, JM, Davies, KE, Changeux, JP & Jasmin, BJ (1999). Induction of utrophin gene expression by heregulin in skeletal muscle cells: role of the N-box motif and GA binding protein. *Proc Natl Acad Sci U S A*, 96, 6, pp. 3223-3227.

Grasa, L, Gil, V, Gallego, D, Martin, MT & Jimenez, M (2009). P2Y(1) receptors mediate inhibitory neuromuscular transmission in the rat colon. *Br J Pharmacol*, 158, 6, pp. 1641-1652.

Grishin, SN, Teplov, AY, Galkin, AV, Devyataev, AM, Zefirov, AL, Mukhamedyarov, MA, Ziganshin, AU, Burnstock, G & Palotas, A (2006). Different effects of ATP on the contractile activity of mice diaphragmatic and skeletal muscles. *Neurochem Int*, 49, 8, pp. 756-763.

Guma, A, Martinez-Redondo, V, Lopez-Soldado, I, Canto, C & Zorzano, A (2010). Emerging role of neuregulin as a modulator of muscle metabolism. *Am J Physiol Endocrinol Metab*, 298, 4, pp. E742-750.

Hack, AA, Groh, ME & McNally, EM (2000). Sarcoglycans in muscular dystrophy. *Microsc Res Tech*, 48, 3-4, pp. 167-180.

Haslett, JN, Sanoudou, D, Kho, AT, Bennett, RR, Greenberg, SA, Kohane, IS, Beggs, AH & Kunkel, LM (2002). Gene expression comparison of biopsies from Duchenne muscular dystrophy (DMD) and normal skeletal muscle. *Proc Natl Acad Sci U S A*, 99, 23, pp. 15000-15005.

Hellsten, Y, Maclean, D, Radegran, G, Saltin, B & Bangsbo, J (1998). Adenosine concentrations in the interstitium of resting and contracting human skeletal muscle. *Circulation*, 98, 1, pp. 6-8.

Hirata, M, Sakuma, K, Okajima, S, Fujiwara, H, Inashima, S, Yasuhara, M & Kubo, T (2007). Increased expression of neuregulin-1 in differentiating muscle satellite cells and in motoneurons during muscle regeneration. *Acta Neuropathol*, 113, 4, pp. 451-459.

Hnia, K, Gayraud, J, Hugon, G, Ramonatxo, M, De La Porte, S, Matecki, S & Mornet, D (2008). L-arginine decreases inflammation and modulates the nuclear factor-kappaB/matrix metalloproteinase cascade in mdx muscle fibers. *Am J Pathol*, 172, 6, pp. 1509-1519.

Hollingworth, S, Zeiger, U & Baylor, SM (2008). Comparison of the myoplasmic calcium transient elicited by an action potential in intact fibres of mdx and normal mice. *J Physiol*, 586, Pt 21, pp. 5063-5075.

Iwata, Y, Katanosaka, Y, Hisamitsu, T & Wakabayashi, S (2007). Enhanced Na+/H+ exchange activity contributes to the pathogenesis of muscular dystrophy via involvement of P2 receptors. *Am J Pathol*, 171, 5, pp. 1576-1587.

Jacobson, KA & Boeynaems, JM (2010). P2Y nucleotide receptors: promise of therapeutic applications. *Drug Discov Today*, 15, 13-14, pp. 570-578.

Jacobson, KA, Ivanov, AA, de Castro, S, Harden, TK & Ko, H (2009). Development of selective agonists and antagonists of P2Y receptors. *Purinergic Signal*, 5, 1, pp. 75-89.

Jaimovich, E, Reyes, R, Liberona, JL & Powell, JA (2000). IP(3) receptors, IP(3) transients, and nucleus-associated Ca(2+) signals in cultured skeletal muscle. *Am J Physiol Cell Physiol*, 278, 5, pp. C998-C1010.

Jarvis, MF & Khakh, BS (2009). ATP-gated P2X cation-channels. *Neuropharmacology*, 56, 1, pp. 208-215.

Jia, M, Li, MX, Fields, RD & Nelson, PG (2007). Extracellular ATP in activity-dependent remodeling of the neuromuscular junction. *Dev Neurobiol*, 67, 7, pp. 924-932.

Jiang, T, Yeung, D, Lien, CF & Gorecki, DC (2005). Localized expression of specific P2X receptors in dystrophin-deficient DMD and mdx muscle. *Neuromuscul Disord*, 15, 3, pp. 225-236.

Jorquera, G, Juretic, N, Jaimovich, E & Riveros, N (2009). Membrane depolarization induces calcium-dependent upregulation of Hsp70 and Hmox-1 in skeletal muscle cells. *Am J Physiol Cell Physiol*, 297, 3, pp. C581-590.

Juretić, N, Jorquera, G, Caviedes, P, Jaimovich, E & Riveros, N (n.d.). Electrical stimulation induces calcium-dependent up-regulation of neuregulin-1β in dystrophic skeletal muscle cell lines. Manuscript in preparation

Juretic, N, Garcia-Huidobro, P, Iturrieta, JA, Jaimovich, E & Riveros, N (2006). Depolarization-induced slow Ca2+ transients stimulate transcription of IL-6 gene in skeletal muscle cells. *Am J Physiol Cell Physiol*, 290, 5, pp. C1428-1436.

Juretic, N, Urzua, U, Munroe, DJ, Jaimovich, E & Riveros, N (2007). Differential gene expression in skeletal muscle cells after membrane depolarization. *J Cell Physiol*, 210, 3, pp. 819-830.

Kapsa, R, Kornberg, AJ & Byrne, E (2003). Novel therapies for Duchenne muscular dystrophy. *Lancet Neurol*, 2, 5, pp. 299-310.

Kargacin, ME & Kargacin, GJ (1996). The sarcoplasmic reticulum calcium pump is functionally altered in dystrophic muscle. *Biochim Biophys Acta*, 1290, 1, pp. 4-8.

Khurana, TS, Hoffman, EP & Kunkel, LM (1990). Identification of a chromosome 6-encoded dystrophin-related protein. *J Biol Chem*, 265, 28, pp. 16717-16720.

Khurana, TS, Rosmarin, AG, Shang, J, Krag, TO, Das, S & Gammeltoft, S (1999). Activation of utrophin promoter by heregulin via the ets-related transcription factor complex GA-binding protein alpha/beta. *Mol Biol Cell*, 10, 6, pp. 2075-2086.

Krag, TO, Bogdanovich, S, Jensen, CJ, Fischer, MD, Hansen-Schwartz, J, Javazon, EH, Flake, AW, Edvinsson, L & Khurana, TS (2004). Heregulin ameliorates the dystrophic phenotype in mdx mice. *Proc Natl Acad Sci U S A*, 101, 38, pp. 13856-13860.

Kumar, A & Boriek, AM (2003). Mechanical stress activates the nuclear factor-kappaB pathway in skeletal muscle fibers: a possible role in Duchenne muscular dystrophy. *FASEB J*, 17, 3, pp. 386-396.

Lang, JM, Esser, KA & Dupont-Versteegden, EE (2004). Altered activity of signaling pathways in diaphragm and tibialis anterior muscle of dystrophic mice. *Exp Biol Med (Maywood)*, 229, 6, pp. 503-511.

Lebrasseur, NK, Cote, GM, Miller, TA, Fielding, RA & Sawyer, DB (2003). Regulation of neuregulin/ErbB signaling by contractile activity in skeletal muscle. *Am J Physiol Cell Physiol*, 284, 5, pp. C1149-1155.

Liberona, JL, Powell, JA, Shenoi, S, Petherbridge, L, Caviedes, R & Jaimovich, E (1998). Differences in both inositol 1,4,5-trisphosphate mass and inositol 1,4,5-trisphosphate receptors between normal and dystrophic skeletal muscle cell lines. *Muscle Nerve*, 21, 7, pp. 902-909.

Liu, HT, Toychiev, AH, Takahashi, N, Sabirov, RZ & Okada, Y (2008). Maxi-anion channel as a candidate pathway for osmosensitive ATP release from mouse astrocytes in primary culture. *Cell Res*, 18, 5, pp. 558-565.

Lopez, JR, Briceno, LE, Sanchez, V & Horvart, D (1987). Myoplasmic (Ca2+) in Duchenne muscular dystrophy patients. *Acta Cient Venez*, 38, 4, pp. 503-504.

Love, DR, Hill, DF, Dickson, G, Spurr, NK, Byth, BC, Marsden, RF, Walsh, FS, Edwards, YH & Davies, KE (1989). An autosomal transcript in skeletal muscle with homology to dystrophin. *Nature*, 339, 6219, pp. 55-58.

Matsumura, K, Ervasti, JM, Ohlendieck, K, Kahl, SD & Campbell, KP (1992). Association of dystrophin-related protein with dystrophin-associated proteins in mdx mouse muscle. *Nature*, 360, 6404, pp. 588-591.

May, C, Weigl, L, Karel, A & Hohenegger, M (2006). Extracellular ATP activates ERK1/ERK2 via a metabotropic P2Y1 receptor in a Ca2+ independent manner in differentiated human skeletal muscle cells. *Biochem Pharmacol*, 71, 10, pp. 1497-1509.

Messina, S, Bitto, A, Aguennouz, M, Vita, GL, Polito, F, Irrera, N, Altavilla, D, Marini, H, Migliorato, A, Squadrito, F & Vita, G (2011). The soy isoflavone genistein blunts nuclear factor kappa-B, MAPKs and TNF-alpha activation and ameliorates muscle function and morphology in mdx mice. *Neuromuscul Disord*, 21, 8, pp. 579-589.

Millay, DP, Sargent, MA, Osinska, H, Baines, CP, Barton, ER, Vuagniaux, G, Sweeney, HL, Robbins, J & Molkentin, JD (2008). Genetic and pharmacologic inhibition of mitochondrial-dependent necrosis attenuates muscular dystrophy. *Nat Med*, 14, 4, pp. 442-447.

Miura, P & Jasmin, BJ (2006). Utrophin upregulation for treating Duchenne or Becker muscular dystrophy: how close are we? *Trends Mol Med*, 12, 3, pp. 122-129.

Mokri, B & Engel, AG (1998). Duchenne dystrophy: electron microscopic findings pointing to a basic or early abnormality in the plasma membrane of the muscle fiber. 1975. *Neurology*, 51, 1, pp. 1 and 10 pages following.

Morine, KJ, Sleeper, MM, Barton, ER & Sweeney, HL (2010). Overexpression of SERCA1a in the mdx diaphragm reduces susceptibility to contraction-induced damage. *Hum Gene Ther*, 21, 12, pp. 1735-1739.

Nakamura, T, Iwanaga, K, Murata, T, Hori, M & Ozaki, H (2011). ATP induces contraction mediated by the P2Y(2) receptor in rat intestinal subepithelial myofibroblasts. *Eur J Pharmacol*, 657, 1-3, pp. 152-158.

Nakata, H, Yoshioka, K & Kamiya, T (2004). Purinergic-receptor oligomerization: implications for neural functions in the central nervous system. *Neurotox Res*, 6, 4, pp. 291-297.

Nguyen, TM, Ellis, JM, Love, DR, Davies, KE, Gatter, KC, Dickson, G & Morris, GE (1991). Localization of the DMDL gene-encoded dystrophin-related protein using a panel of nineteen monoclonal antibodies: presence at neuromuscular junctions, in the sarcolemma of dystrophic skeletal muscle, in vascular and other smooth muscles, and in proliferating brain cell lines. *J Cell Biol*, 115, 6, pp. 1695-1700.

Niebroj-Dobosz, I & Hausmanowa-Petrusewicz, I (2005). The involvement of oxidative stress in determining the severity and progress of pathological processes in dystrophin-deficient muscles. *Acta Biochim Pol*, 52, 2, pp. 449-452.

Noguchi, S, Tsukahara, T, Fujita, M, Kurokawa, R, Tachikawa, M, Toda, T, Tsujimoto, A, Arahata, K & Nishino, I (2003). cDNA microarray analysis of individual Duchenne muscular dystrophy patients. *Hum Mol Genet*, 12, 6, pp. 595-600.

North, RA (2002). Molecular physiology of P2X receptors. *Physiol Rev*, 82, 4, pp. 1013-1067.

Ohlendieck, K, Ervasti, JM, Matsumura, K, Kahl, SD, Leveille, CJ & Campbell, KP (1991). Dystrophin-related protein is localized to neuromuscular junctions of adult skeletal muscle. *Neuron*, 7, 3, pp. 499-508.

Petrof, BJ, Shrager, JB, Stedman, HH, Kelly, AM & Sweeney, HL (1993). Dystrophin protects the sarcolemma from stresses developed during muscle contraction. *Proc Natl Acad Sci U S A*, 90, 8, pp. 3710-3714.

Porreca, E, Guglielmi, MD, Uncini, A, Di Gregorio, P, Angelini, A, Di Febbo, C, Pierdomenico, SD, Baccante, G & Cuccurullo, F (1999). Haemostatic abnormalities, cardiac involvement and serum tumor necrosis factor levels in X-linked dystrophic patients. *Thromb Haemost*, 81, 4, pp. 543-546.

Porter, JD, Guo, W, Merriam, AP, Khanna, S, Cheng, G, Zhou, X, Andrade, FH, Richmonds, C & Kaminski, HJ (2003a). Persistent over-expression of specific CC class chemokines correlates with macrophage and T-cell recruitment in mdx skeletal muscle. *Neuromuscul Disord*, 13, 3, pp. 223-235.

Porter, JD, Khanna, S, Kaminski, HJ, Rao, JS, Merriam, AP, Richmonds, CR, Leahy, P, Li, J, Guo, W & Andrade, FH (2002). A chronic inflammatory response dominates the skeletal muscle molecular signature in dystrophin-deficient mdx mice. *Hum Mol Genet*, 11, 3, pp. 263-272.

Porter, JD, Merriam, AP, Leahy, P, Gong, B, Feuerman, J, Cheng, G & Khanna, S (2004). Temporal gene expression profiling of dystrophin-deficient (mdx) mouse diaphragm identifies conserved and muscle group-specific mechanisms in the pathogenesis of muscular dystrophy. *Hum Mol Genet*, 13, 3, pp. 257-269.

Porter, JD, Merriam, AP, Leahy, P, Gong, B & Khanna, S (2003b). Dissection of temporal gene expression signatures of affected and spared muscle groups in dystrophin-deficient (mdx) mice. *Hum Mol Genet*, 12, 15, pp. 1813-1821.

Powell, JA, Carrasco, MA, Adams, DS, Drouet, B, Rios, J, Muller, M, Estrada, M & Jaimovich, E (2001). IP(3) receptor function and localization in myotubes: an unexplored Ca(2+) signaling pathway in skeletal muscle. *J Cell Sci*, 114, Pt 20, pp. 3673-3683.

Rando, TA (2001). The dystrophin-glycoprotein complex, cellular signaling, and the regulation of cell survival in the muscular dystrophies. *Muscle Nerve*, 24, 12, pp. 1575-1594.

Raqeeb, A, Sheng, J, Ao, N & Braun, AP (2011). Purinergic P2Y2 receptors mediate rapid Ca(2+) mobilization, membrane hyperpolarization and nitric oxide production in human vascular endothelial cells. *Cell Calcium*, 49, 4, pp. 240-248.

Roberds, SL, Leturcq, F, Allamand, V, Piccolo, F, Jeanpierre, M, Anderson, RD, Lim, LE, Lee, JC, Tome, FM, Romero, NB & et al. (1994). Missense mutations in the adhalin gene linked to autosomal recessive muscular dystrophy. *Cell*, 78, 4, pp. 625-633.

Robert, V, Massimino, ML, Tosello, V, Marsault, R, Cantini, M, Sorrentino, V & Pozzan, T (2001). Alteration in calcium handling at the subcellular level in mdx myotubes. *J Biol Chem*, 276, 7, pp. 4647-4651.

Ryten, M, Dunn, PM, Neary, JT & Burnstock, G (2002). ATP regulates the differentiation of mammalian skeletal muscle by activation of a P2X5 receptor on satellite cells. *J Cell Biol*, 158, 2, pp. 345-355.

Ryten, M, Yang, SY, Dunn, PM, Goldspink, G & Burnstock, G (2004). Purinoceptor expression in regenerating skeletal muscle in the mdx mouse model of muscular dystrophy and in satellite cell cultures. *FASEB J*, 18, 12, pp. 1404-1406.

Sabirov, RZ & Okada, Y (2005). ATP release via anion channels. *Purinergic Signal*, 1, 4, pp. 311-328.

Sandona, D, Danieli-Betto, D, Germinario, E, Biral, D, Martinello, T, Lioy, A, Tarricone, E, Gastaldello, S & Betto, R (2005). The T-tubule membrane ATP-operated P2X4 receptor influences contractility of skeletal muscle. *FASEB J*, 19, 9, pp. 1184-1186.

Sandona, D, Gastaldello, S, Martinello, T & Betto, R (2004). Characterization of the ATP-hydrolysing activity of alpha-sarcoglycan. *Biochem J*, 381, Pt 1, pp. 105-112.

Shestopalov, VI & Panchin, Y (2008). Pannexins and gap junction protein diversity. *Cell Mol Life Sci*, 65, 3, pp. 376-394.

Silinsky, EM & Redman, RS (1996). Synchronous release of ATP and neurotransmitter within milliseconds of a motor nerve impulse in the frog. *J Physiol*, 492 (Pt 3), pp. 815-822.

Smith, DO (1991). Sources of adenosine released during neuromuscular transmission in the rat. *J Physiol*, 432, pp. 343-354.

Spencer, MJ, Croall, DE & Tidball, JG (1995). Calpains are activated in necrotic fibers from mdx dystrophic mice. *J Biol Chem*, 270, 18, pp. 10909-10914.

Suadicani, SO, Brosnan, CF & Scemes, E (2006). P2X7 receptors mediate ATP release and amplification of astrocytic intercellular Ca2+ signaling. *J Neurosci*, 26, 5, pp. 1378-1385.

Surprenant, A & North, RA (2009). Signaling at purinergic P2X receptors. *Annu Rev Physiol*, 71, pp. 333-359.

Tinsley, J, Deconinck, N, Fisher, R, Kahn, D, Phelps, S, Gillis, JM & Davies, K (1998). Expression of full-length utrophin prevents muscular dystrophy in mdx mice. *Nat Med*, 4, 12, pp. 1441-1444.

Tinsley, JM, Blake, DJ, Roche, A, Fairbrother, U, Riss, J, Byth, BC, Knight, AE, Kendrick-Jones, J, Suthers, GK, Love, DR & et al. (1992). Primary structure of dystrophin-related protein. *Nature*, 360, 6404, pp. 591-593.

Tinsley, JM, Potter, AC, Phelps, SR, Fisher, R, Trickett, JI & Davies, KE (1996). Amelioration of the dystrophic phenotype of mdx mice using a truncated utrophin transgene. *Nature*, 384, 6607, pp. 349-353.

Turk, R, Sterrenburg, E, de Meijer, EJ, van Ommen, GJ, den Dunnen, JT & t Hoen, PA (2005). Muscle regeneration in dystrophin-deficient mdx mice studied by gene expression profiling. *BMC Genomics*, 6, pp. 98.

Turner, PR, Fong, PY, Denetclaw, WF & Steinhardt, RA (1991). Increased calcium influx in dystrophic muscle. *J Cell Biol*, 115, 6, pp. 1701-1712.

Turner, PR, Schultz, R, Ganguly, B & Steinhardt, RA (1993). Proteolysis results in altered leak channel kinetics and elevated free calcium in mdx muscle. *J Membr Biol*, 133, 3, pp. 243-251.

Turner, PR, Westwood, T, Regen, CM & Steinhardt, RA (1988). Increased protein degradation results from elevated free calcium levels found in muscle from mdx mice. *Nature*, 335, 6192, pp. 735-738.

Vandebrouck, A, Ducret, T, Basset, O, Sebille, S, Raymond, G, Ruegg, U, Gailly, P, Cognard, C & Constantin, B (2006). Regulation of store-operated calcium entries and mitochondrial uptake by minidystrophin expression in cultured myotubes. *FASEB J*, 20, 1, pp. 136-138.

Vandebrouck, C, Martin, D, Colson-Van Schoor, M, Debaix, H & Gailly, P (2002). Involvement of TRPC in the abnormal calcium influx observed in dystrophic (mdx) mouse skeletal muscle fibers. *J Cell Biol*, 158, 6, pp. 1089-1096.

Volonte, C & D'Ambrosi, N (2009). Membrane compartments and purinergic signalling: the purinome, a complex interplay among ligands, degrading enzymes, receptors and transporters. *FEBS J*, 276, 2, pp. 318-329.

von Kugelgen, I (2006). Pharmacological profiles of cloned mammalian P2Y-receptor subtypes. *Pharmacol Ther*, 110, 3, pp. 415-432.

Voss, AA (2009). Extracellular ATP inhibits chloride channels in mature mammalian skeletal muscle by activating P2Y1 receptors. *J Physiol*, 587, Pt 23, pp. 5739-5752.

Winder, SJ, Hemmings, L, Maciver, SK, Bolton, SJ, Tinsley, JM, Davies, KE, Critchley, DR & Kendrick-Jones, J (1995). Utrophin actin binding domain: analysis of actin binding and cellular targeting. *J Cell Sci*, 108 (Pt 1), pp. 63-71.

Woods, CE, Novo, D, DiFranco, M & Vergara, JL (2004). The action potential-evoked sarcoplasmic reticulum calcium release is impaired in mdx mouse muscle fibres. *J Physiol*, 557, Pt 1, pp. 59-75.

Yegutkin, GG (2008). Nucleotide- and nucleoside-converting ectoenzymes: Important modulators of purinergic signalling cascade. *Biochim Biophys Acta*, 1783, 5, pp. 673-694.

Yeung, D, Kharidia, R, Brown, SC & Gorecki, DC (2004). Enhanced expression of the P2X4 receptor in Duchenne muscular dystrophy correlates with macrophage invasion. *Neurobiol Dis*, 15, 2, pp. 212-220.

Yeung, D, Zablocki, K, Lien, CF, Jiang, T, Arkle, S, Brutkowski, W, Brown, J, Lochmuller, H, Simon, J, Barnard, EA & Gorecki, DC (2006). Increased susceptibility to ATP via alteration of P2X receptor function in dystrophic mdx mouse muscle cells. *FASEB J*, 20, 6, pp. 610-620.

Yeung, EW, Whitehead, NP, Suchyna, TM, Gottlieb, PA, Sachs, F & Allen, DG (2005). Effects of stretch-activated channel blockers on [Ca2+]i and muscle damage in the mdx mouse. *J Physiol*, 562, Pt 2, pp. 367-380.

Zhang, BT, Yeung, SS, Allen, DG, Qin, L & Yeung, EW (2008). Role of the calcium-calpain pathway in cytoskeletal damage after eccentric contractions. *J Appl Physiol*, 105, 1, pp. 352-357.

10

Synaptic Changes at the Spinal Cord Level and Peripheral Nerve Regeneration During the Course of Muscular Dystrophy in MDX Mice

Gustavo Ferreira Simões and Alexandre Leite Rodrigues de Oliveira
University of Campinas (UNICAMP),
Brasil

1. Introduction

Muscular dystrophies are part of a group of degenerative diseases of the muscular system, which are characterized by muscle degeneration and structural changes at the neuromuscular junction. The most common form is Duchenne Muscular Dystrophy (DMD) (Whitehead et al., 2006), which affects approximately 1 in every 3500 live births (Balaban et al., 2005; Judge et al., 2005; Withehead et al., 2006; Radley et al., 2007). It is a severe X-linked recessive disorder, where the X chromosome is mutated in the region of the gene Xp21, which encodes for the production of dystrophin (Pearce, 2005).

Dystrophin is a protein located adjacent to the sarcolemma of myocytes (Arahata et al., 1988; Chelly et al., 1988; Carretta et al., 2001). The dystrophin-glycoprotein complex has the functions of maintaining links between the cytoskeleton and the extracellular matrix (Figure 1), maintaining the integrity of the sarcoplasmic membrane, distributing the lateral forces between the muscle fibers and communicating via the intra-and extracellular environment (Lowe et al., 2006). Its absence is characterized by progressive degeneration and weakness of the skeletal muscles, and an inability to properly repair the muscular tissue, which is gradually replaced by fat and connective tissue (Whitehead et al., 2006).

DMD is usually diagnosed between 2 and 5 years old (Balaban et al., 2005), being inexorably fatal, and the patients usually die around the second decade of life due to impairment of the cardiac and diaphragm muscle (Judge et al., 2005; Whitehead et al., 2006).Duchenne muscular dystrophy is characterized in MDX mice (an animal model for the study of Duchenne Muscular Dystrophy) by a set of muscle degeneration fibers with intense infiltrate inflammation (Nonaka, 1998). The MDX mice myonecrosis is often preceded by a collapse and detachment of the basal lamina of the sarcolemma, and subsequent muscle fiber degeneration associated with an extensive inflammatory process. Macrophages, CD4 + and CD8 + T cells represent the main constituents of the population of inflammatory cells that surround the myofiber degeneration process (Mcdowall et al., 1990; Spencer et al., 2001). Concerning this aspect, Lagrota-Candido et al. (2002) revealed that during the process of muscle degeneration, there is an accumulation of CD4 + and CD8 cells in the skeletal muscles of 4-week old MDX mice. Moreover, during the period of muscle regeneration, there is a proliferation of B lymphocytes and secretion of IFN-β by lymphocytes.

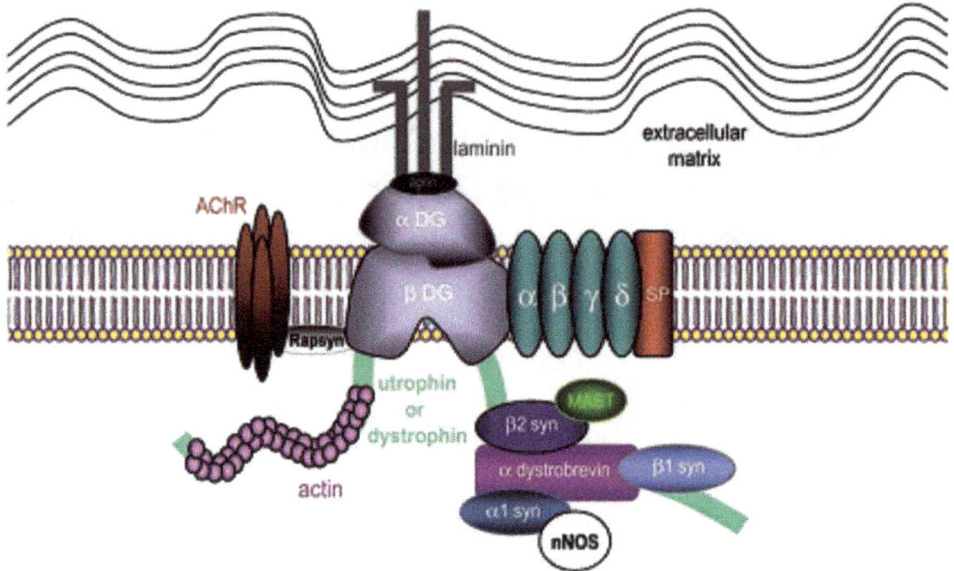

Fig. 1. Composition and schematic organization of the dystrophin glycoprotein complex (DGC) at the neuromuscular junction. Dystrophin or utrophin bind to actin filaments via their N terminus. At the C terminus, dystrophin or utrophin are associated with integral and peripheral membrane proteins that can be classified as the dystroglycan complex, the sarcoglycan-sarcospan complex and the cytoplasmic complex. *Role of dystrophin and utrophin for assembly and function of the dystrophin glycoprotein complex in non-muscle tissue* – review from Cellular and Molecular Life Sciences; 63 (2006) 1614–1631.

Currently, much is known about the muscle involvement during the course of DMD, but few studies have focused on the effects on the CNS, specifically in the microenvironment of the spinal motoneurons. It is known that during the course of the disease, axonal terminals enter a cycle of denervation (retraction) and reinnervation (sprouting), and this cycle can pass in a retrograde manner to the cell bodies of the spinal alpha-motoneurons. After an injury resulting in disruption of the contact between the motoneurons and their target muscle fibers, a series of changes occurs in the cell body of the neuron (for example, the presence of edema in the cell body, displacement of the nucleus to the periphery of the cell body and a decrease in electron density along with the dissolution of Nissl corpuscles), which, together, is called chromatolysis (Romanes, 1946; Lieberman, 1971; Aldskogius & Svensson, 1993) – Figure 2.

Pastoret & Sebille (1994) investigated the cycles of muscle degeneration and regeneration as from the second week and up to 104 weeks of life in MDX mice. Their results showed that in the second week of life, some abnormalities could be found in muscle fibers of the tibialis anterior, extensor digitorum longus, muscle longus plantar and soleus muscle. These changes included small scattered foci of degenerated muscle fibers surrounded by cellular infiltrates, "pale" muscle fibers and small groups of regenerated muscle fibers with a central nucleus. By the third week of life these abnormalities were evident and widespread in all the

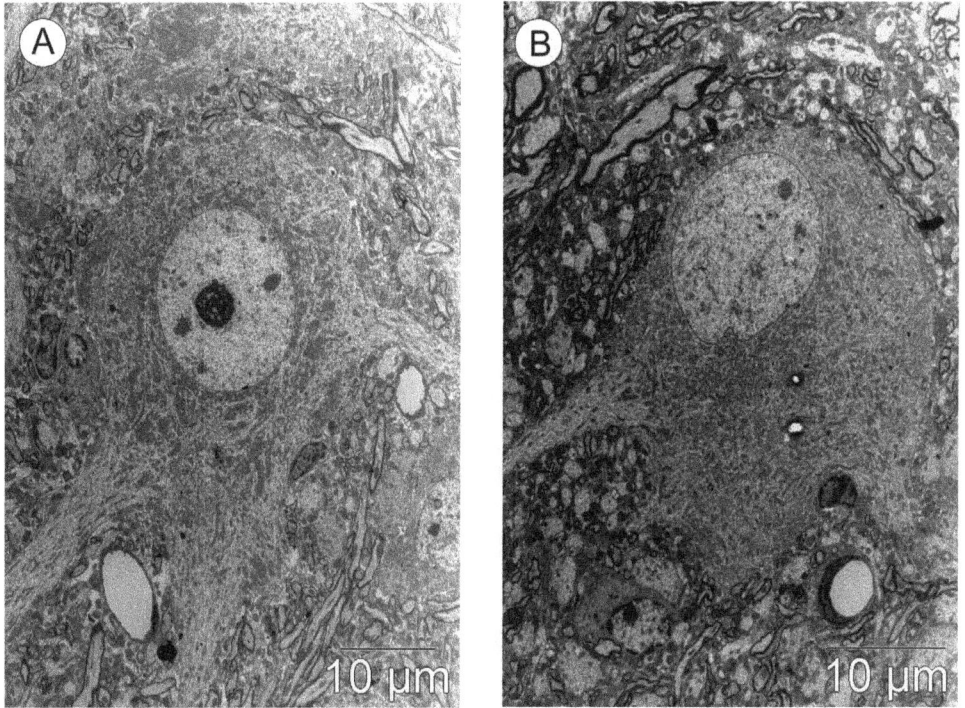

Fig. 2. B and C respectively, a motoneuron subjected to peripheral axotomy and a normal
motoneuron, both observed under transmission electron microscopy. Scale = 10µm.
(Expression of class I major histocompatibility complex (MHC I) in the central nervous system: role
in synaptic plasticity and regeneration – review from Coluna/Columna. 2010; 9(2):193-198).

muscles studied by these authors. These same authors showed that in the sixth week of life,
about 50% of the muscle fibers of the lower limb muscles presented a central nucleus, and
by the eighth week of life, all the muscles showed hypertrophic fibers coexisting with foci of
small fibers in various stages of maturation, providing an increase in the variety of fiber
diameters. Huard et al. (1992) demonstrated the expression of dystrophin in the cerebellum,
cerebral cortex, hippocampus and spinal cord of the central nervous system (CNS) of
humans and monkeys. However, Lidove et al. (1993) demonstrated that in mice, dystrophin
is expressed almost exclusively in the pyramidal cells and in other neurons of the cerebral
cortex and in the Purkinje cells. Sbriccoli et al. (1995) suggested that the dystrophin localized
in the CNS has an important role in developing and maintaining the structural and
functional properties in the interconnections between neurons. Evidence of abnormal
connections in the adult MDX mouse brain has been demonstrated primarily by Carretta et
al. (2001). Sbriccoli et al. (1995) showed that in MDX mice, there are decreased numbers of
cortico-spinal tract axons. This change in the cortico-spinal tract can be justified by the role
of dystrophin in the cerebral cortex, and the complete loss of its expression in MDX mice.
Therefore, it plays an important role in the migration and maturation of neurons in the
cerebral cortex.

Bearing in mind the possible repercussions of the process of muscle degeneration and regeneration in the spinal microenvironment, unilateral axotomy of the sciatic nerve followed by analysis of the spinal motoneurons was used in MDX mice (Figure 3). This experimental model of peripheral nerve injury was chosen, keeping in mind that the transection of a peripheral nerve, such as the sciatic nerve, is a well-established experimental model to study the correlation between glial reactivity and neuronal response to injury at the anterior column level of the spinal cord (Lundberg et al., 2001). This is due to the fact that in this model, the only elements directly affected by the injury are the axons of spinal neurons. Thus any changes observed in the vicinity of motoneuron bodies, including reactive astrogliosis and the activation of MHC I molecules (histocompatibility complex type I), are reflections of direct communication between the neuron and the glia.

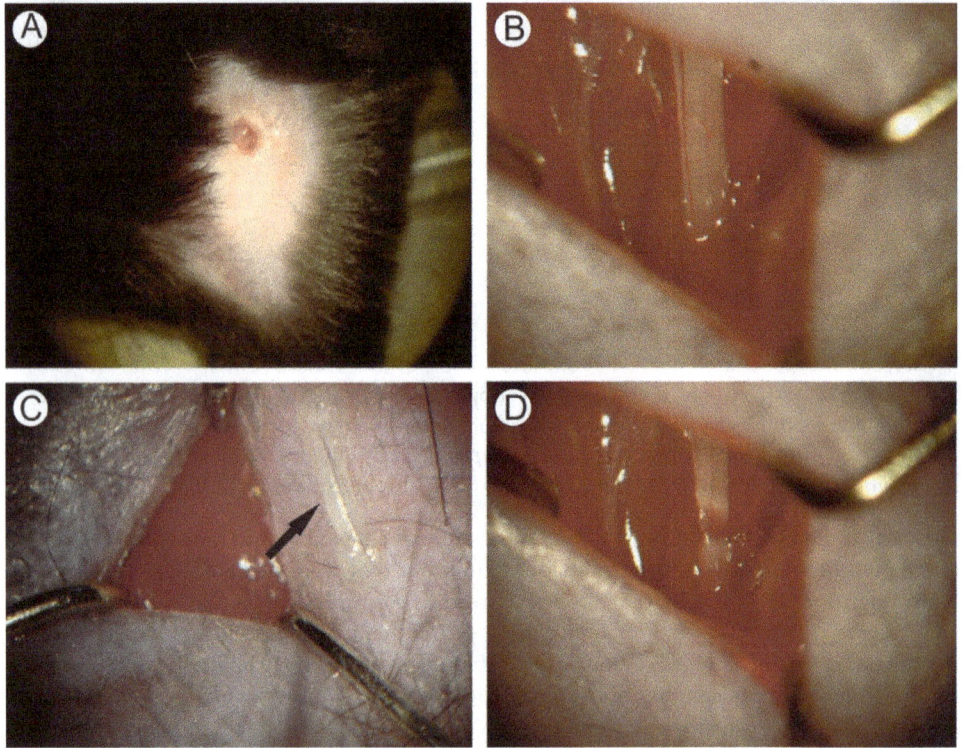

Fig. 3. A - Shaving in the region of the posterior left thigh and an incision in the skin of the mid-thigh, and then parallel to the femur using a scalpel. B - The skin and thigh muscle were carefully retracted, exposing the sciatic nerve to be transected. C - Figure showing the transected sciatic nerve. D – Crushed sciatic nerve.

Distal axotomy also induces, in addition to astroglial activation, the retraction of presynaptic terminals in contact with the cell body (Figure 4) and dendrites of the spinal alpha-motoneurons (Brännström & Kellerth, 1998: Aldskogious et al., 1999). This retraction is more intense in the synaptic terminals of the motoneuron cell body (Brännström & Kellerth, 1998), and occurs in the acute phase of injury, being influenced by the change in physiological state of the neurons, that pass from the transmission state condition to the survival and regeneration condition (Piehl et al., 1998). Reier et al. (1989) have proposed that the astrocytes act as a barrier to axon growth by way of the formation of scar tissue, but may promote its regeneration by releasing neurotrophic factors (Baba, 1998). Therefore the astrocytes directly influence the dynamics of synaptic contacts (Walz, 1989: Araque & Perea, 2004) and may thus influence the processes of synaptic reorganization after injury (Aldskogius et al., 1999).

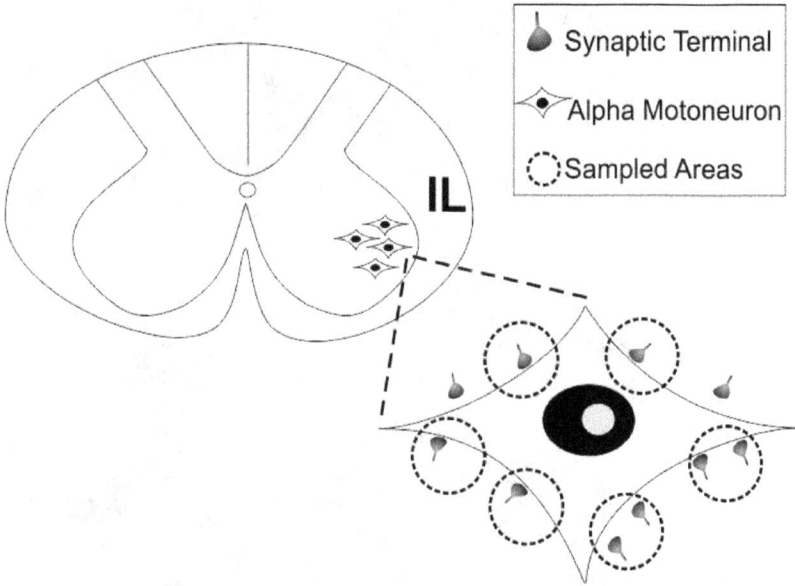

Fig. 4. Schematic representation of the sciatic nerve pool in the ventral horn of the spinal cord. One motoneuron is shown in detail with apposed presynaptic terminals. The dashed circles represent the areas where synaptic retraction is present. 2010 Blackwell Publishing Ltd, *Neuropathology and Applied Neurobiology,* **36** , 55–70.

2. Results and discussion

The immunohistochemistry and transmission electron microscopy results demonstrated that glial reactivity varies between the two strains. In MDX mice with no injury, an increase in GFAP immunoreactivity can be seen as compared to the same group in C57BL/10 mice (Figure 5A and 5B, respectively). The MDX and C57BL/10 ipsilateral groups showed a significant increase in reactive astrogliosis (GFAP) in relation to the contralateral groups in both strains (Figures 5E and 5F, respectively). However, with respect to this, there was evidence of increased astrocyte activity in the MDX contralateral group, as demonstrated by astrogliosis in the region of the spinal alpha-motoneurons (Figure 5D). This increase was approximately 49.5% higher than in the same side of the C57BL/10 strain. The analysis showed a significant increase in ipsilateral activity of the astrocytes in MDX mice, about 65.2% higher as compared to the C57BL/10 mice. Increased astrogliosis at the level of the anterior column of the spinal cord correlates with significant synaptic plasticity in the process of regeneration of injured neurons, as demonstrated by Emirandetti et al. (2006).

However, when the ipsi/contralateral ratio of the GFAP expression was analyzed, it was confirmed that there was no significant difference between the strains studied.

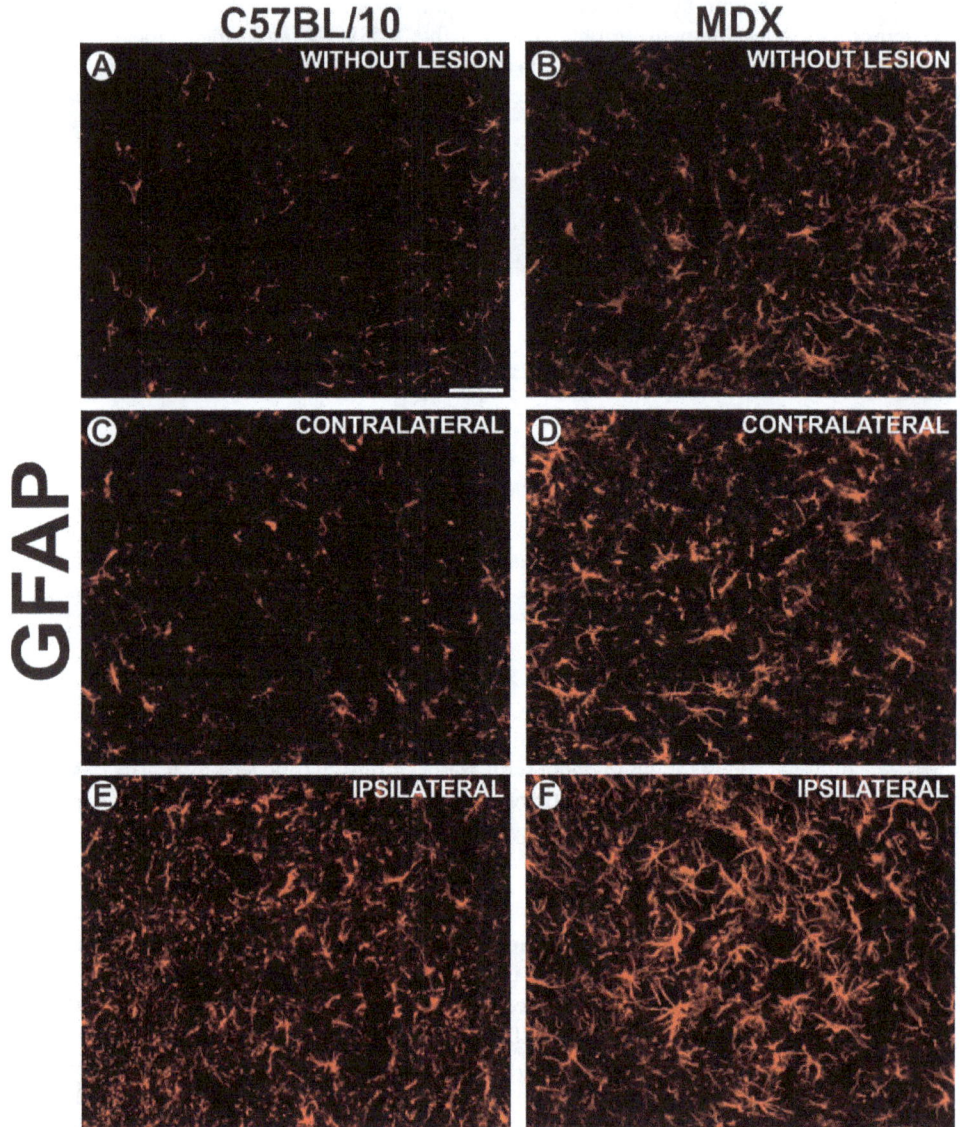

Fig. 5. Anti-GFAP immunostaining. A and B show non-injured animals (C57BL/10 and MDX, respectively). C and D show contralateral groups seven days after axotomy (C57BL/10 and MDX, respectively). E and F show ipsilateral sides, seven days after axotomy (C57BL/10 and MDX, respectively). Note that in general there is a greater expression of GFAP in the MDX strain in relation to the C57BL/10 strain. 2010 Blackwell Publishing Ltd, *Neuropathology and Applied Neurobiology,* **36** , 55–70.

Synaptic Changes at the Spinal Cord Level and Peripheral Nerve Regeneration During the Course of Muscular
Dystrophy in MDX Mice

203

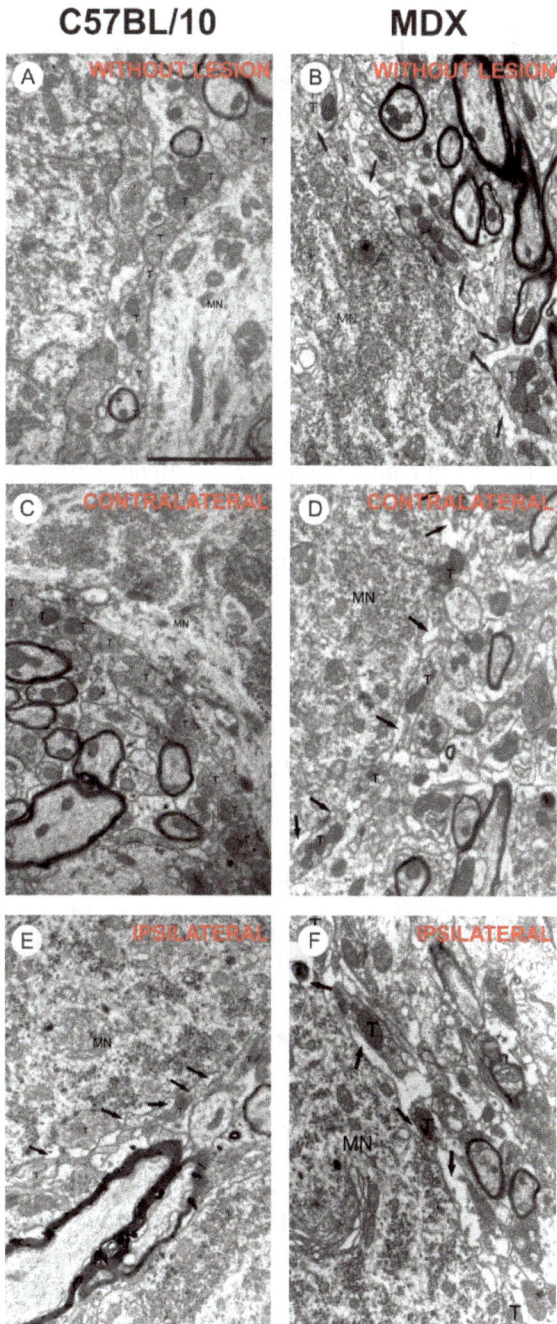

Fig. 6. Ultrastructure of the surface of without lesion spinal cord alpha motoneurons (MN).
A – C57BL/10; B – MDX. Observe the normal C57BL/10 terminal apposition on the

postsynaptic membrane. In contrast, the MDX inputs (presynaptic terminals – T) to the motoneurons are partially detached (arrows), with a reduced area of apposition. C – Synaptic covering in the C57BL/10 contralateral side one week after axotomy. E – Synaptic elimination following axotomy in C57BL/10 mice. The arrows represent astroglial processes and T represents the synaptic boutons. D – Synaptic covering in the MDX contralateral side. F – Synaptic elimination following axotomy in MDX mice. The arrows represent astroglial processes and T represents the synaptic boutons. Observe a more intense synaptic loss in MDX mice, also present on without lesion at the contralateral side of the lesion, indicating that the course of the disease had an impact on the spinal cord circuits. Scale = 2 µm. 2010 Blackwell Publishing Ltd, *Neuropathology and Applied Neurobiology*, **36** , 55–70.

Although there was no statistical difference between the ipsi/contralateral ratios of the two strains, it is evident that the MDX mice present a greater astrocyte response in relation to the C57BL/10 mice, taking into account the difference in astrogliosis between the ipsilateral and contralateral sides of each strain. The fact that the MDX mice showed a superior basal level of GFAP in relation to the C57/BL10 mice, suggests that the effects of Ducehnne Muscular Dystrophy are directly reflected in the spinal cord microenvironment, resulting in significant changes in the spinal circuits. It is suggested that such changes in the MDX mice contribute to the progress of the disease by affecting the functionality of the motoneurons.

An ultrastructural analysis of the alpha-motoneurons plasma membrane showed the presence of synaptic elimination processes in both sides (injured and uninjured) on MDX mice. In the ipsilateral side, the two strains exhibited significant synaptic retraction, and the MDX mice showed less synaptic elimination when evaluating the percentage of synaptic covering before and after axotomy (MDX - 14.61% and C57/BL10 - 23.60 % approximately, Figure 6E and 6F). This fact demonstrates that in addition to the synaptic elimination resulting from the disease, the MDX mice probably have a lower potential for response to peripheral nerve injury. This may be related to the fact that these animals show a lower expression of MHC I (Simões & Oliveira, 2009).

These results show a correlation between glial reactivity, subsequent to the axotomy process, and the synaptic retraction that occurs at the spinal cord (Emirandetti et al., 2006), more evident in the MDX strain.

The communication between neurons and glia through MHC I signaling, probably involves receptors that may be able to translate the signal from MHC I to the neurons, and also from the astrocytes and microglia. In an attempt to understand the functional role of MHC I molecules in the CNS, specifically in synaptic plasticity and the regeneration of neurons in adult animals, Oliveira et al. (2004), performed sciatic nerve transection in knock out mice for the β2 microglobulin protein expression, a subunit of the complex of MHC I. In this study, these authors demonstrated that MHC I plays an important role in maintaining selective inhibitory terminals in apposition to axotomized neurons (Figure 8).

The absence or lower expression of MHC I results in a minor retraction of presynaptic boutons thus reducing the regenerative potential of injured neurons (Oliveira et al., 2004). This fact is consistent with that shown in MDX mice, keeping in view the relative synaptic elimination after axotomy. Similarly, Sabha et al. (2008) showed that the lower expression of

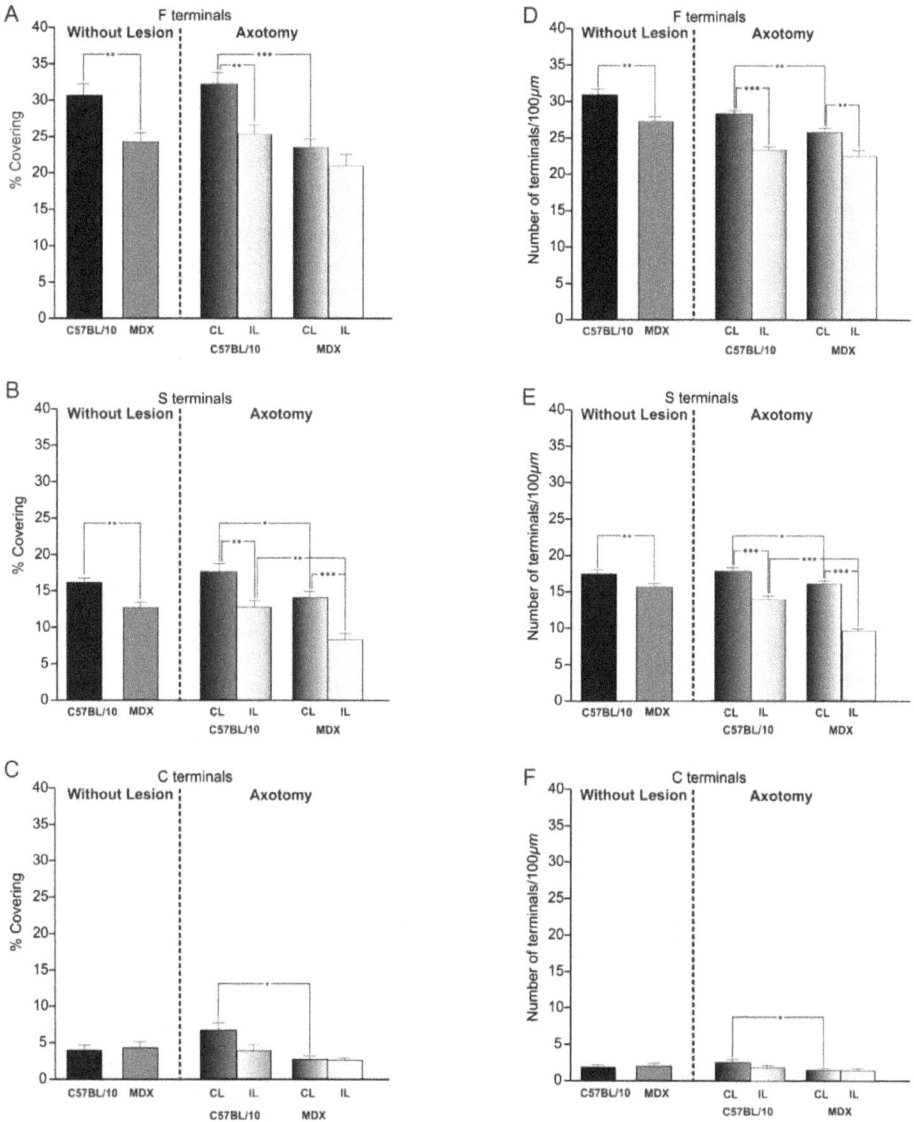

Fig. 7. Representation of the quantitative ultrastructural analysis of the percentage of covering
by F, S and C synaptic terminals, and the quantitative ultrastructural analysis of the number of
terminals (F, S and C) in apposition/100µm. A, B and C - show the covering of the F, S and C
terminals as a percentage, for, respectively, those without injury and the contralateral and
axotomized sides of both strains. D, E and F - show the number of presynaptic F, S and C
terminals, respectively, in apposition to the neuronal membrane/100µm, for those without
injury, and for the control and axotomized groups of both strains. Note that in the MDX mice,
the F and S terminals are reduced before and after axotomy in both groups. 2010 Blackwell
Publishing Ltd, *Neuropathology and Applied Neurobiology, 36 , 55–70.*

MHC I in C57/BL6J mice results in lower regenerative capacity in relation to A/J mice, which showed a higher expression of MHC I. Thus one can suggest that MDX mice show a lower potential axonal regeneration after peripheral nerve injuries, reflecting the evolution of the disease associated with a lower capacity to express MHC I (Figure 9).

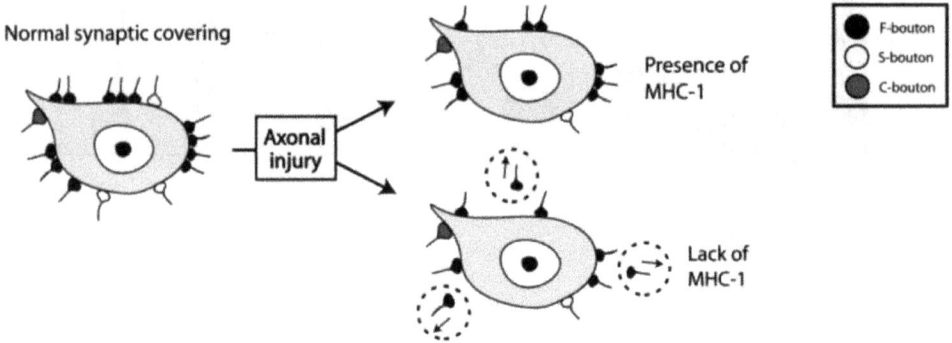

Fig. 8. Scheme showing the synaptic retraction process in motoneurons with the presence and absence of MHC-I. Note the retraction of the boutons in the motoneuron with the absence of MHC-I as compared to the motoneuron with MHC-I. Oliveira et al., *PNAS*, *101(51): 17843-17848, 2004.*

This hypothesis was tested by the sciatic nerve crush, another type of peripheral nerve injury, followed by an analysis of motor recovery using the walking track test (Figure 10). After crushing, the animals were monitored for three weeks, every day up to the tenth day after injury, and then on alternate days from the eleventh to the twenty-first day after injury. The results show that MDX mice have a motor deficit compared with C57BL/10 mice, even before injury (MDX, -35.14 ± 3.82, mean + SD; C57BL/10, -7.63 ± 0.94, p <0.001). The motor recovery curve was similar for the two strains, but the MDX mice showed a significant reduction in motor function after three weeks (MDX, -27.76 ± 5.03; C57BL/10, -7.71 ± 2.99, p <0.01).

With regard to synaptic immunoreactivity, a study of the expression of synaptophysin showed there was reduced immunoreactivity in the MDX strain, both ipsilateral and contralateral to the lesion (Figure 13). A significant decrease in the expression of synaptophysin was observed in the MDX mice contralateral to the lesion, approximately 27% lower as compared to the same side in the C57BL/10 strain.

The immunohistochemical evaluation showed an increase in immunoreactivity for the neurofilaments (Figure 11) and the p75[NTR] – low affinity receptor for neurotrophins – (Figure 12) in both strains after crushing. It can also be seen that the MDX mice showed an increased expression of the neurofilament and p75[NTR] contralateral to the lesion. Similarly, immunostaining showed a better reorganization of regenerated fibers in the C57BL/10 mice. These results suggest that the reduction in motor function in the MDX mice could be related to the cycles of muscle degeneration that directly affect the neuromuscular junctions.

Synaptic Changes at the Spinal Cord Level and Peripheral Nerve Regeneration During the Course of Muscular
Dystrophy in MDX Mice

207

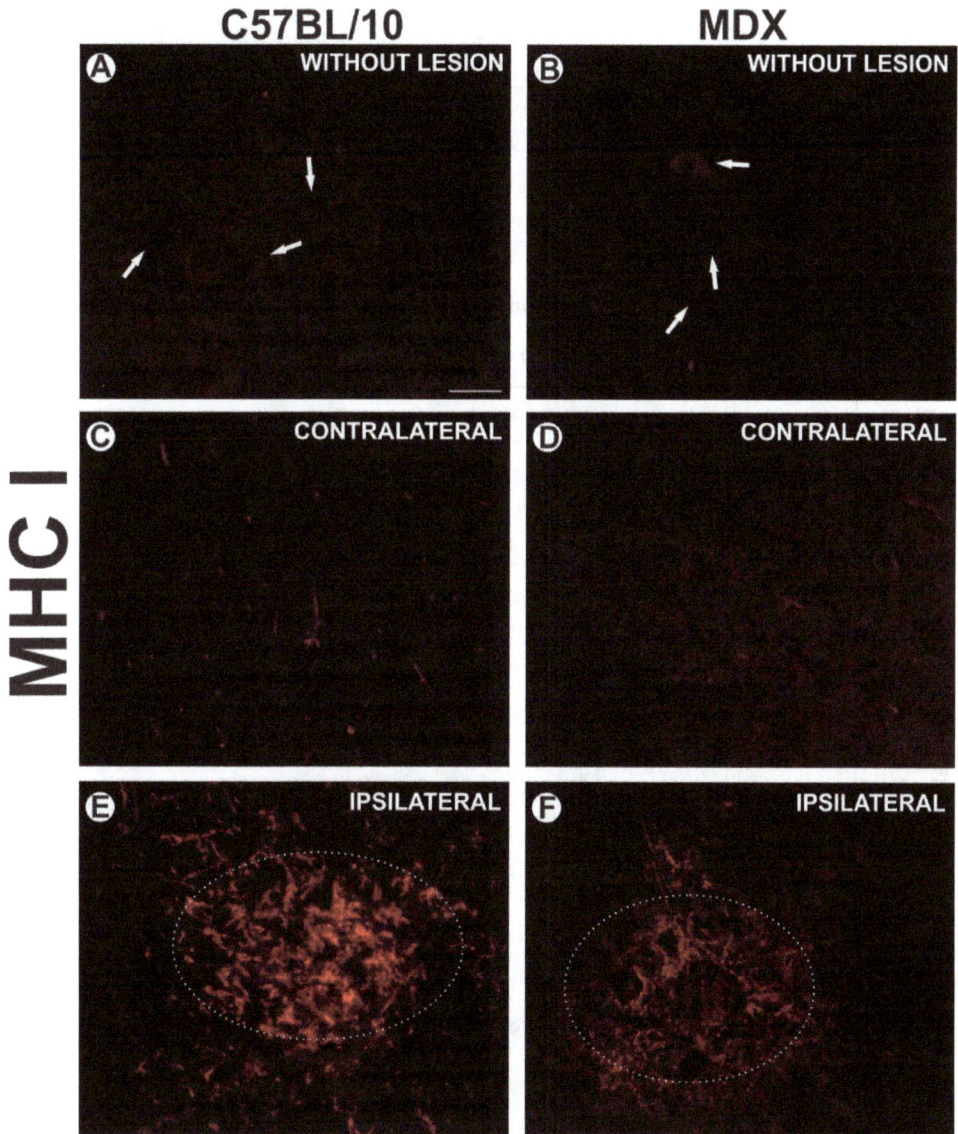

Fig. 9. A and B – Major histocompatibility complex of class I (MHC I) expression in non-injured C57BL/10 and MDX mice, respectively. C and D – Immunolabeling against the MHC I complex on the contralateral (CL) (non-injured) side of the spinal cord. Note the low basal expression of MHC I in both strains. E and F – Immunolabeling against the MHC I protein complex on the ipsilateral (IL) side of the spinal cord 1 week after axotomy, showing an increased expression in both strains, especially in the motoneuron surroundings and adjacent neuropil (dashed areas). The arrows indicate the cell body of the motoneurons. Scale = 50 mm. 2010 Blackwell Publishing Ltd, 9 *Neuropathology and Applied Neurobiology*, 36 , 55–70. 10

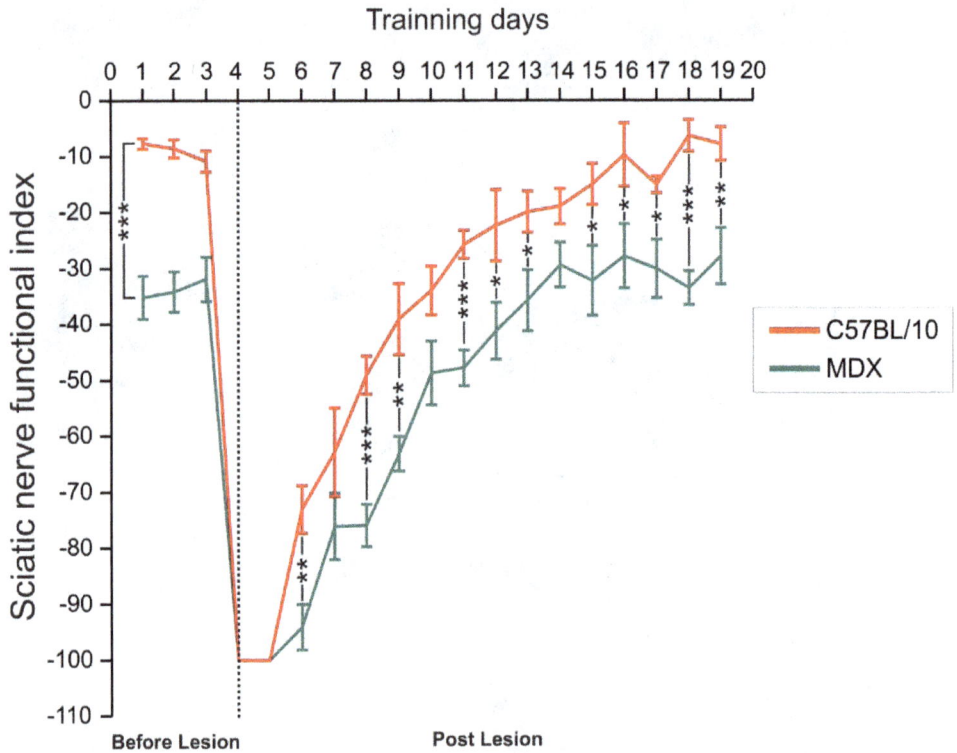

Fig. 10. Graph showing the motor function recovery of the two strains. Note that the MDX mice showed weakened motor function in relation to the C57BL/10 mice, both before and after the sciatic nerve crush.

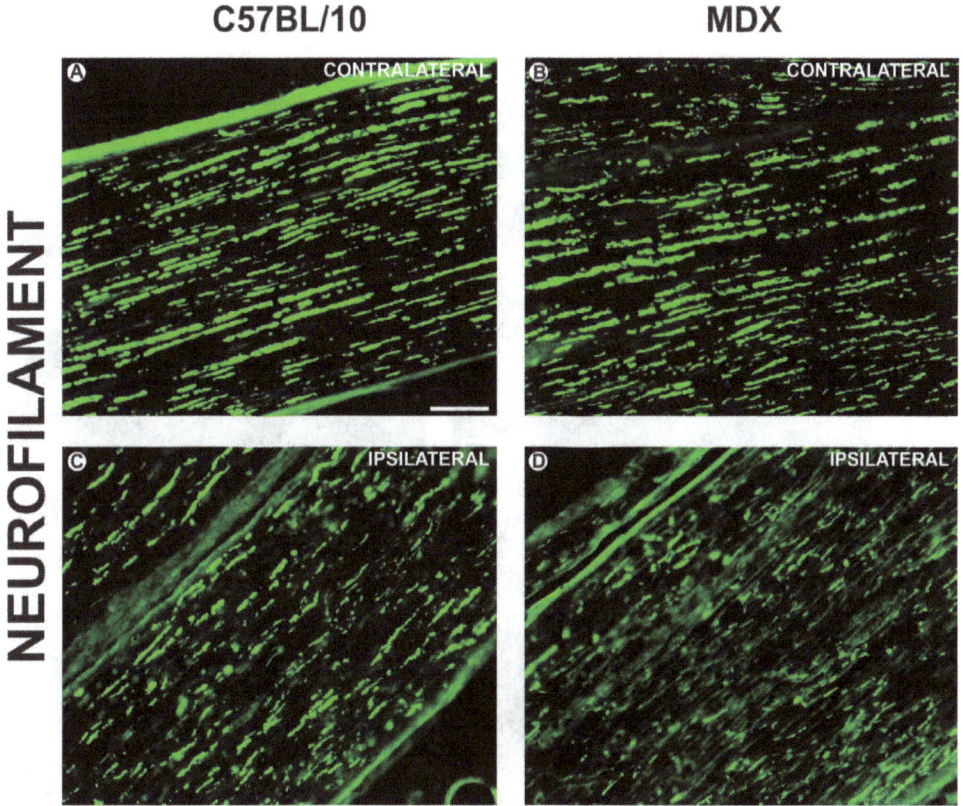

Fig. 11. Anti-neurofilament immunostaining three weeks after the sciatic nerve crush. A and B show the contralateral nerve. C and D show the ipsilateral nerve. Note that there is better organization in the axon fibers after nerve crush in the C57BL/10 mice as compared to the MDX strain.

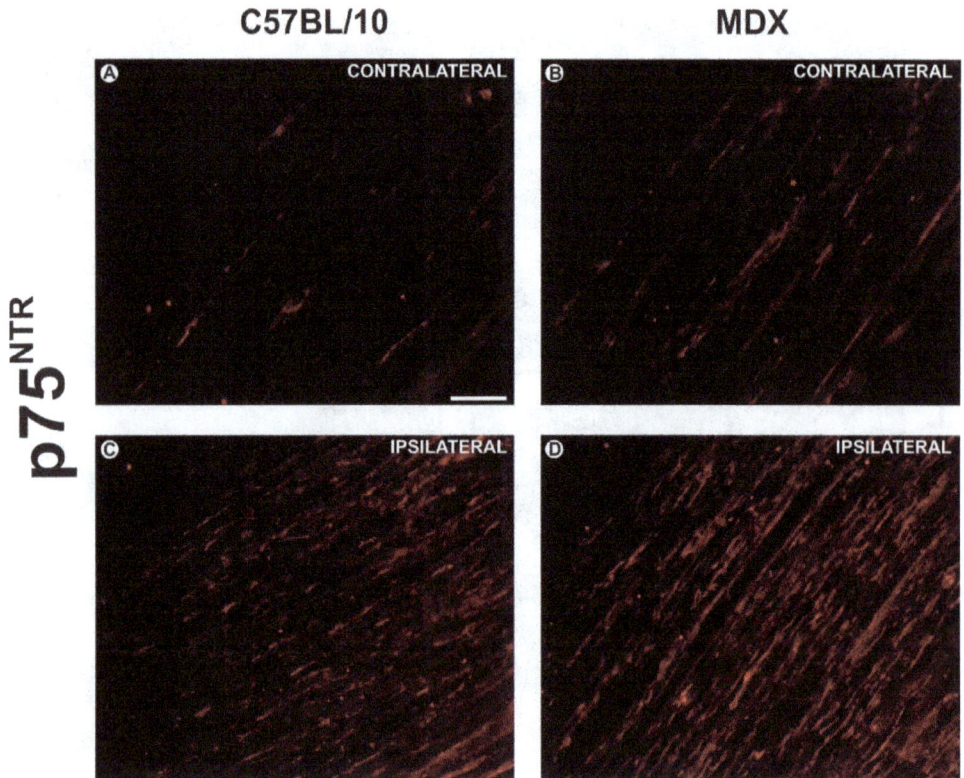

Fig. 12. Immunostaining of the anti- p75NTR (low affinity receptor for neurotrophins) three weeks after sciatic nerve crush. A and B show the contralateral nerves in both strains. C and D show the ipsilateral nerves. Note that there is greater immunoreactivity in the MDX mice as compared to the C57BL/10 mice before and after nerve crushing.

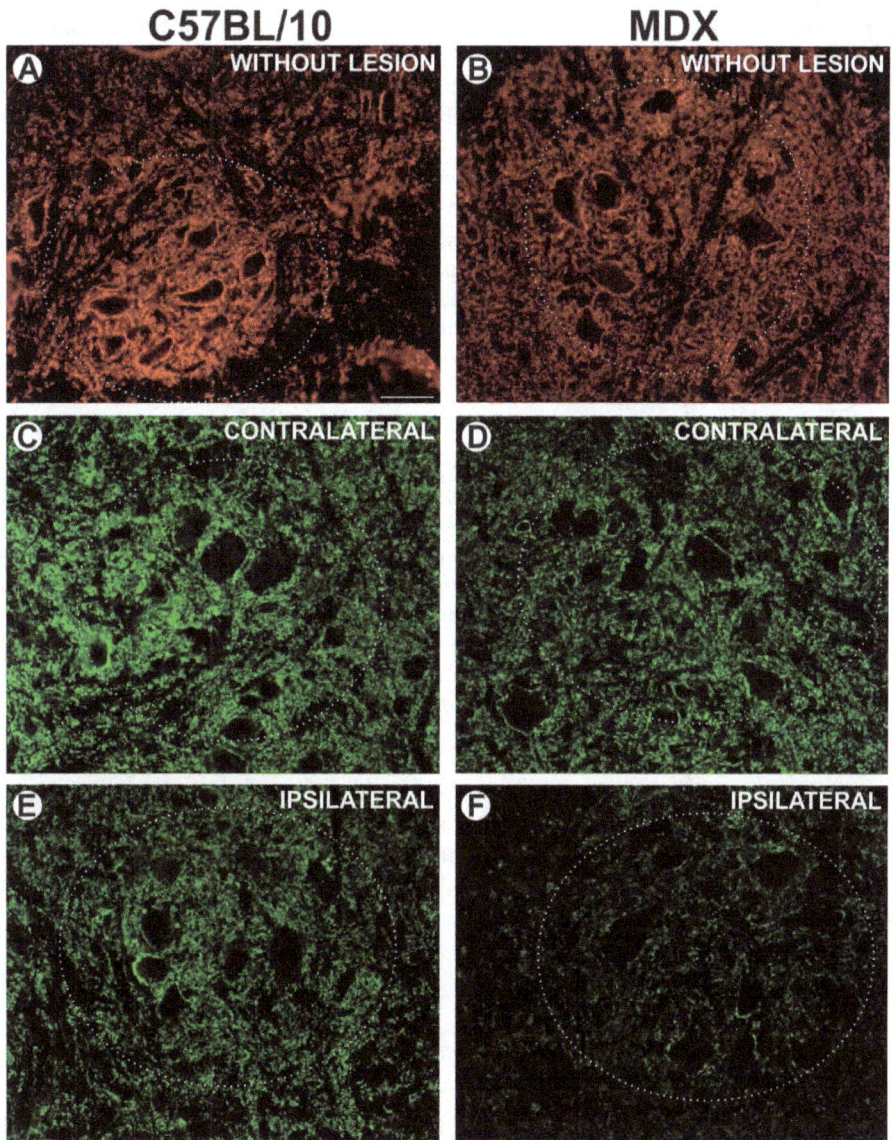

Fig. 13. A and B – Synaptophysin Immunolabeling in non-injured animals. C and D – Synaptophysin immunolabelling of the spinal cord contralateral to the injury 1 week after axotomy. Note the lower synaptic covering in the MDX mice. E and F – the lumbar spinal cord ispsilateral to the injury, 1 week after axotomy, showing an overall decrease in synaptophysin expression around the axotomized motor neuron. The areas containing axotomized motor neurones are highlighted by dashed circles. Scale = 50 mm. 2010 Blackwell Publishing Ltd, *Neuropathology and Applied Neurobiology*, **36** , 55–70.

Altogether, the results described herein indicate that the reduction of inputs in the spinal alpha-motoneurons resulted from a partial disconnection between the motoneuron axon and the muscle targeted during the cycles of muscle degeneration and regeneration that occurred after the second week postnatal. It should be noted that when the animals underwent axotomy at six weeks old, there was a clear central nucleus (indicative of regeneration) in approximately 50% of the muscle fibers (Pastoret & Sebille, 1994). Moreover, in the MDX mice there was a decrease in the number of cells in the cortico-spinal tract (Sbriccoli et al., 1995) and this could also reduce the number of inputs to the spinal alpha-motoneurons and thus cause a decrease in synaptic covering. The present results showing a decrease in protein expression of the synaptophysin and synaptic covering when compared with the findings of Oliveira et al. (2004), are consistent with the idea that the MHC I acts on the stability of the synaptic terminals. Nevertheless, considering its role in signaling between the presynaptic terminals and the motoneurons, as well as taking part in the communication of these with the glia, the greater expression of this protein in the C57BL/10 mice could promote a greater nerve regeneration process as compared to the MDX mice.

As demonstrated by Oliveira et al. (2004), after a nerve injury, MHC I plays a key role in stabilizing the selective inhibitory synapses, which contributes to the presynaptic terminal retraction process occurring in a specific way. Sabha et al. (2008) correlated an increased expression of MHC I with an intensification of the synaptic elimination process seven days after peripheral axotomy in the spinal cord microenvironment. This was evident in both C57BL/10 and MDX strains, but with a lower expression of MHC I in the MDX mice. One hypothesis for this occurrence is that the muscle degeneration and regeneration process already proceeding in these mice at a young age (Pastoret & Sebille, 1994), promotes a "partial disconnection" of the sciatic nerve with its target muscle, possibly stimulating an increased expression of MHC I molecules in these animals. This fact may contribute to the differentiated response of the MDX mice in comparison with that normally seen in the C57BL/10mice, similarly to what was shown in the work of Sabha et al. (2008), where the MHC I expression remained high over a period of up to 3 weeks after axotomy. Thus it is suggested that the lower expression of MHC I in MDX mice may indicate a reduced capacity for adjustment of the inputs by the motoneurons, indicating a lower regenerative potential after nerve injury.

3. References

Aldskogius, H. & Svensson, M. 1993. Neuronal and glial responses to axon injury. In S.K. Malhotra (eds): Advances in structural biology. Greenwich, Connecticut: JAI Press.
Aldskogius, H.; Liu, L.; Svensson, M, 1999. *Glial responses to synaptic damage and plasticity.* Journal Neuroscience Research, 58:33-41.
Arahata, K.: Ishihara, T.; Nonaka, I.; Ozawa, E.; Sugita, H. 1988. *Imunnostaining of skeletal and cardiac muscle surface membrane with antibody against Duchenne muscular dystrophy peptide.* Nature, 333:861-868.
Araque, A. & Perea, G. 2004. *Glial modulation of synaptic transmission in culture.* Glia. 47:241-248.
Baba, A. 1998. *Role of endothelin B receptor signals in reactive astrocytes.* Life Sci., 62 (17/18):1711-1715.

Balaban, B.; Matthews DJ.; Clayton, GH.; Carry T. 2005. *Corticosteroid treatment an functional improvement in Duchenne Muscular Dystrophy: long-term effect*. Am J Phys Med Rehabil., 84:843-850.

Brännström, T. & Kellerth, J.O. 1998. *Changes in synaptology of adult cat spinal alpha-motoneurons after axotomy*. Experimental Brain Research, 118:1-13.

Carreta, D.; Santarelli, M.; Vanni, D.; Carrai, R.; Sbriccoli, A.; Pinto, F.; Minciacchi, D. 2001 *The organization of spinal projecting brainstem neurons in an animal modelo f muscular dystrophy: A retrograde tracinig study on mdx mutante mice*. Brain Research, 895:213-222.

Chelly, J.; Kaplan, J.C.; Maire, P.; Gautron, S.; Kahn, A. 1988. *Transcription of the dystrophy (mdx) in the mouse*. Proc. Natl. Acad. Sci. USA, 81:1189-1192.

Emirandetti, A.; Zanon, R.G.; Sabha, M.J.; Oliveira, A.L.R. 2006. *Astrocyte reactivity influences the number of presynaptic terminals apposed to spinal motoneurons after axotomy*. Brain Research, 1095:35-42.

Haenggi T. & Fritschy J.M. 2006. *Role of dystrophin and utrophin for assembly and function of the dystrophin glycoprotein complex in non-muscle tissue*. Cell Mol Life Sci. 2006 Jul;63(14):1614-31.

Huard, J.; Coté, P.Y.; Parent, A.; Bouchard, J.P.; Tremblay, J.P. 1992. *Dystrophin-like immunoreactivity in monkey and human brain areas involved in learning and motor functions*. Neuroscience Lett., 141:181-186.

Judge, L.M.; Haraguchi, M.; Chamberlain, J.S. 2005. *Dissecting the signaling and mechanical functions of the dystrophin-glycoprotein complex*. Journal of Cell Science., 119:1537-1546.

Lagrota-Candido, J.; Vasconcellos, R.; Cavalcanti, M.; Bozza, M.; Savino, W.; Quirico-Santos, T. 2002. *Resolution of skeletal muscle inflammation in mdx dystrophic mouse is accompanied by increased immunoglobulin and interferon-gama production*. Int. J. Exp. Path., 83:121-132.

Lidov, H.G.; Byers, T.J.; Kunkel, L.M. 1993. *The distribuition of dystrphin in the murine central nervous system: an immunocytochemical study*. Neuroscience, 54:167-187.

Lieberman, A. R. 1971. *The axon reaction: a review of the principal features of perikaryal responses to axon injury*. Int. Rev. Neurobiol., 14:49-124.

Lindå, H.; Piehl, F.; Dagerlind, A.; Verge, V. M.; Arvidsson, U.; Cullheim, S.; Risling, M.; Ulfhake, B.; Hokfelt, T. 1992. *Expression of GAP-43 mRNA in the adult mammalian spinal cord under normal conditions and after different types of lesions, with special reference to motoneurons*. Exp. Brain Res. 91, 284-295.

Lindå, H.; Hammarberg, H.; Cullheim, S.; Levinovitz, A.; Khademi, M.; Olsson, T. 1998. *Expression of MHC class I and β2 – Microglobulin in rat spinal motoneurons: regulatory influences by IFN – gamma and axotomy*. Exp. Neurol., 150, 282-295.

Lowe, Dawn A.; Willians, Brian O.; Thomas, David D. and Grange, Robert. 2006. *Molecular and cellular contractile dysfunction of dystrophic muscle from young mice*. Muscle & Nerve., 34:92-100.

Lundberg, C.; Lidman, O.; Holmdahl, R; Olsson, T; Piehl, F.2001. *Neurodegeneration and glial activation patterns after mechanical nerve injury are differentially regulated by non-MHC genes in congenic inbred rat strains*. J Comp Neurol., 26;431(1):75-87.

Mcdowall, R.M.; Dunn, M.J.; Billiau, A. 1990. *Nature of the mononuclear infiltrate and the mechanism of muscle damage in juvenile dermatomyositis and Duchenne muscular dystrophy*. J. Neurol. Science, 99:199-217.

Nonaka, I. 1998. Animals models of muscular dystrophies. Loboratory Anim. Sci. 48:8-16.

Oliveira, A.L.; Thams, S.; Ldman, O.; Piehl, F.; Hökfelt, T.; Kärre, Lindå, H.; Cullhem, 2004. *A role for MHC class I molecules in synaptic plasticity and regeneration of neurons after axotomy.* PNAS. 101(51):17843-17848.

Pastoret, C. & Sebille, A. 1994. *MDX mice show progressive weakness and muscle deterioration whith age.* Journal of Neurological Sciences, 129:97-105.

Pearce, J.M.S. 2005. *Early Observations on Duchenne-Meryon muscular dystrophy.* Eur Neurol., 54: 46-48.

Piehl, F.; Hammarberg, H.; Hokfelt, T.; Cullheim, S. 1998. *Regulatory effects of trophic factors on expression and distribuition of CGRP and GAP-43 in rat motoneurons.* J. Neurosci., 5:1321-1333.

Radley, H.G.; Davies, M.J.; Grounds, M.D. 2007. *Reduced muscles necrosis and long-term benefits in dystrophic mdx mice after cV1q (blockade of TNF) treatment.* Neuromuscular Disorders, 18:227-238

Reier, P.J.; Eng, L.F.; Jakeman, L. 1989. *Reactive astrocyte and axonal outgrowth in the injured CNS: is gliosis really an impediment to regeneration?* Neur. Reg. Transpl. Front. Clinical Neuroscience, 6;193-209.

Romanes, G. 1946. *Motor localization and the effects of nerve injury on the ventral horn cells of the spinal cord.* J Anat., 80:117-131.

Sabha, M.JR.; Emirandetti, A.; Cullheim, S.; Oliveira, A.L.R. 2008. *MHC I expression and synaptic plasticity ind different mice strains after axotomy.* Synapse, 62:137-148.

Sbriccoli, A.; Santarelli, M.; Carreta, D.; Pinto, F.; Granato, A.; Minciacchi, D. 1995. Architectural changes of the cortiço-spinal system in the dystrophin defective mdx mice. Neuroscience Letters, 200:53-56.

Simões G.F. & Oliveira, A.L. 2010. *Alpha motoneurone input changes in dystrophic MDX mice after sciatic nerve transection.* Neuropathol Appl Neurobiol., 36(1):55-70.

Spencer, M.J.; Montecino-Rodrigues, E.; Dorshkind, K.; Tidball, J.G. 2001. *Helper (CD4+) and cytotoxic (CD8+) T cells promote the pathology of dystrophin-deficient muscle.* Clin. Immunol., 989:235-243.

Wals, W. 1989 Role of glial cells in the regulation of the brain ion microenvironment. Prog. Neurobiol., 33(4):309-333.

Whitehead, N.P.; Yeung, E.W. and Allen, D. 2006. *Muscle damage in MDX (dystrophic) mice: role of calcium and reactive oxygen species.* Clinical and Experimental Pharmacology and Physiology. 33:657-662.

Zanon, R.G.; Emirandetti, A.; Simões, G.F.; Freria, C.M.; Victório, S.C.; Cartarozzi, L.P.; Barbizan, R.; Oliveira, A.L.R. 2010. *Expressão do complexo de histocompatilidade principal de classe I (MHC I) no sistema nervoso central: plasticidade sináptica e regeneração.* COLUNA/COLUMNA.; 9(2):193-198

Section 3

Disease Diagnosis and Management

11

Rehabilitation in Muscular Dystrophies: Changing Approach

Imelda J.M. de Groot, Nicoline B.M. Voet,
Merel Jansen and Lenie van den Engel-Hoek
Radboud University Nijmegen Medical Centre
The Netherlands

1. Introduction

Life expectancy is increasing in muscular dystrophies: as an example due to technical medical interventions like spine surgery and home ventilation, boys with Duchenne muscular dystrophy become men. Increasing evidence concerning retarding drugs becomes available for muscular dystrophies. Cardiac symptoms can effectively be treated with drugs and also cardioprotective drugs are tested. New retarding treatments, like exon skipping, stem cell treatment or vector-gene transfer, are in the phase of animal studies or already in randomized clinical trials. Together these treatments are changing the course of the muscular dystrophies.

In line with these developments rehabilitation management is also changing. In the past the treatment was focused on maintaining walking abilities as long as possible with physiotherapy, stretching, and with or without braces. However, due to the slower progression of the disorder and the technical possibilities of home ventilation the focus is changing to arm- and hand-function. There are good technical solutions for the loss of ambulation as there are many type of electrical wheelchairs. All kind of technical and electronic supports are available to operate telephone, television, radio etc. However, in all kind of daily activities a certain ability of the arm and hand is necessary. Training and support of these functions in muscular dystrophies come into prominence.

New symptoms or symptoms not noticed in the past are becoming more apparent. This can be due to the increasing age that they are now identified or augment during the longer course of the disease, such as feeding and swallowing problems, gastrointestinal and urogenital problems.

Already known symptoms like osteoporosis in muscular dystrophies also increase if corticosteroids are used. For example vertebral fractures are more seen in boys with Duchenne muscular dystrophy. The question is whether we can retard osteoporosis by means of supported physical activities with weight load on the bones. In the light of increasing life expectancy and the possibilities to use sophisticated orthoses or exoskeletons, it is important to maintain the physical capacities with balanced training.

Also due to increasing life expectancy an unforeseen population emerges who want to participate in social life in broad sense: education, jobs, friends, relationships, marriage, children. This desire is in slight contrast to adults who received the diagnosis muscular dystrophy in adulthood, they are attempting to maintain their participation in social life. Possibilities to live independent with supportive devices need to be established, robotics as support in daily activities will develop, and with the possibilities of the world wide web and computer technology education and jobs become available.

In this chapter we will not describe the established rehabilitation managements, but will describe the new focuses on training, the new or less noticed symptoms, and the development of new devices.

2. Training

2.1 Physical training for children with a muscular dystrophy

2.1.1 Disuse

Muscular dystrophies in children comprise a heterogeneous group of myopathies that appear during childhood. The most common muscular dystrophy in children is Duchenne Muscular Dystrophy (DMD) affecting 1/4200 life-born boys. Other muscular dsytrophies are Myotonic Dystrophy (MD), Becker Muscular Dystrophy (BMD), Limb Girdle Muscular Dystrophy (LGMD) and FacioScapuloHumeral muscular Dystrophy (FSHD). All muscular dystrophies are characterized by progressive loss of muscle function and only symptomatic treatments (such as corticosteroids and assisted mechanical ventilation) are currently available. An important aim in the management of muscular dystrophies is to delay the loss of functional abilities and to maintain independency. Physical training could retard the loss of physical abilities as a result of disuse.

Children with a muscular dystrophy are less physically active compared to age-matched healthy controls in their daily life (McDonald et al 2005). The more sedentary lifestyle can be explained primarily by the disease, but also by disuse(McDonald 2002, Bar-or and Rowland 2004). Disuse can be defined a discrepancy between children's capacity and performance, and gradually causes a secondary reduction of physical activity. Indeed, the increasing amount of energy a certain activity costs, and the fear of falls with the need for help to stand up, make children move less. An early decline of the physical activity level enhances the loss of functional abilities. This appears from the loss of arm functions that occurs fast after the onset of wheelchair-dependency(McDonald et al. 1995). An electric wheelchair limits arm functions (like lifting and reaching), since a top blade and a central operating joystick force children to function within the outlines of the wheelchair. Another example is the high number of children with DMD (20-40%) that loses the ability to walk as a result of a fracture of the lower extremity(Vestergaard et al , 2001). From this perspective, the saying "use it or lose it" is certainly applicable to children with a muscular dystrophy and encourages physical training.

2.1.2 Evidence for training

The number of studies that investigated the effects of physical training in children with a muscular dystrophy is limited (Voet et al. 2010). None of them were performed in a randomized controlled setting and most studies focused on DMD. Furthermore, clinical trials in children only investigated the effect of resistance exercises. This is remarkable, as recent studies in adults with BMD and the mdx mice (a mouse model for DMD) encourage aerobic exercises.

Previous clinical trials among boys with DMD showed that (sub)maximal resistance exercises have limited positive effects on muscle strength and time functional tests (such as the time it takes to walk 10m) but, importantly, are not harmful. In a study by Vignos et al. (1966), the effects of a one-year maximum resistance exercise program (i.e. the maximum load that could be lifted through ten repetitions) were examined(Vignos, Jr. and Watkins, 1966). Fourteen ambulatory children with DMD exercised their legs, arms and abdominal muscles and were compared with a control group of children with DMD who did not exercise. Results from this study showed that muscle strength decreased in control group, while strength was maintained during the training period in the exercise group. However, children were not randomly allocated to the exercise or non-exercise (natural cohort) group. Another study by De Lateur et al. (1979) showed that a six-month submaximal isokinetic exercise program could be of limited value in increasing strength in DMD (de Lateur and Giaconi, 1979). In this study, four ambulatory children with DMD performed quadriceps exercises with one leg (4 to 5 days per week), while the other leg was not trained at all. Finally, Scott et al. (1981) investigated the effects of six months manually applied resistance exercises and "free exercises" in eighteen boys with DMD(Scott et al., 1981). At six months, no statistically differences were found between the two groups at the level of muscle strength, locomotor abilities and functional abilities. No evidence for training-induced physical deterioration was found.

With respect to aerobic exercises, recent studies in mdx mice (an animal model for DMD) showed that voluntary wheel running had positive effects on muscle strength and fatigue resistance and non-weight bearing exercises (such as swimming) had no detrimental effects 1998; Hayes and Williams 1996). Dynamic exercises (bicycle training) improved endurance and muscles strength in adult BMD patients as well(Sveen et al. 2008) . In this study of Sveen et al. (2008), eleven ambulatory BMD patients, and seven healthy age-matched controls, participated in a 12-weeks cycling training. Participants cycled thirty minutes at 65% of their maximal oxygen uptake (VO_{2max}). At 12 weeks, workload and VO_{2max} were improved without an increase in CK level. Although this study was conducted among adults, the results of this study might be applicable for children with a muscular dystrophy as well.

Results of recently published clinical trial protocols, such as the protocol of the randomized controlled trials No Use is Disuse (NUD)(Jansen et al. 2010), will increase insight into what type of physical training (type, intensity, frequency, duration) should be recommended to children with a muscular dystrophy. The NUD study investigates whether an assisted bicycle training is beneficial and does not cause any harm for boys with DMD. Motor-assistance allowed cycling with the legs and arms (arm cranking) even when muscle strength was insufficient to achieve fully active movements. In another part of the study, the effect of an arm training with arm support is investigated. Both ambulatory and wheelchair-dependent children participate in this study. Preliminary data show that assisted training is effective in boys with DMD in maintaining functional capacities.

2.1.3 Training mechanisms

The mechanism by which training could oppose the physical deterioration in children with a muscular dystrophy is still unclear. Muscle fibers in muscular dystrophy patients are abnormally vulnerable to contraction-induced injury due to the absence, or lack, of mechanical reinforcement of the sarcolemmal membrane(Petrof 1998). Eccentric exercises should therefore be avoided(Lim et al 2004). Conversely, a recently published review by Markert et al. (2011) described that enhancing myofiber repair, decreasing muscle fibrosis and the production of antioxidants against oxidative damage are potential explainable factors for exercise-induced improvements(Markert et al. 2011). Work-induced damage could enhance muscle regeneration and repair(Okano et al. 2005), and low-stress exercise may produce beneficial effects on myofiber contractility and energetic efficiency(Petrof 1998).

2.1.4 International training guidelines

International training guidelines for children with a muscular dystrophy are preferably disease-specific and should be adapted to the individual child(Edouard et al. 2007). Based on the currently available evidence, guidelines for ambulatory boys with DMD recommend voluntary active exercises (such as swimming) and to avoid eccentric exercises(Eagle 2002). For wheelchair-dependent children, passive or actively-assisted mobilizing exercises to maintain comfort and symmetry are advised(Eagle 2002). A cardiomyopathy could be a contraindication to participate in any physical training programs(Edouard et al. 2007). It is suggested that the training intensity could be based on children's perceived exertion instead of maximum heart rate when performance is predominantly limited by the peripheral capacity instead of the oxygen transport(Jansen et al. 2010).

To conclude, physical training could delay the physical deterioration as a result of disuse in children with a muscular dystrophy. Disuse enhances the loss of functional abilities, whereas physical training could be beneficial. Currently available evidence is limited to uncontrolled clinical trials and further research is required to develop specific training prescriptions. At this moment, international guidelines recommend voluntary (dynamic) exercises to maintain comfort and symmetry, and to avoid eccentric exercises.

2.2 Training and fatigue in adult muscular dystrophies

2.2.1 Physical exercise

In a study by McDonald the three problems most frequently cited as "very significant" by patients with slowly progressive neuromuscular disease were muscle weakness (57%), difficulty exercising (43%) and fatigue (40%) {McDonald 2002}. Two main types of fatigue can be distinguished. Physiological fatigue, or muscle fatigue, has been defined as a reduction in maximal voluntary muscle force (MVC) during exercise. Experienced fatigue, on the other hand, is the subjective feeling of fatigue. Muscle fatigue is not necessarily accompanied by experienced fatigue, or vice versa. Distinguishing experienced fatigue from muscle weakness, the key feature in muscular dystrophy, may be difficult. In a study by Kalkman 61% of patients with facioscapulohumeral dystrophy (FSHD) (n = 139) and 74% of patients with myotonic dystrophy (MD) (n = 322) were "severely fatigued" {Kalkman et al, 2005 }. Patients with MD had higher scores for experienced fatigue, reported greater problems with concentration and had more difficulties with initiative and planning than patients with FSHD. In FSHD patients and MD patients, social functioning was related to fatigue severity. Apparently, fatigue is not only a frequent, but also a relevant problem in muscular dystrophy. In a subsequent longitudinal study Kalkman built a model of perpetuating factors, which contribute to the continuation of experienced fatigue {Kalkman et al, 2007 }. In FSHD, the level of physical (in)activity has a central place in the model. Due to fatigue, patients often alter their lifestyles and reduce their activities. Low physical activity levels may lead to even greater weakness and atrophy of skeletal muscles, which causes a vicious circle of disuse and weakness. Physical inactivity in turn can lead to chronic cardiovascular and muscle deconditioning and increased cardiovascular health risks {McDonald, 2002 }. In addition, pain complaints influence levels of experienced fatigue both directly and indirectly by decreasing physical activity (see figure below). In MD, physical activity and pain did not significantly contribute to experienced fatigue. Yet, sleep disturbances lead to higher levels of experienced fatigue in both FSHD and MD patients. The observed patterns of perpetuating factors can be used as a basis to develop evidence-based interventions to reduce fatigue. Specific attention should be paid to sleep disturbances in both patient groups. Specifically in FSHD, treatment of fatigue should also be directed at increasing physical activity and reducing pain complaints. Irrespective of its cause, physical inactivity should be discouraged in muscular dystrophy patients because of an increasing risk of cardiovascular disease and muscle deconditioning.

In the past, many patients with muscular dystrophy were advised not to exercise because of the belief that too much exercise might lead to overuse weakness {Johnson, 1971;Johnson, 1971;Carter, 1995;Fowler, 1984;Petrof, 1998}. Yet, in their Cochrane review on muscle strength training and aerobic exercise training for patients with muscle diseases, Voet concluded that moderate-intensity strength training in MD and FSHD appeared not to be harmful, although there was insufficient evidence to establish its benefit {Voet et al , 2010}. This conclusion was based on merely two randomised clinical trials {Lindeman et al , 1995;van der Kooi et al, 2004}. For this reason, Cup reviewed not only randomised clinical trials, but also controlled clinical trials and other designs of sufficient quality {Cup et al, 2007}. All types of exercise therapy and other physical therapy modalities were included for patients with muscular dystrophy, among which were patients with FSHD, LGMD, MD and DMD. Cup *et al.* also concluded that exercise training is not harmful in muscular dystrophies. However, based on the reviewed studies, there was insufficient evidence for the effectiveness of muscle strengthening exercises, although there were some indications that aerobic exercises may have a positive effect on body functions, as well as on activities and participation. Because of the weakness of the muscle membrane there is concern about the potentially damaging effects of eccentric and high-intensity muscle contractions during strength training. In animal models of muscular dystrophy, there is evidence that eccentric contractions, known to stress muscle fibers, cause greater cell injury to these dystrophic muscle fibers. Although transferring results from animal studies to humans must be done with caution, eccentric training studies in muscular dystrophy patients are so far being avoided.

To conclude, although the current scientific evidence is scarce, aerobic exercise training appears not to be harmful in muscular dystrophies and could have a positive effect on functioning, activities and participation, but the number of high-quality studies is low. When prescribing exercise training, the recommendations from the ACSM Position Stand can be used as requirements to achieve an effective, safe and individualised exercise prescription {1998}.

2.2.2 Alternative training

Muscular dystrophies have a large impact on psychosocial functioning as patients must continuously adapt to their progressive illness. Illness cognitions and coping styles influence the level of physical activity and, consequently, experienced fatigue and health status. Hence, changing illness cognitions and coping style may lead to a better quality of life. A cognitive behaviour approach has been proven successful in the chronic fatigue syndrome {Prins et al, 2001;Chambers et al, 2006} and for post-cancer fatigue {Gielissen et al, 2007;Gielissen et al, 2006} and may be effective in patients with muscular dystrophy as well.

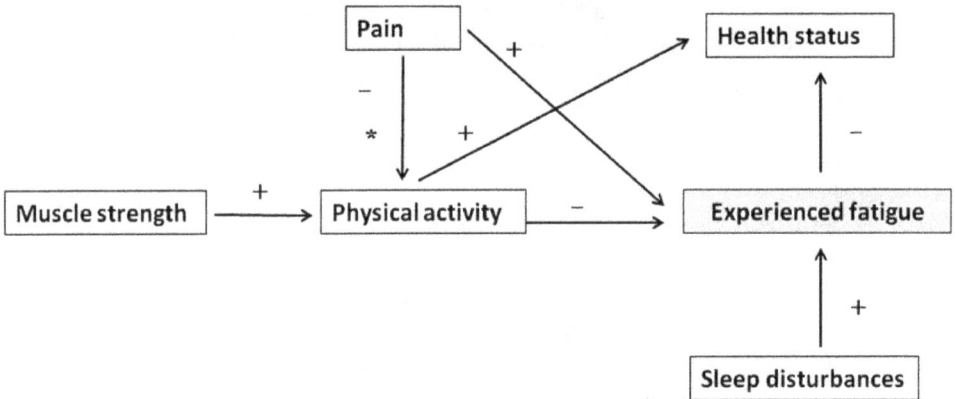

Pain   +   Health status

−   *   +   −

Muscle strength   +   Physical activity   −   Experienced fatigue

+

Sleep disturbances

Fig. 1. Cognitive behaviour therapy in FSHD should, for instance, be focused on the known perpetuating factors of experienced fatigue as described by Kalkman i.e. sleep disturbances, pain complaints and physical inactivity (Della et al. 49-53;Kalkman et al. 571-79). Therapy should be adapted to the life of each individual, resulting in an individualised treatment approach. Altogether, cognitive behaviour therapy seems a rational, promising treatment for fatigue in muscular dystrophies.

3. Feeding problems and dysphagia

3.1 Swallowing

Swallowing is a complex sensorimotor process that depends on information from multiple levels of the central and peripheral nervous system. Descending excitatory and inhibitory signals from the cortex and subcortex and ascending signals from the oropharyngeal area trigger the central pattern generator (CPG) in the bulbar reticular formation (Jean 2001, Leopold 2010). This network of premotor neurons and interneurons drives the motor neurons of swallowing in cranial nerves (CN) V, VII, IX, X and XII. Muscles of lips, submental muscle group, tongue, palate, larynx, pharynx and esophagus, innervated by these CNs, are excited and inhibited sequentially, when a person forms a bolus and swallows (Ertekin 2003). The oral phase and the initiation of the pharyngeal phase are under voluntary neural control, whereas the completion of the pharyngeal phase and the esophageal phase are under involuntary neural control (Miller 2008). In dysphagia, problems may occur in the oral, pharyngeal, esophageal phase, or in more than one phase (Arvedson 2008). In children with neurologic etiologies from different origins, dysphagia is often reported with variable signs and symptoms. The dysphagia of children with CP is characterized by oral motor problems and frequent aspiration of thin liquid with no observable response (silent aspiration) (Rogers 1994). In neuromuscular disorders (NMD), weakness of the muscles is due to damage along the course of the peripheral nerve (lower motor neuron) or the muscle itself (Dubowitz 2000). Feeding and swallowing problems are not uncommon in muscular dystrophies, which can lead to dehydration, malnutrition or aspiration pneumonia.In patients with chronic muscle disease a prevalence of 35% of feeding problems and dysphagia was reported (Kumin 1994).

3.2 Problems in the oral phase

In NMD chewing problems and the need to multiple swallows to clear the oral cavity (piecemeal deglutition) are the main problems in the oral phase of swallowing. Reduced bite force and weakness of the masticatory muscles (Morel-Verdebout 2007) causes chewing problems and the inability to eat solid or firm food. The reduced range of mandibular motion, reported in SMA type II (Van Bruggen 2011) and DMD (Botteron 2009) may reduce the quality of chewing and results in a hampered food comminution, inadequate food bolus formation, and oral transport. Moreover, the limited mandibular range of motion has an impact on oral hygiene and dental care. Facial muscle weakness can lead to craniofacial and dental malocclusion (Kumin 1994; Pane 2006) which aggravates the chewing problems.

Reduced strength of the tongue muscles causes piecemeal deglutition, especially with thick liquid and solid food (van den Engel-Hoek 2009). This results in prolonged oral transit time and oral residue after swallowing.

3.3 Problems in the pharyngeal phase

The initiation of the pharyngeal phase is typically normal in patients with NMD, but problems with solid food and residue after swallow are reported in patients with SMA type II (van den Engel-Hoek 2009), DMD (Aloysius 2008;Shinonaga 2008), in MD (Leonard 2001) and congenital myopathies (Mehta 2006;de Swart 2002). In all patient groups the problems occurred more in advanced stages. Dysphagia and feeding problems were also reported in nemaline myopathy, but more in the neonatal period and infancy than in adults (Bagnall 2006). Residue after swallow is caused a combination of reduced strength of the tongue and submental muscle group, and reduced opening of the upper esophageal sphincter. In patients with oculopharyngeal muscular dystrophy (OPMD) the dysphagia was aggravated by the retroflexion of the head, caused by ptosis (de Swart 2002). In patients with SMA II a retracted position of the head, due to a lumbar lordosis and a diminished head balance, caused reduced movement of the submental muscle group resulting in more post swallow residue with thick liquid and solid food than with thin liquid. The post swallow residue places patients at risk for aspiration the airway reopens (Arvedson 1998)

3.4 Swallowing assessments

A videofluroscopic swallow study (VFSS) is generally considered as the gold standard method for diagnosing dysphagia in adults (Logemann 2000) and children (Hiorns 2006), especially to detect aspiration. However, a VFSS was not considered as additional benefit to a careful feeding history in patients with DMD (Aloysius 2008). Other assessments are available to describe oral structures and biomechanical oral functions needed for feeding and swallowing to better understand the nature and clinical course of dysphagia in NMD. Surface EMG (sEMG) of the submental muscle group, tongue pressure, ultrasonographic and manometric assessments during swallowing can be used to understand the nature and clinical course of dysphagia in NMD.

Patients are not always mentioning swallowing difficulties (Leonard 2001;Stubgen 2008). They should also always be carefully interviewed for symptoms of swallowing difficulties that may require a swallowing assessment and a careful observation of oral motor abilities during mealtime (Messina 2008; Manzur 2008).

3.5 Recommendations

To improve their quality of life and nutritional state, NMD patients with swallowing difficulties benefit from dietetic and swallowing recommendations. This can be nutritional, related to consistencies, safe swallowing techniques or advices about postural management and feeding aids . The dysphagia in NMD show different patterns in flaccid bulbar paresis like NMD than in neuromuscular disorders. In contrast to the usual advice for thickening the food, in NMD more liquid food is advised or alternating thick with thin consistencies. Strategies are recommended to reduce problems in chewing and oral and pharyngeal post swallow residue. Careful chewing and bolus preparation to a liquid consistency, effortful swallowing and double swallows can reduce problems of reduced pharyngeal clearing. In case of post swallow residue it is also advised to clear the oral and pharyngeal cavity with water after mealtime. Positioning of the head in sitting position can also be important to prevent residue. In case of a retracted head position, like in SMA II (van den Engel 2009) a more flexed head position prevented laryngeal post swallow residue. Also in patients with OPMD a slightly flexed head improved swallowing (de Swart 2002).

4. Gastrointestinal problems

If swallowing and chewing gets more difficult, eating takes too much time or energy, enteral tube feeding is a possibility. The percutaneous gastrostomy is quite regular, although there are also complications described during (re)placement. In myotonic dystrophy impairment of gastrointestinal motility is known and seems to be gradual worsening(Bellini et al 2006), probably related to gastrointestinal symptoms like regurgitation, dyspepsia, abodominal pain, bloating, and changes in bowl habits. Although there is only a low correlation between the degree of skeletal muscle involvement and the presence and severity of gastrointestinal disturbances it is a positive correlation (Bellini et al 2006). Also in boys with Duchenne and Becker muscular dystrophy abnormalities in gastric motility are seen and the possibility of progressive failure in neuromuscular function is put forward (Borelli et al 2005). Promotility agents are advised as are good diet, stool softeners, and hydration (Bellini et al 2006, Wagner et al 2007). There is little evidence on the benefits of exercise and chronic constipation (Leung et al 2011), but practical experience often reported is that doing exercise or standing in a standing table or frame does seem to help. This would be in line with the former recommendations for exercise.

5. Urogenital problems in muscular dystrophies

Lower urinary tract symptoms are described in boys with Duchenne muscular dystrophy and seem not to be rare (van Wijk et al 2009). Nearly 85 % of the boys/men with Duchenne muscular dystrophy reported lower urinary tract symptoms, and 51 % had more than 3 problems. The main problems were post micturation dribble, straining, (urge) incontinence, and feeling of incomplete emptying. There is a very low correlation between age and functional abilities and lower urinary tract problems; these problems seem not to worsen with disease progression. In 42 % the boys/men mentioned that the complaints influenced their social life, and 25 % reported a decrease in quality of life. Also in myotonic dystrophy urinary tract symptoms are reported but only anecdotal. This is probably an underreported symptom and should have attention in the management.

It is recommended to ask for lower urinary tract symptoms, use a micturation questionnaire if there are concerns, and register for several days the pattern. Up till now no pathophysiological studies are available, the possibility of a bladder-sphincter dys-synergy is suggested, and the symptoms are treated symptomatically by medication.

6. Technical possibilities

New very sophisticated devices are being developed like exoskeletons, robot arms and motion controlled orthoses (see for example websites of www.Flextension.nl and www.FocalMeditech.nl). Not only can these devices support a natural function, but they can also simulate a natural movement. It is possible that with an exoskeleton a person with severe paresis can still move in a rather natural way. In an earlier stage these devices can also be used for assisted training and it is theoretically possible that by regular use one can prevent contractures. Robotica can potentially reduce the extent of personal help needed, thus making an adjusted independent life possible and making participation in social life possible.

7. References

1998, American College of Sports Medicine Position Stand. The recommended quantity and quality of exercise for developing and maintaining cardiorespiratory and muscular fitness, and flexibility in healthy adults: Med.Sci.Sports Exerc., v. 30, no. 6, p. 975-991.

Aloysius A., P. Born, M. Kinali, T. Davis, M. Pane, E. Mercuri, 2008, Swallowing difficulties in Duchenne muscular dystrophy: indications for feeding assessment and outcome of videofluroscopic swallow studies, Eur. J. Paediatr. Neurol., v.12, n. 3, p. 239-45.

Arvedson J.C., M.A. Lefton-Greif, 1998, Pediatric videofluoroscopic swallow studies: a professional manual with caregiver guidelines, San Antonio, Texas: Communication Skill Builders, Psychological Corporation.

Arvedson J.C., 2008, Assessment of pediatric dysphagia and feeding disorders: clinical and instrumental approaches. Dev Disabil Res Rev, v. 12, no. 2, p. 118-27.

Bagnall A.K., M.A. Al-Mahaizea, A.Y. Manzur, 2006, Feeding and speech difficulties in typical congenital Nemaline myopathy, Advances in Speech-Language Pathology, v. 8, n. 1, p. 7-16.

Bellini M., S. Biagi, C. Stasi, F. Costa, M.G. Mumolo, A. Ricchiutti, S. Marchi, 2006, Gastrointestinal manifestations in myotonic dystrophy, World J Gastroenterol v. 28, n.12, p.1821-1828

Borrelli O., G. Salvi, V. Mancini, L. Santoro, F. Tagliente, E.F. Romeo, S. Cucchiara, 2005, Evolution of gastric electrical features and gastric emptying in children with Duchenne and Becker Muscular Dystrophy, Am.J.Gastroenterol, v. 100, p. 695-702

Botteron S., C.M. Verbout, P.Y. Jeannet, S. Kiliaridis, 2009, Orofacial dysfunction in Duchenne muscular dystrophy, Arch. Oral. Biol., v. 54, n. 1, p. 26-31

Carter, G. T., M. A. Wineinger, S. A. Walsh, S. J. Horasek, R. T. Abresch, and W. M. Fowler, Jr., 1995, Effect of voluntary wheel-running exercise on muscles of the mdx mouse: Neuromuscul.Disord., v. 5, no. 4, p. 323-332.

Chambers, D., A. M. Bagnall, S. Hempel, and C. Forbes, 2006, Interventions for the treatment, management and rehabilitation of patients with chronic fatigue syndrome/myalgic encephalomyelitis: an updated systematic review: J.R.Soc.Med., v. 99, no. 10, p. 506-520.

Cup, E. H., A. J. Pieterse, J. M. Ten Broek-Pastoor, M. Munneke, B. G. van Engelen, H. T. Hendricks, G. J. van der Wilt, and R. A. Oostendorp, 2007, Exercise therapy and other types of physical therapy for patients with neuromuscular diseases: a systematic review: Arch.Phys.Med.Rehabil., v. 88, no. 11, p. 1452-1464.

De Lateur B.J., R.M. Giaconi. 1979. Effect on maximal strength of submaxiaml exercise in Duchenne muscular dystrophy. Am J Phys Med 58 (1): 26-36

Della, M. G. et al., 2007, Sleep quality in Facioscapulohumeral muscular dystrophy: J.Neurol.Sci., v. 263, no. 1-2, p. 49-53.

De Swart B.J., G. W. Padberg, B.G. van Engelen, 2002, Less is more: treatment of aggravating behaviour in myasthenia gravis patients with dysphagia, Eur. J. Neurol., v. 9, n. 6, p. 688-9.

Dubowitz V., 2000, Muscle disorders in childhood. London: W.B.Saunders Company LTD.

Dupont-Versteegden E.E., R.J. McCarter, M.S. Katz. 1994. Voluntary exercise decreases progression of muscular dystrophy in diaphragm of mdx mice. J Appl Physiol 77 (4): 1736-41

Eagle M. 2002. Report on the muscular dystrophy campaign workshop: exercise in neuromuscular diseases. Neuromuscul Disord 12 (10): 975-83

Edouard P, et a;. 2007. Training programs for children: literature review. Ann Readapt Med Phys 50 (6): 510-09.

Ertekin C, I. Aydogdu, 2003, Neurophysiology of swallowing, Clin Neurophysio, v. 114, no. 12, p. 2226-44

Fowler, W. M., Jr., 1984, Importance of overwork weakness: Muscle Nerve, v. 7, no. 6, p. 496-499.

Gielissen, M. F., C. A. Verhagen, and G. Bleijenberg, 2007, Cognitive behaviour therapy for fatigued cancer survivors: long-term follow-up: Br.J.Cancer, v. 97, no. 5, p. 612-618.

Gielissen, M. F., S. Verhagen, F. Witjes, and G. Bleijenberg, 2006, Effects of cognitive behavior therapy in severely fatigued disease-free cancer patients compared with patients waiting for cognitive behavior therapy: a randomized controlled trial: J.Clin.Oncol., v. 24, no. 30, p. 4882-4887.

Hayes A, D.A. Williams. 1996. Beneficial effects of voluntary wheel running on the properties of dystrophic mouse muscle. J Appl Physiol 80 (2): 670-79

Hayes A et al 1998. Contractile function and low-intensity exercise effects of old dystrophic (mdx) mice. Am J Physiol 274 (4): C1138-C1144.

Hiorns M.P., M.M. Ryan, 2006, Current practice in paediatric videofluoroscopy, Pediatr. Radiol., v. 36, n. 9, p. 911-9.

Janssen M. I.J.M. de Groot, N. van Alfen, A.C.H. Geurts. 2010 Physical training in boys with Duchenne Muscular Dystrophy: the protocol of the No Use is Disuse study. BMC Pediatr. 10: 55

Jean A, 2001, Brain stem control of swallowing: neuronal network and cellular mechanisms, Physiol. Rev., v 81, no 2, p. 929-69

Johnson, E. W., and R. Braddom, 1971, Over-work weakness in facioscapulohuumeral muscular dystrophy: Arch.Phys.Med.Rehabil., v. 52, no. 7, p. 333-336.

Kalkman, J. S., M. L. Schillings, S. P. van der Werf, G. W. Padberg, M. J. Zwarts, B. G. van Engelen, and G. Bleijenberg, 2005, Experienced fatigue in facioscapulohumeral dystrophy, myotonic dystrophy, and HMSN-I: J.Neurol.Neurosurg.Psychiatry, v. 76, no. 10, p. 1406-1409.

Kalkman, J. S., M. L. Schillings, M. J. Zwarts, B. G. van Engelen, and G. Bleijenberg, 2007, The development of a model of fatigue in neuromuscular disorders: a longitudinal study: J.Psychosom.Res., v. 62, no. 5, p. 571-579.

Kumin L., 1994, Intelligibility of speech in children with Down syndrome in natural settings: parents' perspective, Percept Mot Skills, v.78, n. 1, p. 307-13

Leopold N.A, S.K. Daniels, 2010, Supranuclear control of swallowing., Dyspahgia, v. 25, no. 3, p. 250-7.

Leonard R.J., K.A. Kendall, R. Johnson, S. McKenzie, 2001, Swallowing in myotonic muscular dystrophy: a videofluoroscopic study, Arch. Phys. Med. Rehabil., v. 82, n. 7, p. 979-85.

Leung L., T. Riutta, J. Kotecha, W. Rosser, 2011, Chronic constipation: an evidence-based review, J.Am.Board Fa,. Med., v. 24, no.4, p. 436-451

Lim, J.H., D.Y Kim, M.S. Bang, 2004, Effects of exercise and steroid on skeletal muscle apoptosis in the mdx mouse. Muscle Nerve 30, no 4, p 456-62

Lindeman, E., P. Leffers, F. Spaans, J. Drukker, J. Reulen, M. Kerckhoffs, and A. Koke, 1995, Strength training in patients with myotonic dystrophy and hereditary motor and sensory neuropathy: a randomized clinical trial: Arch.Phys.Med.Rehabil., v. 76, no. 7, p. 612-620.

Logemann J.A., B.R. Pauloski, A.W. Rademaker, L.A. Colangelo, P.J. Kahrilas, C.H. Smith, 2000, Temporal and biomechanical characteristics of oropharyngeal swallow in younger and older men, J. Speech Lang. Hear. Res., v, 43, n. 5, p. 1264-74.

Manzur A.Y., M. Kinali, F. Muntoni, 2008, Update on the management of Duchenne muscular dystrophy, Arch. Dis. Child., v.93, n. 11, p. 986-90.

Markert, C.D. et al , 2011Exercise and Duchenne muscular dystrophy: toward evidence-based exercise prescription, Muscle Nerve 43, no 4, p 464-78

McDonald, C.M., et al , 1995, Profiles on neuromuscular diseases. Duchenne muscular dystrophy. Am. J. Phys Med. Rehabil. 74, no 5 suppl, p S70-92

McDonald, C. M., 2002, Physical activity, health impairments, and disability in neuromuscular disease: Am.J.Phys.Med.Rehabil., v. 81, no. 11 Suppl, p. S108-S120.

Mehta S.G., G. D. Watts, B. McGillivray, S. Mumm, S.J. Hamilton, S. Ramdeen, D. Novack, C. Briggs, M.P. Whyte, V.E. Kimonis, 2006, Manifestations in a family with autosomal dominant bone fragility and limb-girdle myopathy, Am. J. Med. Genet., v. 140, n. 4, p. 322-30.

Messina S., M. Pane, P.D. Rose, I. Vasta, D. Sorleti, A.Aloysius, F. Sciarra, F. Mangiola, M. Kinali, E. Bertini, E. Mercuri, 2008, Feeding problems and malnutrition in spinal muscular atrophy type II, Neuromuscul. Disord., v. 18, n.5, p. 389-93.

Miller A.J., 2008, The neurobiology of swallowing and dysphagia. Dev Disabil Res Rev, v. 14, no. 2, p. 77-86.

Morel-Verdebout c., S. Botteron, S. Killiaridis, 2007, Dentofacial characteristics of growing patients with Duchenne muscular dystrophy: a morphological study, Eur. J. Orthod., v. 29, n. 5, p. 500-7.

Okano, T, et al , 2005, Chronic exercise accelerates the degeneration-regeneration cycle and down regulates insulin-like growth factor-1 in muscle of mdx mice. Muscle Nerver 32, no 2, p 1991-99.

Pane M., I. Vaste, S. Messina, D. Sorletti, A. Aloysius, F. Sciarra, F. Mangiola, M. Kinali, E. Ricci, E. Mercuri, 2006, Feeding problems and weight gain in Duchenne muscular dystrophy, Eur. J. Paediatr. Neurol., v. 10, n. 5-6, p. 231-6.

Petrof, B. J., 1998, The molecular basis of activity-induced muscle injury in Duchenne muscular dystrophy: Mol.Cell Biochem., v. 179, no. 1-2, p. 111-123.

Prins, J. B., G. Bleijenberg, E. Bazelmans, L. D. Elving, T. M. de Boo, J. L. Severens, G. J. van der Wilt, P. Spinhoven, and J. W. van der Meer, 2001, Cognitive behaviour therapy for chronic fatigue syndrome: a multicentre randomised controlled trial: Lancet, v. 357, no. 9259, p. 841-847.

Rogers B, J. Arvedson, G. Buck, P. Smart, M. Msall, 1994, Characteristics of dysphagia in children with cerebral palsy, Dysphagia, v. 9, n.1, p. 69-73.

Scott, O. M., et al. , 1981, Effect of exercise in Duchenne muscular dystrophy, Physiotherapy, 67, no 6, p174-76.

Shinonaga C., M. Fukuda, Y. Suzuki, T. Higaki, Y. Ischida, E. Ischii, M. Hyodo, T. Morimoto, N. Sano, 2008, Evaluations of swallowing function in Duchenne muscular dystrophy, Dev. Med. Child Neurol., v. 50, n. 6, p. 478-80.

Stubgen J.P., 2008, Facioscapulohumeral muscular dystrophy: a radiologic and manometric study of the pharynz and esophagus, Dysphagia, v. 23, n. 4, p. 341-7.

Sveen, M.L. et al ,2008, Endurance training improves fitness and strength in patients with Becker muscular dystrophy, Brain, 131, pt 11, p 2824-31.

Van Bruggen H.W., L. van den Engel-Hoek, W.L. van der Pol, A. de Weier, I.J.M. de Groot, M.H. Steenks, 2011, Impaired mandibular function in Spinal Muscular Atrophy type II: need for early recognition, J. Child Neurol., e-pud ahead

van den Engel-Hoek L., C.E. .Erasmus, H.W. van Bruggen, B.J.M. de Swart,L.T. Sie, M.H. Steenks, I.J.M. de Groot IJM, 2009, Dysphagia in spinal muscular atrophy type II, more than a bulbar problem?, Neurology; v. 73, p.1787-1791

van der Kooi, E. L., O. J. Vogels, R. J. van Asseldonk, E. Lindeman, J. C. Hendriks, M. Wohlgemuth, S. M. van der Maarel, and G. W. Padberg, 2004, Strength training and albuterol in facioscapulohumeral muscular dystrophy: Neurology, v. 63, no. 4, p. 702-708.

Van Wijk E., B.J. Messelink, L. Heijnen, I.J.M. de Groot, 2009, Prevalence and psychosocial impact of lower urinary tract symptoms in patients with Duchenne muscular dystrophy, Neuromusc.Disord, v. 19, p.754-758

Vestergaard, P, et al , 2001, Fracture risk in patients with muscular dystrophy and spinal muscular atrophy, J. Rehabil. Med, 33, no 4, p. 150-55

Vignos P.J., M.P. Watkins, 1966, The effect of exercise in muscular dystrophy, JAMA, 197, no 11, p. 843-48

Voet, N. B., E. L. van der Kooi, I. I. Riphagen, E. Lindeman, B. G. van Engelen, and A. C. Geurts, 2010, Strength training and aerobic exercise training for muscle disease: Cochrane.Database.Syst.Rev., no. 1, p. CD003907.

Wagner K.R., N. Lechtzin, D.P. Judge, 2007, Current treatment of adult Duchenne muscular dystrophy, Bioch.Biophys.Acta, v. 1772, p.229-237

12

Diagnosis of the Muscular Dystrophies

Leigh B. Waddell, Frances J. Evesson, Kathryn N. North,
Sandra T. Cooper and Nigel F. Clarke
*Institute for Neuroscience and Muscle Research,
Children's Hospital at Westmead and Discipline of Paediatrics & Child Health,
University of Sydney,
Australia*

1. Introduction

The diagnosis of muscular dystrophies (MDs) has advanced considerably since these disorders were first described in the 1800s, due to characterisation of phenotypes and advances in biochemical and molecular analyses. Over the last ten years in particular, there has been a rapid expansion in the list of genes that are known to cause MD. Providing a specific genetic diagnosis to a patient is important for many reasons. It resolves many uncertainties for families, enables accurate genetic counselling and options for prevention and prenatal diagnosis, and provides doctors and families with information about prognosis, which allows medical care to be individualised. In some cases, a genetic diagnosis prompts the clinician to begin surveillance and/or interventions that may be life-saving, such as aggressive cardiac surveillance in disorders associated with cardiac arrhythmias or cardiomyopathy. In addition, knowledge of the primary genetic cause will be an essential prerequisite to prescribe specific gene-based or biochemical therapies when they are developed in the future. Making a genetic diagnosis should now be the universal goal for all patients with MD.

Diagnosis of the three most common forms of MD, Duchenne muscular dystrophy (DMD), myotonic dystrophy and Facioscapulohumeral muscular dystrophy (FSHD) MD, is now straightforward in most patients, as clinical features guide the appropriate genetic tests to be requested. However, establishing the specific diagnosis in many patients with other forms of MD remains difficult. The main reasons are the large number of potential genetic causes in several subgroups of MD, a lack of specific features to guide diagnosis and the wide range of phenotypes that are possible with many genetic forms. These combine to make it a challenge for the clinician to predict the correct genetic cause from the patient's clinical presentation and history, or from standard clinical tests alone. Laboratory investigations, including muscle histopathology and protein analysis (immunohistochemistry and Western blotting), are useful to guide genetic testing in many situations. However, even in well-resourced diagnostic services, the genetic cause remains unknown in a large proportion of MD patients. It is likely that many of these patients have as yet undiscovered genetic forms of MD.

This chapter summarises the most important clinical and laboratory information to consider when diagnosing MDs, and the approach to diagnosing the different forms. This includes an appreciation of clinical presentations, the use of specialised muscle imaging, muscle histopathology, laboratory protein analysis and specific genetic tests. We also discuss the challenges when diagnosing many rare forms of MD, and how new technologies may aid this process.

2. The different forms of muscular dystrophy

The MDs are a genetically and phenotypically diverse group of disorders. In children, the most common form of MD is Duchenne MD (DMD), caused by mutations in the *DMD* gene that encodes dystrophin, with an estimated prevalence of 1 in 3000 males (Jones and North 1997). Most affected boys lose ambulation around 10 years of age and die from respiratory or cardiac complications in the third or fourth decades of life. Becker MD (BMD) is a less severe condition associated with a later age of onset and slower disease progression that is also caused by mutations in the dystrophin protein.

In adults, the most common forms of MD are myotonic dystrophy type 1 (DM1) and facioscapulohumeral MD (FSHD). The average estimated prevalence of DM1 is ~1 in 10,000 (Norwood, Harling et al. 2009; Turner and Hilton-Jones 2010) and for FSHD it is 1 in 20,000 (Norwood, Harling et al. 2009; Statland and Tawil 2011). DM1 is a multi-system disorder caused by a trinucleotide repeat expansion (CTG) in the *DMPK* gene on chromosome 19 and there is a wide range of severity that partially correlates with the size of the repeat expansion (McNally and Pytel 2007; Turner and Hilton-Jones 2010). The classical form of DM1 is characterised by progressive muscle weakness that begins in the muscles of the face, ankle, hands and neck and myotonia, a delayed relaxation of muscles after contraction. Patients also have an increased risk of cardiac conduction defects, cataracts, type 2 diabetes, daytime somnolence and balding (males especially). Congenital onset DM1 is strongly associated with respiratory difficulties at birth and intellectual disabililty (Turner and Hilton-Jones 2010). A second form of myotonic dystrophy (DM2) is due to mutations in the *ZNF9* gene, does not have a congenital onset form, and is probably less common. FSHD is characterised by weakness of the facial, scapular, ankle and upper arm muscles and is caused by deletions of large D4Z4 DNA repeats in the sub-telomeric region of chromosome 4q (McNally and Pytel 2007; Pandya, King et al. 2008).

Disease	Gene	Chromosome	Protein	Year Identified
FSHD	*DUX4*	4q35	Double homeobox 4	1990 [1]
Myotonic Dystrophy (DM1)	*DMPK*	19q13	*Expansion of non-coding triplet (CTG) repeat*	1992 [2,3]
Myotonic Dystrophy (DM2)	*ZNF9*	3q21	*Expansion of non-coding quadruplet (CCTG) repeat*	2001 [4,5]
Oculopharyngeal MD	*PABPN1*	14q11.2-q13	Poly(A) binding protein, nuclear 1	1998 [6-8]
MD with Lipodystrophy	*PTRF*	17q21-23	Cavin-1	2009 [9]
DMD/BMD	*DMD*	Xp21.2	Dystrophin	1986/87 [10-14]

Disease	Gene	Chromosome	Protein	Year Identified
EDMD	EMD	Xq28	Emerin	1994 [15]
	FHL1	Xq27.2	Four and a half LIM domain 1	2009 [16]
	LMNA	1q21.2	Lamin A/C	1999 [17]
	SYNE1	6q25	Nesprin-1	2007 [18]
	SYNE2	14q23	Nesprin-2	2007 [18]
LGMD1A	MYOT	5q31	Myotilin	2000 [19]
LGMD1B	LMNA	1q22	Lamin A/C	2000 [20]
LGMD1C	CAV3	3p25	Caveolin-3	1998 [21,22]
LGMD1D	*	7q36.3		[23]
LGMD1E	*	6q23		[24]
LGMD1F	*	7q32		[25]
LGMD1G	*	4q21		[26]
LGMD2A	CAPN3	15q15.1	Calpain-3	1995 [27,28]
LGMD2B	DYSF	2p13	Dysferlin	1998 [29,30]
LGMD2C	SGCG	13q12	γ-sarcoglycan	1995 [31]
LGMD2D	SGCA	17q12-21.33	α-sarcoglycan	1994 [32]
LGMD2E	SGCB	4q12	β-sarcoglycan	1996 [33]
LGMD2F	SGCD	5q33	δ-sarcoglycan	1996 [34]
LGMD2G	TCAP	17q12	Telethonin	2000 [35]
LGMD2H	TRIM32	9q31-34	Tripartite motif-containing 32	2002 [36,37]
LGMD2I	FKRP	19q13.3	Fukutin related protein	2001 [38,39]
LGMD2J	TTN	2q31	Titin	2002 [40]
LGMD2K	POMT1	9q34	Protein O-mannosyl-transferase 1	2005 [41]
LGMD2L	ANO5	11p14.3	Anoctamin 5	2010 [42]
LGMD2M	FKTN	9q31-33	Fukutin	2006 [43,44]
LGMD2N	POMT2	14q24	Protein O-mannosyl-transferase 2	2007 [45]
LGMD2O	POMGnT1	1p34	Protein O-linked mannose beta 1,2-N-acetylglucosaminyl transferase 1	2007 [46]
MDC1A	LAMA2	6q2	Laminin α2 chain of merosin	1995 [47-49]
MDC1B	*	1q42		[50]
MDC1C	FKRP	19q13	Fukutin related protein	2001 [51]
MDC1D	LARGE	22q12	Like-glycosyltransferase	2003 [52]
FCMD	FCMD	9q31-33	Fukutin	1998 [53,54]
WWS	FCMD	9q31-33	Fukutin	2003 [55]
	POMT1	9q34	Protein O-mannosyl-transferase 1	2002 [56]
	POMT2	14q24.3	Protein O-mannosyl-transferase 2	2005 [57]
	FKRP	19q13	Fukutin related protein	2005 [58]
	POMGnT1	1p3	Protein O-linked mannose beta 1,2-N-acetylglucosaminyl transferase 1	2003 [59]

Disease	Gene	Chromosome	Protein	Year Identified
MEB	POMGnT1	1p3	Protein O-linked mannose beta 1,2-N-acetylglucosaminyl transferase 1	2001 [60]
	FKRP	19q13	Fukutin related protein	2005 [58]
	POMT2	14q24.3	Protein O-mannosyl-transferase 2	2006 [61]
Rigid Spine Syndrome	SEPN1	1p36	Selenoprotein N1	2001 [62,63]
UCMD	COL6A1	21q22.3	Collagen VI, subunit α1	2003 [64,65]
	COL6A2	21q22.3	Collagen VI, subunit α2	2001 [66,67]
	COL6A3	2q37	Collagen VI, subunit α3	2002 [68]
Bethlem myopathy	COL6A1	21q22.3	Collagen VI, subunit α1	1996 [69]
	COL6A2	21q22.3	Collagen VI, subunit α2	1996 [69]
	COL6A3	2q37	Collagen VI, subunit α3	1998 [70,71]
CMD integrin defect	ITGA7	12q13	Integrin α7	1998 [72]
CMD dynamin 2 defect	DNM2	19p13.2	Dynamin 2	2008 [73]
CMD joint hyperlaxity	*	3p23-21		[74]

Adapted from the NMD Gene Table 2011 (Kaplan 2010). * = no gene discovered yet. **Abbreviations:** FSHD: Facio-scapulo-humeral MD, MD: muscular dystrophy, DMD: Duchenne MD, BMD: Becker MD, EDMD: Emery-Dreifuss MD, LGMD: limb-girdle MD, MDC: MD congenital, FCMD: Fukuyama congenital MD, WWS: Walker-Warburg Syndrome, MEB: Muscle-eye-brain disease, UCMD: Ullrich congenital MD and CMD: congenital MD. References: 1(Wijmenga, Frants et al. 1990), 2(Brook, McCurrach et al. 1992), 3(Renwick, Bundey et al. 1971), 4(Liquori, Ricker et al. 2001), 5(Ranum, Rasmussen et al. 1998), 6(Brais, Bouchard et al. 1998), 7(Brais, Xie et al. 1995), 8(Robinson, Hammans et al. 2005), 9(Hayashi, Matsuda et al. 2009), 10(Burghes, Logan et al. 1987), 11(Hoffman, Brown et al. 1987), 12(Koenig, Hoffman et al. 1987), 13(Koenig, Monaco et al. 1988), 14(Monaco, Neve et al. 1986), 15(Bione, Maestrini et al. 1994), 16(Gueneau, Bertrand et al. 2009), 17(Bonne, Di Barletta et al. 1999), 18(Zhang, Bethmann et al. 2007), 19(Hauser, Horrigan et al. 2000), 20(Muchir, Bonne et al. 2000), 21(McNally, de Sa Moreira et al. 1998), 22(Minetti, Sotgia et al. 1998), 23(Speer, Vance et al. 1999), 24(Messina, Speer et al. 1997), 25(Palenzuela, Andreu et al. 2003), 26(Starling, Kok et al. 2004), 27(Richard, Brenguier et al. 1997), 28(Richard, Broux et al. 1995), 29(Bashir, Britton et al. 1998), 30(Liu, Aoki et al. 1998), 31(Noguchi, McNally et al. 1995), 32(Roberds, Leturcq et al. 1994), 33(Bonnemann, Passos-Bueno et al. 1996), 34(Nigro, de Sa Moreira et al. 1996), 35(Moreira, Wiltshire et al. 2000), 36(Frosk, Weiler et al. 2002), 37(Weiler, Greenberg et al. 1998), 38(Brockington, Blake et al. 2001), 39(Driss, Amouri et al. 2000), 40(Hackman, Vihola et al. 2002), 41(Balci, Uyanik et al. 2005), 42(Bolduc, Marlow et al. 2010), 43(Godfrey, Escolar et al. 2006), 44(Murakami, Hayashi et al. 2006), 45(Biancheri, Falace et al. 2007), 46(Godfrey, Clement et al. 2007), 47(Helbling-Leclerc, Zhang et al. 1995), 48(Hillaire, Leclerc et al. 1994), 49(Tome, Evangelista et al. 1994), 50(Brockington, Sewry et al. 2000), 51(Brockington, Blake et al. 2001), 52(Longman, Brockington et al. 2003), 53(Kobayashi, Nakahori et al. 1998), 54(Toda, Segawa et al. 1993), 55(de Bernabe, van Bokhoven et al. 2003), 56(Beltran-Valero de Bernabe, Currier et al. 2002), 57(van Reeuwijk, Janssen et al. 2005), 58(Beltran-Valero de Bernabe, Voit et al. 2004), 59(Taniguchi, Kobayashi et al. 2003), 60(Yoshida, Kobayashi et al. 2001), 61(Mercuri, D'Amico et al. 2006), 62(Moghadaszadeh, Desguerre et al. 1998), 63(Moghadaszadeh, Petit et al. 2001), 64(Giusti, Lucarini et al. 2005), 65(Pan, Zhang et al. 2003), 66(Camacho Vanegas, Bertini et al. 2001), 67(Higuchi, Shiraishi et al. 2001), 68(Demir, Sabatelli et al. 2002), 69(Jobsis, Keizers et al. 1996), 70(Pan, Zhang et al. 1998), 71(Speer, Tandan et al. 1996), 72(Hayashi, Chou et al. 1998), 73(Susman, Quijano-Roy et al. 2010), 74(Tetreault, Duquette et al. 2006) and 75(Kaplan 2010).

Table 1. Table of muscular dystrophy genes and proteins.

The other major forms of MD are grouped by age of onset or clinical phenotype (see Table 1). Each specific genetic form of MD has a characteristic pattern of disease onset, severity, clinical course and involvement of particular muscle groups, although there is marked overlap between phenotypes (see Table 2). The congenital MDs (CMD) are characterised by onset of muscle weakness within the first year of life (often at birth) and usually have a slowly progressive disease course. In the limb girdle MDs (LGMD), patients can present during childhood or adulthood with weakness that is most prominent in proximal limb or shoulder and/or pelvic girdle muscles. They are subdivided based on mode of inheritance into LGMD type 1 (autosomal dominant) and LGMD type 2 (autosomal recessive); DMD and BMD can be considered as X-linked forms of LGMD. Emery Dreifuss MD (EDMD) is a clinical syndrome with several possible genetic causes characterised by prominent weakness in the upper arm and ankle dorsiflexor muscles, early contractures of the elbows, ankles and neck and cardiac involvement. Other forms of MD with notable phenotypes are oculopharyngeal MD, where mainly the muscles of the eye and throat are affected, and the distal myopathies which mainly affect the muscles of the hands and feet.

In addition to the different forms of MD listed so far, a wide range of muscle conditions have clinical and histological features that overlap with the MDs and these should be kept in mind whenever a diagnosis of a MD is considered. The most important differential diagnoses are the myofibrillar myopathies (characterised by desmin-positive inclusions in muscle fibres, prominent distal limb muscle involvement, cardiomyopathy and peripheral neuropathy) and some severe forms of congenital myopathy (especially those due to *RYR1* and *DNM2* mutations).

3. Overview of the approach to diagnosis

A diagnosis of MD usually begins with a patient presenting with muscle weakness, muscle pain, reduced stamina; or in children, delayed motor development. Occasionally a raised serum creatine kinase (CK) level is the first sign of a MD and an incidental finding during investigation of other symptoms. A detailed clinical history and examination can provide important clues about the diagnosis and the most appropriate path of investigation. Muscle imaging is a non-invasive option that may be helpful in particular situations. A muscle biopsy is still required for the diagnosis of many types of MD. In most children and some adults a skin biopsy is taken for fibroblast cell culture at this time. Standard muscle histopathology provides information about muscle architecture and frozen portions of the muscle biopsy can be used for a range of protein analyses. Information from all of these sources is used to direct genetic testing, which usually provides the definitive diagnosis. This process is outlined in Figure 1.

3.1 Clinical information

Clinical information remains of paramount importance in the diagnostic process, even with recent advances in genetics (Bushby, Norwood et al. 2007; Norwood, de Visser et al. 2007; Guglieri and Bushby 2008). Each MD has a characteristic clinical pattern in terms of age of onset, rate of progression, severity and range of muscles involved. In some forms of MD, the pattern of clinical features is sufficiently distinct for a relatively accurate provisional

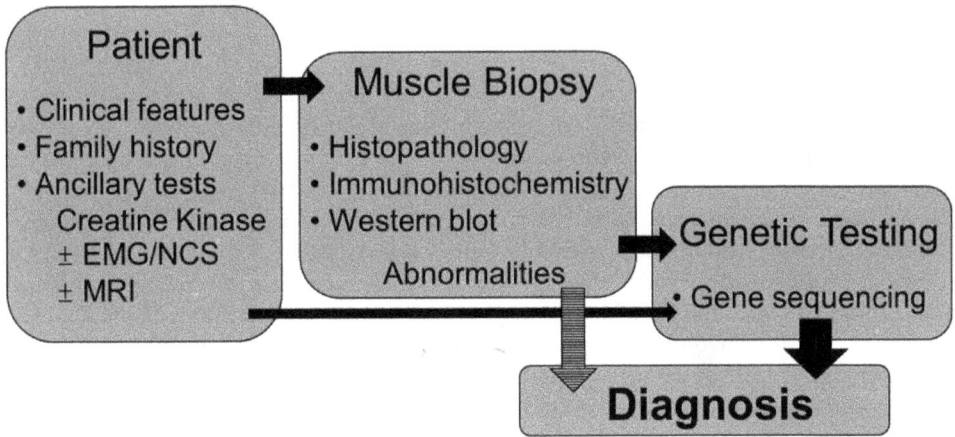

Abbreviations: EMG: Electromyography, NCS: nerve conduction studies, MRI: magnetic resonance imaging.

Fig. 1. Overview of MD diagnostic process.

diagnosis to be made on the basis of clinical history, examination and some basic clinical tests. This is the case for the three most common forms of MD - myotonic dystrophy, FSHD and DMD. It is recommended that clinician spends time familiarising themselves with these three disorders in particular, as they are the most common conditions encountered. Genetic testing is widely available for these conditions and many patients no longer require a muscle biopsy, so long as the clinician can make an accurate provisional diagnosis from clinical features.

Age of disease onset is a key feature that is used to classify major subgroups of MD. The congenital muscular dystrohies (CMDs) present in the first two years of life, most often at birth. The limb girdle MDs (LGMDs) begin after age 2 years. Onset can vary between the first decade of life to old age depending on the specific form of LGMD and its severity.

The pattern of weakness may also provide clues to the MD subtype. For example while LGMDs are characterised by proximal weakness, some subtypes may also have significant involvement of scapular stabilisers or distal limb muscles (see Table 2). Other important variables include the presence or absence of brain, cardiac or respiratory muscle involvement, calf muscle hypertrophy, contractures and skin abnormalities (see Table 2).

The level of creatine kinase (CK) in blood, which is thought to be a marker of ongoing muscle necrosis or damage, can also help to differentiate between forms of MD. While some fluctuation in CK levels from day to day occurs and there is a tendency for CK levels to drop with disease progression, categorising CK results into broad ranges such as normal, mildly raised, moderately raised and markedly elevated is useful.

Disease	Gene	Prevalence*	Age of onset (yrs)	CK	Distal	Cardiac	Respiratory	Muscle hypertrophy	Spine	Contractures	Useful diagnostic information	References
FSHD	DUX4	Common	10-50	↑-↑↑							CE, FHx, GT	1,2
Myotonic Dystrophy (DM1)	DMPK	Common	0-80	↑-↑↑	✓	✓	✓				CE, FHx, EMG, GT	3
Myotonic Dystrophy (DM2)	ZNF9	Probably uncommon	10-60	↑-↑↑	✓	✓		✓			CE, FHx, EMG, GT	3
DMD-BMD	DMD	Common	DMD: 2-6 BMD:>5	↑↑-↑↑↑		✓	✓	✓	✓	✓	CE, FHx, IHC, WB, GT, SEQ	4,5
EDMD	EMD	Uncommon	>3	↑-↑↑		✓			✓	✓✓	IHC, WB, SEQ	6,7
	FHL1	Rare	4-48	N-↑↑		✓			✓	✓	SEQ	8
	LMNA	Uncommon	>3	N-↑↑		✓✓			✓	✓✓	SEQ	
LGMD1A	MYOT	Rare	>25	↑-↑↑	✓	✓					SEQ	9
LGMD1B	LMNA	Uncommon	>3	↑-↑↑	✓	✓✓			✓		SEQ	10
LGMD1C	CAV3	Uncommon	>4	↑↑-↑↑↑				✓			IHC, WB, SEQ	11
LGMD2A	CAPN3	Common	2-40	↑-↑↑↑			✓		✓	✓	± WB, SEQ	12,13
LGMD2B	DYSF	Moderately common^	12-25	↑↑↑	✓						IHC, WB, SEQ	14-16
LGMD2C	SGCG	Rare	>3	↑↑-↑↑↑		✓	✓	✓	✓	✓	IHC, WB, SEQ	17-21
LGMD2D	SGCA	Rare	>3	↑↑-↑↑↑		✓	✓	✓	✓	✓	IHC, WB, SEQ	17-21
LGMD2E	SGCB	Rare	>3	↑↑-↑↑↑		✓	✓	✓	✓	✓	IHC, WB, SEQ	17-21
LGMD2F	SGCD	Rare	>3	↑↑-↑↑↑		✓	✓	✓	✓	✓	IHC, WB, SEQ	17-21
LGMD2G	TCAP	Rare	9-20	↑-↑↑↑	✓	?			✓	✓	IHC, SEQ	22,23
LGMD2H	TRIM32	Rare‡	8-30	↑↑-↑↑↑				✓			SEQ	24
LGMD2I	FKRP	Common	2-40	↑↑-↑↑↑		✓	✓	✓	✓	✓	IHC+, WB+, SEQ	25
LGMD2J	TTN	Rare	8-30	N-↑	✓						MRI, (SEQ)	26
LGMD2L	ANO5	Common	>17	↑↑↑	✓			✓			SEQ	27,28
MDC1A	LAMA2	Common	0	↑↑-↑↑↑			✓		✓	✓	IHC, WB, SEQ	29-32
MDC1C	FKRP	Rare	0	↑↑↑		✓	✓	✓	✓	✓	IHC+, WB+, SEQ	33
FCMD	FKTN	Common†	0	↑↑-↑↑↑		✓	✓	✓	✓	✓	IHC+,	34

Disease	Gene	Prevalence*	Age of onset (yrs)	CK	Distal	Cardiac	Respiratory	Muscle hypertrophy	Spine	Contractures	Useful diagnostic information	References
Rigid Spine Syndrome	*SEPN1*	Uncommon	0-2	N-↑			✓✓		✓✓		WB+, SEQ SEQ	35
UCMD	*COL6A1-3*	Common	0	N-↑↑			✓		✓	✓✓	IHC, FIBS, SEQ	36-38
Bethlem myopathy	*COL6A1-3*	Common	2-20	N-↑↑			✓		✓	✓✓	FIBS, SEQ	36,38

This table does not include the rarest forms of muscular dystrophy. Brain involvement can be seen in congenital myotonic dystrophy (DM1), DMD, the α-dystroglycanopathies and MDC1A. * = Prevalence varies for some disorders in different populations. Distal = prominent distal limb muscle involvement. CK = creatine kinase. Spine = prominent scoliosis or spinal rigidity. N = CK within normal range, ↑ = CK level 1 to 4 times upper limit of normal, ↑↑ = CK 4 to 15 times upper limit of normal, ↑↑↑ = CK > 15 times upper limit of normal. ✓ = commonly associated, ✓✓ = key feature for diagnosis and/or management. ^ = in Indian subcontinent especially, ‡ = mainly reported in Manitoba Hutterites, † = mainly reported in Japanese. CE = important clinical examination findings, FHx = clues from family history, GT = specific genetic test (other tthan full gene sequencing), EMG = Electromyography, IHC = immunohistochemistry, WB = Western blot, SEQ = direct gene sequencing, MRI = magnetic resonance imaging, FIBS = fibroblast culture, + = protein studies assess levels of glycolsylated α-dystroglycan. References: 1(Statland and Tawil 2011), 2(Sorrel-Dejerine and Fardeau 1982), 3(Turner and Hilton-Jones 2010), 4(Bushby, Finkel et al. 2010), 5(Jones and North 1997), 6(Bonne, Mercuri et al. 2000), 7(Emery 1989), 8(Gueneau, Bertrand et al. 2009), 9(Hauser, Horrigan et al. 2000), 10(van der Kooi, van Meegen et al. 1997), 11(Minetti, Sotgia et al. 1998), 12(Fardeau, Hillaire et al. 1996), 13(Piluso, Politano et al. 2005), 14(Bushby, Bashir et al. 1996), 15(Guglieri, Magri et al. 2008), 16(Zatz, de Paula et al. 2003), 17(Azibi, Bachner et al. 1993), 18(Bonnemann, Passos-Bueno et al. 1996), 19(Jones, Kim et al. 1998), 20(Lim, Duclos et al. 1995), 21(Passos-Bueno, Moreira et al. 1996), 22(Moreira, Vainzof et al. 1997), 23(Moreira, Wiltshire et al. 2000), 24(Borg, Stucka et al. 2009), 25(Brockington, Yuva et al. 2001), 26(Udd, Partanen et al. 1993), 27(Bolduc, Marlow et al. 2010), 28(Hicks, Sarkozy et al. 2011), 29(Allamand and Guicheney 2002), 30(Jones, Morgan et al. 2001), 31(North, Specht et al. 1996), 32(Tome 1999), 33(Brockington, Blake et al. 2001), 34(Toda and Kobayashi 1999), 35(Moghadaszadeh, Petit et al. 2001), 36(Bertini and Pepe 2002), 37(Nadeau, Kinali et al. 2009),and 38(Peat, Smith et al. 2008).

Table 2. Discriminating clinical features in genetically characterised muscular dystrophies.

3.2 Muscle pathology

The MDs are characterised by the presence of 'dystrophic' changes on muscle biopsy and one should be cautious about making a diagnosis of a MD if these are not present. The specific pathological features that in combination signify a dystrophy include variation in fibre size, increased internal nuclei, increased connective and adipose tissue, (Norwood, de Visser et al. 2007) and the presence of regenerating and degenerating fibres (see Figure 2). In addition, fibre splitting and inflammatory cell infiltrates are sometimes seen in MDs but are less specific for these disorders. These histological features likely arise from recurrent episodes of muscle fibres necrosis and regeneration that occur because fibres are more prone to damage than normal during muscle contraction (Jones and North 1997; Voit 2001). The relative prominence of different dystrophic features varies depending on the specific type of dystrophy, the age of the patient and the muscle biopsied (since the degree of involvement varies among different muscle groups in different dystrophies).

It is rarely possible to define the genetic cause of a MD from biopsy features alone but the pattern of dystrophic features can provide clues about the diagnosis. For example, dystrophic changes are often mild in the caveolinopathies (Minetti, Sotgia et al. 1998; Waddell, Lemckert et al. 2011), and the laminopathies (Quijano-Roy, Mbieleu et al. 2008; Rankin, Auer-Grumbach et al. 2008) compared to the dystrophinopathies and sarcoglycanopathies (Bonnemann, Passos-Bueno et al. 1996; Eymard, Romero et al. 1997). LGMD2B (dysferlin) (Norwood, de Visser et al. 2007) and LGMD2L (anoctamin-5) (Hicks, Sarkozy et al. 2011) often have an infiltration of inflammatory cells as an additional feature, and patients can be initially misdiagnosed with polymyositis (Norwood, de Visser et al. 2007). Young patients with Ullrich congenital muscular dystrophy (UCMD) (collagen VI) may only show non-specific myopathic changes or congenital fibre type disproportion (CFTD) (Peat, Smith et al. 2008; Schessl, Goemans et al. 2008). Mutations in *SEPN1* can cause various changes on muscle pathology including those resembling CMD, multiminicore disease or CFTD (Ferreiro, Quijano-Roy et al. 2002; Clarke, Kidson et al. 2006). The presence of other pathological abnormalities can be a clue to specific disorders, such as rimmed vacuoles which are associated with LGMD2G (telethonin) (Moreira, Vainzof et al. 1997) and LGMD2J (Udd, Partanen et al. 1993).

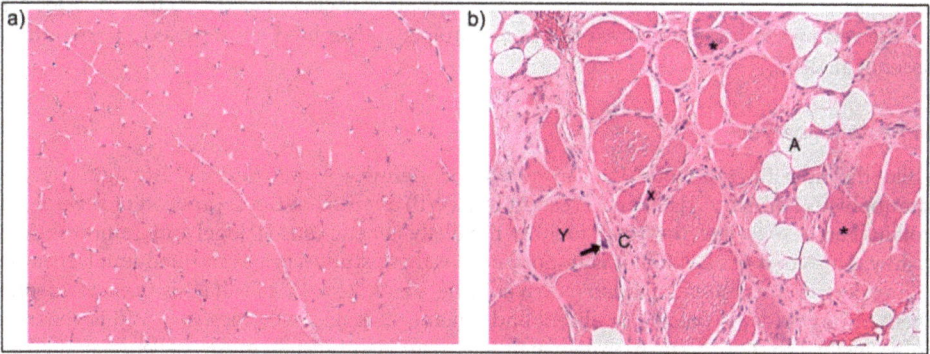

Human muscle in cross section stained with Haematoxylin and Eosin. a) Normal muscle. b) Dystrophic muscle showing a large variation in fibre size with both atrophic (X) and hypertrophic (Y) fibres, increased internal nuclei (*), increased connective (C) and adipose tissue (A) and the presence of regenerating and degenerating fibres (arrow pointing to likely degenerating fibre).

Fig. 2. Healthy and dystrophic human muscle.

3.3 Muscle imaging – MRI and ultrasound

Muscle magnetic resonance imaging has long been used as an adjunct to the diagnosis of inflammatory myopathies, but its usefulness in other neuromuscular disorders is increasingly recognized (Himmrich, Popov et al.). MRI is able to define the pattern of muscle involvement more precisely than clinical examination. Some dystrophies are associated with consistent and relatively specific patterns of abnormality on T1-weighted MRI scans of the thighs, calves and pelvis. For example, muscle MRI of patients with LGMD2I (*FKRP*) and LGMD2A (calpain-3) show marked signal changes in the adductor muscles, posterior thigh muscles and posterior calf muscles, with additional signal changes of medial gastrocnemius and soleus muscles in LGMD2A patients, differentiating these disorders from the other forms of LGMD (Fischer, Walter et al. 2005). Muscle MRI in combination with detailed clinical information and biochemical analysis is now being used increasingly to guide genetic investigations (Mercuri, Pichiecchio et al. 2002; Mercuri, Jungbluth et al. 2005).

Relatively distinct patterns of muscle involvement have also been described for the dystrophinopathies (Lamminen 1990; Lamminen, Tanttu et al. 1990), the sarcoglycanopathies (α, β and γ) (Eymard, Romero et al. 1997; Lodi, Muntoni et al. 1997), dysferlinopathy (Meola, Sansone et al. 1996; Cupler, Bohlega et al. 1998; Suzuki, Aoki et al. 2004; Paradas, Llauger et al. 2010), Bethlem myopathy (Mercuri, Cini et al. 2002; Mercuri, Cini et al. 2003; Mercuri, Lampe et al. 2005), and for mutations in *ANO5* (Hicks, Sarkozy et al. 2011), *LMNA*, *EMD* (Mercuri, Counsell et al. 2002), and *TTN* (Udd, Vihola et al. 2005).

Muscle MRI has been used to direct investigations in older patients with CMD, since distinctive patterns of muscle involvement are described for Ullrich CMD (Mercuri, Cini et al. 2002; Mercuri, Cini et al. 2003; Mercuri, Lampe et al. 2005) and *SEPN1*-related myopathies (Flanigan, Kerr et al. 2000; Mercuri, Talim et al. 2002; Mercuri, Clements et al. 2010). The need for a general anaesthetic to perform an MRI scan on patients less than age 5 years makes it a less attractive investigation for young patients.

Muscle MRI can also assist in choosing an appropriate muscle to biopsy, so that muscles that are affected by the disease process but not completely atrophied are targeted (Norwood, de Visser et al. 2007).

3.4 Protein analysis

While the specific type of MD can rarely be defined from routine histological stains, immunohistochemistry (IHC) and Western blot (WB) analysis of the expression of several MD proteins can be extremely useful to identify the likely genetic cause (Vogel and Zamecnik 2005; Bushby, Norwood et al. 2007). It is important that these studies are performed in a laboratory with expertise in these techniques (Norwood, de Visser et al. 2007). IHC is used to identify whether the protein is present or absent and whether it is normally localised. WB is generally more sensitive to reductions in protein expression but is technically more challenging. IHC has well-established roles in the diagnosis of the CMDs (Peat, Smith et al. 2008), the dystrophinopathies (Bonilla, Samitt et al. 1988; Hoffman, Fischbeck et al. 1988; Jones, Kim et al. 1998) and the sarcoglycanopathies (Vainzof, Passos-Bueno et al. 1996; Bonnemann, Wong et al. 2002) in particular. However, IHC is not helpful in all forms of MD. For example, in some dominant LGMDs such as LGMD1B, lamin A/C staining usually appears normal by IHC (Lo, Cooper et al. 2008). Mild to moderate 'secondary' staining abnormalities can arise in association with a primary abnormality in another protein or due to the disease process itself. Therefore the results of a single stain should always be considered in the context of other IHC results, the clinical situation and ideally protein quantification on Western blot (Ohlendieck, Matsumura et al. 1993; Mizuno, Yoshida et al. 1994; Vainzof, Passos-Bueno et al. 1996; Jones, Kim et al. 1998 (Lo, Cooper et al. 2008). For example, absence of dystrophin in DMD often results in partial loss of staining of other components of the dystrophin-associated protein complex (e.g. the sarcoglycans) and merosin. Reduced or abnormal localisation of dysferlin by IHC occurs in ~45% of all dystrophic muscle biopsies (Lo, Cooper et al. 2008), and it is only the absence of dysferlin by IHC and WB that indicates a primary dysferlinopathy.

Obtaining a muscle biopsy from a patient is an invasive procedure and biopsies are precious resources for both diagnosis and research. The single section WB technique (Cooper, Lo et al. 2003) has been an important advance on traditional methods by significantly reducing the amount of muscle biopsy used for each blot, from 20 - 100 mg down to one 8 μm cryosection. WB analysis has been found to be more effective for diagnosis than IHC for several forms of LGMD, such as LGMD2B (dysferlin) (Vainzof, Anderson et al. 2001; Nguyen, Bassez et al. 2005; Lo, Cooper et al. 2008), LGMD1C (caveolin-3) (Minetti, Sotgia et al. 1998; Carbone, Bruno et al. 2000; Herrmann, Straub et al. 2000; Lo, Cooper et al. 2008) , Becker MD (dystrophin) (Voit, Stuettgen et al. 1991) and arguably the alpha-dystroglycanopathies (Peat, Smith et al. 2008). However the sensitivity and specificity of WB is relatively poor for LGMD2A (calpain-3) (Fanin, Fulizio et al. 2004; Saenz, Leturcq et al. 2005; Groen, Charlton et al. 2007; Lo, Cooper et al. 2008) and the laminopathies (Menezes et al. 2011).

3.5 Genetic analysis

A provisional diagnosis can often be made by considering the clinical information, muscle pathology and protein studies, which can then be confirmed by direct gene sequencing (Bushby, Norwood et al. 2007; Norwood, de Visser et al. 2007). Even with recent advances, it is often difficult to correctly predict the correct LGMD sub-type and several genes may need to be tested before a definitive diagnosis is made. If genetic testing identifies mutations previously published or listed in on-line databases, a firm diagnosis can be made. However, if previously unreported genetic changes are found, then further functional protein studies may be useful to differentiate pathogenic mutations from rare harmless sequence variants.

Even in the best diagnostic centres, establishing a genetic cause for MD is only possible in around 90% of patients. Likely reasons are that the full phenotypic spectrum of many known genes is still being clarified and many MD genes likely remain unidentified. Whole exome or whole genome sequencing and other techniques that capitalise on recent advances in gene sequencing are likely to provide new opportunities to diagnose patients with MD. These approaches also have the capacity to identify new MD disease genes, which may account for many of the currently undiagnosed patients worldwide.

4. Diagnosis in specific forms of muscular dystrophy

4.1 Myotonic dystrophy

Myotonic dystrophy can usually be suspected from clinical examination and family history (see Section 2) and the clinician should have a low threshold for requesting genetic testing for DM1 since it is so common. Electromyography (EMG) is useful for showing characteristic myotonic discharges although these may not be present in young children with DM1 and in the occasional adult patient with DM2. Both DM1 and DM2 are multi-system disorders and involve predisposition to cataracts, cardiac conduction defects, cardiomyopathy, testicular failure and diabetes, as well as myotonia and muscle weakness. In myotonic dystrophy, muscle biopsy histopathology lacks specific diagnostic features but common features include smallness of a particular fibre type (type 1 atrophy in DM1 and type 2 atrophy in DM2), prominent internal nuclei and mild dystrophic changes. Genetic testing for DM1 is widely available and involves assessment of the size of a triplet repeat (CTG) in the *DMPK* gene (normal 5-34 repeats, asymptomatic/premutation 35-49 repeats, mild DM1 phenotype 50-~150, classical DM1 ~100-1000, congenital DM1 > 2000 repeats), (2000; Turner and Hilton-Jones 2010). Repeat numbers correlate only approximately with the severity of the phenotype and a normal genetic test excludes this condition. There is a tendency for the disease severity of DM1 to worsen when inherited by descendents due to further expansion in the size of the *DMPK* gene CTG repeat, a phenomenon called *anticipation*.

DM2 should be considered as a diagnosis if there are strong clinical clues for DM1 in an adult but genetic testing for DM1 is normal. In DM2, proximal limb weakness is more prominent than in DM1, weakness of facial and ankle dorsiflexor muscles may be less prominent and a congenital-onset form has not been described (Turner and Hilton-Jones 2010). Genetic testing for DM2, which is caused by an expansion of a quadruplet repeat (CCTG) the *ZNF9* gene, is technically more challenging and is less widely performed.

4.2 Facioscapulohumeral MD (FSHD)

A diagnosis of FSHD should be suspected when there is prominent (often asymmetric) weakness of muscles of the face, scapular stabilisers, upper arms and ankle dorsiflexor muscles that begins in late childhood to young adulthood on clinical examination (Sorrel-Dejerine and Fardeau 1982). With disease progression many other muscle groups become involved such as neck extensors, abdominal and pelvic muscles. Although FSHD follows an autosomal dominant pattern of inheritance, a negative family history does not exclude the condition as reduced penetrance (~10% especially in women) and *de novo* mutations (~20%) are relatively common. If a diagnosis of FSHD is considered possible on the basis of a clinical examination, genetic testing is the first investigation of choice since muscle biopsy usually shows non-specific dystrophic abnormalities and no protein studies are helpful. FSHD has a complex genetic cause that is not yet fully understood, but is associated with reduced numbers of large scale D4Z4 repeats in the subtelomeric region of chromosome 4. Genetic testing for the 4q deletion is technically challenging and is only 95% sensitive for the condition with the possibility of intermediate results, which are often difficult to interpret. As a result, testing is best conducted in an experienced laboratory, and family studies and the input of a clinical geneticist may assist when results are unclear.

4.3 Duchenne muscular dystrophy (DMD)

The diagnosis of DMD can usually be suspected on the basis of family history, age of onset, and clinical examination. DMD is an X-linked disorder that usually only affects males. Serum CK levels are markedly elevated in all male patients from birth. DMD gene testing using multiplex ligation-dependent probe amplification (MLPA) is a useful preliminary test that detects exon deletions or duplications and is diagnostic in about 75% of DMD patients (and in around 90% of BMD patients). If MLPA is negative, a muscle biopsy is often requested for protein studies. Marked dystrophic features are usually present and absence of dystrophin protein using IHC and/or WB is also diagnostic for DMD (Figure 3). These methods can also be used to detect reduced protein levels or the presence of a truncated protein product in patients with the milder form of the condition, Becker MD (BMD). Dystrophin sequencing may be required to determine point mutations that cannot be detected with MLPA. Around two-thirds of women who have a son with DMD are carriers of the mutation and gonadal mosaicism is relatively common in women who test negative for the mutation in DNA from blood leukocytes. Identifying the mutation causing DMD in

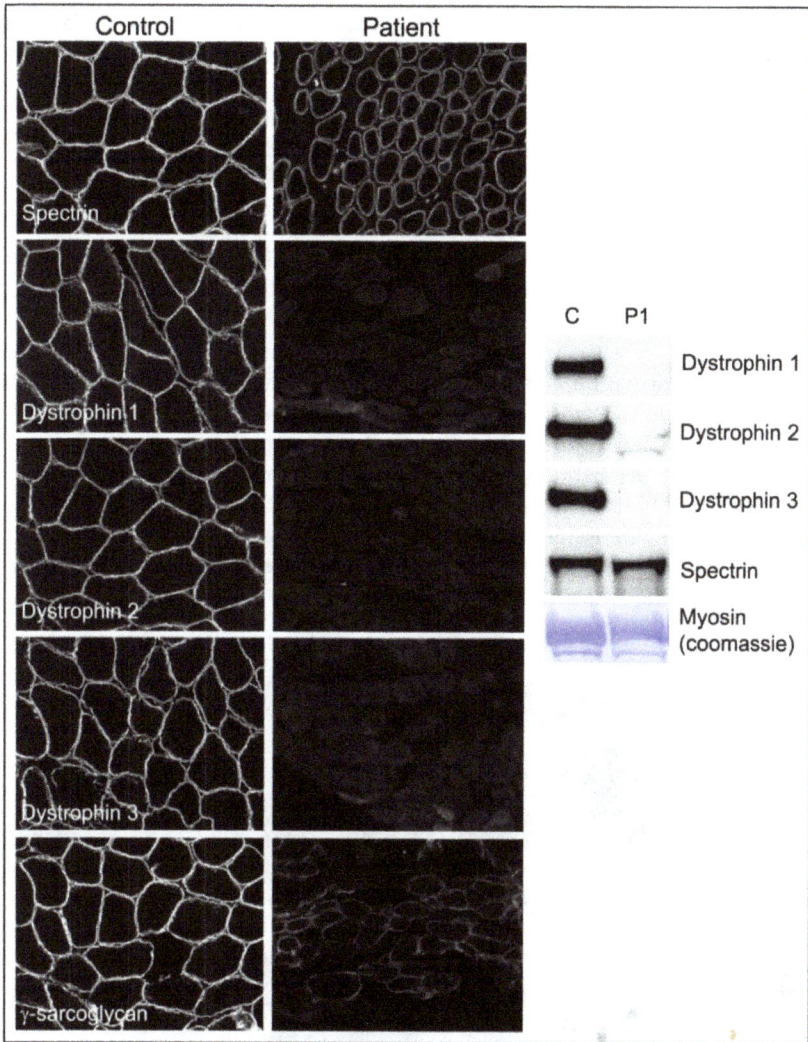

IHC and WB confirm dystrophin-deficiency in a patient with suspected DMD (P1). All patient muscle is stained with spectrin (NCL-SPEC1, Leica Microsystems, Wetzlar, Germany) as a control for membrane integrity. Three antibodies raised to different epitopes spanning the large dystrophin protein are used to help distinguish between total absence of dystrophin (DMD) and reduction or truncation of dystrophin (BMD) (NCL-Dys1, 2 & 3, Leica Microsystems, Wetzlar, Germany). Primary loss of dystrophin can result in secondary reductions in other members of the dystrophin-protein complex (sarcoglycans, dystroglycans) as shown here by a secondary reduction in γ-sarcoglycan (NCL-γ SARC, Leica Microsystems, Wetzlar, Germany), compared to control muscle. Western blot confirms absence of dystrophin protein when probed with the three dystrophin antibodies, strongly suggesting a primary abnormality in dystrophin which was confirmed by DMD gene analysis. Coomassie staining of myosin is used to show that equal amounts of protein are loaded for both patient and control in the WB.

Fig. 3. Immunohistochemistry and Western blot analysis of dystrophin and γ-sarcoglycan in the diagnosis of a patient with DMD.

each family is extremely useful so that highly accurate genetic testing is available for other women in the family who may be at risk of having affected sons. Approximately 10% of females with *DMD* gene mutations will show signs of muscle weakness (manifesting carriers) due to skewing of their ratio of X-chromosome inactivation, but most only become symptomatic during adulthood with mild muscle weakness and/or cardiomyopathy.

4.4 LGMD2B (dysferlinopathy)

A diagnosis of LGMD2B, due to autosomal recessive mutations in the *DYSF* gene, should be considered in patients with muscle weakness that begins in the late teenage years or early adulthood. It is common for *DYSF* patients to present with early involvement of calf muscles (also called Miyoshi myopathy) and difficulty standing on tip-toes. However, some *DYSF* patients present with a classical LGMD pattern of weakness involving the hip and shoulder girdles. Early calf wasting markedly raised serum CK levels (often 5000 – 20 000 U/ml) are distinguishing features of a primary dysferlinopathy, in contrast to many other forms of MD with calf hypertrophy. *DYSF* patient biopsy samples often display a prominent inflammatory cell infiltrate, sometimes leading to misdiagnosis of polymyositis. A range of abnormal dysferlin staining patterns are seen in many types of MD as non-specific secondary abnormalities (see Figure 4b), but complete absence of staining by IHC and WB (Figure 4a) is specific for LGMD2B.

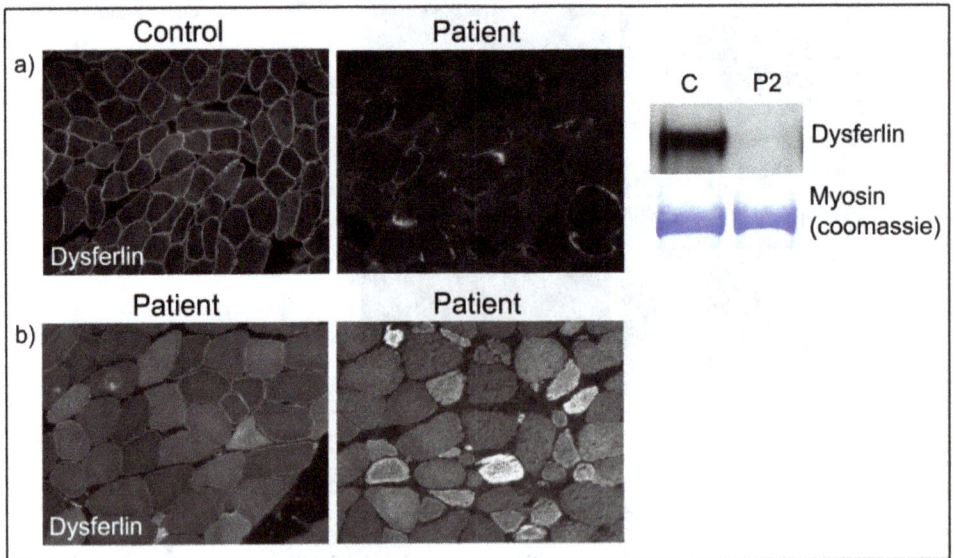

a) IHC of LGMD2B patient muscle shows a severe reduction in dysferlin (NCL-Hamlet, Leica Microsystems) staining at the muscle membrane compared to control muscle, and a corresponding loss of dysferlin by WB (P2). Genetic analysis of this patient confirmed mutations in the *DYSF* gene.
b) Secondary reductions and abnormal dysferlin protein localisation by IHC occur commonly as secondary abnormalities in many dystrophies but absence on WB is specific to dysferlinopathies.

Fig. 4. Immunohistochemistry and Western blot analysis of dysferlin in the diagnosis of LGMD2B.

4.5 LGMD2I

Patients with LGMD2I, due to autosomal recessive mutations in *FKRP*, usually present with a classical LGMD pattern of weakness, often with greater involvement of the lower limbs, and calf hypertrophy. Some patients also have macroglossia (an enlarged tongue) and ankle contractures. α-dystroglycan staining by IHC is usually reduced in LGMD2I patients (see Figure 5), although the reduction may be subtle and is rarely absent. WB can be used to look for reduction of glycosylated α-dystroglycan, which usually appears as a smeared band at ~156 kDa due to variable glycosylation of the core protein which results in a range of final molecular weights (Figure 5). Almost all LGMD2I patients have at least one copy of the c.826C>A (L276I) mutation, a founder mutation that is particularly common in Northern European populations (Walter, Petersen et al. 2004). Severe reductions in α-dystroglycan by IHC and WB can also be associated with other mutations in *FKRP*, or with mutations in the other 'alpha-dystroglycanopathy' genes encoding glycosylation enzymes that result in CMD, WWS or MEB phenotypes (see Table 1).

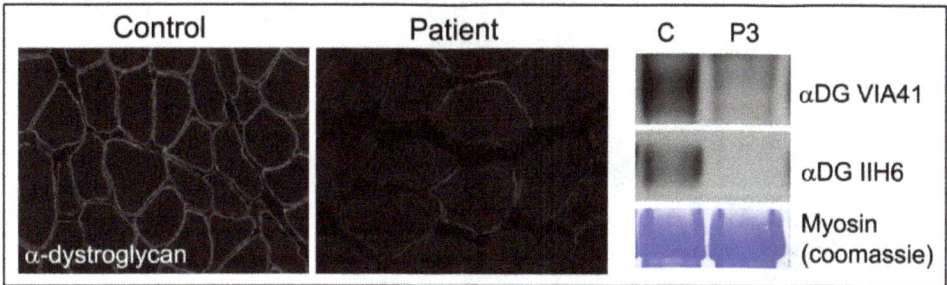

α-dystroglycan levels are reduced by IHC and WB (using both VIA41 (Millipore, CA, USA) and IIH6 (kind gift from Dr Kevin Campbell) antibodies that recognize glycosylated α-dystroglycan, in a number of glycosyltransferase disorders. Specific genetic testing is required to determine the particular genetic cause. In this case the patient was found to have recessive mutations in the *FKRP* gene, causing LGMD2I.

Fig. 5. Immunohistochemistry and Western blot analysis of α-dystroglycan in a patient with LGMD2I.

4.6 Emery-Dreifuss muscular dystrophy (EDMD)

EDMD should be suspected in patients who develop early joint contractures, particularly of the elbows, neck extensors and tendo-Achilles. Patients present with progressive muscle weakness and wasting particularly of the upper arm and ankle dorsiflexor muscles, and often develop cardiac abnormalities (heart block, arrhythmias or cardiomyopathy). Mutations in three genes are associated with this phenotype, *LMNA* (which follows autosomal dominant inheritance), *EMD* and *FHL1* (both X-linked genes), but further genetic causes are likely. IHC for emerin in skeletal muscle shows from the nuclear envelope in X-linked EDMD due to *EMD* mutations and is specific for this condition (see Figure 6). Emerin is also completely absent by WB in these patients (Figure 6). Finding mutations on *EMD* gene sequencing confirms the diagnosis and allows for carrier testing of at-risk females. There are no robust protein-based screening tests for *LMNA* mutations and direct sequencing is required to exclude the diagnosis. Clinicians should have a low threshold for testing both the *EMD* and *LMNA* genes if a diagnosis of EDMD is possible, due to the risk of developing potentially lethal cardic arrhythmias. Early diagnosis allows for introduction of close cardiac surveillance by electrocardiogram (ECG), Holter ambulatory ECG monitoring, echocardiography and the early use of implantable cardiac defibrillators to reduce morbidity and mortality.

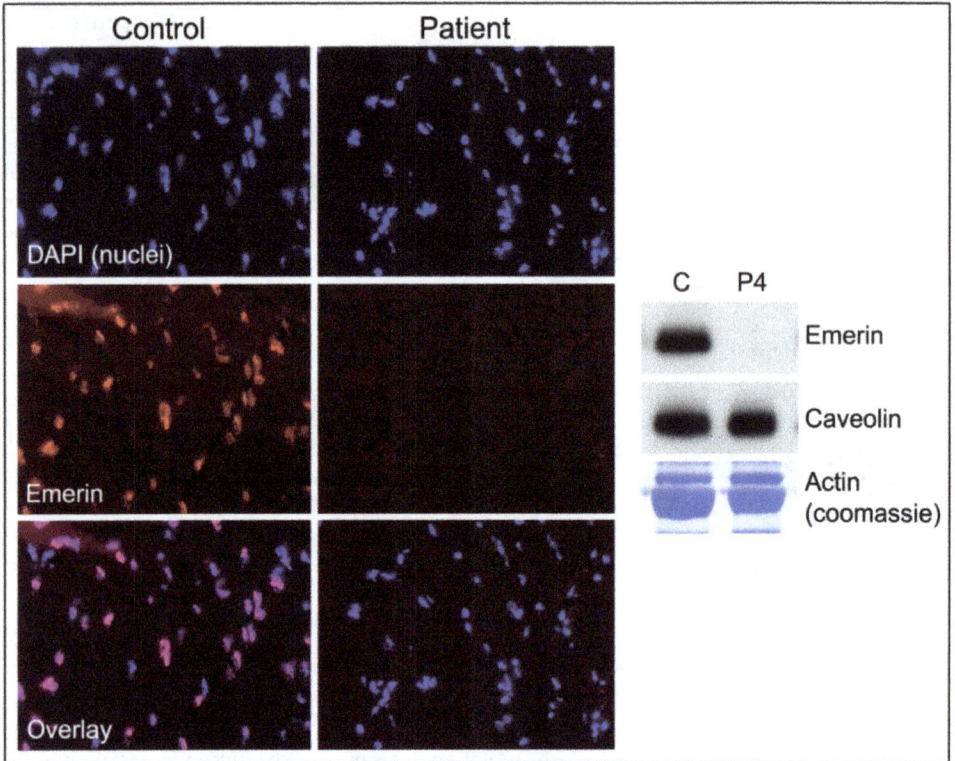

Examples of Emerin immunostaining is absent from the nuclear envelope in muscle from a patient with X-linked EDMD (nuclei are stained by DAPI (4',6-diamidino-2-phenylindole, dihydrochloride), Invitrogen, CA, USA). WB analysis shows absent staining for emerin (P4), and a genetic mutation (c.651_655dupGGGCC) was later identified. Immunoblot for caveolin-3 and coomassie staining of actin are used to show equal protein loading.

Fig. 6. Immunohistochemistry and Western blot analysis of emerin in the diagnosis of EDMD.

4.7 Ullrich congenital muscular dystrophy (UCMD) and Bethlem myopathy

Patients with UCMD usually present with generalised muscle weakness, wasting, hypotonia and marked distal laxity from birth (Nonaka, Une et al. 1981; De Paillette, Aicardi et al. 1989; Mercuri, Yuva et al. 2002). Clinically, patients often have a distinctive sandpaper-like skin rash, congenital hip dislocation, scoliosis, a high arched palate and prominent heels. IHC is a useful diagnostic test, and staining of muscle sections with collagen VI in combination with a muscle membrane marker, e.g. perlecan or collagen IV, can highlight a characteristic loss of collagen VI at the muscle membranes even though collagen VI staining may be retained in connective tissue between fibres (Figure 7). Reduced secretion of collagen VI by cultured

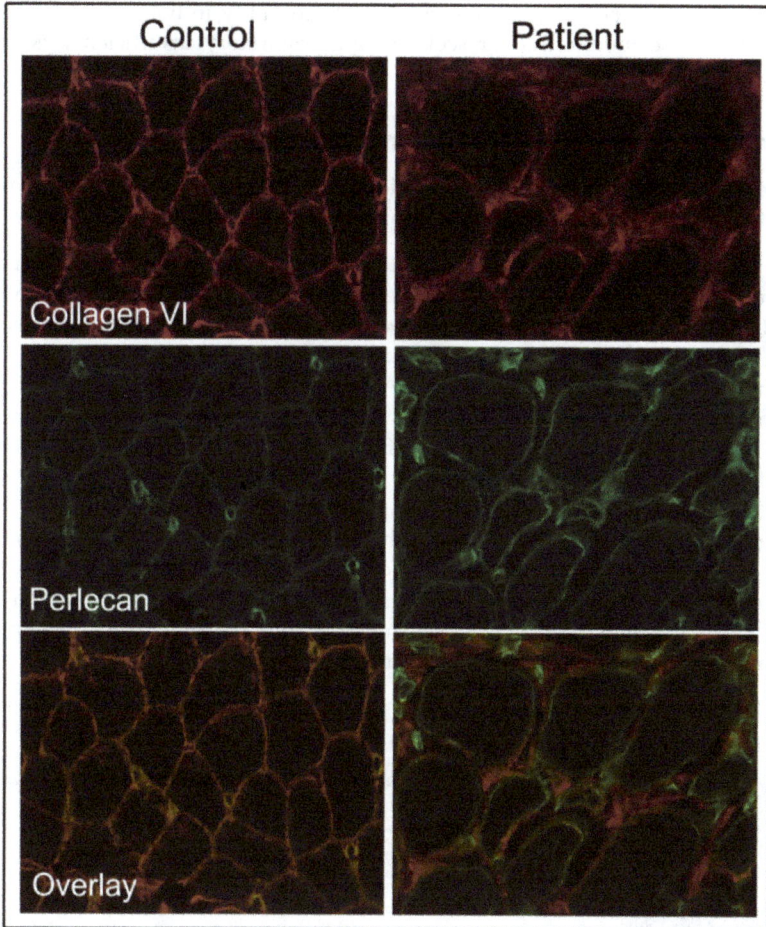

In UCMD and Bethlem myopathy, collagen VI is reduced or lost at the plasma membrane of muscle fibres but may be present in interstitial connective tissue. After carefully optimising conditions to achieve equal intensity of collagen VI (70-XR95, Fitzgerald Industries International Inc, MA, USA) and perlecan (A7L6, MAB1948, Miilipore, CA, USA) staining in control muscle, an overlay image can identify a reduction in collagen VI, relative to perlecan, at the muscle sarcolemmal membrane. In this example, an overlay image from control muscle appears mostly yellow/orange, with broadly equal intensities of perlecan (green) and collagen VI (red) staining. In contrast, an overlay image from a UCMD patient, reveals a dominance of perlecan (green labelling), indicating a relative deficiency of collagen VI (red label) at the muscle membrane. These results are consistent with a primary collagenopathy, and a dominant mutation was identified in the *COL6A2* gene.

Fig. 7. Immunohistochemistry analysis of collagen VI in the diagnosis of UCMD.

patient fibroblasts strongly supports a diagnosis of UCMD or Bethlem myopathy but genetic testing of the three genes that code for collagen VI chains (see Table 1) is required to confirm the diagnosis. Collagen VI gene mutations that do not result in severe protein abnormalities usually present in childhood with a less severe phenotype called Bethlem myopathy.

Progressive joint contractures are major sources of morbidity in both UCMD and Bethlem myopathy and close monitoring for scoliosis and respiratory insufficiency is important, particularly in UCMD.

5. Frequency of diagnosis of less common types of MD

The frequency of some forms of MD varies widely in different parts of the world, which can influence the most appropriate diagnostic approach to follow in different countries.

LGMD2A accounted for 50% of all LGMD patients in a Turkish study (Dincer, Leturcq et al. 1997), around 25% of patients in Italy (Guglieri, Magri et al. 2008; Fanin, Nascimbeni et al. 2009) and the United Kingdom (UK) (Norwood, Harling et al. 2009) but only 5-8% in American (Moore, Shilling et al. 2006), Brazilian (Vainzof, Passos-Bueno et al. 1999) and Australian (Lo, Cooper et al. 2008) studies. Although different diagnostic techniques may account for some of the variability, this finding points to major regional differences in the frequency of *CAPN3* gene mutations in different populations. Similarly LGMD2I seems particularly prevalent in Scandinavia (Sveen, Schwartz et al. 2006) and the UK (Norwood, Harling et al. 2009) compared with other populations (see Table 3). High rates of known genetic forms of LGMD likely contribute to a high overall rate of LGMD diagnosis in Turkey (Dincer, Leturcq et al. 1997), the UK (Norwood, Harling et al. 2009) and Denmark (Sveen, Schwartz et al. 2006). The rates identified for many forms of LGMD are similar in Australia (Lo, Cooper et al. 2008) to the USA (Moore, Shilling et al. 2006) and it is interesting that both populations are comprised of a mixture of ethnicities.

	LGMD								Total Diagnosis
	1A	1B	1C	2A	2B	2C,D,E,F	2G	2I	
Denmark [1]	NA	NA	NA	12%	2%	22%	NA	37%	73%
Turkey [2]	NA	NA	NA	50%	5%	20%	NA	NA	75%
Italy [3]	0%	0%	1.3%	28%	19%	18%	0%	6%	73%
Northern England [4]		9%		26%	6%	12%		19%	72%
USA [5]	0.6%	7%	0%	9%	3%	19%	NA	7%	46%
Italy [6]	NA	1%	1.5%	19%	8%	11%	NA	3%	43%
Brazil [7]	NA	NA	NA	5%	3%	17%	NA	NA	24%
Australia [8]	NA	1%	2.6%	8%	5%	2.6%	NA	2.6%	23%
Brazil [9]	NA	NA	NA	32%	22%	32%	3%	11%	N/A

LGMD = limb-girdle muscular dystrophy. NA = not assessed, N/A = retrospective review, no total diagnosis stated. References: 1(Sveen, Schwartz et al. 2006), 2(Dincer, Leturcq et al. 1997), 3(Guglieri, Magri et al. 2008), 4(Norwood, Harling et al. 2009), 5(Moore, Shilling et al. 2006), 6(Fanin, Nascimbeni et al. 2009), 7(Vainzof, Passos-Bueno et al. 1999), 8(Lo, Cooper et al. 2008) and 9(Zatz, de Paula et al. 2003).

Table 3. Diagnoses in LGMD cohort studies.

As for LGMD, the proportions of some forms of CMD have varied widely between studies in different countries. A Brazilian study diagnosed merosin-deficiency in around 40% of CMD patients (Ferreira, Marie et al. 2005), while this diagnosis accounted for only 8% of CMD patients in an Australian study (Peat, Smith et al. 2008). Differences in CMD ascertainment criteria may be partly responsible but it is likely there are true differences in disease incidence in different populations. Similarly, different rates of collagen VI diagnoses have been observed, ranging from 8% in Australia (Peat, Smith et al. 2008) to 1.7% in Brazil (Ferreira, Marie et al. 2005).

6. Future directions

In the past, genetic testing for MD has involved the sequencing of individual genes that were considered likely causes based on clinical presentation and screening tests. The large number of possible genetic causes with overlapping phenotypes has made it difficult to predict the correct genetic cause in many MD patients and consequently, finding the causative mutation in many families has often been a prolonged, expensive exercise. Recent advances in gene sequencing are likely to have a major impact on the diagnosis of MD in the near future. It is now possible to sequence multiple muscle disease genes and even the whole genome relatively cheaply in a single experiment (Metzker 2010). Next generation sequencing technologies will also facilitate the discovery of new MD genes, leading to increased rates of patient diagnosis. As thesetechnologies become more routinely used and costs reduce, the approach to diagnosing forms of MD such as, LGMD, that have many possible genetic causes is likely to move from the sequencing of individual candidate genes towards a multi-gene or genome-wide sequencing approach. Some diagnostic centres worldwide are already implementing this technology for the diagnosis of MDs. These methods bring new challenges, such as distinguishing genetic sequence variants that are the primary cause of the disease from variants that modify a phenotype or are harmless polymorphisms. It is likely that there will always be a need for centres with expertise in clinical phenotyping and protein studies to clarify the diagnosis when genetic analysis alone cannot confirm whether a sequence variant in a gene is truly disease-causing or not.

7. Glossary

BMD   Becker muscular dystrophy
CK   Creatine kinase
CMD   Congenital muscular dystrophy
DMD   Duchenne muscular dystrophy
DM   Myotonic dystrophy (DM1 Type 1, DM2 Type 2)
ECG   Electrocardiogram
EDMD   Emery Dreifuss muscular dystrophy
FCMD   Fukuyama congenital muscular dystrophy
FSHD   Facioscapulohumeral muscular dystrophy
IHC   Immunohistochemistry
LGMD   Limb girdle muscular dystrophy (Type 1 dominant, Type 2 recessive)
MD   Muscular dystrophy
MEB   Muscle-eye-brain disease
MLPA   Multiplex Ligation-dependent Probe Amplification
MRI   Magnetic resonance imaging
UCMD   Ullrich congenital muscular dystrophy
UK   United Kingdom
WB   Western blot
WWS   Walker-Warburg Syndrome

8. References

(2000). "New nomenclature and DNA testing guidelines for myotonic dystrophy type 1 (DM1). The International Myotonic Dystrophy Consortium (IDMC)." *Neurology* 54(6): 1218-1221.

Allamand, V. and P. Guicheney (2002). "Merosin-deficient congenital muscular dystrophy, autosomal recessive (MDC1A, MIM#156225, LAMA2 gene coding for alpha2 chain of laminin)." *Eur J Hum Genet* 10(2): 91-94.

Azibi, K., L. Bachner, et al. (1993). "Severe childhood autosomal recessive muscular dystrophy with the deficiency of the 50 kDa dystrophin-associated glycoprotein maps to chromosome 13q12." *Hum Mol Genet* 2(9): 1423-1428.

Balci, B., G. Uyanik, et al. (2005). "An autosomal recessive limb girdle muscular dystrophy (LGMD2) with mild mental retardation is allelic to Walker-Warburg syndrome (WWS) caused by a mutation in the POMT1 gene." *Neuromuscul Disord* 15(4): 271-275.

Bashir, R., S. Britton, et al. (1998). "A gene related to Caenorhabditis elegans spermatogenesis factor fer-1 is mutated in limb-girdle muscular dystrophy type 2B." *Nat Genet* 20(1): 37-42.

Beltran-Valero de Bernabe, D., S. Currier, et al. (2002). "Mutations in the O-mannosyltransferase gene POMT1 give rise to the severe neuronal migration disorder Walker-Warburg syndrome." *Am J Hum Genet* 71(5): 1033-1043.

Beltran-Valero de Bernabe, D., T. Voit, et al. (2004). "Mutations in the FKRP gene can cause muscle-eye-brain disease and Walker-Warburg syndrome." *J Med Genet* 41(5): e61.

Bertini, E. and G. Pepe (2002). "Collagen type VI and related disorders: Bethlem myopathy and Ullrich scleroatonic muscular dystrophy." *Eur J Paediatr Neurol* 6(4): 193-198.

Biancheri, R., A. Falace, et al. (2007). "POMT2 gene mutation in limb-girdle muscular dystrophy with inflammatory changes." *Biochem Biophys Res Commun* 363(4): 1033-1037.

Bione, S., E. Maestrini, et al. (1994). "Identification of a novel X-linked gene responsible for Emery-Dreifuss muscular dystrophy." *Nat Genet* 8(4): 323-327.

Bolduc, V., G. Marlow, et al. (2010). "Recessive mutations in the putative calcium-activated chloride channel Anoctamin 5 cause proximal LGMD2L and distal MMD3 muscular dystrophies." *Am J Hum Genet* 86(2): 213-221.

Bonilla, E., C. E. Samitt, et al. (1988). "Duchenne muscular dystrophy: deficiency of dystrophin at the muscle cell surface." *Cell* 54(4): 447-452.

Bonne, G., M. R. Di Barletta, et al. (1999). "Mutations in the gene encoding lamin A/C cause autosomal dominant Emery-Dreifuss muscular dystrophy." *Nat Genet* 21(3): 285-288.

Bonne, G., E. Mercuri, et al. (2000). "Clinical and molecular genetic spectrum of autosomal dominant Emery-Dreifuss muscular dystrophy due to mutations of the lamin A/C gene." *Ann Neurol* 48(2): 170-180.

Bonnemann, C. G., M. R. Passos-Bueno, et al. (1996). "Genomic screening for beta-sarcoglycan gene mutations: missense mutations may cause severe limb-girdle muscular dystrophy type 2E (LGMD 2E)." *Hum Mol Genet* 5(12): 1953-1961.

Bonnemann, C. G., J. Wong, et al. (2002). "Primary gamma-sarcoglycanopathy (LGMD 2C): broadening of the mutational spectrum guided by the immunohistochemical profile." *Neuromuscul Disord* 12(3): 273-280.

Borg, K., R. Stucka, et al. (2009). "Intragenic deletion of TRIM32 in compound heterozygotes with sarcotubular myopathy/LGMD2H." *Hum Mutat*.

Brais, B., J. P. Bouchard, et al. (1998). "Short GCG expansions in the PABP2 gene cause oculopharyngeal muscular dystrophy." *Nat Genet* 18(2): 164-167.

Brais, B., Y. G. Xie, et al. (1995). "The oculopharyngeal muscular dystrophy locus maps to the region of the cardiac alpha and beta myosin heavy chain genes on chromosome 14q11.2-q13." *Hum Mol Genet* 4(3): 429-434.

Brockington, M., D. J. Blake, et al. (2001). "Mutations in the fukutin-related protein gene (FKRP) cause a form of congenital muscular dystrophy with secondary laminin alpha2 deficiency and abnormal glycosylation of alpha-dystroglycan." *Am J Hum Genet* 69(6): 1198-1209.

Brockington, M., C. A. Sewry, et al. (2000). "Assignment of a form of congenital muscular dystrophy with secondary merosin deficiency to chromosome 1q42." *Am J Hum Genet* 66(2): 428-435.

Brockington, M., Y. Yuva, et al. (2001). "Mutations in the fukutin-related protein gene (FKRP) identify limb girdle muscular dystrophy 2I as a milder allelic variant of congenital muscular dystrophy MDC1C." *Hum Mol Genet* 10(25): 2851-2859.

Brook, J. D., M. E. McCurrach, et al. (1992). "Molecular basis of myotonic dystrophy: expansion of a trinucleotide (CTG) repeat at the 3' end of a transcript encoding a protein kinase family member." *Cell* 68(4): 799-808.

Burghes, A. H., C. Logan, et al. (1987). "A cDNA clone from the Duchenne/Becker muscular dystrophy gene." *Nature* 328(6129): 434-437.

Bushby, K., R. Bashir, et al. (1996). "The molecular biology of LGMD2B--towards the identification of the LGMD gene on chromosome 2p13." *Neuromuscul Disord* 6(6): 491-492.

Bushby, K., R. Finkel, et al. (2010). "Diagnosis and management of Duchenne muscular dystrophy, part 1: diagnosis, and pharmacological and psychosocial management." *Lancet Neurol* 9(1): 77-93.

Bushby, K., F. Norwood, et al. (2007). "The limb-girdle muscular dystrophies--diagnostic strategies." *Biochim Biophys Acta* 1772(2): 238-242.

Camacho Vanegas, O., E. Bertini, et al. (2001). "Ullrich scleroatonic muscular dystrophy is caused by recessive mutations in collagen type VI." *Proc Natl Acad Sci U S A* 98(13): 7516-7521.

Carbone, I., C. Bruno, et al. (2000). "Mutation in the CAV3 gene causes partial caveolin-3 deficiency and hyperCKemia." *Neurology* 54(6): 1373-1376.

Clarke, N. F., W. Kidson, et al. (2006). "SEPN1: associated with congenital fiber-type disproportion and insulin resistance." *Ann Neurol* 59(3): 546-552.

Cooper, S. T., H. P. Lo, et al. (2003). "Single section Western blot: improving the molecular diagnosis of the muscular dystrophies." *Neurology* 61(1): 93-97.

Cupler, E. J., S. Bohlega, et al. (1998). "Miyoshi myopathy in Saudi Arabia: clinical, electrophysiological, histopathological and radiological features." *Neuromuscul Disord* 8(5): 321-326.

de Bernabe, D. B., H. van Bokhoven, et al. (2003). "A homozygous nonsense mutation in the fukutin gene causes a Walker-Warburg syndrome phenotype." *J Med Genet* 40(11): 845-848.

De Paillette, L., J. Aicardi, et al. (1989). "Ullrich's congenital atonic sclerotic muscular dystrophy. A case report." *J Neurol* 236(2): 108-110.

Demir, E., P. Sabatelli, et al. (2002). "Mutations in COL6A3 cause severe and mild phenotypes of Ullrich congenital muscular dystrophy." *Am J Hum Genet* 70(6): 1446-1458.

Dincer, P., F. Leturcq, et al. (1997). "A biochemical, genetic, and clinical survey of autosomal recessive limb girdle muscular dystrophies in Turkey." *Ann Neurol* 42(2): 222-229.

Driss, A., R. Amouri, et al. (2000). "A new locus for autosomal recessive limb-girdle muscular dystrophy in a large consanguineous Tunisian family maps to chromosome 19q13.3." *Neuromuscul Disord* 10(4-5): 240-246.

Emery, A. E. (1989). "Emery-Dreifuss syndrome." *J Med Genet* 26(10): 637-641.

Eymard, B., N. B. Romero, et al. (1997). "Primary adhalinopathy (alpha-sarcoglycanopathy): clinical, pathologic, and genetic correlation in 20 patients with autosomal recessive muscular dystrophy." *Neurology* 48(5): 1227-1234.

Fanin, M., L. Fulizio, et al. (2004). "Molecular diagnosis in LGMD2A: mutation analysis or protein testing?" *Hum Mutat* 24(1): 52-62.

Fanin, M., A. C. Nascimbeni, et al. (2009). "Frequency of LGMD gene mutations in Italian patients with distinct clinical phenotypes." *Neurology* 72(16): 1432-1435.

Fardeau, M., D. Hillaire, et al. (1996). "Juvenile limb-girdle muscular dystrophy. Clinical, histopathological and genetic data from a small community living in the Reunion Island." *Brain* 119 (Pt 1): 295-308.

Ferreira, L. G., S. K. Marie, et al. (2005). "Dystrophin-glycoproteins associated in congenital muscular dystrophy: immunohistochemical analysis of 59 Brazilian cases." *Arq Neuropsiquiatr* 63(3B): 791-800.

Ferreiro, A., S. Quijano-Roy, et al. (2002). "Mutations of the selenoprotein N gene, which is implicated in rigid spine muscular dystrophy, cause the classical phenotype of multiminicore disease: reassessing the nosology of early-onset myopathies." *Am J Hum Genet* 71(4): 739-749.

Fischer, D., M. C. Walter, et al. (2005). "Diagnostic value of muscle MRI in differentiating LGMD2I from other LGMDs." *J Neurol* 252(5): 538-547.

Flanigan, K. M., L. Kerr, et al. (2000). "Congenital muscular dystrophy with rigid spine syndrome: a clinical, pathological, radiological, and genetic study." *Ann Neurol* 47(2): 152-161.

Frosk, P., T. Weiler, et al. (2002). "Limb-girdle muscular dystrophy type 2H associated with mutation in TRIM32, a putative E3-ubiquitin-ligase gene." *Am J Hum Genet* 70(3): 663-672.

Giusti, B., L. Lucarini, et al. (2005). "Dominant and recessive COL6A1 mutations in Ullrich scleroatonic muscular dystrophy." *Ann Neurol* 58(3): 400-410.

Godfrey, C., E. Clement, et al. (2007). "Refining genotype phenotype correlations in muscular dystrophies with defective glycosylation of dystroglycan." *Brain* 130(Pt 10): 2725-2735.

Godfrey, C., D. Escolar, et al. (2006). "Fukutin gene mutations in steroid-responsive limb girdle muscular dystrophy." *Ann Neurol* 60(5): 603-610.

Groen, E. J., R. Charlton, et al. (2007). "Analysis of the UK diagnostic strategy for limb girdle muscular dystrophy 2A." *Brain* 130(Pt 12): 3237-3249.

Gueneau, L., A. T. Bertrand, et al. (2009). "Mutations of the FHL1 gene cause Emery-Dreifuss muscular dystrophy." *Am J Hum Genet* 85(3): 338-353.

Guglieri, M. and K. Bushby (2008). "How to go about diagnosing and managing the limb-girdle muscular dystrophies." *Neurol India* 56(3): 271-280.

Guglieri, M., F. Magri, et al. (2008). "Clinical, molecular, and protein correlations in a large sample of genetically diagnosed Italian limb girdle muscular dystrophy patients." *Hum Mutat* 29(2): 258-266.

Hackman, P., A. Vihola, et al. (2002). "Tibial muscular dystrophy is a titinopathy caused by mutations in TTN, the gene encoding the giant skeletal-muscle protein titin." *Am J Hum Genet* 71(3): 492-500.

Hauser, M. A., S. K. Horrigan, et al. (2000). "Myotilin is mutated in limb girdle muscular dystrophy 1A." *Hum Mol Genet* 9(14): 2141-2147.

Hayashi, Y. K., F. L. Chou, et al. (1998). "Mutations in the integrin alpha7 gene cause congenital myopathy." *Nat Genet* 19(1): 94-97.

Hayashi, Y. K., C. Matsuda, et al. (2009). "Human PTRF mutations cause secondary deficiency of caveolins resulting in muscular dystrophy with generalized lipodystrophy." *J Clin Invest* 119(9): 2623-2633.

Helbling-Leclerc, A., X. Zhang, et al. (1995). "Mutations in the laminin alpha 2-chain gene (LAMA2) cause merosin-deficient congenital muscular dystrophy." *Nat Genet* 11(2): 216-218.

Herrmann, R., V. Straub, et al. (2000). "Dissociation of the dystroglycan complex in caveolin-3-deficient limb girdle muscular dystrophy." *Hum Mol Genet* 9(15): 2335-2340.

Hicks, D., A. Sarkozy, et al. (2011). "A founder mutation in Anoctamin 5 is a major cause of limb-girdle muscular dystrophy." *Brain* 134(Pt 1): 171-182.

Higuchi, I., T. Shiraishi, et al. (2001). "Frameshift mutation in the collagen VI gene causes Ullrich's disease." *Ann Neurol* 50(2): 261-265.

Hillaire, D., A. Leclerc, et al. (1994). "Localization of merosin-negative congenital muscular dystrophy to chromosome 6q2 by homozygosity mapping." *Hum Mol Genet* 3(9): 1657-1661.

Himmrich, E., S. Popov, et al. (2000). "[Hidden intracardiac conduction disturbances and their spontaneous course in patients with progressive muscular dystrophy]." *Z Kardiol* 89(7): 592-598.

Hoffman, E. P., R. H. Brown, Jr., et al. (1987). "Dystrophin: the protein product of the Duchenne muscular dystrophy locus." *Cell* 51(6): 919-928.

Hoffman, E. P., K. H. Fischbeck, et al. (1988). "Characterization of dystrophin in muscle-biopsy specimens from patients with Duchenne's or Becker's muscular dystrophy." *N Engl J Med* 318(21): 1363-1368.

Jobsis, G. J., H. Keizers, et al. (1996). "Type VI collagen mutations in Bethlem myopathy, an autosomal dominant myopathy with contractures." *Nat Genet* 14(1): 113-115.

Jones, K. J., S. S. Kim, et al. (1998). "Abnormalities of dystrophin, the sarcoglycans, and laminin alpha2 in the muscular dystrophies." *J Med Genet* 35(5): 379-386.

Jones, K. J., G. Morgan, et al. (2001). "The expanding phenotype of laminin alpha2 chain (merosin) abnormalities: case series and review." *J Med Genet* 38(10): 649-657.

Jones, K. J. and K. N. North (1997). "Recent advances in diagnosis of the childhood muscular dystrophies." *J Paediatr Child Health* 33(3): 195-201.

Kaplan, J. C. (2010). "The 2011 version of the gene table of neuromuscular disorders." *Neuromuscul Disord* 20(12): 852-873.

Kobayashi, K., Y. Nakahori, et al. (1998). "An ancient retrotransposal insertion causes Fukuyama-type congenital muscular dystrophy." *Nature* 394(6691): 388-392.

Koenig, M., E. P. Hoffman, et al. (1987). "Complete cloning of the Duchenne muscular dystrophy (DMD) cDNA and preliminary genomic organization of the DMD gene in normal and affected individuals." *Cell* 50(3): 509-517.

Koenig, M., A. P. Monaco, et al. (1988). "The complete sequence of dystrophin predicts a rod-shaped cytoskeletal protein." *Cell* 53(2): 219-228.

Lamminen, A. E. (1990). "Magnetic resonance imaging of primary skeletal muscle diseases: patterns of distribution and severity of involvement." *Br J Radiol* 63(756): 946-950.

Lamminen, A. E., J. I. Tanttu, et al. (1990). "Magnetic resonance of diseased skeletal muscle: combined T1 measurement and chemical shift imaging." *Br J Radiol* 63(752): 591-596.

Lim, L. E., F. Duclos, et al. (1995). "Beta-sarcoglycan: characterization and role in limb-girdle muscular dystrophy linked to 4q12." *Nat Genet* 11(3): 257-265.

Liquori, C. L., K. Ricker, et al. (2001). "Myotonic dystrophy type 2 caused by a CCTG expansion in intron 1 of ZNF9." *Science* 293(5531): 864-867.

Liu, J., M. Aoki, et al. (1998). "Dysferlin, a novel skeletal muscle gene, is mutated in Miyoshi myopathy and limb girdle muscular dystrophy." *Nat Genet* 20(1): 31-36.

Lo, H. P., S. T. Cooper, et al. (2008). "Limb-girdle muscular dystrophy: diagnostic evaluation, frequency and clues to pathogenesis." *Neuromuscul Disord* 18(1): 34-44.

Lodi, R., F. Muntoni, et al. (1997). "Correlative MR imaging and 31P-MR spectroscopy study in sarcoglycan deficient limb girdle muscular dystrophy." *Neuromuscul Disord* 7(8): 505-511.

Longman, C., M. Brockington, et al. (2003). "Mutations in the human LARGE gene cause MDC1D, a novel form of congenital muscular dystrophy with severe mental retardation and abnormal glycosylation of alpha-dystroglycan." *Hum Mol Genet* 12(21): 2853-2861.

McNally, E. M., E. de Sa Moreira, et al. (1998). "Caveolin-3 in muscular dystrophy." *Hum Mol Genet* 7(5): 871-877.

McNally, E. M. and P. Pytel (2007). "Muscle diseases: the muscular dystrophies." *Annu Rev Pathol* 2: 87-109.

Menezes, M.P., L.B. Waddell, et al. (2011) "The importance and challenge of making an early diagnosis in LMNA-related muscular dystrophy." *Neurol.* (Accepted 14th Dec 2011).

Meola, G., V. Sansone, et al. (1996). "Computerized tomography and magnetic resonance muscle imaging in Miyoshi's myopathy." *Muscle Nerve* 19(11): 1476-1480.

Mercuri, E., C. Cini, et al. (2002). "Muscle MRI findings in a three-generation family affected by Bethlem myopathy." *Eur J Paediatr Neurol* 6(6): 309-314.

Mercuri, E., C. Cini, et al. (2003). "Muscle magnetic resonance imaging in patients with congenital muscular dystrophy and Ullrich phenotype." *Neuromuscul Disord* 13(7-8): 554-558.

Mercuri, E., E. Clements, et al. (2010). "Muscle magnetic resonance imaging involvement in muscular dystrophies with rigidity of the spine." *Ann Neurol* 67(2): 201-208.

Mercuri, E., S. Counsell, et al. (2002). "Selective muscle involvement on magnetic resonance imaging in autosomal dominant Emery-Dreifuss muscular dystrophy." *Neuropediatrics* 33(1): 10-14.

Mercuri, E., A. D'Amico, et al. (2006). "POMT2 mutation in a patient with 'MEB-like' phenotype." *Neuromuscul Disord* 16(7): 446-448.

Mercuri, E., H. Jungbluth, et al. (2005). "Muscle imaging in clinical practice: diagnostic value of muscle magnetic resonance imaging in inherited neuromuscular disorders." *Curr Opin Neurol* 18(5): 526-537.

Mercuri, E., A. Lampe, et al. (2005). "Muscle MRI in Ullrich congenital muscular dystrophy and Bethlem myopathy." *Neuromuscul Disord* 15(4): 303-310.

Mercuri, E., A. Pichiecchio, et al. (2002). "A short protocol for muscle MRI in children with muscular dystrophies." *Eur J Paediatr Neurol* 6(6): 305-307.

Mercuri, E., B. Talim, et al. (2002). "Clinical and imaging findings in six cases of congenital muscular dystrophy with rigid spine syndrome linked to chromosome 1p (RSMD1)." Neuromuscul Disord 12(7-8): 631-638.

Mercuri, E., Y. Yuva, et al. (2002). "Collagen VI involvement in Ullrich syndrome: a clinical, genetic, and immunohistochemical study." Neurology 58(9): 1354-1359.

Messina, D. N., M. C. Speer, et al. (1997). "Linkage of familial dilated cardiomyopathy with conduction defect and muscular dystrophy to chromosome 6q23." Am J Hum Genet 61(4): 909-917.

Metzker, M. L. (2010). "Sequencing technologies - the next generation." Nat Rev Genet 11(1): 31-46.

Minetti, C., F. Sotgia, et al. (1998). "Mutations in the caveolin-3 gene cause autosomal dominant limb-girdle muscular dystrophy." Nat Genet 18(4): 365-368.

Moghadaszadeh, B., I. Desguerre, et al. (1998). "Identification of a new locus for a peculiar form of congenital muscular dystrophy with early rigidity of the spine, on chromosome 1p35-36." Am J Hum Genet 62(6): 1439-1445.

Moghadaszadeh, B., N. Petit, et al. (2001). "Mutations in SEPN1 cause congenital muscular dystrophy with spinal rigidity and restrictive respiratory syndrome." Nat Genet 29(1): 17-18.

Monaco, A. P., R. L. Neve, et al. (1986). "Isolation of candidate cDNAs for portions of the Duchenne muscular dystrophy gene." Nature 323(6089): 646-650.

Moore, S. A., C. J. Shilling, et al. (2006). "Limb-girdle muscular dystrophy in the United States." J Neuropathol Exp Neurol 65(10): 995-1003.

Moreira, E. S., M. Vainzof, et al. (1997). "The seventh form of autosomal recessive limb-girdle muscular dystrophy is mapped to 17q11-12." Am J Hum Genet 61(1): 151-159.

Moreira, E. S., T. J. Wiltshire, et al. (2000). "Limb-girdle muscular dystrophy type 2G is caused by mutations in the gene encoding the sarcomeric protein telethonin." Nat Genet 24(2): 163-166.

Muchir, A., G. Bonne, et al. (2000). "Identification of mutations in the gene encoding lamins A/C in autosomal dominant limb girdle muscular dystrophy with atrioventricular conduction disturbances (LGMD1B)." Hum Mol Genet 9(9): 1453-1459.

Murakami, T., Y. K. Hayashi, et al. (2006). "Fukutin gene mutations cause dilated cardiomyopathy with minimal muscle weakness." Ann Neurol 60(5): 597-602.

Nadeau, A., M. Kinali, et al. (2009). "Natural history of Ullrich congenital muscular dystrophy." Neurology 73(1): 25-31.

Nguyen, K., G. Bassez, et al. (2005). "Dysferlin mutations in LGMD2B, Miyoshi myopathy, and atypical dysferlinopathies." Hum Mutat 26(2): 165.

Nigro, V., E. de Sa Moreira, et al. (1996). "Autosomal recessive limb-girdle muscular dystrophy, LGMD2F, is caused by a mutation in the delta-sarcoglycan gene." Nat Genet 14(2): 195-198.

Noguchi, S., E. M. McNally, et al. (1995). "Mutations in the dystrophin-associated protein gamma-sarcoglycan in chromosome 13 muscular dystrophy." Science 270(5237): 819-822.

Nonaka, I., Y. Une, et al. (1981). "A clinical and histological study of Ullrich's disease (congenital atonic-sclerotic muscular dystrophy)." Neuropediatrics 12(3): 197-208.

North, K. N., L. A. Specht, et al. (1996). "Congenital muscular dystrophy associated with merosin deficiency." J Child Neurol 11(4): 291-295.

Norwood, F., M. de Visser, et al. (2007). "EFNS guideline on diagnosis and management of limb girdle muscular dystrophies." *Eur J Neurol* 14(12): 1305-1312.

Norwood, F. L., C. Harling, et al. (2009). "Prevalence of genetic muscle disease in Northern England: in-depth analysis of a muscle clinic population." *Brain* 132(Pt 11): 3175-3186.

Palenzuela, L., A. L. Andreu, et al. (2003). "A novel autosomal dominant limb-girdle muscular dystrophy (LGMD 1F) maps to 7q32.1-32.2." *Neurology* 61(3): 404-406.

Pan, T. C., R. Z. Zhang, et al. (1998). "CA repeat polymorphism of the COL6A3 gene on chromosome 2q37." *Hum Hered* 48(4): 235-236.

Pan, T. C., R. Z. Zhang, et al. (2003). "New molecular mechanism for Ullrich congenital muscular dystrophy: a heterozygous in-frame deletion in the COL6A1 gene causes a severe phenotype." *Am J Hum Genet* 73(2): 355-369.

Pandya, S., W. M. King, et al. (2008). "Facioscapulohumeral dystrophy." *Phys Ther* 88(1): 105-113.

Paradas, C., J. Llauger, et al. (2010). "Redefining dysferlinopathy phenotypes based on clinical findings and muscle imaging studies." *Neurology* 75(4): 316-323.

Passos-Bueno, M. R., E. S. Moreira, et al. (1996). "Linkage analysis in autosomal recessive limb-girdle muscular dystrophy (AR LGMD) maps a sixth form to 5q33-34 (LGMD2F) and indicates that there is at least one more subtype of AR LGMD." *Hum Mol Genet* 5(6): 815-820.

Peat, R. A., J. M. Smith, et al. (2008). "Diagnosis and etiology of congenital muscular dystrophy." *Neurology* 71(5): 312-321.

Piluso, G., L. Politano, et al. (2005). "Extensive scanning of the calpain-3 gene broadens the spectrum of LGMD2A phenotypes." *J Med Genet* 42(9): 686-693.

Quijano-Roy, S., B. Mbieleu, et al. (2008). "De novo LMNA mutations cause a new form of congenital muscular dystrophy." *Ann Neurol* 64(2): 177-186.

Rankin, J., M. Auer-Grumbach, et al. (2008). "Extreme phenotypic diversity and nonpenetrance in families with the LMNA gene mutation R644C." *Am J Med Genet A* 146A(12): 1530-1542.

Ranum, L. P., P. F. Rasmussen, et al. (1998). "Genetic mapping of a second myotonic dystrophy locus." *Nat Genet* 19(2): 196-198.

Renwick, J. H., S. E. Bundey, et al. (1971). "Confirmation of linkage of the loci for myotonic dystrophy and ABH secretion." *J Med Genet* 8(4): 407-416.

Richard, I., L. Brenguier, et al. (1997). "Multiple independent molecular etiology for limb-girdle muscular dystrophy type 2A patients from various geographical origins." *Am J Hum Genet* 60(5): 1128-1138.

Richard, I., O. Broux, et al. (1995). "Mutations in the proteolytic enzyme calpain 3 cause limb-girdle muscular dystrophy type 2A." *Cell* 81(1): 27-40.

Roberds, S. L., F. Leturcq, et al. (1994). "Missense mutations in the adhalin gene linked to autosomal recessive muscular dystrophy." *Cell* 78(4): 625-633.

Robinson, D. O., S. R. Hammans, et al. (2005). "Oculopharyngeal muscular dystrophy (OPMD): analysis of the PABPN1 gene expansion sequence in 86 patients reveals 13 different expansion types and further evidence for unequal recombination as the mutational mechanism." *Hum Genet* 116(4): 267-271.

Saenz, A., F. Leturcq, et al. (2005). "LGMD2A: genotype-phenotype correlations based on a large mutational survey on the calpain 3 gene." *Brain* 128(Pt 4): 732-742.

Schessl, J., N. M. Goemans, et al. (2008). "Predominant fiber atrophy and fiber type disproportion in early ullrich disease." *Muscle Nerve* 38(3): 1184-1191.

Sorrel-Dejerine, Y. and M. Fardeau (1982). "[Birth and metamorphosis of Landouzy-Dejerine progressive atrophic myopathy]." *Rev Neurol (Paris)* 138(12): 1041-1051.

Speer, M. C., R. Tandan, et al. (1996). "Evidence for locus heterogeneity in the Bethlem myopathy and linkage to 2q37." *Hum Mol Genet* 5(7): 1043-1046.

Speer, M. C., J. M. Vance, et al. (1999). "Identification of a new autosomal dominant limb-girdle muscular dystrophy locus on chromosome 7." *Am J Hum Genet* 64(2): 556-562.

Starling, A., F. Kok, et al. (2004). "A new form of autosomal dominant limb-girdle muscular dystrophy (LGMD1G) with progressive fingers and toes flexion limitation maps to chromosome 4p21." *Eur J Hum Genet* 12(12): 1033-1040.

Statland, J. M. and R. Tawil (2011). "Facioscapulohumeral muscular dystrophy: molecular pathological advances and future directions." *Curr Opin Neurol.*

Susman, R. D., S. Quijano-Roy, et al. (2010). "Expanding the clinical, pathological and MRI phenotype of DNM2-related centronuclear myopathy." *Neuromuscul Disord* 20(4): 229-237.

Suzuki, N., M. Aoki, et al. (2004). "Novel dysferlin mutations and characteristic muscle atrophy in late-onset Miyoshi myopathy." *Muscle Nerve* 29(5): 721-723.

Sveen, M. L., M. Schwartz, et al. (2006). "High prevalence and phenotype-genotype correlations of limb girdle muscular dystrophy type 2I in Denmark." *Ann Neurol* 59(5): 808-815.

Taniguchi, K., K. Kobayashi, et al. (2003). "Worldwide distribution and broader clinical spectrum of muscle-eye-brain disease." *Hum Mol Genet* 12(5): 527-534.

Tetreault, M., A. Duquette, et al. (2006). "A new form of congenital muscular dystrophy with joint hyperlaxity maps to 3p23-21." *Brain* 129(Pt 8): 2077-2084.

Toda, T. and K. Kobayashi (1999). "Fukuyama-type congenital muscular dystrophy: the first human disease to be caused by an ancient retrotransposal integration." *J Mol Med* 77(12): 816-823.

Toda, T., M. Segawa, et al. (1993). "Localization of a gene for Fukuyama type congenital muscular dystrophy to chromosome 9q31-33." *Nat Genet* 5(3): 283-286.

Tome, F. M. (1999). "The Peter Emil Becker Award lecture 1998. The saga of congenital muscular dystrophy." *Neuropediatrics* 30(2): 55-65.

Tome, F. M., T. Evangelista, et al. (1994). "Congenital muscular dystrophy with merosin deficiency." *C R Acad Sci III* 317(4): 351-357.

Turner, C. and D. Hilton-Jones (2010). "The myotonic dystrophies: diagnosis and management." *J Neurol Neurosurg Psychiatry* 81(4): 358-367.

Udd, B., J. Partanen, et al. (1993). "Tibial muscular dystrophy. Late adult-onset distal myopathy in 66 Finnish patients." *Arch Neurol* 50(6): 604-608.

Udd, B., A. Vihola, et al. (2005). "Titinopathies and extension of the M-line mutation phenotype beyond distal myopathy and LGMD2J." *Neurology* 64(4): 636-642.

Vainzof, M., L. V. Anderson, et al. (2001). "Dysferlin protein analysis in limb-girdle muscular dystrophies." *J Mol Neurosci* 17(1): 71-80.

Vainzof, M., M. R. Passos-Bueno, et al. (1996). "The sarcoglycan complex in the six autosomal recessive limb-girdle muscular dystrophies." *Hum Mol Genet* 5(12): 1963-1969.

Vainzof, M., M. R. Passos-Bueno, et al. (1999). "Sarcoglycanopathies are responsible for 68% of severe autosomal recessive limb-girdle muscular dystrophy in the Brazilian population." *J Neurol Sci* 164(1): 44-49.

van der Kooi, A. J., M. van Meegen, et al. (1997). "Genetic localization of a newly recognized autosomal dominant limb-girdle muscular dystrophy with cardiac involvement (LGMD1B) to chromosome 1q11-21." *Am J Hum Genet* 60(4): 891-895.

van Reeuwijk, J., M. Janssen, et al. (2005). "POMT2 mutations cause alpha-dystroglycan hypoglycosylation and Walker-Warburg syndrome." *J Med Genet* 42(12): 907-912.

Vogel, H. and J. Zamecnik (2005). "Diagnostic immunohistology of muscle diseases." *J Neuropathol Exp Neurol* 64(3): 181-193.

Voit, T. (2001). Congenital Muscular Dystrophies. *Disorders of voluntary muscle.* H.-J. D. Karpati G, Griggs RC. Cambridge, UK, Press Syndicate of the University of Cambridge: 503-524.

Voit, T., P. Stuettgen, et al. (1991). "Dystrophin as a diagnostic marker in Duchenne and Becker muscular dystrophy. Correlation of immunofluorescence and western blot." *Neuropediatrics* 22(3): 152-162.

Waddell, L. B., F. A. Lemckert, et al. (2011). "Dysferlin, annexin A1, and mitsugumin 53 are upregulated in muscular dystrophy and localize to longitudinal tubules of the T-system with stretch." *J Neuropathol Exp Neurol* 70(4): 302-313.

Walter, M. C., J. A. Petersen, et al. (2004). "FKRP (826C>A) frequently causes limb-girdle muscular dystrophy in German patients." *J Med Genet* 41(4): e50.

Weiler, T., C. R. Greenberg, et al. (1998). "A gene for autosomal recessive limb-girdle muscular dystrophy in Manitoba Hutterites maps to chromosome region 9q31-q33: evidence for another limb-girdle muscular dystrophy locus." *Am J Hum Genet* 63(1): 140-147.

Wijmenga, C., R. R. Frants, et al. (1990). "Location of facioscapulohumeral muscular dystrophy gene on chromosome 4." *Lancet* 336(8716): 651-653.

Yoshida, A., K. Kobayashi, et al. (2001). "Muscular dystrophy and neuronal migration disorder caused by mutations in a glycosyltransferase, POMGnT1." *Dev Cell* 1(5): 717-724.

Zatz, M., F. de Paula, et al. (2003). "The 10 autosomal recessive limb-girdle muscular dystrophies." *Neuromuscul Disord* 13(7-8): 532-544.

Zhang, Q., C. Bethmann, et al. (2007). "Nesprin-1 and -2 are involved in the pathogenesis of Emery Dreifuss muscular dystrophy and are critical for nuclear envelope integrity." *Hum Mol Genet* 16(23): 2816-2833.

13

Database of Wards for Patients with Muscular Dystrophy in Japan

Toshio Saito[1] and Katsunori Tatara[2]

[1]*Division of Neurology, National Hospital Organization Toneyama National Hospital,*
[2]*Division of Pediatrics, National Hospital Organization Tokushima National Hospital,*
Japan

1. Introduction

Twenty-seven hospitals in Japan specialize in treatment of muscular dystrophy patients, including inpatient care, of which 26 belong to the National Hospital Organization, and the other is the National Center of Neurology and Psychiatry. Since 1999, Japanese muscular dystrophy research groups investigating nervous and mental disorder have been developing a database of cases treated at these 27 institutions. In that regard, we conducted a survey of inpatients with muscular dystrophy and other neuromuscular disorders based on data collected by the National Hospital Organization and National Center of Neurology and Psychiatry. Herein, we examined data obtained between 1999 and 2010 in order to evaluate the medical condition of inpatients with muscular dystrophy in Japan.

2. Subjects and methods

The database includes numbers of inpatients, gender, age, diagnosis, respiratory condition, nutritional state, number of death cases, causes of death, and other relevant findings from data collected annually on October 1 every year since 1999. We examined these data using longitudinal and horizontal analyses.

3. Sequential changes in total numbers of inpatients treated at muscular dystrophy wards of National Hospital Organization and National Center of Neurology and Psychiatry

The total numbers of inpatients treated at the muscular dystrophy wards of the National Hospital Organization and National Center of Neurology and Psychiatry were quite consistent during the examination period. The lowest number of inpatients was 2066 in 2007 and the highest was 2193 in 2003 (Fig. 1).

3.1 Details regarding number of inpatients

The number of inpatients with Duchenne muscular dystrophy gradually decreased (882~770) every year (Fig. 2), whereas that of those with myotonic dystrophy gradually increased (327~411) (Fig. 3). The numbers of inpatients with other types of muscular dystrophy, such

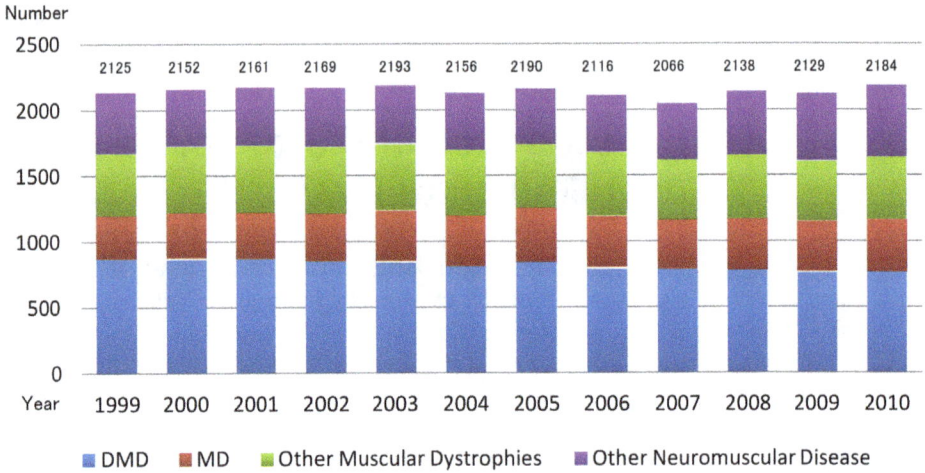

"Other muscular dystrophies" includes Becker muscular dystrophy, Fukuyama congenital muscular dystrophy, limb-girdle muscular dystrophy, facio-scapulo-humeral muscular dystrophy, Ullrich muscular dystrophy, and others.
"Other neuromuscular disease" includes amyotrophic lateral sclerosis, spinal muscular atrophy, hereditary sensory motor neuropathy, congenital myopathy, and others.
DMD, Duchenne muscular dystrophy; MD, myotonic dystrophy

Fig. 1. Total numbers of inpatients in muscular dystrophy wards of National Hospital Organization and National Center of Neurology and Psychiatry.

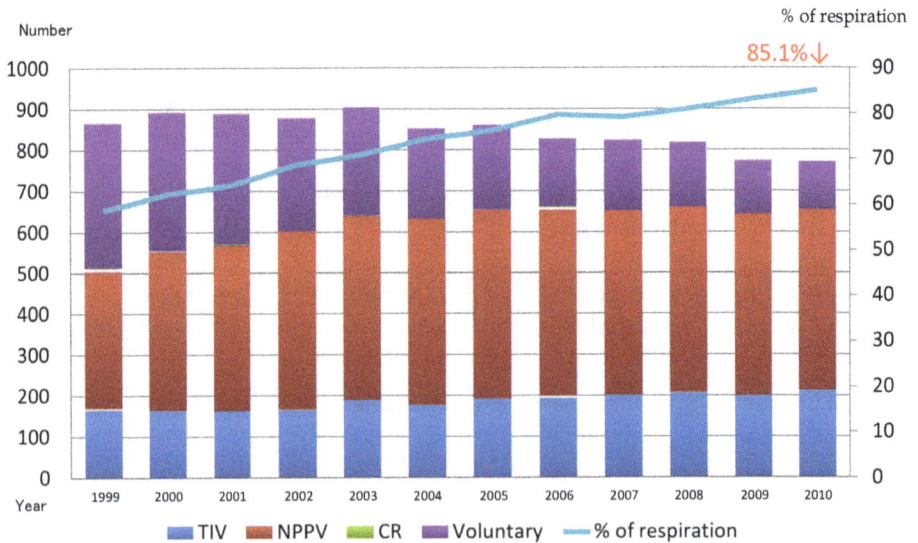

The number with Duchenne muscular dystrophy has gradually decreased every year.
TIV,tracheostomy intermittent ventilation; NPPV, non-invasive positive pressure ventilation

Fig. 2. Sequential changes in number of inpatients with Duchenne muscular dystrophy and rate of mechanical ventilation dependence.

as Becker muscular dystrophy (94~105), Fukuyama congenital muscular dystrophy (50~64), limb-girdle type muscular dystrophy (185~216), and facio-scapulo-humeral muscular dystrophy (64~72) showed some fluctuations. Inpatients with spinal muscular atrophy showed a gradual decreasing tendency from 73 in 1999 to 56 in 2010, while those with amyotrophic lateral sclerosis increased every year from 29 to 132 (Fig. 4). Other diseases encountered in these patients included congenital metabolic disease, mitochondrial disease, various types of myopathy, peripheral nerve disease, bone disease, chromosomal abnormalities, spinocerebellar ataxia, neonatal period disease sequelae, infectious diseases, and others, though their numbers were small and equalled around 10% of all diseases.

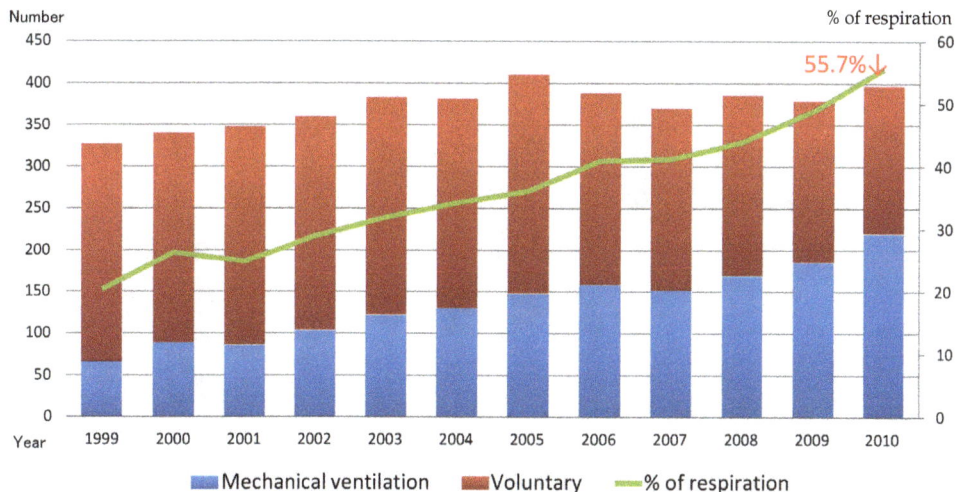

The number with myotonic dystrophy has gradually increased every year.

Fig. 3. Sequential changes in number of inpatients with myotonic dystrophy and rate of mechanical ventilation dependence.

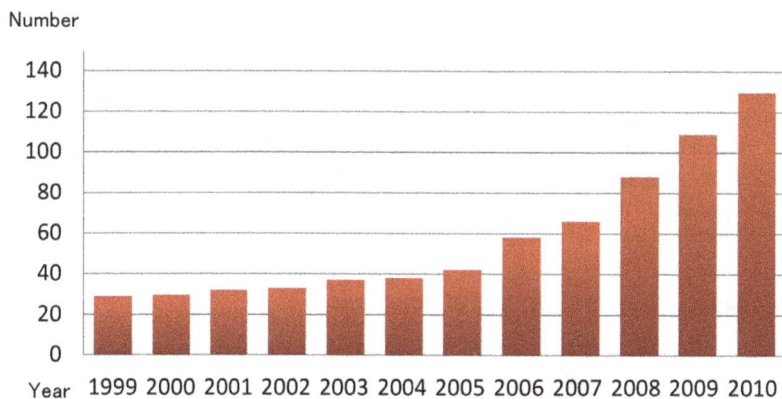

The number with amyotrophic lateral sclerosis has gradually increased every year.

Fig. 4. Sequential changes in number of inpatients with amyotrophic lateral sclerosis.

3.2 Sequential changes in respiratory care for inpatients and rate of mechanical ventilation dependence

The rate of mechanical ventilation use in 1999 was 37.9%, which gradually increased to 62.9% in 2010 (Fig. 5), while that for Duchenne muscular dystrophy patients in 1999 was 58.7% and gradually increased to 85.1% in 2010 (Fig. 2). Although the total number of inpatients with Duchenne muscular dystrophy gradually decreased, cases of non-invasive ventilation gradually increased and tracheostomy cases were also slightly increased. The rate of mechanical ventilation use for myotonic dystrophy patients in 1999 was 20.3%, which gradually increased to 55.7% in 2010 (Fig. 3).

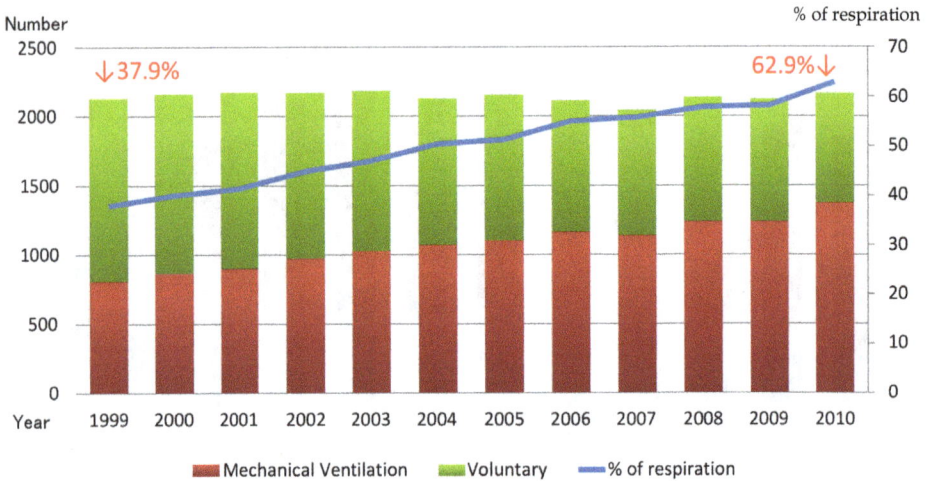

The rate of mechanical ventilation use in 1999 was 37.9%, which gradually increased to 62.9% in 2010.

Fig. 5. Sequential changes in respiratory care for inpatients and rate of mechanical ventilation dependence.

3.3 Analysis of mean age of inpatients

3.3.1 Changes in age distribution of inpatients in muscular dystrophy wards

The age distribution of inpatients in muscular dystrophy wards in 1999 showed 2 peaks. Those with Duchenne muscular dystrophy largely constituted the younger age peak in the 20s, while those with myotonic dystrophy larger constituted the older age peak in the 50s. These age peaks shifted to a higher range and became slightly flattened in 2009 (Fig. 6).

3.3.2 Sequential changes in mean age of inpatients

The mean age of the inpatients in 1999 was 36.6 years old, which gradually increased to 45.3 years old in 2010. That of Duchenne muscular dystrophy patients in 1999 was 23.6 years old, which gradually increased to 29.4 years old in 2010, while that of myotonic dystrophy patients changed only slightly from 51.4 years old in 1999 to 53.6 years old in 2010 (Fig. 7).

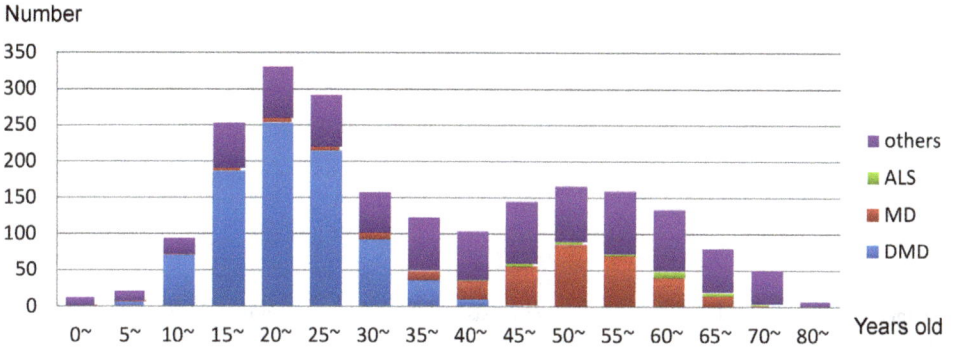

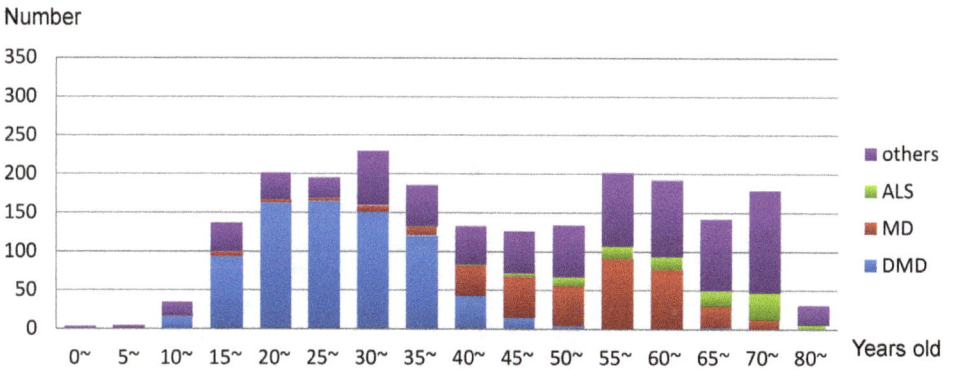

Upper: 1999. Lower: 2009. The age distribution of inpatients in muscular dystrophy wards shifted to a higher range over time.

Fig. 6. Changes in age distribution of inpatients in muscular dystrophy wards.

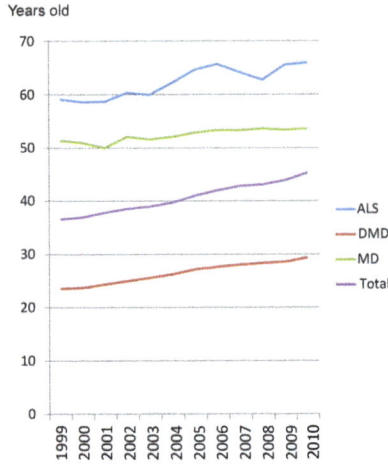

The mean age of the inpatients was gradually increased. DMD, Duchenne muscular dystrophy; MD, myotonic dystrophy; ALS, amyotrophic lateral sclerosis

Fig. 7. Sequential changes in mean age of inpatients.

Gradual changes in age distribution of inpatients with Duchenne muscular dystrophy was observed. The age peak in 1999 shifted to a higher range and became slightly flattened in 2009 (Fig. 8).

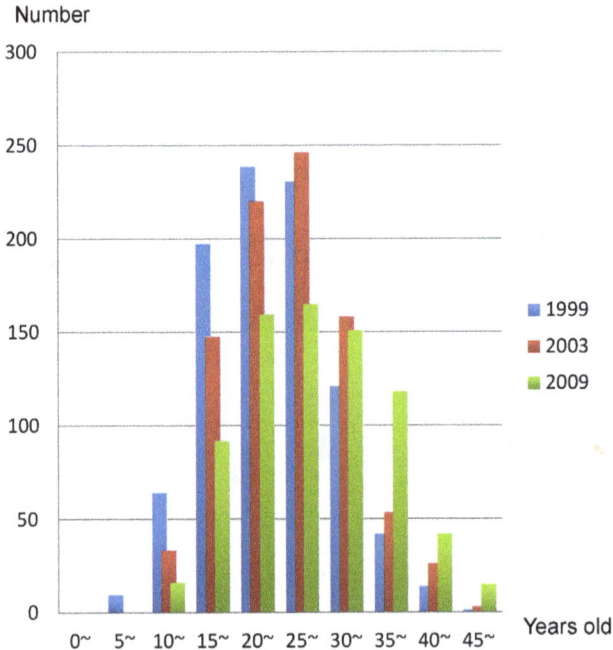

Fig. 8. Changes in age distribution of inpatients with Duchenne muscular dystrophy.

3.4 Sequential changes in numbers of patients receiving oral nutrition and those with Duchenne muscular dystrophy who underwent a percutaneous endoscopic gastrostomy

The proportion of patients with Duchenne muscular dystrophy receiving oral nutrition in 1999 was 95.1%, which gradually decreased to 70.6% in 2010. In contrast, the number who required tube feeding, including a nasal nutrition tube and undergoing a percutaneous endoscopic gastrostomy, gradually increased to 107 in 2010.

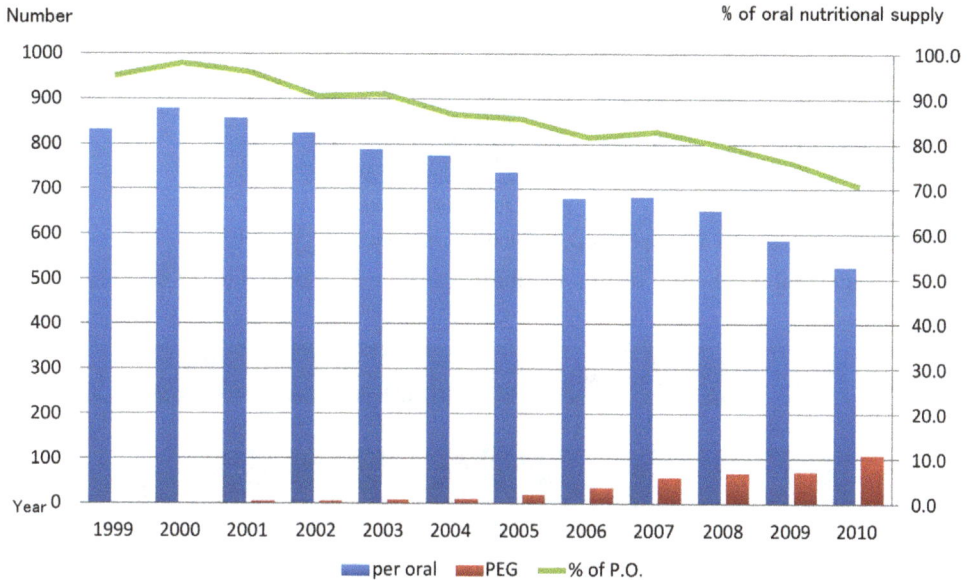

PEG, percutaneous endoscopic gastrostomy

Fig. 9. Sequential changes in numbers of Duchenne muscular dystrophy patients and those who underwent an endoscopic gastrostomy patients receiving oral nutrition.

3.5 Death case analysis

The total number of deaths reported from 2000 to 2010 was 1307, which ranged from 95-174 annually in a variable pattern (Fig. 10). The number of Duchenne muscular dystrophy patients who died was 409, while that of myotonic dystrophy patients was 363.

The mean age of death among Duchenne muscular dystrophy patients was 26.7 years old in 2000, which gradually increased to 35.1 years old by 2010. On the other hand, the mean age of death for myotonic dystrophy patients was 59.0 years old in 2000 and 59.1 years old in 2010, which was not significantly different (Fig. 10).

The most frequent cause of death among Duchenne muscular dystrophy patients was heart failure, accounting for 47%. As for myotonic dystrophy patients, the most frequent cause was respiratory disorders, such as respiratory failure and respiratory tract infection, which accounted for 64% (Fig. 11).

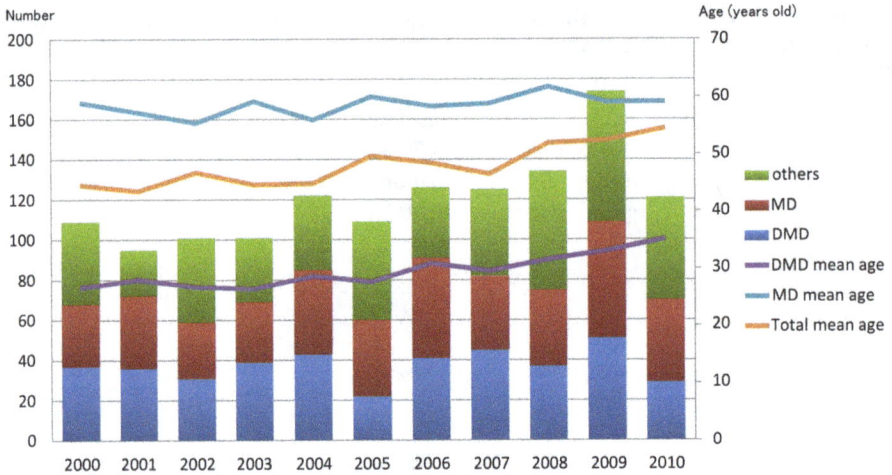

DMD, Duchenne muscular dystrophy; MD, myotonic dystrophy

Fig. 10. Sequential numbers of deaths and mean age at death reported to the database.

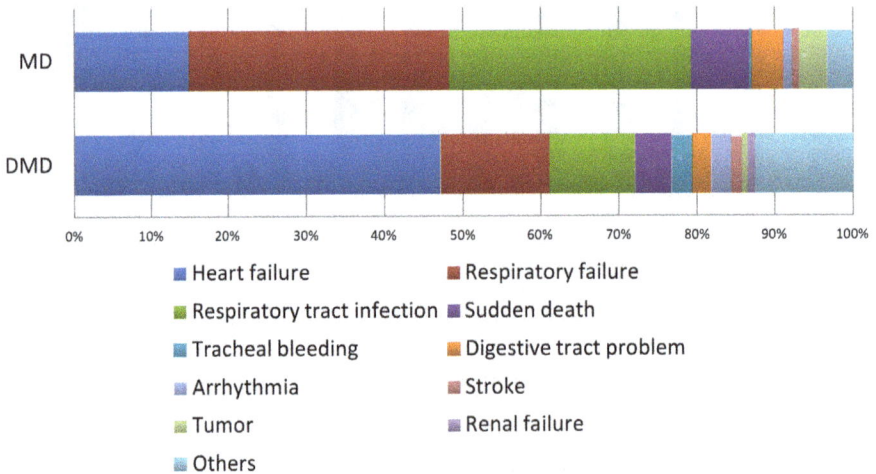

The most frequent cause of death among Duchenne muscular dystrophy patients was heart failure. In contrast, that of myotonic dystrophy patients was respiratory disorder.
DMD, Duchenne muscular dystrophy; MD, myotonic dystrophy

Fig. 11. Causes of death among Duchenne muscular dystrophy and myotonic dystrophy patients (2000~2010).

3.6 Proportional changes in numbers of inpatients in muscular dystrophy wards of each institution

Twenty-seven hospitals in Japan specialize in treatment of muscular dystrophy patients are not same in terms of types of muscular dystrophy of inpatient, disease severity, and actual care. Fig. 12 shows the proportion of inpatients by each institution. The upper figure, which shows the proportion in 1999, is arranged according to rate of Duchenne muscular dystrophy inpatients. There were significant differences in regard to the proportion of inpatients among the institutions in 1999, which changed over time. In 2009, the proportion of inpatients with amyotrophic lateral sclerosis was notable.

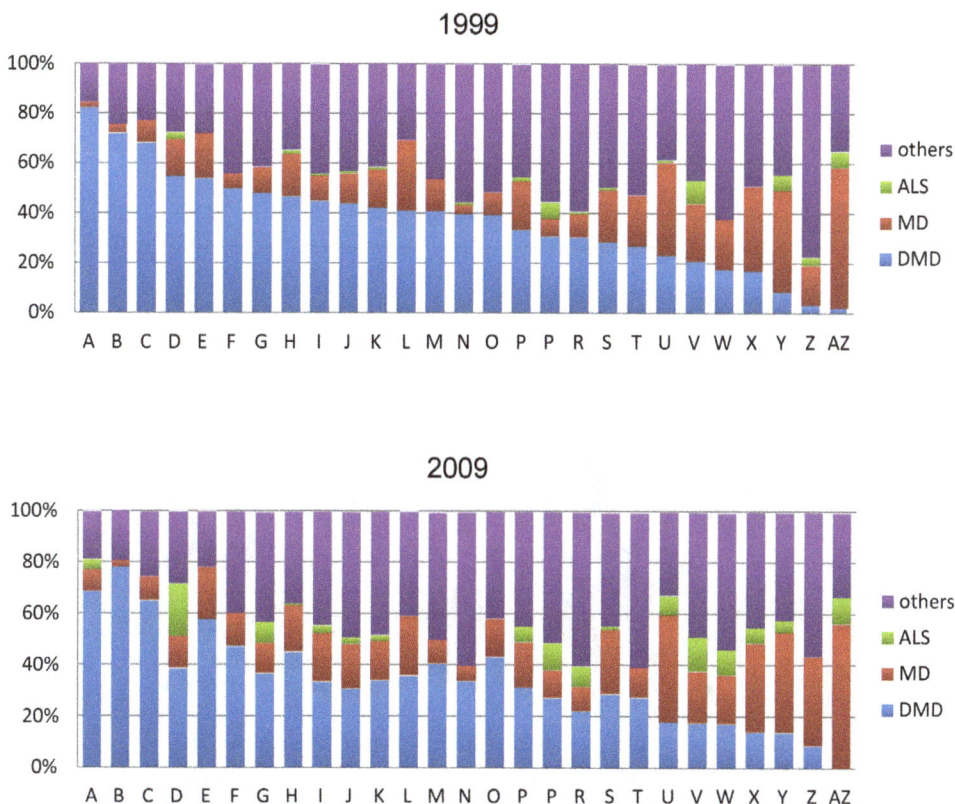

Upper: 1999. Lower: 2009. A~AZ represent the individual institution. Institute AZ, which had lowest rate of DMD patients among institutions in 1999, has no DMD patient in 2009.
DMD, Duchenne muscular dystrophy; MD, myotonic dystrophy; ALS, amyotrophic lateral sclerosis

Fig. 12. Changes in proportions of inpatients in muscular dystrophy wards of each institution

3.7 Sequential changes in respiratory conditions of Duchenne muscular dystrophy patients at each institution (1999~2009).

The total number of Duchenne muscular dystrophy patients treated from 1999 to 2009 was 1427. The changes in motor function of the patients were nearly uniform, whereas the therapeutic respiratory conditions varied among the institutions.

Figure 13 presents the respiratory conditions of the patients for the 11-year period from 1999 to 2009. In the 10s, almost patients keep voluntary respiratory function. In the 20s, various respiratory patterns are observed, which seem not to be different among the institutions. In more than 30s, there were apparent differences among the institutions. Some institutes have no tracheostomy older patients, which generation is generally supposed not to be compensated by non-invasive positive pressure ventilation and use tracheotomy ventilation.

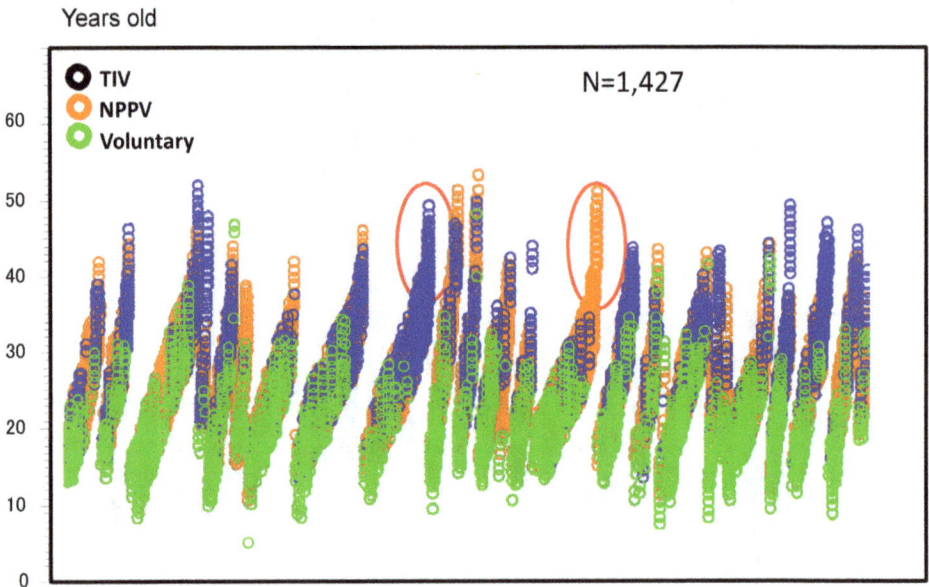

Each cluster indicates a single institution. The vertical axis indicates the course of a single Duchenne muscular dystrophy patient. The respiratory conditions of older patients differed among the institutions. For example, the left oval indicates a tracheostomy case and the right oval a non-invasive positive pressure ventilation case.
TIV,tracheostomy intermittent ventilation; NPPV, non-invasive positive pressure ventilation

Fig. 13. Sequential changes in respiratory conditions of Duchenne muscular dystrophy patients treated at each institution (1999~2009).

4. Conclusion

Wards for patients with muscular dystrophy were originally established in Japan in 1964 and then gradually expanded throughout the country. As a result, approximate 2500 beds are now provided among 27 institutions. In the early days, many of the patients were boys with Duchenne muscular dystrophy, who received education in schools near the hospital where they received care. However, over time, regular public elementary and junior high schools began to accept disabled children, and such patients were then able to receive an education at schools in their home town. Thus, cases of admission for the purpose of education gradually decreased.

On the other hand, progress in therapeutic strategies for respiratory failure (American Thoracic Society Documents, 2004), heart failure (Ishikawa, 1999; Matsumura, 2010) and other complications associated with muscular dystrophy prolonged the life span of affected individuals (Bushby 2010a, b). Now, most inpatients admitted to a muscular dystrophy ward have a severe general condition and many are assisted by mechanical ventilation (Tatara, 2008). In addition, in terms of nutritional control (American Thoracic Society Documents, 2004; Bushby 2010b), the number of percutaneous endoscopic gastrostomy patients with Duchenne muscular dystrophy has gradually increased.

Thus, the age and disease severity of inpatients have been gradually progressed with this changing environment. And social welfare systems related to muscular dystrophy wards in Japan also have been changing during this research. The social role of wards for inpatients with muscular dystrophy has been changing. The gradual increase of number of inpatients with amyotrophic lateral sclerosis means that the ward for patients with muscular dystrophy is no longer only for patients with muscular dystrophy. Present wards have purpose for care and treatment for severe disabilities, not limited to patients with muscular dystrophy.

There are some reports concerned with prognosis of patients with Duchenne muscular dystrophy from single institution belonging to the National Hospital Organization (Ishikawa, 2011; Matsumura, 2011). Just as these reports, we showed the increasing mean age of death among Duchenne muscular dystrophy patients. Although the most frequent cause of death among Duchenne muscular dystrophy patients was heart failure, the progression for cardioprotection therapy to cardiomyopathy (Ishikawa, 1999; Matsumura, 2010) improved the prognosis.

However, the present findings showed that there are apparent differences in regard to the proportion of inpatients and therapeutic conditions among institutions. Hereafter, these differences will be more remarkable. So far almost same therapy has been offered among the National Hospital Organization and National Center of Neurology and Psychiatry. However, these conditions will not continue and may influence the prognosis of patients with muscular dystrophy in Japan.

Social role of wards for patients with muscular dystrophy at establishment, offering patients with muscular dystrophy opportunities of education and treatment, has changed into offering severe disabilities care and treatment. We should consider how to manage these conditions.

5. Acknowledgments

This study was supported by a Research Grant for Nervous and Mental Disorders from the Ministry of Health, Labour and Welfare of Japan.

We are grateful to Dr. Mitsuru Kawai for the kind advice, as well as the members of the FUKUNAGA (1999-2005) and SHINNO (2006-2011) muscular dystrophy research groups of the National Hospital Organization for the data collection.

Institutions specializing in muscular dystrophy treatment in Japan (Fig.14)

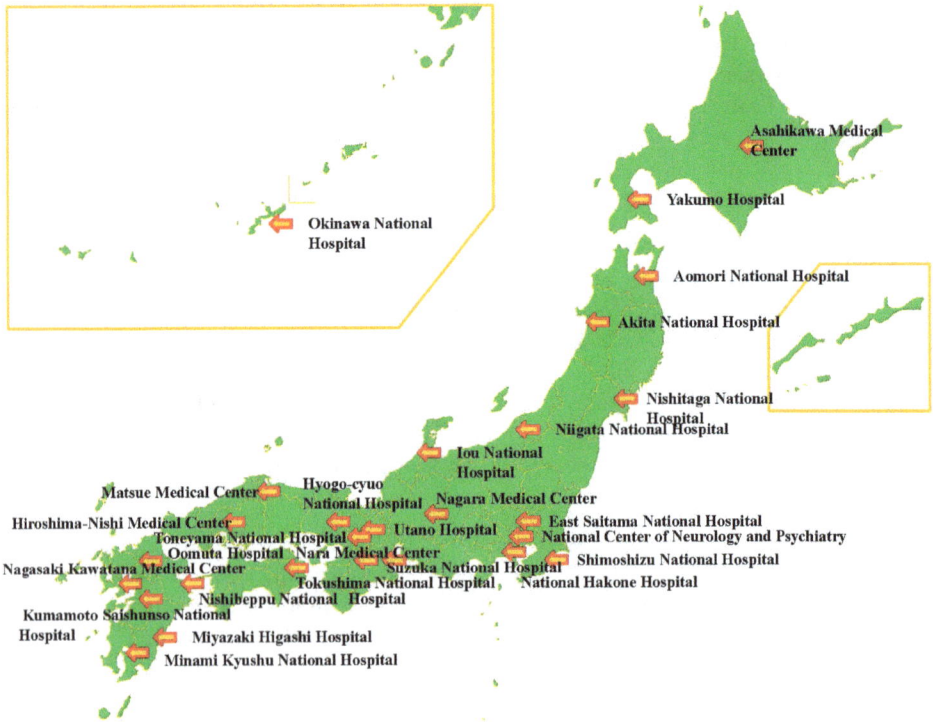

Fig. 14. Institutions specializing in muscular dystrophy treatment in Japan

National Hospital Organization:

- Asahikawa Medical Center, Yakumo Hospital, Aomori National Hospital,

- Akita National Hospital, Nishitaga National Hospital, East Saitama National Hospital,

- Shimoshizu National Hospital, National Hakone Hospital, Niigata National Hospital,

- Iou National Hospital, Nagara Medical Center, Suzuka National Hospital,

- Nara Medical Center, Utano Hospital, Toneyama National Hospital,

- Hyogo-cyuo National Hospital, Hiroshima-Nishi Medical Center, Matsue Medical Center,

- Tokushima National Hospital, Oomuta Hospital, Nagasaki Kawatana Medical Center,

- Kumamoto Saishunso National Hospital, Nishibeppu National Hospital,

- Miyazaki Higashi Hospital, Minami Kyushu National Hospital, Okinawa National Hospital

National Center of Neurology and Psychiatry

6. References

American Thoracic Society Documents (2004). Respiratory Care of the Patient with Duchenne Muscular Dystrophy. ATS Consensus Statement · *American Journal of Respiratory and Critical Care Medicine*, Vol 170, pp 456–465.

Bushby K, Finkel R, Birnkrant DJ, Case LE, Clemens PR, Cripe L, Kaul A, Kinnett K, McDonald C, Pandya S, Poysky J, Shapiro F, Tomezsko J, Constantin C, for the DMD care considerations working group (2010a). Diagnosis and management of Duchenne muscular dystrophy, part 1: diagnosis, and pharmacological and psychosocial management. *The Lancet Neurology*, Vol.9, pp 77-93.

Bushby K, Finkel R, Birnkrant DJ, Case LE, Clemens PR, Cripe L, Kaul A, Kinnett K, McDonald C, Pandya S, Poysky J, Shapiro F, Tomezsko J, Constantin C, for the DMD care considerations working group (2010b). Diagnosis and management of Duchenne muscular dystrophy, part 2: implementation of multidisciplinary care. *The Lancet Neurology*, Vol.9, pp 177–189.

Ishikawa Y, Bach JR, Minami R (1999). Cardioprotection for Duchenne's muscular dystrophy.*American Heart Journal* Vol.137, pp 895–902.

Ishikawa Y, Miura T, Ishikawa Y, Aoyagi T, Ogata H, Hamada S, Minami R (2011). Duchenne muscular dystrophy: Survival by cardio-respiratory interventions. *Neuromuscular Disorders* Vol. 21, pp 47–51.

Matsumura T, Tamura T, Kuru S, Kikuchi Y, Kawai M (2010) · Carvedilol can prevent cardiac events in Duchenne muscular dystrophy. *Internal Medicine* Vol. 49, pp 1357-1363.

Matsumura T, Saito T, Fujimura H, Shinno S, Sakoda S (2011). A longitudinal cause-of-death analysis of patients with Duchenne muscular dystrophy.*Rinsho-shinkeigaku* Vol. 51, pp743-750.

Tatara K, Shinno S (2008). Management of mechanical ventilation and prognosis in Duchenne muscular dystrophy. *IRYO*, Vol. 62, pp 566–571.

14

Effects of Dietary Phosphate on Ectopic Calcification and Muscle Function in mdx Mice

Eiji Wada, Namiko Kikkawa, Mizuko Yoshida,
Munehiro Date, Tetsuo Higashi and Ryoichi Matsuda
The University of Tokyo,
Japan

1. Introduction

Calcium deposits in extra-skeletal tissues are highly correlated with lifestyle diseases. The mechanisms and clinical effects of such deposition have been widely studied due to increase mortality rate. Vascular calcification is a major complication in a number of diseases, including chronic kidney disease (CKD) and diabetes (Giachelli, 2009). The number of regulation mechanisms affecting calcium precipitation in soft tissues remains underestimated, as many regulators are considered to be involved in this complex process (Hu et al., 2010; Kendrick et al., 2011). Elevated serum phosphate levels which leads hyperphosphatemia is one of the prevalent factors of vascular calcification in CKD (El-Abbadi et al., 2009). The kidneys play a central role in the regulation of phosphate homeostasis. In individuals with normal renal function, serum phosphate levels are strictly controlled through dietary intake, intestinal absorption, renal excretion, and bone metabolism. When the kidneys are either mechanically or functionally impaired, phosphate metabolism is imbalanced. Abnormalities of phosphate metabolism related to kidney malfunction may play a central role in the deposition of calcium and phosphate in extra-skeletal tissues. Ectopic calcification in skeletal muscle has been reported to occur in three Duchenne muscular dystrophy (DMD) animal models; mdx mice (Coulton et al., 1987; Kikkawa et al., 2009), dystrophic puppies (Nguyen et al., 2002), and hypertrophic muscular dystrophy cats (Gaschen et al., 1992). In this chapter, we review the mechanisms of ectopic calcification in mdx mice and report a new finding of effects of dietary phosphate intake on calcium deposits and muscle function in mdx mice.

2. Ectopic calcification in animal models of muscular dystrophy

The mdx mouse, dystrophic canine, and hypertrophic muscular dystrophy feline develop progressive muscle lesions and calcium deposits in skeletal muscle during muscle regeneration. The pathological features of dystrophic golden retriever puppies are particularly severe and are similar to those of DMD boys, who are characterized by progressive muscle necrosis that leads to early death. Nguyen et al. (2002) detected early ectopic calcification in muscles from 4-day-old and 2-month-old puppies. Thus calcium deposition in skeletal muscle appears to be an early event associated with muscle degeneration.

In mdx mice, the observed muscle pathology is relatively mild compared with DMD patients but calcifying lesions are commonly seen in the lower limbs and diaphragm of mice from approximately five weeks of age. Recently, ectopic calcification (Fig. 1) has been reported to be a characteristic feature of muscular pathology (Korff et al., 2006; Verma et al., 2010). For example, Korff et al. (2006) found that myocardial calcification commonly occurs in mice following necrosis induced by mechanical stresses and proposed that calcification in the heart is dependent upon genetic background. Verma et al. (2010) suggested that the absence of ectopic calcification in the diaphragm serves as a marker of amelioration of mdx pathology. In addition, one of the prednisone-induced side effects in a canine model of DMD is skeletal muscle calcification (Liu et al., 2004). However, a palliative glucocorticoid therapy using prednisone is a feasible and effective treatment approach for DMD despite of the serious potential side effects (Wong et al., 2002; Khan, 1993). Studies in these animals have revealed that the percentages of calcified myofibers in necrotic lesions increase dose dependently. It is speculated that calcium deposits in skeletal muscle are occurred as results of abnormal calcium and phosphate homeostasis and delayed muscle degeneration and regeneration cycle.

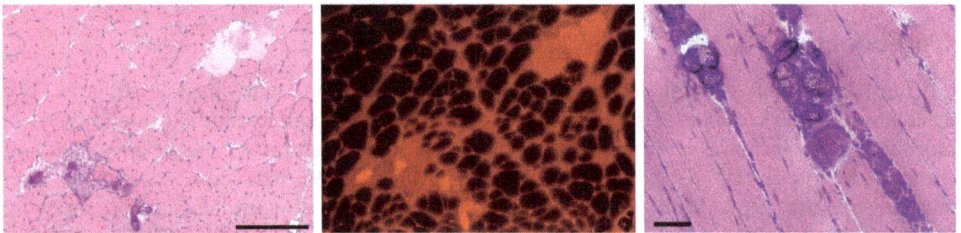

Fig. 1. Ectopic calcification in mdx mice (90 days old). Transverse (left and center) and longitudinal (right) sections, stained with H&E (left and right) and Evans blue (center). The bar represents 100 μm.

3. Identification of calcium deposits in mdx mice skeletal muscle

Our group is actively studying ectopic calcification in mdx mice skeletal muscle (Kikkawa et al., 2009). We performed experiments with 90-day-old mdx and control mice (C57BL/10: B10) fed a commercial standard chow (CE-2; Clea Japan, Tokyo, Japan) and water *ad libitum*. Following sacrificed of the mice, high-resolution X-ray micro-computed tomography (CT) imaging of the hind limbs of mdx and B10 mice using a SkyScan-1074 scanner (SkyScan, Kontich, Belgium) revealed that all mdx mice had muscle calcification in the hind limb, whereas no calcium precipitation was observed in the control mice (Fig. 2).

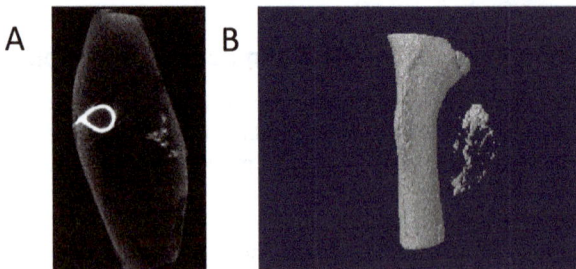

Fig. 2. Images of the hind limb of a two-month-old mdx mouse. X-ray-absorbing materials are shown as gray shadows and the femeur can be seen in the center of the X-ray image. (A) CT image. (B) Reconstructed 3D image. (Kikkawa et al., 2009)

The main composition of calcium deposits in the skeletal muscle was identified using an back-scattered electron imaging and energy-dispersive X-ray spectrometry (EDS) analysis by S-4500 SEM (Hitachi, Tokyo, Japan). In a cross-section of the muscle from an mdx mouse, spotty and bright crystals were observed. The EDS spectra obtained from the crystals indicated the presence of both calcium and phosphorus (Fig. 2A-B). To determine whether the composition of the deposits consisted of a calcium phosphate phase, muscle samples were analyzed using a JEM-2010 TEM (JEOL, Tokyo, Japan) equipped with an EDS detector. The electron diffraction pattern from an obtained TEM image of the specimen nearly was an identical match with a simulated diffraction pattern of hydroxyapatite ($Ca_5(PO_4)_3OH$; HA) (Fig. 3C). Based on these results, we concluded that the calcification of mdx skeletal muscles is due to the precipitation of hydroxyapatite.

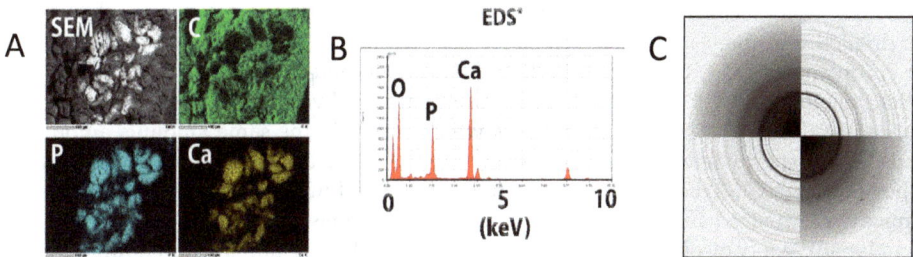

Fig. 3. SEM and TEM analyses of ectopic calcification in mdx mice skeletal muscle. (A) Electron probe microanalysis identified the particles as calcium phosphate. (B) Energy dispersive X-ray spectroscopy. (C) Identical match of X-ray diffraction of the particles and HA. (Kikkawa et al., 2009).

4. Serum biochemistry of mdx and B10 mice fed a commercial diet

As we determined that ectopic calcification is composed of HA, the main component of bones, we suspected that mdx mice have a metabolic disorder of calcium (Ca) and phosphate (Pi) homeostasis. To examine the levels of Ca and Pi in blood, serum samples were collected from two-month-old mdx and B10 mice fed a commercial diet (CE-2 containing 1.0 g/100 g Pi and 1.0 g/100 g Ca) and water *ad libitum*. The two minerals were measured using an automated clinical chemistry analyzer Fuji Dri-chem 4000 (Fujifilm, Tokyo, Japan). Comparison of the serum mineral components of mdx and B10 mice revealed that mdx mice had significantly higher serum Pi levels (1.41 fold; $P < 0.05$) than the control mice, whereas no significant differences in serum Ca levels were detected. These results are supported by a previous study in mdx and B10 mice by Brazeau et al. (1992).

The concentrations of serum fibroblast growth factor-23 (FGF-23), which is an important regulator of phosphorus, were also measured using an FGF-23 ELISA kit (Kainos Laboratories, Tokyo, Japan). The serum level of FGF-23 of mdx mice was significantly higher (1.5 fold; $P < 0.05$) than that of B10 mice.

Nearly all of the identified functions of FGF-23 are activated or operate through Klotho, a single transmembrane protein of the β-glycosidase family that is expressed in the distal kidney tubules and parathyroid gland (Kuro-o, 2010). Both FGF-23 and Klotho have emerged as responsible factors for mediating phosphate homeostasis. It has been reported that soft tissue calcification and hyperphosphatemia are observed in mice lacking either FGF-23 (Razzaque et al., 2006) or Klotho (Kuro-o et al., 1997). Klotho mutant mice also exhibit multiple age-associated disorders, such as arteriosclerosis, osteoporosis, short-life span, and ectopic calcification. However, as these phenotypes are rescued by the restriction of dietary phosphorus alone in male Klotho mice (Morishita et al., 2010) we predicted that the amount of dietary Pi intake influences the precipitation of calcium in mdx mice, and that the restriction of dietary Pi may improve mdx muscle pathology and function.

5. Influence of phosphate diet

Based on our findings that mdx mice have calcium deposits composed of HA and exhibit higher serum phosphate levels, we speculated that dietary phosphate intake might modulate ectopic calcification in mdx mice. To test this speculation, mdx mice and B10 mice were divided into three diet groups (n=30) from weaning (20 days old) that were fed diets with Pi contents of 2.0 g/100 g (high-Pi diet), 1.0 g/100 g (mid-Pi diet), and 0.7 g/100 g (low-Pi diet) manufactured by Oriental Yeast Company (Tokyo, Japan). Other ingredients, including calcium (1.2 g/100 g) in the diets were present in the same amounts among the groups. The experimental diets were based on the CE-2 and mid-Pi diet was a same composition with CE-2 diet which was fed to pregnant and nursing mice of both genotypes. All mice were housed in cages with pulp bedding (Palmas-µ; Material Research Center, Tokyo, Japan) in a controlled room with a 12-h light/dark cycle and a temperature of 25℃. The experimental chows and water were available *ad libitum*. Mice were either sacrificed with an overdose of diethylether at age 30, 60, or 90 days or used for measurements of muscular function at age 60 days. Twenty-four hours before euthanasia, mice were received an intraperitoneal injection of Evans blue dye (EBD, 100 mg/kg) which incorporates into regenerating myofibers with permeable membranes (Matsuda et al., 1995). All procedures were performed in accordance with the ethical guidelines of the University of Tokyo.

5.1 Changes in ectopic calcification in skeletal muscle

Changes in ectopic calcification in mdx mice skeletal muscle induced by dietary phosphate content were observed using a modified whole body double-staining method involving alizarin red S and alcian blue, which stain bones and cartilage respectively (Dingerkus et al., 1977; McLeod, 1980; Webb et al., 1994). Briefly, 90-day-old mice were sacrificed and fixed in 95% ethanol (EtOH) for 7 days after the skin and organs were removed. The EtOH was then replaced in acetone and the samples were further incubated for 3~4 days. After partial drying, samples were stained in a mixed solution of 0.3% alcian blue 8GX (Fluka, Germany) in 70% EtOH, 0.1% alizarin red S (WAKO, Osaka, Japan) in 95% EtOH, and 2.0% potassium hydrogen phthalate in 70% EtOH for 3 days. Each stained mouse was washed in distilled water and placed in 0.75% potassium hydroxide (KOH) in MilliQ water for 2 days to initiated maceration and clearing. Clearing was continued by adding increasing concentration of glycerol (20%, 50%, 70% and 100%) in 0.75% KOH to obtain a completely cleared specimen (Fig. 4A). Calcified regions were stained reddish violet, similar to appearance of stained bones.

Imaging of the stained and cleared samples showed that no bone-like red staining was present in the skeletal muscles of B10 mice fed any of the three phosphate diets (Fig. 4A-a). However, in mid-Pi fed mdx mice, striped and spotty red stained areas, particularly in the back, gluteus, and lower limbs muscles, were detected (Fig. 4A-b), while excessive calcification was clearly observed in the samples from high-Pi fed mdx mice (Fig. 4A-c, Fig. 4B). The staining revealed severe calcification, particularly in the diaphragm, back, gluteus, and lower limbs muscles, where severely degenerated muscle fibers were visible macroscopically by EBD staining (Fig. 4C). In contrast, bone–like red staining was rarely seen in the whole bodies of the low-Pi fed mdx mice (Fig. 4A-d, Fig. 4B).

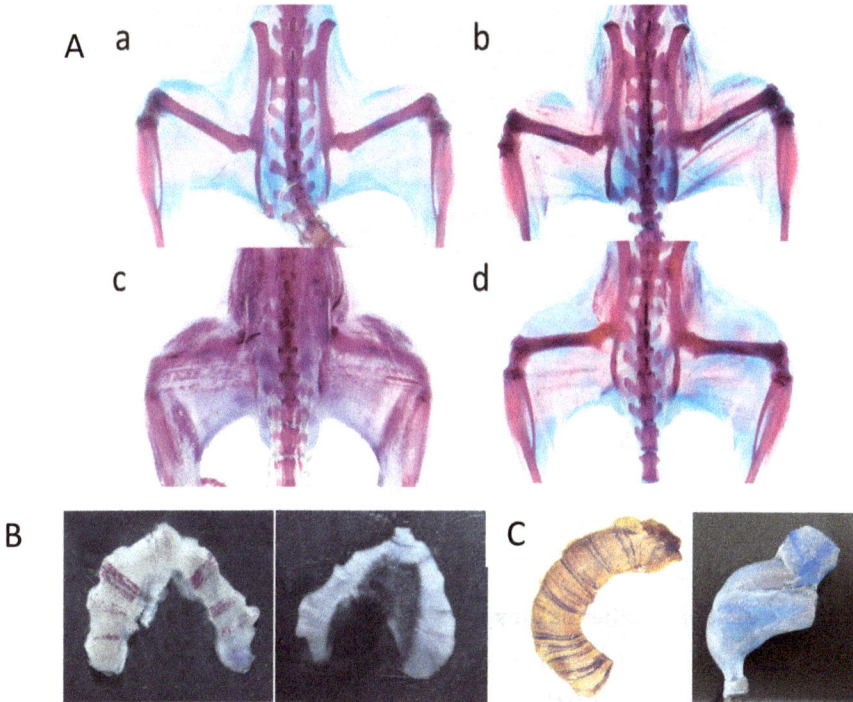

Fig. 4. Results of whole-body double staining of mdx and B10 mice, and Evans blue dye staining of mdx mice. (A) Images of the whole-body double staining of the lower body. (A-a) Lower body of a B10 mouse fed a high-Pi diet. The lower body of mdx mice (A-b) fed a mid-Pi diet, (A-c) high-Pi diet and (A-d) low-Pi diet. (B) Pictures of the whole body double staining of diaphragm. Diaphragm of an mdx mouse fed a high-Pi diet (left) and low-Pi diet (right). (C) Evans blue dye in the diaphragm (left) and lower limb (right) of an mdx mouse. Evans blue-positive lesions are seen in blue.

Quadriceps muscle samples from low-Pi, mid-Pi, and high-Pi fed mdx mice at 30, 60, and 90 days of age were sectioned at 8 μm thickness to determine the onset of calcifying lesions. Hematoxylin and eosin (H&E) and alizarin red S (1%) staining were used to observe pathology and detect calcification in the samples (Fig. 5). Histology showed early mineralization in degenerating myofibers in high-Pi fed mdx mice at 30 days of age (only fed a high-Pi diet only for 10 days), whereas no alizarin red-positive areas were present in either mid-Pi or low-Pi fed mdx mice of the same age. In addition, few calcium deposits were seen in mid-Pi fed mdx mice by the age of 60 days or in low-Pi fed mdx mice even by

90 days of age. Calcium deposits were extensive throughout the entire sections of high-Pi fed mdx mice at 90 days of age.

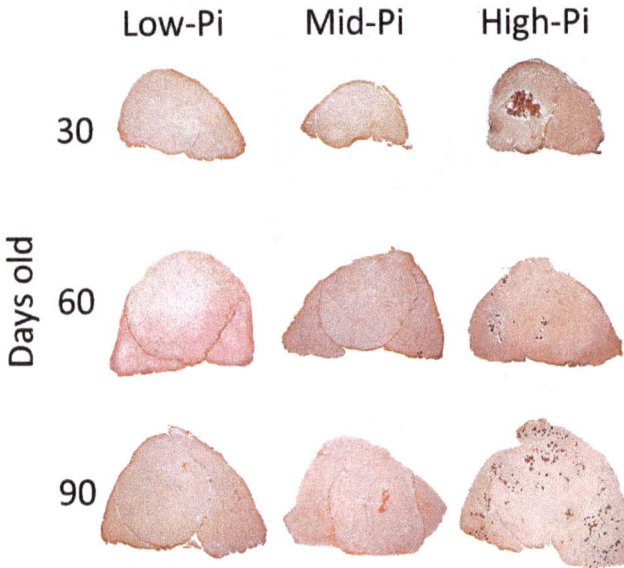

Fig. 5. Alizarin red S-stained cryosections of mdx mice quadriceps muscle. Calcium deposits are stained red.

5.2 Ectopic calcification in other tissues

Although the presence of calcification is rarely reported in organs of mdx mice other than skeletal muscle, including the heart and kidneys, these mice exhibit abnormal cardiac pathology and function (Zhang et al., 2008) and their myocardium is vulnerable (Costas et al., 2010). Rodent models of muscular dystrophies may have potential for sensitivity to myocardial calcification when challenged by mechanical or chemical stressors, because such calcification is commonly observed in the hamster model of muscular dystrophy (Burbach, 1987). For instance, Elsherif et al. (2008) found that dystrophin and $\beta 1$ integrin double-knockout mice ($\beta 1KOmdx$) show exacerbated myocardiopathy and extensive calcification in the heart, particularly under pregnancy-induced stress. Thus we predicted that high-Pi intake would also affect calcification in the myocardium of mdx mice.

Calcification in the heart was evaluated by 8 μm cryosections of samples from the three Pi-diet group mice. We found that high-Pi intake induced relatively few cases of myocardial calcification in mdx mice at both 60 and 90 days of age (4 of 30 samples). The form of the crystallization observed in the heart was similar to that of myofiber calcification, although the amount was considerably less (Fig. 6A, C). The incidence of calcification in the heart was absent in mdx fed mid-Pi or low-Pi diets. None of B10 mice fed any of the three types of phosphate diets exhibited myocardial calcification.

As previously described, klotho mutant mice display a number of age-related diseases, including soft tissue calcification. Morishita et al. (2010) reported that klotho mice fed a normal diet show kidney calcification, whereas mice fed a low-Pi diet have reduced precipitation of calcium in the kidneys. We found that a high-Pi intake results in slight ectopic calcification in kidneys of mdx mice (Fig. 6B, D) whereas mdx mice fed mid-Pi or low-Pi diets showed no evidence of calcium deposition in the kidneys. Similar to the findings in the heart, B10 mice under all phosphate diets also showed no calcification in the kidneys.

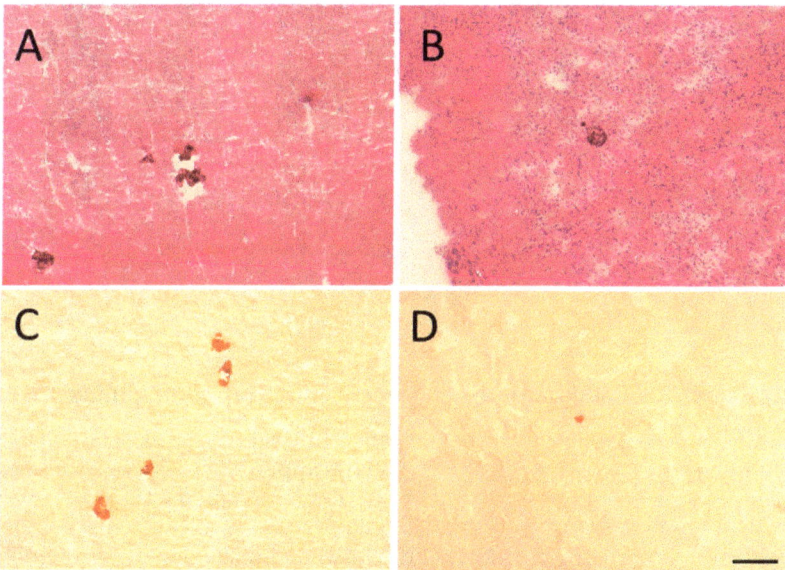

Fig. 6. H&E and alizarin red S-stained cryosections of the heart and kidneys of an mdx mouse fed a high-Pi diet. H&E-stained cryosections of the heart (A) and kidney (B). Alizarin red S-stained cryosections of the heart (C) and kidney (D). The bar represents 100 μm.

5.3 Changes in serum biochemistry

We also examined the serum calcium and phosphate concentrations of B10 and mdx mice fed the three types of Pi diets. The serum phosphate levels of high-Pi fed mdx mice were significantly higher than those of B10 mice fed the same diet, and mdx mice under mid-Pi and low-Pi diets (Fig. 7). However, no marked differences in serum calcium concentrations of mdx mice were detect in the different diet groups. Serum phosphate concentration is largely influenced by dietary intake, with the over-consumption of phosphate often resuting to cause hyperphosphatemia (Calvo et al., 1994), secondary hyperparathyroidism with bone re-sorption (Lutwak et al., 1975), and bone loss (Draper et al., 1979). It is likely that high phosphate intake leads to overworked kidneys and a reduced rate of calcium and phosphate filtration.

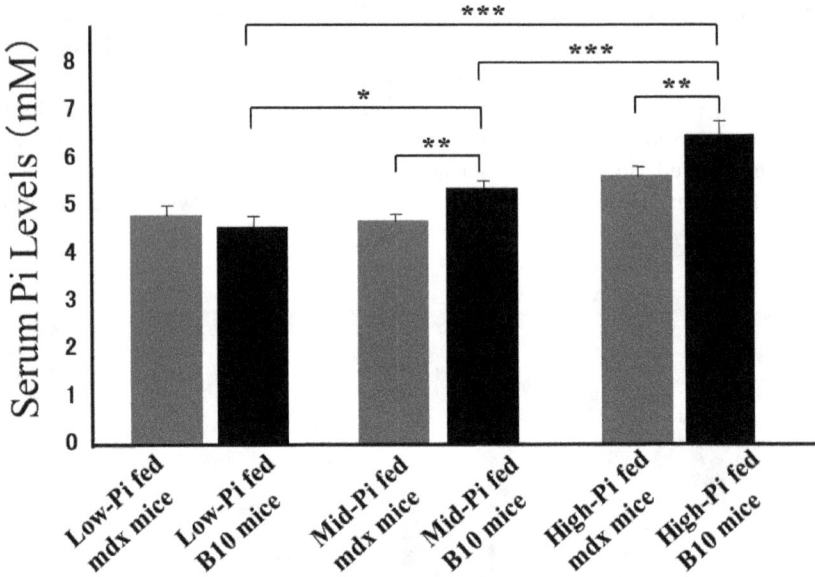

Fig. 7. Serum Pi levels of three-month-old B10 and mdx mice fed three types of Pi diets. Comparison of B10 and mdx mice fed the three Pi diets. (*: p<0.05; **: p<0.01; ***: p<0.001).

6. Effects of ectopic calcification on muscle function of mdx mice

High-Pi intake induced severe ectopic calcification throughout the skeletal muscle of mdx mice. The presence of ectopic calcification in muscles appeared to have a negative impact on the force output of skeletal muscle. To date, no studies have reported the pathophysiological effects of the accumulation of calcium phosphate in muscles. For this reason, we have investigated the effects of ectopic calcification on skeletal muscle contraction of mdx mice.

For muscle force measurements, *in situ* maximal isometric twitch force and tetanic force of right triceps surae muscle (TSM) were recorded. The isometric force recording system was custom-made and the experimental protocols were based on the design of Dorchies et al. (2006). Sixty-day-old B10 and mdx mice fed the three phosphate diets were lightly anesthetized by diethylether gas and then immobilized on a cork board by covering the bodies with Novix-II (Asahi Techno Glass, Chiba, Japan). A confined area of skin and myofasia of the right hindlimb was cut and exposed, and the sciatic nerve was dissected to induce the analgesic conditions. The knee joint was firmly immobilized by a needle that served as the fulcrum and the Achilles tendon of the leg was then severed and connected to a platinum electrode clip associated with a force transducer (DS2-50N Digital Force Gauge; Imada, Aichi, Japan). A second platinum electrode was directly inserted into the TSM. Experimental trials were started after the animals recovered from anesthesia. Using this procedure, we avoided negative effects (*i.e.* muscle relaxation) of the anesthetic regimen, which we previously confirmed and were able to collect real data without any disturbances. For the measurement of maximal single twitch, muscles were stimulated with a square wave pulse (0.5-msec duration) of stimulation voltage. Tetanic force was measured with 200-msec bursts of frequency set to 100 Hz. Muscle length and weight of TSM were measured to estimate the cross-sectional area

(CSA) of the muscle (in mm^2). The specific twitch and tetanic force were normalized by dividing the measured force by the CSA. Using manual settings of the optimal muscle length, maximal twitch contractions were measured within trials up to 20 contractions and all tetanic force measurements were made at locations where the single twitch force was the greatest.

6.1 Results of maximal single force (MSF) and maximal tetanic force (MTF) measurements

Pre-tests results revealed that B10 mice fed the normal CE-2 diet had significantly stronger maximal single force in response to single-pulse stimulation than that of mdx mice (data not shown). This result is consistent with a previous study by Dorchies et al. (2006). Furthermore, although mdx mice have a heavier body weight and muscle mass of the TSM, they exhibited weaker muscle force compared with the control mice. This finding was also consisted with that reported previously (Quinlan et al., 1992), although the muscle mass of anterior tibial muscle was compared, rather than TSM. Therefore, we are confident that our isometric force recording system can be used to evaluate and compare muscle forces between B10 and mdx mice fed the different phosphate diets (Table 1).

We did not detect any significant differences in twitch force between B10 mice of the three phosphate diets groups. However, the high-Pi diet mdx mice had significantly lower (p<0.001) single force than that of mdx mice fed a mid-Pi diet (Fig. 8A), while maximal single force was significantly higher in mdx mice fed a low-Pi diet compared with mid-Pi diet mdx mice. Notably, however, this value was still lower (25% less) than the corresponding value of B10 mice fed a low-Pi diet.

The maximal tetanic force in response to burst stimulation was also measured for all mice. Similar to the results of twitch force, B10 mice had significantly higher tetanic force than mdx mice for all three phosphate diets, whereas no marked differences were detected among B10 mice. Mdx mice fed a high-Pi diet produced significantly less (p<0.001) tetanic force than the other mdx mice (Fig. 8B). Based on these findings, we conclude that high-Pi diet has a greater influence on generating the tetanic force in mdx mice than producing twitch force. These results strongly suggest that calcium deposits in muscles interfere with muscle function. The improvement of muscle forces was likely due to the reduction of ectopic calcification because low Pi-diet did not have a positive effect on force generation in B10 mice, which have no ectopic calcification. However, it is also likely that other factors related to dietary phosphate restriction also contribute to improving muscle function.

Mouse	#	Weight (g)	MSF (mN/mm²)	MTF (mN/mm²)
Low-Pi B10	7	23.1±1.0	102.5±4.6	344.8±15.2
Low-Pi mdx	7	23.8±1.4	74.2±2.4	254.9±14.6
Mid-Pi B10	7	22.3±0.7	100.0±4.1	341.0±11.1
Mid-Pi mdx	7	25.2±0.5	66.8±1.5	246.4±7.2
High-Pi B10	7	22.8±0.7	101.0±3.3	335.6±6.3
High-Pi mdx	7	23.6±0.7	59.6±2.0	193.9±9.6

Table 1. Results of MSF and MTFmeasurements of B10 and mdx mice for the three Pi diet conditions.

MSF

MTF

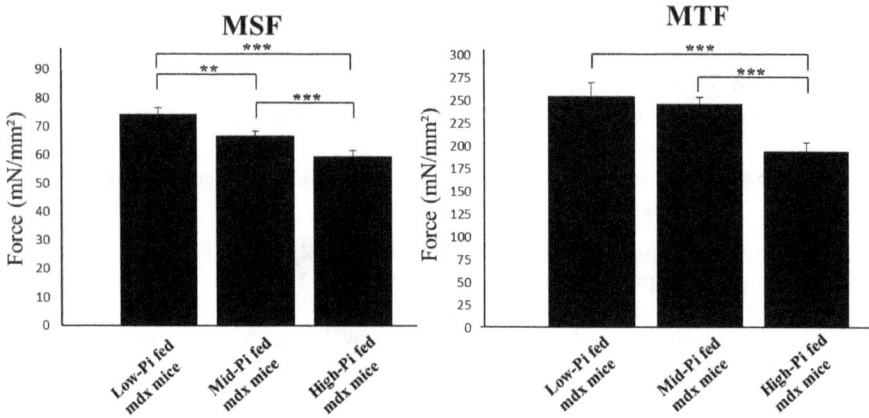

Fig. 8. MSF and MTF measurements of mdx mice for the three Pi diet conditions. (A) Results of MSF. (B) Results of MTF (**: p<0.01; ***: p<0.001).

7. Reduced calcification by low Pi diet in a longitudinal study

Although the influence of dietary phosphate intake on the precipitation of calcium in mdx mice skeletal muscles has been clarified, the effects of phosphate restriction on severe ectopic calcification remained unclear. To understand the impact of phosphate restriction on the deposition of calcium, a longitudinal study was conducted for four mdx mice raised on high-Pi diet from weaning to 60 days of age. At age of 60 days, whole-body images of the mdx mice were taken by noninvasive CT scanning using a Latheta LTC-200 X-ray micro CT scanner (Hitachi Aloka Medical, Tokyo, Japan) (Fig. 9). The mdx mice were then divided into two groups, a continuously fed high-Pi diet group and a low-Pi diet group, until the age of 90 days, at which point whole-body images of the mice were taken again. The whole-body images and volume density of ectopic calcification in the lower body (from the top of os coxae to ankle joint) were compared (Fig. 10). Mice fed a high-Pi diet displayed an increased volume (0.066 cm^3) of ectopic calcification from 60 to 90 days of age, whereas mdx mice fed a low-Pi diet had a reduced (-0.007 cm^3). Thus, it was concluded that the restriction the restriction of dietary phosphate from the age of 60 days reduced the pre-formed ectopic calcification within one month, while continuously feeding the mice a high-Pi diet led to more severe calcium deposits.

8. Mechanisms of calcification

The complete mechanism underlying progressive muscle degeneration due to dystrophin deficit is unclear. Dystrophin-deficient muscles are highly susceptible to the oxidative stress that results from the early onset of muscle degeneration. Muscle necrosis actively occurs following the degeneration, leading to fibrosis and calcification of muscle fibers (Vercherat et al., 2009). It has been suggested that vascular calcification is actively regulated by osteogenic gene expression in vascular smooth muscle cells (Giachelli, 1999). Attention has been focused on inorganic phosphate as one of the potential factors regulating the observed cellular phenotypic changes, as smooth muscle cells *in vitro* cultured under high-Pi conditions undergo osteogenesis and form calcium deposits (Jono et al., 2000). As skeletal muscle satellite cells possess multilineage potential (Asakura et al., 2001; Wada et al., 2002), they might also undergo osteogenic differentiation under high-Pi conditions.

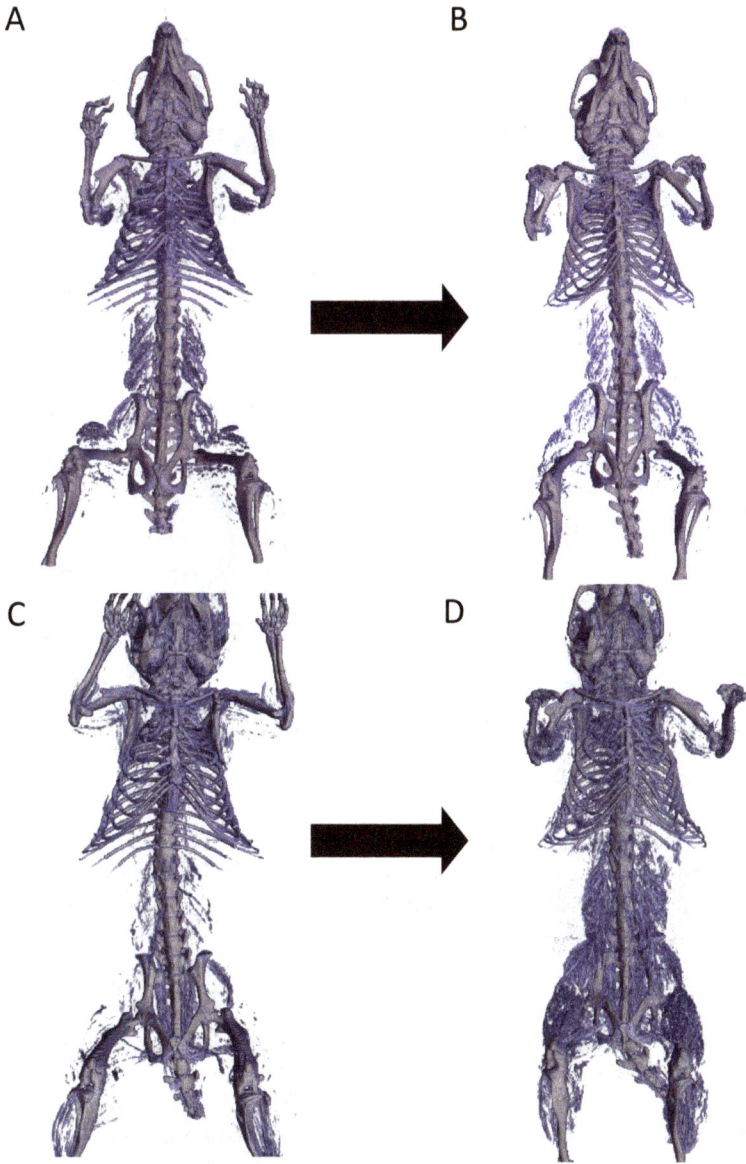

Fig. 9. 3D images of 60-day-old mdx mice fed a high-Pi diet (left) and the images of the same mice after 30 days. (A, B) Sixty-day-old mdx mice fed a high-Pi diet. (C) The same mdx mice (90-day-old) fed a low-Pi diet for 30 days. (D) The same mdx mice (90-day-old) fed a high-Pi diet for 30 days. Bones are shown in grey and ectopic calcification is in light blue.

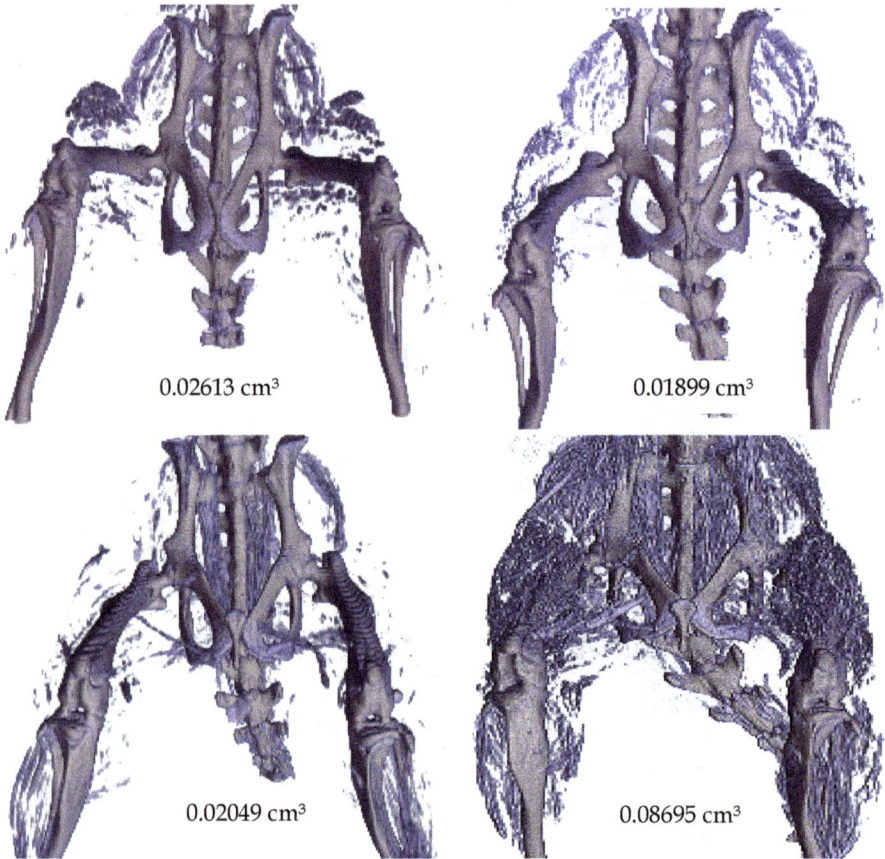

Fig. 10. Enlarged 3D images of the lower limbs of mdx mice fed a high-Pi diet (left) and the images of the same mice fed either low-Pi (top right) or high-Pi diets (bottom right) for 30 days. The numbers represent the volume densities of ectopic calcification in the lower body (from the top of os coxae to ankle joint).

8.1 Pi-induced osteogenesis and reduced myogenesis in C2C12 cells

To study the effects of Pi on muscle cell differentiation, murine myoblast-derived C2C12 cells were cultured for four days under various Pi concentrations and then immunostained for the presence of myogenic (myosin heavy chain; MyHC) and osteogenic (Matrix Gla Protein; MGP) markers. When cultured in normal differentiation medium (Pi=1 mM), the cells underwent muscle differentiation and formed myotubes. Myogenesis proceeded until the Pi concentration of the differentiation medium reached 5 mM, while myotube formation was strongly suppressed at 7 mM. (Fig. 11).

The expression of Runx2, a transcription factor of osteogenesis, increased with the rise of the Pi concentration (Fig. 12A). The retardation of myogenesis caused by the high Pi concentration was also evident by the decrease in both the fusion index and myogenin expression (Fig. 12A). It was notable that in medium containing 5 mM Pi, myogenesis was not inhibited and the C2C12 cells differentiated into myotubes, while the expression Runx2 was augmented (Fig. 12B). Further observation revealed that myogenin and Runx2 did not colocalize in the nuclei of myotubes, rather, Runx2 was localized in the cytoplasm. This finding suggests that Runx2 is inactive in myogenic cells, as it has been reported that Runx2 activity is regulated by translocation between the nucleus and cytoplasm (Zaidi et al., 2001). Upregulation of Runx2 expression was observed by Western blotting not only when the C2C12 cells were cultured under high-Pi conditions, but also when cultured in the presence of calcium deposits, which were generated by the addition of sodium phosphate and calcium chloride to the medium (Fig. 12C). Osteocalcin, another osteogenic marker which is a secreted protein whose expression is regulated by Runx2, was also examined (Fig 12D). RT-PCR was performed with RNA samples prepared from C2C12 cells cultured under the various Pi concentrations for four days. Osteocalcin expression was undetectable when the cells were cultured with 1 mM Pi, but increased with the elevation of the Pi concentration. We also measured calcium deposition in C2C12 cells cultured under the various Pi concentrations and found that although the cells did not deposit calcium under normal Pi conditions, cells cultured in medium containing 3 mM Pi or higher deposited calcium (alizarin red S-positive cells; Fig. 12E). The amount of calcium deposits increased significantly at higher Pi concentrations.

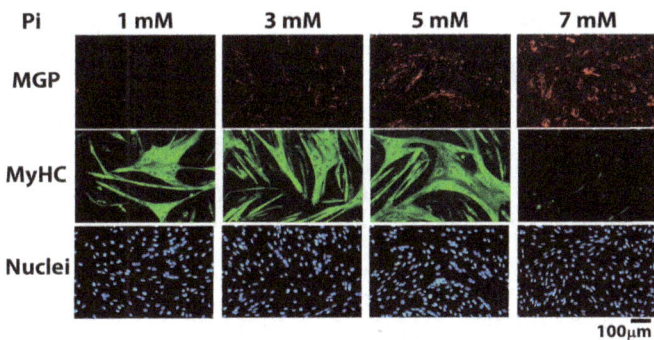

Fig. 11. Immunocytochemistry of C2C12 cells cultured under various Pi concentrations. Cells were immunostained for MyHC (green), MGP (red), and nuclei (blue).

8.2 Pi-induced calcification in primary cultures of skeletal muscle cells

Cells isolated from mdx skeletal muscle tissue were cultured in normal Pi (1.3 mM) to high-Pi (5 mM) medium to study the effects of Pi in primary culture cells. The cells formed myotubes when cultured in normal medium, whereas myotube formation was strongly inhibited under high-Pi conditions. The results of both alizarin red S and von Kossa staining revealed that numerous calcium deposits were present in cells after ten days of culture in high-Pi medium, but none detected in cells cultured in normal medium (Fig. 13). Therefore, Pi induces osteogenesis in myoblasts, resulting in calcification while inhibiting myogenesis. We conclude that the calcification of skeletal muscle is mainly due to the elevation of intracellular Pi levels.

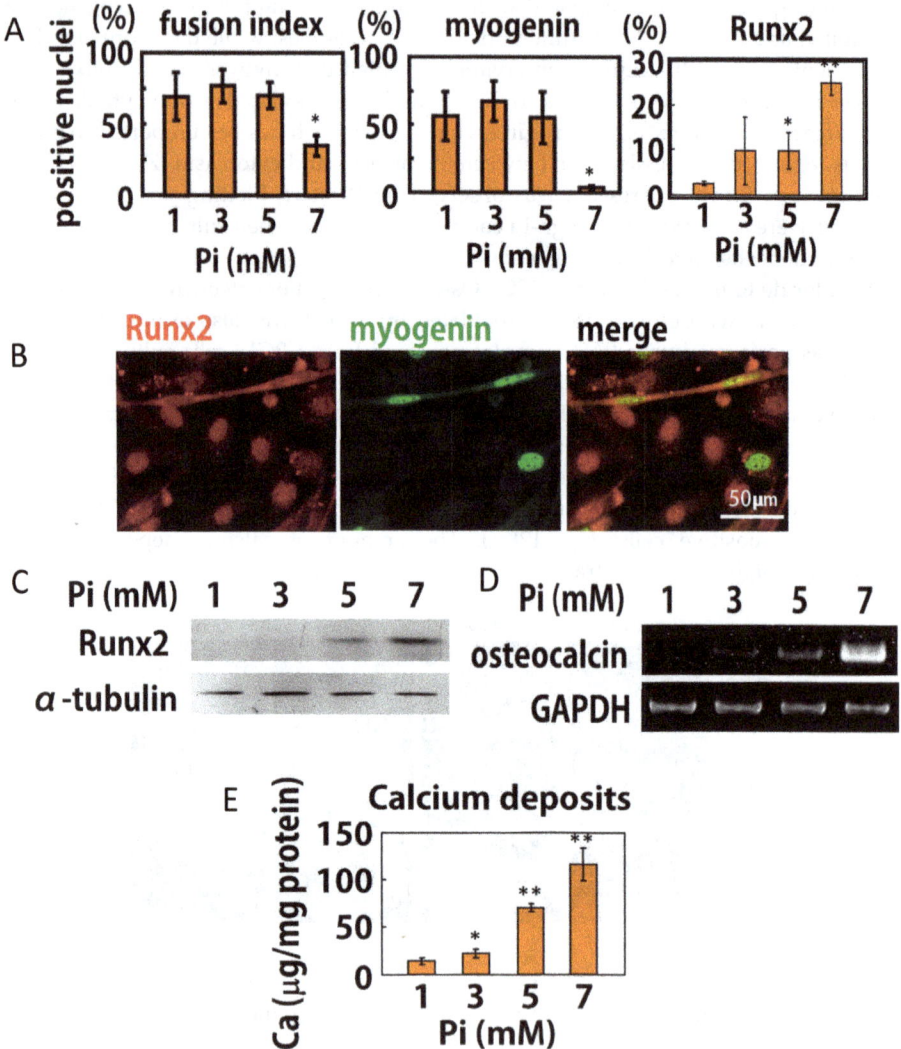

Fig. 12. Immunocytochemistry and RT-PCR of C2C12 cells cultured under various Pi concentrations (1, 3, 5, and 7 m). (A) The fusion index, myogenin expression, and expression of Runx2 were quantified. The fusion index and ratio of nuclei expressing myogenin decreased, while the ratio of Runx2-expressing nuclei increased with increasing Pi concentration. (B) Close observation of cells cultured in medium containing 5 mM Pi by staining with Hoechst 33258 to show the nuclei, or immunostained for myogenin or Runx2. (C) Western blotting of C2C12 cells cultured under increased Pi or Ca concentrations. (D) RT-PCR for osteocalcin in C2C12 cells cultured under various Pi concentrations. (E) Quantification of calcium deposites generated by C2C12 cells cultured under various Pi concentrations. (*: $p < 0.05$; **: $p < 0.01$).

Phase Contrast Image	Alizarin red S	Kossa

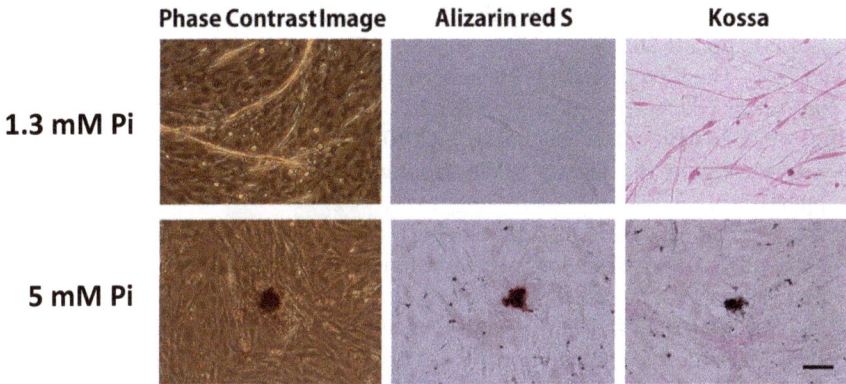

Fig. 13. Calcification of mdx mouse muscle-derived primary culture cells. Calcium deposits were stained red or black with alizarin red S and von Kossa staining, respectively. No calcification was observed when cells were cultured in normal medium containing 1.3 mM Pi. The von Kossa-stained samples were counterstained with nuclear fast red, and myotubes appear pink. The bar represents 100μm.

9. Conclusion

In this study, we reviewed the mechanisms underlying calcification in skeletal muscle cells following the elevation of intracellular Pi concentrations and revealed the effects of dietary phosphate intake on ectopic calcification in mdx mice. Both *in vivo* and *in vitro*, high-Pi conditions lead to the precipitation of calcium in mdx mice. We have demonstrated that the presence of ectopic calcification in skeletal muscle exacerbates the impaired muscle function of mdx mice, which represents a novel finding. The main goal of our studies is to understand the effects and efficacy of nutritional components on muscular dystrophy as a prior therapy. The effects of dietary phosphate intake on muscle pathology and kidney function need to further elucidated in future studies. Furthermore, the therapeutic potential of nutrition, particularly phosphate intake, should be considered when treating patients with DMD.

10. Acknowledgement

This work has been supported by Health and Labour Sciences Research Grant (19A-020) for Research on Psychiatric and Neurological Diseases and Mental Health, Intramural Research Grant(23-5) for Neurological and Psychiatric Disorders of NCNP and a Research Grant for Nervous and Mental Disorders [20B-13] from the Ministry of Health, Labour and Welfare, Japan.

11. References

Asakura, A.; Komaki, M. & Rudnicki, M. (2001). Muscle Satellite Cells are Multipotential Stem Cells that Exhibit Myogenic, Osteogenic, and Adipogenic Differentiation. Differentiation, Vol.68, pp.245-253.

Burbach, J. (1987). Ultrastructure of Cardiocyte Degeneration and Myocardial Calcification in the Dystrophic Hamster. *The American Journal of Anatomy*, Vol.179, pp.291-307.

Calvo, M. (1994). The Effects of High Phosphoru Intake on Calcium Homeostasis. *Advances in Nutritional Researches*, Vol.9, pp.183-207.

Costas, J.; Nye, D.; Henley, J. & Plochocki, J. (2010). Voluntary Exercise Induces Structural Remodeling in the Hearts of Dystrophin-deficient Mice. *Muscle Nerve*, Vol.42, pp.881-885.

Coulton, G.; Morgan, J.; Partridge, T. & Sloper, J. (1988). The mdx Mouse Skeletal Muscle Myopathy: I. A Histological, Morphometric and Biochemical Investigation. *Neuropathology and Applies Neurobiology*, Vol.14, pp.53-70.

Dingerkus, G. & Uhler, L. (1977). Enzyme Clearing of Alcian Blue Stained Whole Small Vertebrates for Demonstration of Cartilage. *Biotechnic & Histochemistry*, Vol.52, pp.229-232.

Dorchies, O.; Wagner, S.; Vuadens, O.; Waldhauser, K.; Buetler, T.; Kucera, P. & Ruegg, U. (2006). Green Tea Extract and Its Major Polyphenol(-)-epigallocatechin Gallate Improve Muscle Function in a Mouse Model of Duchenne Muscular Dystrophy. *American Journal of Physiology. Cell Physiology*, Vol.290, pp.616-625.

Draper, H. & Bell, R. (1979). Nutrition and Osteoporosis. *Advances in Nutritional Researches*, Vol.145, pp.389-391.

El-Abbadi, M.; Pai, A.; Leaf, E.; Yang, H.; Bartley, B.; Quan, K.; Ingalls, C.; Liao, H. & Giachelli, C. (2009). Phosphate Feeding Induces Arterial Medial Calcification in Uremic Mice: Role of Serum Phosphorus, Fibroblast Growth Factor-23, and Osteopontin. *Kidney International*, Vol.75, pp.1297-1307.

Elsherif, L.; Huang, M.; Shai, S.; Yang, Y.; Li, R.; Chun, J.; Mekany, M.; Chu, A.; Kaufman, S. & Ross, R. (2008). Combined Deficiency of Dystrophin and $\beta 1$ Integrin in Cardiac Myocyte Causes Myocardial Dysfunction, Fibrosis and Calcification. *Circulation Research*, Vol.102, pp.1109-1117.

Gaschen, F.; Hoffman, E.; Gorospe, J.; Uhl, E.; Senior, D.; Cardinet, G. & Pearce, L. (1992). Dystrophin Deficiency Causes Lethal Muscle Hypertrophy in Cats. *Journal of the Neurological Sciences*, Vol.110, pp.149-159.

Giachelli, C. (2009). The Emerging Role of Phosphate in Vascular Calcification. Kidney International, V0l75, pp.890-897.

Hu, M.; Kuro-o,M. & Moe, O. (2010). Klotho and Kidney Disease. *Journal of Nephrology*, Vol.16, pp.136-144.

Kendrick, J.; Kestenbaum, B. & Chonchol, M. (2011). Phosphate and Cardiovascular Disease. *Advances in Chronic Kidney Disease*, Vol.18, pp.113-119.

Khan, M. (1993). Corticosteroid Therapy in Duchenne Muscular Dystrophy. *Journal of the Neurological Sciences*, V0l.120, pp.8-14.

Kikkawa, M.; Ohno, T.; Nagata, Y.; Shiozuka, M.; Kogure, T. & Matsuda, R. (2009). Ectopic Calcification is Caused by Elevated Levels of Serum Inorganic Phosphate in Mdx Mice. *Cell Structure and Function*, Vol.34, pp.77-88.

Korff, S.; Riechert, N.; Schoensiegel, F.; Weichenhan, D.; Autschbach, F.; Katus, H. & Ivandic, B. (2006). Calcification of Myocardial Necrosis is Common in Mice. *Virchows Archiv*, Vol.448, pp.630-638.

Kuro-o. (2010). Overview of the FGF-23-Klotho Axis. *Pediatric Nephrology*, Vol.25, pp.583-590.

Kuro-o, M.; Matsumura, Y.; Aizawa, H.; Kawaguchi, H.; Suga, T.; Utsugi, T.; Ohyama, Y.; Kurabayashi, M.; Kaname, T.; Kume, E.; Iwasaki, H.; Iida, A.; Shiraki-Iida, T.; Nishikawa, S.; Nagai, R. & Nabeshima, Y. (1997). Mutation of the Mouse *Klotho* Gene Leads to a Syndrome Resembling Ageing. *Nature*, Vol.309, pp.45-51.

Liu, J.; Okamura, C.; Bogan, D.; Bogan, J.; Childers, M. & Kornegay. J. (2004). Effects of Prednisone in Canine Muscular Dystrophy. *Muscle Nerve*, Vol.30, pp.767-773.

Lutwak, L. (1975). Metabolic and Biochemical Considerations of Bone. *Annals of Clinical and Laboratory Science*, Vol.5, pp.185-194.

Matsuda, R.; Nishikawa, A. & Tanaka, H. (1995). Visualization of Dystrophic Muscle Fibers in Mdx Mouse by Vital Staining with Evans Blue: Evidence of Apoptosis in Dystrophin-Deficient Muscle. *Journal of Biochemistry*, Vol.118, pp.959-964.

McLeod, M. (1980). Differential Staining of Cartilage and Bone in Whole Mouse Fetuses by Alcian Blue and Alizarin Red S. *Teratology*, Vol.22, pp.229-301.

Morishita, K.; Shirai, A.; Kubota, M.; Katakura, Y.; Nabeshima, Y.; Takeshige, K. & Kamiya, T. (2010). The Progression of Aging in *Klotho* Mutant Mice Can Be Modified by Dietary Phosphorus and Zinc. *The Journal of Nutrition*, Vol.131, pp.3182-3188.

Nguyen, F.; Cherel, L.; Guigand, I.; Goubault-Leroux & Myers, M. (2002). Muscle Lesions Associated with Dystrophin Deficiency in Neonatal Golden Retriever Puppies. *Journal of Comparative Pathology*, Vol.126, pp.100-108.

Quinlan, J.; Johnson, S.; McKee, M. & Lyden, S. (1992). Twitch and Tetanus in mdx Mouse Muscle. *Muscle Nerve*, Vol.15, pp.837-842.

Razzaque, M.; Sitara, D.; Taguchi, T.; St-Arnaud, R. & Lanske, B. (2006). Premature Aging-like Phenotype in Fibroblast Growth Factor 23 Null Mice is a Vitamin D Mediated Process. *The FASEB Journal*, Vol.20, pp.720-722.

Vercherat, C.; Chung, T.; Yalcin, S.; Gulbagci, N.; Gopinadhan, S.; Ghaffari, S. & Taneja, R. (2009). Stra13 Regulates Oxidative Stress Mediated Skeletal Muscle Degeneration. *Human Molecular Genetics*, Vol.18, pp.4304-4316.

Verma, M.; Asakura, Y.; Hirai, H.; Watanabe, S.; Tastad, C.; Fong, G.; Ema, M.; Call, J.; Lowe, D. & Asakura, A. (2010). *Fit-1* Haploinsufficiency Ameliorates Muscular Dystrophy Phenotype by Developmentally Increased Vasculature in Mdx Mice. *Human Molecular Genetics*, Vol.19, pp.4145-4159.

Wada, M.; Inagawa-Ogashiwa, M.; Shimizu, S.; Yasumoto, S. & Hashimoto, N. (2002). Generation of Different Fates from Multipotent Muscle Stem Cells. *Development*, Vol.129, pp.2987-2995.

Webb, G. & Byrd, R. (1994). Simultaneous Differential Staining of Cartilage and Bone in Rodent Fetuses: an Alcian Blue and Alizarin Red S Procedure Without Glacial Acetic Acid. *Biotechnic and Histochemistry*, Vol.64, pp.181-185.

Wong, B. & Christopher, C. (2002). Corticosteroids in Duchenne Muscular Dystrophy: a Reappraisal. *Journal of Child Neurology*, Vol.17, pp.183-190.

Zaidi, S.; Javed, A.; Choi, J.; van Wijnen, A.; Stein, J.; Lian, J. & Stein, G. (2001). A Specific Targeting Signal Directs Runx2/Cbfa1 to Subnuclear Domains and Contributes to Transactivation of the Osteocalcin Gene. *Journal of Cell Sciences*, Vol.114, pp.3093-3102.

Zhang, W.; Hove, M.; Schneider, J.; Stuckey, D.; Sebag-Montefiore, L.; Bia, B.; Radda, G.; Davis, K.; Neubauer, S. & Clarke, K. (2008). Abnormal Cardiac Morphology, Function and Energy Metabolism in the Dystrophic mdx Mouse: An MRI and MRS Study. *Journal of Molecular and Cellular Cardiology*, Vol.45, pp.754-760.

15

Advances in Molecular Analysis of Muscular Dystrophies

Arunkanth Ankala and Madhuri R. Hegde
Emory University
USA

1. Introduction

Molecular genetic testing began in the mid-1980's in research laboratories which involved linkage analysis to aid disease gene discovery (Petersen 2000; Ensenauer, Michels et al. 2005). With the identification of novel disease causing genes, genetic tests became available and were launched in clinical testing laboratories in both academic and commercial settings. Unlike complex diseases such as cardiovascular diseases and cancers, diagnostic assays for monogenic Mendelian genetic disorders are relatively easy to design and use in a clinical diagnostic setting. Muscular dystrophies which affect muscles are mostly monogenic diseases and are either dominantly or recessively inherited. However, due to overlapping phenotype or similar clinical presentations of several disorders caused by closely associated genes, the diagnosis may often be elusive. Muscular dystrophies (MD) are a group of genetically and clinically heterogeneous hereditary myopathies characterized by hypotonia, skeletal muscle weakness, contractures, and delayed motor development. They are broadly classified into nine different types including Duchenne (DMD), Becker (BMD), limb girdle (LGMD), congenital (CMD), facioscapulohumeral (FCMD), myotonic (MD), oculopharyngeal (OPMD), distal and Emery-Dreifuss (EMD), some of which have several subtypes based on the gene involved. The clinical manifestations and severity of the various types and subtypes of muscular dystrophies vary widely, ranging from mild myopathy to even cardiac failure. Because of the heterogeneity and overlapping phenotype the patients often face a diagnostic odyssey before receiving the appropriate clinical and molecular diagnosis (Mendell, Sahenk et al. 1995; Mendell 2001). Given the recent improvement of molecular technologies, the classification of MDs in specific, has significantly changed from phenotype driven towards a more molecular based categorization. Therefore it is of pivotal importance to diagnose the molecular basis for the disease which includes determination of the gene and the genotype involved. Molecular diagnosis of the disease is important not only for subsequent patient follow-up but also for choosing the appropriate personalized therapy. Single gene sequencing is considered effective when a single missing protein is identified by a muscle biopsy and loss of that protein fits the phenotype. However, a comprehensive gene sequencing panel is necessary when ambiguous results arise or when muscle biopsies are difficult to obtain. Recent technological advances in sequencing using next generation sequencing and microarrays has made it possible to screen a large number of genes for causative mutations at a fairly low cost and in a reasonably less time. In this book chapter we will discuss the various technological advancements in the molecular diagnosis of various muscular dystrophies and its impact in the clinical world.

2. Mutation spectrum in genes associated with MD

As discussed in other chapters in this book, each type and subtype of MD is caused by mutations in different genes associated with muscle structure and function. Therefore identifying the gene is critical to diagnosis and treatment. Molecular approach to disease diagnosis is highly dependent on the mutation spectrum of the disease causing gene. For example, while *DMD* associated with Duchenne and Becker dystrophies has a high frequency of intragenic deletions (65%), mutation spectrum of *CAPN3* involved in LGMD2A shows a high frequency of point mutations (76%) (Figure 1). Based on these mutation spectrums, deletion-duplication analysis is suggested prior to sequencing analysis for *DMD* while the inverse is suggested for *CAPN3*.

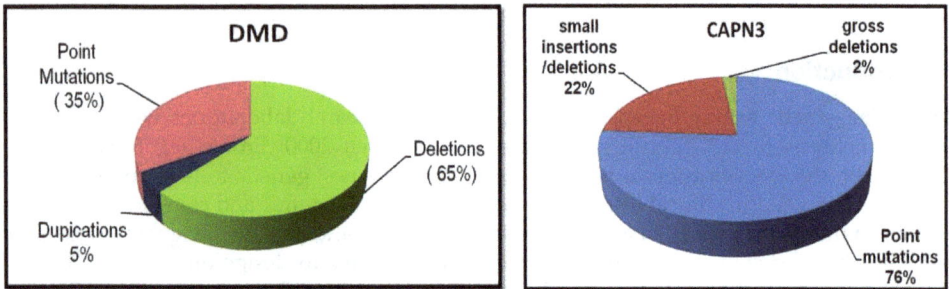

Fig. 1. Mutation spectrum of *DMD* and *CAPN3*

3. Traditional methods used for molecular diagnosis

Since the early practice of genetic testing for diseases that started in mid-1980, several DNA and protein based diagnostic methods have been developed. These traditional methods of diagnosis for muscular dystrophies include linkage analysis, multiplex PCR, Multiplex ligation-dependent probe amplification (MLPA), quantitative PCR, Southern blotting, Immunoblotting (IB) and Immunohistochemical (IHC) analysis. While MLPA, PCR and southern blotting involve DNA analysis, IHC and IB involve protein expression and require muscle biopsies. However, since performing a muscle biopsy is highly invasive it is not preferred both by the patients as well as physicians. Recent advances in molecular analysis for mutation detection have revolutionized the approach to diagnosing these patients (Witkowski 1989; Gangopadhyay, Sherratt et al. 1992; Whittock, Roberts et al. 1997; Ginjaar, Kneppers et al. 2000; Beroud, Carrie et al. 2004).

3.1 Immunohistochemistry

Prior to the development of gene based mutation-detection analysis, disease diagnosis for various MDs was through conventional screening of affected individuals by clinical examination which involved assessment of creatine phosphokinase (CPK) levels and immuno-histological examination of muscle tissue obtained only through an invasive biopsy (Love and Davies 1989; Love, Forrest et al. 1989). As can be seen in the figure below, dystrophic muscle fibers can be easily distinguished from control or normal fibers. These distinguishable characteristics include the high variation in the fiber size and shape, high frequency of internal nuclei, increased connective and adipose tissue in between fibers, as well as presence of large number of regenerating and degenerating fibers in dystrophic musculature (Norwood, de Visser et al. 2007). However these pathological findings vary widely based on the protein involved or disease associated and age of the patient during biopsy. Though immuno-histochemical findings may lead a way to the confirmation of muscular dystrophy, identifying the exact protein (or gene) involved and therefore the specific subtype of muscular dystrophy may always be elusive. This is because of the secondary reduction in protein levels of other closely integrated proteins (Hack, Ly et al. 1998). For example, a mutation in one sarcoglycan can often lead to reduced expression of other sarcoglycans as well (Hack, Ly et al. 1998). Therefore, molecular diagnosis is highly recommended for confirmation of the involved gene and therefore the specific subtype of MD.

Shown in the figure below, are the immunological findings of an individual with mutations in calpain3 (*CAPN3*) which causes LGMD2A (Figure 2). Though calpain3 analysis is not shown here, it can be observed that there is a secondary reduction in β-sarcoglycan. Moreover, in the same patient, Immunoblotting analysis showed occasional reduction of dysferlin protein levels as well. This suggests the importance of molecular diagnosis through DNA analysis, for proper management and therapy.

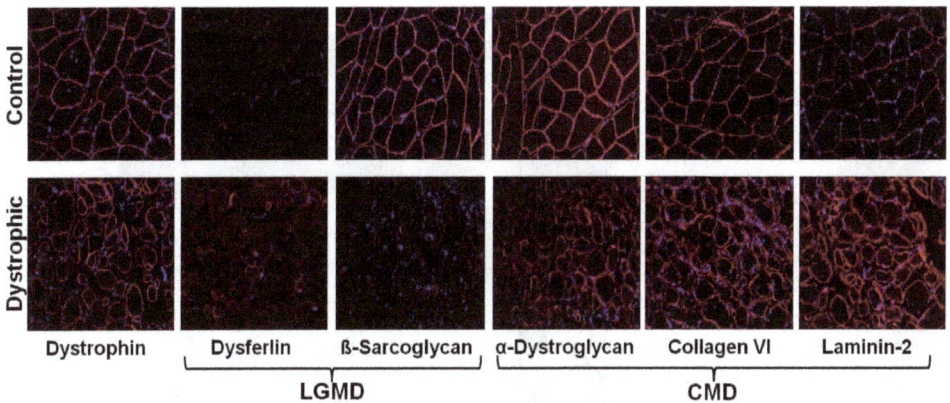

Fig. 2. Immunohistochemical findings in healthy and dystrophic muscle tissue

3.2 Multiplex western blotting

Immunoblotting or western blotting provides an alternative to IHC. IB provides more information regarding the expression and mutation of the protein compared to IHC. Skeletal muscle proteins such as dystrophin, dystroglycans, sarcoglycans and laminin-2 that are associated with Duchenne/Becker muscular dystrophies and different LGMDs as well as CMDs, physically interact and integrate to provide structural stability to the muscle fiber cells. Therefore mutation in one protein may result in altered expressions or stability of these closely associated proteins leading to overlapping phenotypes. Hence, looking at the expression levels of all proteins simultaneously may help better diagnose the disease. Instead of analyzing each protein individually as in IHC and regular IB, a multiplex WB using a cocktail of antibodies can be adopted (Anderson and Davison 1999). This is facilitated by the difference in the molecular sizes of the different proteins. In our laboratory, a variety of antibodies covering different domains of the proteins have been selected to avoid any variability in the hybridization and analyzed as shown (Figure 3).

In the figure below (Figure 3A), at least seven different proteins involved in various MDs were simultaneously analyzed in a set of clinically diagnosed dystrophic patients. Two different cocktails, each made of a set of antibodies targeting different proteins have been optimized for such diagnosis in our laboratory. As can be seen in the figure below, controls (lanes to the left) significantly express dystrophin while no detectable levels could be observed in the patients (lanes to the right). Though there appears to be a secondary reduction in the sarcoglycans as previously described, the complete absence of dystrophin strongly indicates that the causative protein (or gene) is perhaps dystrophin. Further molecular analysis involving deletion-duplication analysis or sequencing of the entire gene is required to confirm the exact mutation. Similarly, carrier and disease status can be inferred by immunoblotting analysis for other MDs like the limb girdle muscular dystrophy type 2 B (LGMD2B) by comparison of dysferlin protein expression (Figure 3B and C). The low expression of dysferlin protein in lane 2 (figure 3B) indicates probable carrier status while the relatively smaller bands in lane 2 (Figure 3C) indicates a probable functional dysferlin protein with a deletion. Both these findings were later confirmed by sequencing analysis.

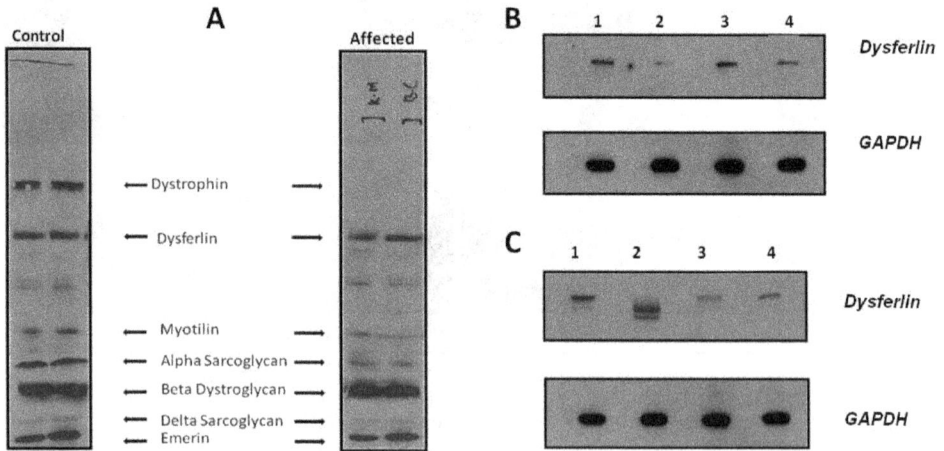

Fig. 3. Immunoblotting analysis of MD proteins. A) A multiplex immunoblot showing the differential expression of various muscle proteins with a clear indication of absence of dystrophin expression in the affected individual when compared to the control. B) Comparison of dysferlin expression in controls and unknowns for carrier and disease status. Lane 1, control healthy individual; lane 2-4 were unknowns C) Comparison of dysferlin expression in controls and unknowns for carrier and disease status. Lane 1, control healthy individual; lane 2-4 were unknowns.

3.3 Multiplex PCR

Multiplex PCR amplification of genomic DNA is a conventional and cost-effective method for identifying deletions in hot spot regions of the gene in affected individuals and involves visualization of bands through regular agarose gels stained with ethidium bromide. Using a combination of several primer pairs in 2-3 reactions, most of the exons including hot-spot regions for *DMD* would be tested for, at a reasonable expense (Beggs, Koenig et al. 1990). However dosage analysis is required for carrier females and is performed through quantitative PCR (qPCR) in which the copy number of the target sequence is directly proportional to the fluorescence of SYBR Green dye during the logarithmic phase. Both deletions and duplications can be identified by qPCR. For example, there would be no amplification of the target product in a male individual with deletion, while in carriers, the amount of product amplified would be half the amount observed in normals carrying two copies of the target sequence to start with. Similarly, in case of a duplication carrier, this ratio would be 3:2 compared to normal. Though these PCR based tools were useful for Duchenne and Becker muscular dystrophies where a majority (70-75%) of disease causing mutations were either deletions or duplications, they were not preferred for other muscular dystrophies.

3.4 Southern blotting

Southern blotting is an alternative technique for screening deletions and duplications in large genes like *DMD*. It involves gel electrophoresis combined with transfer of separated fragments on to membrane and subsequent target fragment detection by hybridization to known probes. It is used in clinical laboratories to confirm deletion and duplication mutations identified by multiplex PCR as well as to determine the extent of the deletion/duplication. Dosage analysis of copy number can also be performed through southern blotting by subsequent densitometry but can be challenging for carrier females (Medori, Brooke et al. 1989).

3.5 MLPA

Multiplex ligation-dependent probe amplification is a variation of conventional PCR and a significant advancement over the multiplex PCR method that permits multiple different targets to be amplified with only a single primer pair (Schouten, McElgunn et al. 2002). Clinically applicable MLPA based simultaneous screening of all 79 exons of DMD gene for deletions and duplications in Duchenne and Becker muscular dystrophy patients was developed around year 2005 and is widely used till date in several clinical laboratories around the world (Schwartz and Duno 2004; Janssen, Hartmann et al. 2005; Lalic, Vossen et al. 2005). It does not require costly equipments and is a very cost-effective method and has therefore been widely accepted by several diagnostic labs. In addition to deletions and duplications it may also identify point mutations. Since MLPA is highly dependant on hybridization of a single probe false positive results can occur in presence of a variation (single nucleotide, deletion or insertion) in the sequence hybridizing to the probe. For this reason single exon deletion need to be investigated further. The presence of variation may also hinder the precise definition of end points of deletions.

3.6 Sequencing

While most of the above mentioned DNA based methods are effective for deletion and duplication detection, they are not preferred for analysis of point mutations. As discussed earlier, majority of the smaller genes associated with MDs have a high frequency of point mutations than for deletions and duplications. Only *DMD* has a high frequency of deletions and duplications while point mutations still account for atleast 35%. Therefore thorough diagnosis of such MDs requires sequence analysis of the exonic regions. PCR amplification of each exon of the suspected gene with exon-specific primer pairs followed by Sanger sequencing is therefore practiced. Patient sequences obtained thus, are then compared to reference sequences and sequence variations as fine as single base-pair change (point mutations) and small indels are efficiently identified (Figure 4).

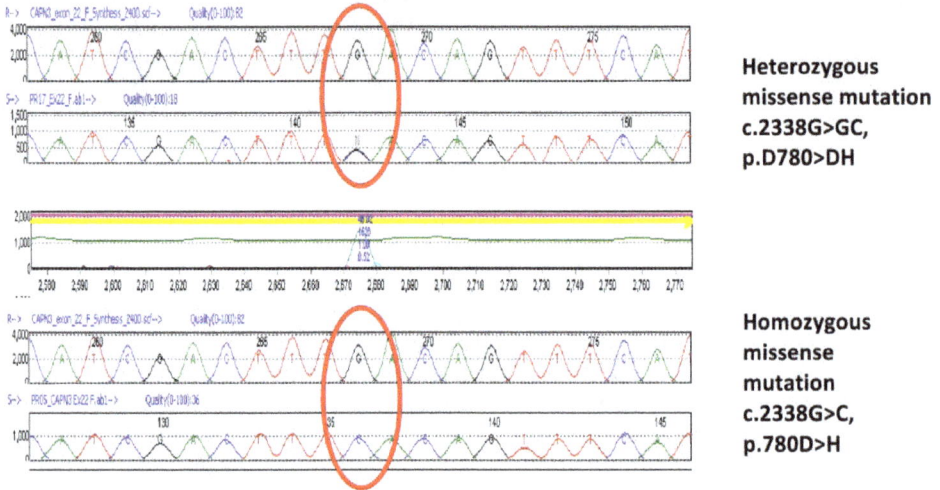

Heterozygous missense mutation c.2338G>GC, p.D780>DH

Homozygous missense mutation c.2338G>C, p.780D>H

Fig. 4. Detection of Point mutations by Sanger sequencing. The upper half of the figure shows a heterozygous point mutation (missense mutation) as detected by a double peak at the corresponding nucleotide when sequenced by Sanger sequencing. The lower half of the figure shows the same point mutation to be present on both alleles making it a homozygous missense mutation.

However, such PCR amplification and sequence analysis may be feasible for small genes that have only few exons. Further, thorough characterization of the clinical presentations need to be performed to narrow down the possible causative gene. Overlapping clinical phenotype and heterogeneity of MDs leads to a suspicion of more than one gene. In such scenario, analysis of more than one gene, some of which have a large number of exons (79 in *DMD*, 55 in *DYSF*, 24 in *CAPN3*) may be very tedious and expensive for clinical diagnosis. Therefore high-throughput, cost effective methods for disease diagnosis have always been in demand.

4. New technological advances in molecular diagnosis

The completion of human genome project has revolutionized the field of human genetics and more specifically human medical genetics (Venter, Adams et al. 2001). High-throughput mutation detection methods such as comparative genomic hybridization arrays (aCGH) and target capture based next generation sequencing panels have been developed. This topic will focus on the various rapidly emerging comprehensive technologies and their advantages over traditional methods. This will include detailed discussion of the microarray based gene panels and next generation sequencing.

4.1 Application of microarrays to detect copy number variation in MD genes

Microarray based comparative genomic hybridization (aCGH), also called molecular karyotyping, is a recently developed technique that enables high-resolution, genome-wide analysis of genomic copy number variations (CNVs). The assay has become a powerful routine clinical diagnostic tool and its increasing resolution and accuracy is gradually replacing traditional cytogenetic approaches for CNV determination. Earlier, the detection potential of genomic imbalances was limited to >5-10Mb with even the highest quality G-banded chromosome analysis. However, with the advent of aCGH, deletions and duplications, as small as 50-100 kb in size are now routinely detected throughout the genome (Stankiewicz, Pursley et al. 2010). The wide-spread application of aCGH has also facilitated the identification of various recurrent CNVs and eventual characterization of several microdeletion and microduplication syndromes.

In a typical aCGH measurement, total genomic DNA is isolated from test (patient) and reference cell populations (or biological sample such as blood or saliva), differentially labeled and hybridized to oligonucleotide arrays. The relative hybridization intensity which is ideally proportional to the relative copy number of target sequence regions is then measured and calculated. The reference genome being normal, any increases and decreases in the intensity ratio directly indicate DNA copy-number variations (deletions or duplications) in the test or patient genome. The intensity data is typically normalized so that the modal ratio for the reference genome is set to a standard value of 0.0, and any decrease is inferred as deletion while an increase in signal in the test genome is inferred as duplication (Figure 5).

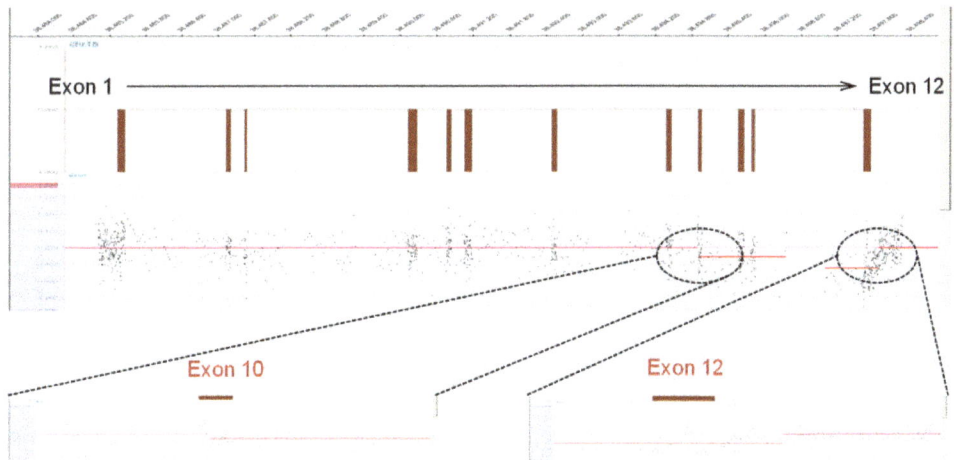

Fig. 5. The figure shows aCGH data for *IVD* gene locus (chr15:40,697,686-40,713,512) using a custom-designed 385K high-density array from NimbleGen. The zoomed in view of the corresponding array highlights the breakpoints for a patient with a deletion mutation encompassing exon 10 to exon 12 with breakpoints in intron 9 and the 3′ UTR. As can be seen in the above figure, the target sequence with normal copy number normalizes to value 0.0, while the deleted regions of exon 10 and exon 12 fall below 0.0 inferrring a loss of a copy number (deletion) compared to reference genome.

In our laboratory, gene-targeted high-resolution oligonucleotide CGH array was custom designed on a NimbleGen 385K platform (till June 2010) or OGT 44K platform (July 2010 onwards) to detect deletions and duplications in 450 genes associated with various genetic disorders. The NimbleGen 385K platform used long oligonucleotides (45–60 mer) to achieve isothermal Tm across the array, with repeat sequence masking implemented to ensure greater sensitivity and specificity. The OGT 44K platform has 44,000 unique sequence probes tiled on the array. Both arrays were designed with average spacing of 10 bp within coding regions and 25 bp within promoter, intronic regions, and 3' UTR, with repeat sequence masking. Use of intronic oligonucleotide probes allows robust detection of dosage changes of the gene within the entire genomic region, as well as determination of approximate breakpoints. The breakpoints for various deletions and duplications detected by the high-resolution aCGH analysis were as close as 500bp to the exact breakpoint determined by conventional sanger sequencing (Ankala, Kohn et al. 2012). Shown below is a figure with aCGH data for several patients with DMD (Figure 6). Deletion-duplication analysis for the entire *DMD* gene by aCGH shows the various intragenic regions that were found deleted in the patients. The zoomed in view of the data also shows the specific exons that were found deleted in these patients thus confirming the molecular diagnosis.

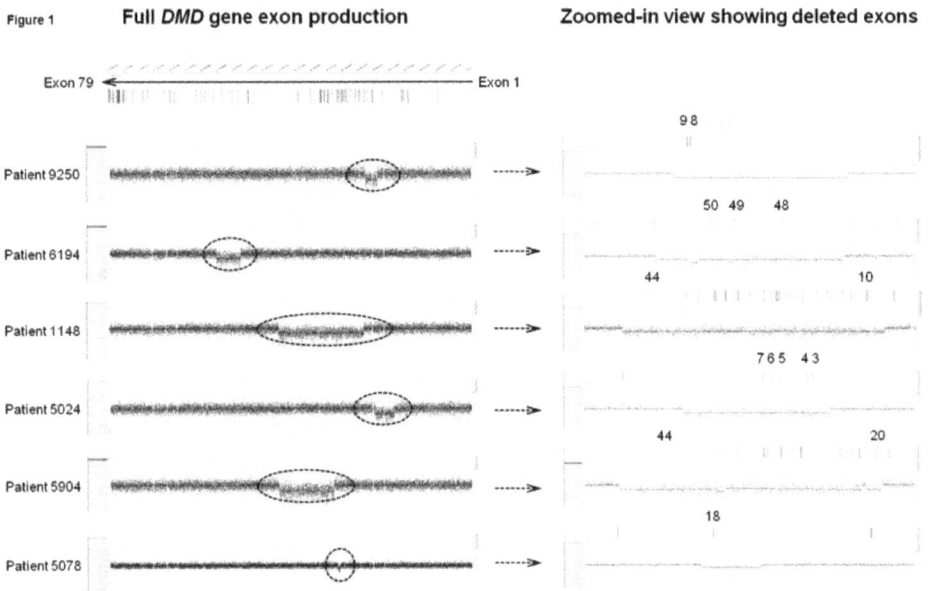

Fig. 6. The column on the left shows comparative genomic hybridization data for DMD gene locus (chrX:31,137,345-33,229,673) for six patient's DNA, using a custom-designed 385K high-density array from NimbleGen. Right column shows the zoomed in view of the corresponding array on the left, with the deleted exons highlighted in red. Each row refers to a patient.

Such a robust, diagnostic test capable of determining disease causing copy number variations (deletions or duplications) in one single assay makes clinical diagnosis rapid and economic. Almost all known MD associated genes can be analyzed simultaneously for mutations through one single affordable test which proves useful especially when the clinical phenotype is very overlapping and narrowing down of genes seems difficult.

4.2 Panel based approach for mutation detection in MDs for example CMD and LGMD

As subtypes of MD caused by different genes share similar clinical presentations simultaneous sequencing of all associated genes as a panel reduces costs and provides quick diagnosis. Several such sequencing panels of different MDs are currently offered in clinical diagnostic laboratories for molecular diagnosis. At least four different sequencing panels are offered at Emory Genetics Laboratory (EGL), which include LGMD, CMD and DMD. Table 1 summarizes the different genes involved in LGMD and the different number of exons in each of these genes.

4.3 Application of next generation sequencing to molecular diagnosis

The high demand for low-cost sequencing has instigated the development of high-throughput sequencing technologies that parallelize the sequence process, producing several thousands of reads or sequences simultaneously in a single reaction (Church 2006; Hall 2007). These high-throughput sequencing technologies have lowered the cost of DNA sequencing beyond what has been possible with the standard sanger sequencing methods (Mardis 2008; Mardis 2008; Schuster 2008). A variety of technologies called next-generation sequencing technologies emerged, each with a unique biochemical strategy (Brenner, Johnson et al. 2000; Church 2006; Mardis 2008; Valouev, Ichikawa et al. 2008; Drmanac, Sparks et al. 2010; Porreca 2010). In general, most of these approaches use an *in vitro* clonal amplification or PCR step to amplify the DNA molecules present in the sample. Illumina or Solexa sequencing, Applied Biosystem's SOLiD sequencing and Ion semiconductor sequencing developed by Ion Torrent Systems Inc are most recent and popular next generation sequencing techniques that are currently being used in clinical laboratories for molecular diagnosis. The sensitivity and specificity of these sequences or the next generation sequencing method is further improved by target capturing the regions of genomic interest from a biological sample or DNA. Particularly when specific regions of the genome need to be targeted or when the gene of interest has been narrowed down to a specific region of the chromosome, then target enrichment methods may be used to enrich the samples in these genomic regions and processed for further analysis of variants or mutations by next generations sequencing. Several capture technologies namely microarray based capture for DMD, RainDance (ten Bosch and Grody 2008) and Fluidigm PCR based capture, Agilent SureSelect and Nimblegen Sequence capture (ten Bosch and Grody 2008) are available in the market. Our comprehensive and comparative analysis of these capture technologies has suggested that RainDance and Fluidigm PCR- based strategies are ideal for clinical panels as they are robust and give a coverage of ~100X whereas in-solution sequence capture protocols from Agilent and Nimblegen are ideal for research based approaches to identify novel genes due to the ability to capture a large number of genes (exome) in a single experiment (Bainbridge, Wang et al. ; Cirulli, Singh et al.).

These target enrichment methods are used both in research and clinical laboratories. In research laboratories, this allows for new gene discovery when CNVs in a particular genomic region correlate with a recurrent clinical phenotype. However, clinical laboratories have a different application where a certain set of disease genes (such as those discussed in

Subtype	Gene Location	Inheritance mode	Gene	Protein	No. of exons
LGMD1A	5q31	AD	MYOT	Myotilin	10
LGMD1B	1q21.2-21.3	AD	LMNA	Progerin, lamin A/C	12
LGMD1C	3p25	AD	CAV3	Caveolin 3	2
LGMD2A	15q15	AR	CAPN3	Calpain 3	24
LGMD2B	2p13	AR	DYSF	Dysferlin	55
LGMD2C	13q12	AR	SGCG	Gamma Sarcoglycan	8
LGMD2D	17q21	AR	SGCA	Alpha Sarcoglycan	10
LGMD2E	4q12	AR	SGCB	Beta Sarcoglycan	6
LGMD2F	5q33	AR	SGCD	Delta Sarcoglycan	8
LGMD2G	17q12	AR	TCAP	telethonin, Titin Cap	2
LGMD2H	9q33.1	AR	TRIM32	TAT-interactive protein, tipartite motif containing 32	2
LGMD2I	19q13.33	AR	FKRP	Fukutin-related protein	4
LGMD2J	2q31	AR	TTN	titin	312
LGMD2K	9q34.1	AR	POMT1	protein-O-mannosyl transferase 1	20
LGMD2L	11p14.3	AR	ANO5	anoctamin 5	22
LGMD2M	9q31-33	AR	FKTN	Fukutin	10
LGMD2N	14Q24.3	AR	POMT2	protein O-mannosyltransferase 2	21
LGMD2O	1p34.1	AR	POMGNT1	protein-O-mannose B1,2-N-acetylglucosaminyl transferase 1	22

Table 1. **Known LGMD subtypes and causative genes.** Shown are the various subtypes of LGMDs and causative genes that have been found to be associated with each of these types of limb girdle muscular dystrophies. Also listed are the number of exons that make up each of these genes to give an overview of the number of sequencing reactions that may be required to sequence and analyze the entire list of genes. Titin alone has 312 exons, and combined with all other genes the number of exons total 550 which may require more than 550 PCR reactions to sequence amplification considering that some exons may be too long for one single sequencing reaction.

gene panels above) are targeted for mutation detection in patient sample. For example, in our clinical laboratory at Emory Genetics Laboratories, target enrichment is performed for a set of 91 genes associated with X-linked Intellectual Disability (XLID) to identify the causative gene and mutation in XLID patients. These two technologies in combination stand the most successful and economic diagnostic tool currently in use both in research and clinical laboratories.

4.4 Whole exome and whole genome sequencing

Whole genome sequencing refers to re-sequencing of the entire genome of the individual while whole exome sequencing refers to selective sequencing of only the coding regions of the genome namely exons. Both strategies may be applied to identifying causal genes and associated mutations for any genetic disorder. However, routine whole genome sequencing is still not feasible due to the high cost associated with the technology. On the other hand, whole exome sequencing is quite affordable as it involves targeted sequencing of all the exons (around 300,000) accounting for only about 1% (36.5 Mb) of the entire human genome (Senapathy, Bhasi et al. 2010). Since it is estimated that these protein coding regions of the human genome account for at least 85% of the disease-causing mutations, the technology is highly appreciable (Choi, Scholl et al. 2009). Currently, whole exome sequencing is being used in research labs for identification of new genes associated with diseases. It involves extensive data mining, validation and confirmation analysis which makes it quite expensive for clinical applications. Whole exome sequencing for mutation detection is currently offered in only one or two clinical labs.

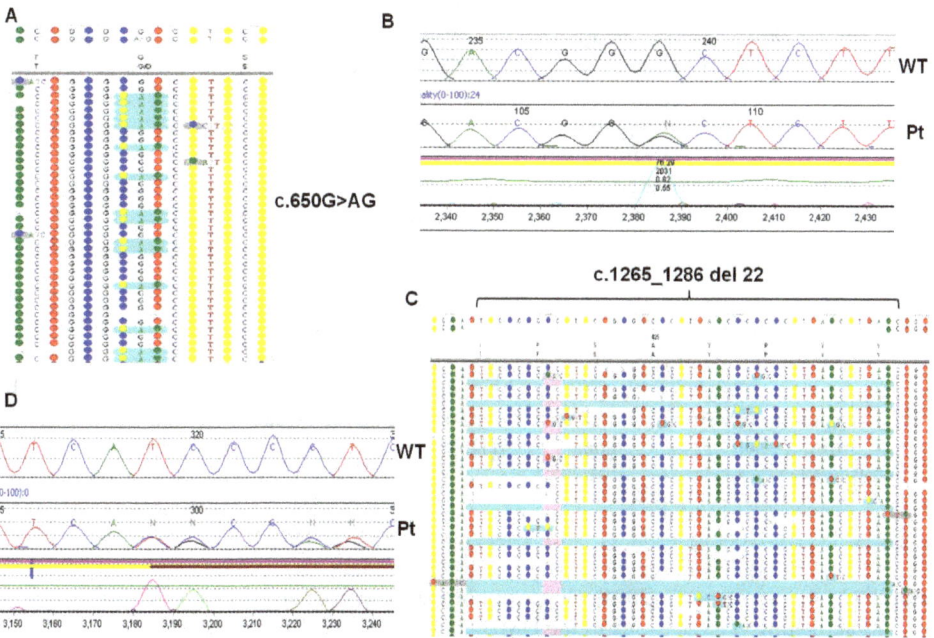

Fig. 7. Sequencing analysis and variant detection A) Next-generation sequencing analysis showing the sequence variants B) Sanger sequence analysis by mutation surveyor software showing the sequence variants and possible pathogenic mutations in the coding region of the gene C) Next-generation sequencing analysis showing a 22bp deletion D) Corresponding sanger sequence analysis by mutation surveyor software showing the start site of the 22bp deletion.

Using whole exome sequencing new candidate genes for several Mendelian disorders have been identified, demonstrating its potential (Ng, Turner et al. 2009; Jones, Ng et al. 2012). To demonstrate the potential of whole exome sequencing, we discuss a patient case that we analyzed through whole exome sequencing and identified pathogenic mutations in a novel gene. This particular patient was tested for all known genes associated with his clinical presentations but was found negative for any pathogenic mutations. We then performed whole exome analysis which gave a large number of variants. Using several filters such as score, coverage and allele percentages we narrowed down the variants. We found two novel mutations that were later confirmed through sanger sequencing (Figure 7).

5. Summary and future directions

We believe whole exome sequencing will become more feasible in the near future and will allow easy identification of disease associated genes and mutations. This definitely needs more sophisticated algorithms to filter the false-positives leaving fewer variants for confirmation and validation. Further, studies involving genotype-phenotype correlation will be very useful and will allow teasing out the various subtypes of the disease (Straub, Rafael et al. 1997; Culligan, Mackey et al. 1998; Gullberg, Tiger et al. 1999; Yurchenco, Cheng et al. 2004; Vainzof, Ayub-Guerrieri et al. 2008). This may be achieved through an integrated approach involving gene expression studies (geneST arrays) and protein antibody arrays. GeneST arrays are expected to give global muscle expression profile and indicate the variability in gene expression by identifying the up and down regulated genes (Vachon, Loechel et al. 1996; Tsao and Mendell 1999; Yamamoto, Kato et al. 2004; Wakayama, Inoue et al. 2008). Also active patient registries should be maintained for each disease type to provide ready access to a pool of information including clinical presentations and causative mutations. This will allow better understanding of the genotype-phenotype correlation and provide more focused approach for molecular diagnosis of the disease.

6. References

Anderson, L. V. and K. Davison (1999). "Multiplex Western blotting system for the analysis of muscular dystrophy proteins." *Am J Pathol* 154(4): 1017-1022.

Ankala, A., J. N. Kohn, et al. (2012). "Aberrant firing of replication origins potentially explains intragenic nonrecurrent rearrangements within genes, including the human DMD gene." *Genome Res* 22(1): 25-34.

Bainbridge, M. N., M. Wang, et al. "Whole exome capture in solution with 3 Gbp of data." *Genome Biol* 11(6): R62.

Beggs, A. H., M. Koenig, et al. (1990). "Detection of 98% of DMD/BMD gene deletions by polymerase chain reaction." *Hum Genet* 86(1): 45-48.

Beroud, C., A. Carrie, et al. (2004). "Dystrophinopathy caused by mid-intronic substitutions activating cryptic exons in the DMD gene." *Neuromuscul Disord* 14(1): 10-18.

Brenner, S., M. Johnson, et al. (2000). "Gene expression analysis by massively parallel signature sequencing (MPSS) on microbead arrays." *Nat Biotechnol* 18(6): 630-634.

Choi, M., U. I. Scholl, et al. (2009). "Genetic diagnosis by whole exome capture and massively parallel DNA sequencing." *Proc Natl Acad Sci U S A* 106(45): 19096-19101.

Church, G. M. (2006). "Genomes for all." *Sci Am* 294(1): 46-54.

Cirulli, E. T., A. Singh, et al. "Screening the human exome: a comparison of whole genome and whole transcriptome sequencing." *Genome Biol* 11(5): R57.

Culligan, K. G., A. J. Mackey, et al. (1998). "Role of dystrophin isoforms and associated proteins in muscular dystrophy (review)." *Int J Mol Med* 2(6): 639-648.

Drmanac, R., A. B. Sparks, et al. (2010). "Human genome sequencing using unchained base reads on self-assembling DNA nanoarrays." *Science* 327(5961): 78-81.

Ensenauer, R. E., V. V. Michels, et al. (2005). "Genetic testing: practical, ethical, and counseling considerations." *Mayo Clin Proc* 80(1): 63-73.

Gangopadhyay, S. B., T. G. Sherratt, et al. (1992). "Dystrophin in frameshift deletion patients with Becker muscular dystrophy." *Am J Hum Genet* 51(3): 562-570.

Ginjaar, I. B., A. L. Kneppers, et al. (2000). "Dystrophin nonsense mutation induces different levels of exon 29 skipping and leads to variable phenotypes within one BMD family." *Eur J Hum Genet* 8(10): 793-796.

Gullberg, D., C. F. Tiger, et al. (1999). "Laminins during muscle development and in muscular dystrophies." *Cell Mol Life Sci* 56(5-6): 442-460.

Hack, A. A., C. T. Ly, et al. (1998). "Gamma-sarcoglycan deficiency leads to muscle membrane defects and apoptosis independent of dystrophin." *J Cell Biol* 142(5): 1279-1287.

Hall, N. (2007). "Advanced sequencing technologies and their wider impact in microbiology." *J Exp Biol* 210(Pt 9): 1518-1525.

Janssen, B., C. Hartmann, et al. (2005). "MLPA analysis for the detection of deletions, duplications and complex rearrangements in the dystrophin gene: potential and pitfalls." *Neurogenetics* 6(1): 29-35.

Jones, M. A., B. G. Ng, et al. (2012). "DDOST Mutations Identified by Whole-Exome Sequencing Are Implicated in Congenital Disorders of Glycosylation." *Am J Hum Genet*.

Lalic, T., R. H. Vossen, et al. (2005). "Deletion and duplication screening in the DMD gene using MLPA." *Eur J Hum Genet* 13(11): 1231-1234.

Love, D. R. and K. E. Davies (1989). "Duchenne muscular dystrophy: the gene and the protein." *Mol Biol Med* 6(1): 7-17.

Love, D. R., S. M. Forrest, et al. (1989). "Molecular analysis of Duchenne and Becker muscular dystrophies." *Br Med Bull* 45(3): 659-680.

Mardis, E. R. (2008). "The impact of next-generation sequencing technology on genetics." *Trends Genet* 24(3): 133-141.

Mardis, E. R. (2008). "Next-generation DNA sequencing methods." *Annu Rev Genomics Hum Genet* 9: 387-402.

Medori, R., M. H. Brooke, et al. (1989). "Genetic abnormalities in Duchenne and Becker dystrophies: clinical correlations." *Neurology* 39(4): 461-465.

Mendell, J. R. (2001). "Congenital muscular dystrophy: searching for a definition after 98 years." *Neurology* 56(8): 993-994.

Mendell, J. R., Z. Sahenk, et al. (1995). "The childhood muscular dystrophies: diseases sharing a common pathogenesis of membrane instability." *J Child Neurol* 10(2): 150-159.

Ng, S. B., E. H. Turner, et al. (2009). "Targeted capture and massively parallel sequencing of 12 human exomes." *Nature* 461(7261): 272-276.

Norwood, F., M. de Visser, et al. (2007). "EFNS guideline on diagnosis and management of limb girdle muscular dystrophies." *Eur J Neurol* 14(12): 1305-1312.

Petersen, G. M. (2000). "Genetic testing." *Hematol Oncol Clin North Am* 14(4): 939-952.

Porreca, G. J. (2010). "Genome sequencing on nanoballs." *Nat Biotechnol* 28(1): 43-44.

Schouten, J. P., C. J. McElgunn, et al. (2002). "Relative quantification of 40 nucleic acid sequences by multiplex ligation-dependent probe amplification." *Nucleic Acids Res* 30(12): e57.

Schuster, S. C. (2008). "Next-generation sequencing transforms today's biology." *Nat Methods* 5(1): 16-18.

Schwartz, M. and M. Duno (2004). "Improved molecular diagnosis of dystrophin gene mutations using the multiplex ligation-dependent probe amplification method." *Genet Test* 8(4): 361-367.

Senapathy, P., A. Bhasi, et al. (2010). "Targeted genome-wide enrichment of functional regions." *PLoS One* 5(6): e11138.

Stankiewicz, P., A. N. Pursley, et al. (2010). "Challenges in clinical interpretation of microduplications detected by array CGH analysis." *Am J Med Genet A* 152A(5): 1089-1100.

Straub, V., J. A. Rafael, et al. (1997). "Animal models for muscular dystrophy show different patterns of sarcolemmal disruption." *J Cell Biol* 139(2): 375-385.

ten Bosch, J. R. and W. W. Grody (2008). "Keeping up with the next generation: massively parallel sequencing in clinical diagnostics." *J Mol Diagn* 10(6): 484-492.

Tsao, C. Y. and J. R. Mendell (1999). "The childhood muscular dystrophies: making order out of chaos." *Semin Neurol* 19(1): 9-23.

Vachon, P. H., F. Loechel, et al. (1996). "Merosin and laminin in myogenesis; specific requirement for merosin in myotube stability and survival." *J Cell Biol* 134(6): 1483-1497.

Vainzof, M., D. Ayub-Guerrieri, et al. (2008). "Animal models for genetic neuromuscular diseases." *J Mol Neurosci* 34(3): 241-248.

Valouev, A., J. Ichikawa, et al. (2008). "A high-resolution, nucleosome position map of C. elegans reveals a lack of universal sequence-dictated positioning." *Genome Res* 18(7): 1051-1063.

Venter, J. C., M. D. Adams, et al. (2001). "The sequence of the human genome." *Science* 291(5507): 1304-1351.

Wakayama, Y., M. Inoue, et al. (2008). "Reduced expression of sarcospan in muscles of Fukuyama congenital muscular dystrophy." *Histol Histopathol* 23(12): 1425-1438.

Whittock, N. V., R. G. Roberts, et al. (1997). "Dystrophin point mutation screening using a multiplexed protein truncation test." *Genet Test* 1(2): 115-123.

Witkowski, J. A. (1989). "Dystrophin-related muscular dystrophies." *J Child Neurol* 4(4): 251-271.

Yamamoto, T., Y. Kato, et al. (2004). "Expression of genes related to muscular dystrophy with lissencephaly." *Pediatr Neurol* 31(3): 183-190.

Yurchenco, P. D., Y. S. Cheng, et al. (2004). "Loss of basement membrane, receptor and cytoskeletal lattices in a laminin-deficient muscular dystrophy." *J Cell Sci* 117(Pt 5): 735-742.

16

Strength and Functional Measurement for Patients with Muscular Dystrophy

Yen-Mou Lu[1] and Yi-Jing Lue[2,3,4]
[1]Department of Orthopedics, Kaohsiung Medical University Hospital,
[2]Department of Physical Therapy, College of Health Science,
[3]Department of Rehabilitation, Kaohsiung Medical University Hospital,
[4]Department and Graduate Institute of Neurology, School of Medicine, College of Medicine,
[1,2,3,4]Kaohsiung Medical University, Kaohsiung,
Taiwan

1. Introduction

Progressive muscle weakness is the major symptom of patients with muscular dystrophy.

The aims of the chapter are to introduce the strength decrease pattern and functional assessment, and to exam the advantages and disadvantages of these measurements applied to various types of muscular dystrophy. Three parts of the measurement for muscular dystrophy are included: the strength decrease pattern, the common general functional scales, and the disease specific scale.

This chapter places emphasis on patients with more weakness in proximal than distal parts. The most common type of proximal muscular dystrophy is Duchenne muscular dystrophy (DMD). Due to rapid deterioration, DMD can be seen as a severe form of muscular dystrophy. Other types of proximal muscular dystrophies have a slower rate of disease progression compared to DMD, such as Beck muscular dystrophy (BMD), limb girdle muscular dystrophy (LGMD), facioscapulohumeral muscular dystrophy (FSHD) and others.

2. Strength measurement

Muscle strength can be assessed by many methods, such as manual muscle testing (MMT) and using the quantitative methods by instrument. Common instruments include the handheld dynamometer (HHD), and the isokinetic dynamometry or other fixation instruments.

For MMT method, the Medical Research Council (MRC) Scale is the most often used system, with the procedures detecting the magnitude of strength by grading muscle strength from 0 to 5. The MRC scale is an ordinal scale, with grades 0-5 also named as "Zero, Trace, Poor, Fair, Good, and Normal". Grade 0 (Zero) cannot be palpated in muscle contraction. Grade 1 (Trace) has some evidence of slight muscle contraction but the strength is too weak to move the joint. Grade 2 (Poor) strength can move the joint (full range of motion) when gravity is eliminated during the test. The Poor grade is sub-graded as Poor minus (2-), Poor, and Poor plus (2+). The 2- indicates strength able to move the joint but unable to complete the range of motion. The 2+ indicates strength to complete the range of motion and also the ability to resist slight force made by the rater. Grade 3 (Fair) strength can be tested at the antigravity position. Similar to Poor grade, the Fair grade is sub-graded as Fair minus (3-: cannot complete the range of motion), Fair (3: can complete the range of motion), and Fair plus (3+: can against gravity with minimal resistance). Grade 4 (Good) completes the range of motion against gravity with moderate resistance, and Grade 5 (Normal) can resist with strong resistance. We recommend using the MMT method to measure the strength decrease pattern for patients with muscular dystrophy especially in clinical applications. The MMT grading system can clearly provide information as to whether patients can move their body in an antigravity position, and even if the strength is very weak, the strength can be discriminated by grade Poor, Trace or Zero. The weakness strength of patients with muscular dystrophy may be unable to be measured by some instrumentation, as most of these are designed to be measured in an antigravity position and the resistance is added during the measurement. The grading system is also graded (recorded) as different symbol methods. For example, the Kendall system ranked the grade from 0 to 10: it leaves the 0 as Zero, and 10 as Normal, and transforms the strength to a percentage, with a range from 0 to 100 %; the 100% being the grade of "Normal" strength. The percentages of Normal grade strength can be used for calculating the mean strength from many muscles. (Kendall et al., 1993)

For isokinetic dynamometer or other fixation methods in strength measurement, complicated procedures are often not practicable due to the expense and time required to prepare the instruments. Although inconvenient, isokinetic dynamometry has been considered to be the gold standard for assessing dynamic muscle strength and provides much information of various muscle performance characteristics (Mark et al., 2004). The isokinetic strength has been studied in patients with mild or moderate strength impairment (Kilmer et al., 1994; Tiffreau et al., 2007). The patient with DMD with severe progressive muscle weakness highlights the method's limitations for assessment of very weak strength (Bäckman, 1988).

For HHD, it is a convenient, portable and inexpensive device for assessing isometric strength in a clinical setting. The rater handholds the device and presses it against the force that subjects exert with maximal effort. The make test and break test are two methods for HHD. In the make test, the rater resists the patient's maximal isometric contraction, whereas in the break test the rater overcomes the force of the patient produced in eccentric contraction (Bohannon, 1988; Stratford & Balsor, 1994). Both methods have their advantage and disadvantages. To measure the weakness strength of patients with muscular dystrophy, we suggest using the make method. The HHD has been studied in DMD; the strength measured by a force transducer and the data presented in Newtons or kilograms has been seen as real compared to the MMT method where the strength record is in ratio-level parametric data (Scott & Mawson, 2006; Brussock et al., 1992; Stuberg & Metcalf, 1988) However, the main disadvantage of the HHD is the unsure reliability of some muscle strength on the tester when stabilizing the dynamometer (Bohannon, 1999).

3. Strength decrease pattern of various types of muscular dystrophy

3.1 Methods of strength measurement

We previously measured the strength decrease pattern of some common types of muscular dystrophy, such as Duchenne muscular dystrophy (DMD), limb girdle muscular dystrophy

(LGMD) and facioscapulohumeral muscular dystrophy (FSHD) (Lue et al., 1992; Lue & Chen, 2000a; Lue & Chen, 2000b). Patients had been diagnosis by two qualified neurologists and followed up for at least two years. Before the strength measurement, they did not receive medication or a strengthening program for improving muscle strength.

The manual muscle test was used by well trained physical therapists. Thirty-two muscle groups were examined on both sides; the muscle groups included neck and trunk muscles, and upper and lower extremities. The neck and trunk muscles included neck flexors/extensor and the trunk flexors/extensors. In the upper extremities, the shoulder (flexors, extensors, and abductors), elbow (flexors and extensors) and wrist (flexors and extensors) muscle strength were measured. In the lower extremities, the hip (flexors, extensors, and abductors), knee (flexors and extensors) and ankle (dorsi- and plantar-flexors) muscle strength were measured. To calculate the mean strength, we used Kendall's percentage method (Kendall et al., 1993).

3.2 Natural strength decrease pattern of patients with DMD

DMD is a quick deterioration muscular dystrophy, with the strength decrease in a linear pattern positively correlated with age. For every year increment in age, the average strength decreases by about 3.9 percent of normal strength. About half of normal strength will be retained at the age of 12 years. The lower extremities are weaker than the upper extremities. The proximal parts are weaker than distal parts; the weakness of the elbow and wrist extensors is more dominant than that of the flexors. In the lower extremities, hip and knee extensors are weaker than hip and knee flexors. If the strengths of agonist and antagonist muscles of a joint are significantly different, the part of the stronger side becomes shorter and joint contracture easily develops. Therefore, in the upper extremities, elbow and wrist flexion contracture is easily found. Routine active or passive range of motion exercise for patients to maintain the full range of motion is a very important part of any rehabilitation program. Similar to the upper extremities, in the lower extremities, hip flexor contracture is commonly found in early stages of DMD; after the patients are unable to walk, the knee joints may develop severe flexion contracture as the joints are not routinely performing the (normal) range of motion exercises. At the end of life of a patient with DMD, the strength of finger flexors can manage some activities, even though at the age of twenty. Therefore, we recommend using computer games as finger exercises or a leisure activity for patients with DMD, and the keyboard may or may not need modification.

3.3 Natural strength decrease pattern of patients with LGMD

LGMD is also named limb girdle muscular dystrophy syndrome, which is combined with various types of limb girdle muscular dystrophy. Therefore, the strength decrease pattern has greater variation than other types of muscular dystrophy. The speed of muscle strength decrease will become slower than the onset after long disease duration. The strength decrease patterns do not fit well in a linear regression model (R^2 only 0.074), and fit better in an inverse regression model (R^2 equal to 0.154), with the equation as follows: mean muscle strength = 0.61+(0.63/disease duration). No significantly stronger strength in flexor than extensor muscles for extremities are found in patients with LGMD. The limitation of this study needs to be mentioned, as these patients with LGMD may or may not have only one type of LGMD. For more precise study in the future, the gene deficit should be confirmed and including the same type of LGMD for strength study is essential.

3.4 Natural strength decrease pattern of patients with FSHD

Comparing the severity of the strength decrease, the strength decrease of patients with FSHD is the mildest compared to the strength decrease of patients with LGMD or DMD. The shoulder muscle strength is the weakest, followed by elbow muscle strength. The strengths of the trunk area and lower extremities are the best. A special pattern of the strength asymmetry is found in patients with FSHD, as the average right side muscle strength is weaker than the left side. Most of the subjects included in this study were right-handed. The dominant side may increase the use and lead to more prominence of strength decrease, therefore, in clinical applications for patients with FSHMD, too many strengthening programs or overload activity for the upper extremities may not suit such patients. The mechanism for asymmetry of strength found in patients with FSHD still requires further studies to be elucidated.

4. Functional measurements

4.1 The brooke and vignos scales

The common functional scales to rate the grade of disease severity are the Brooke Scale and the Vignos Scale. Both scales were firstly designed for DMD, and nowadays have been used in many neuromuscular diseases. The Brooke scale was designed to assess the upper extremity function. The grades of the Brooke scale range from 1 to 6; 1 means that the subject can elevate their arms full range to the head with the arms straight; while 2 means that the shoulder strength is insufficient to elevate their arms and the subject needs to flex the elbow to elevate the arms; in grades 3 and 4, the subject is unable to elevate the shoulders but can raise hands to the mouth with or without weight respectively; grade 5 refers to the subject being unable to raise hands to the mouth and only some hand movement exists, while grade 6 refers to no useful function of hands (Table 1).

Grade	Description
1	Starting with arms at the sides, the patient can abduct the arms in a full circle until they touch above the head
2	Can raise arms above head only by flexing the elbow (shortening the circumference of the movement) or using accessory muscles
3	Cannot raise hands above head, but can raise an 8-oz glass of water to the mouth
4	Can raise hands to the mouth, but cannot raise an 8-oz glass of water to the mouth
5	Cannot raise hands to the mouth, but can use hands to hold a pen or pick up pennies from the table
6	Cannot raise hands to the mouth and has no useful function of hands

Table 1. Grading system for the Brooke scale.

The Vignos scale was designed to assess the lower extremity function. The grades of the Vignos scale range from 1 to 10; 1 means that the subject can walk and climb stairs without assistance; 2 and 3 means that the strength is insufficient to walk upstairs without assistance as they need to use a rail for climbing stairs (grade 2: in a normal speed; grade 3: slowly);

grades 4 and 5 refer to subjects still having the ability to walk unassisted but unable to climb stairs (grade 4 also can rise from a chair but grade 5 cannot); grades 6 to 8 refer to patients using the long leg brace for walking or standing (grade 6: walk without assistance; grade 7: walk with assistance for balance; grade 8: cannot walk, only for standing); grade 9 refers to the subject being unable to stand, but can sit in a wheelchair; and the final grade 10 refers to the subject being confined to a bed (Table 2).

Grade	Description
1	Walks and climbs stairs without assistance
2	Walks and climbs stair with aid of railing
3	Walks and climbs stairs slowly with aid of railing (over 25 seconds for eight standard steps)
4	Walks unassisted and rises from chair but cannot climb stairs
5	Walks unassisted but cannot rise from chair or climb stairs
6	Walks only with assistance or walks independently with long leg braces
7	Walks in long leg braces but requires assistance for balance
8	Stands in long leg braces but unable to walk even with assistance
9	Is in a wheelchair
10	Is confined to a bed

Table 2. Grading system for the Vignos scale.

4.2 Timed tests

Some studies also record the time needed for some activities as a functional testing for patients with muscular dystrophy. The raters measure the time need for a person to complete the activity. The example of these common activities are climbing some steps of stairs, walking a fixed distance, sitting to standing from a chair, rising from the floor, dressing a cloth and cutting a square.

5. Advantages and disadvantage of the common functional scales of various types of muscular dystrophy

The Brooke and Vignos scales are easy to rate the severity of the patients, but the study found some disadvantages (Lue et al., 2009). We assessed the acceptability of the Brooke and Vignos scales in patients with DMD, BMD, FSHMD, and LGMD from a multi-center study. The patients with DMD were classified as severely progressive group, while the others (BMD, FSHD, and LGMD) were classified as slowly progressive group.

The results showed that the Brooke and Vignos scales were easy to assess, and it took a little time to complete the tests, and the patients did not feel uncomfortable. The Brooke scale is acceptable to grade arm function of the severely progressive group; the DMD, each grade of the Brooke scale is distributed with the acceptable percentage (ranging from 7.1% to 33.3%). However, it is insufficient to discriminate differing levels of severity of the slowly progressive group (BMD, FSHMD, and LGMD). No subject was graded at 4, and only one was graded at 6. The floor effect was large in all types of the slowly progressive group (ranging from 20.0% to 61.9%), especially high in BMD.

In the Vignos scale, using the long leg brace to grade the lower limb function may be a major problem for this scale. Grades 6 to 8 are items using long leg braces for walking or standing; these grades are inapplicable, because some cases did not use long leg braces for walking or standing. The floor effect of the Vignos scale was also large in BMD (23.8%) and in FSHD (50.0%). Among the slowly progressive muscular dystrophies, the function of patients with FSHD was the best; they had better leg function and were less influenced in their daily living activities than other types of slowly progressive muscular dystrophy. Using the two scales in combination with other measures (or instead, to use a complicated instrument for various types of muscular dystrophy) to calculate their function is suggested.

6. The muscular dystrophy functional rating scale

The Muscular Dystrophy Functional Rating Scale (MDFRS) is a disease specific scale designed for various muscular dystrophies. The MDFRS was developed by Lue et al. in 2006. Four domains are included in MDFRS. It was developed in many stages: the preliminary pool of items, the admission of various types of muscular dystrophies and the reliability, validity and responsiveness studies (Lue et al. 2006). The results showed the MDFRS is a reliable and valid disease-specific measure of functional status for patients with muscular dystrophy. The internal consistency was excellent, with the value of the Cronbach' alpha ranging from 0.84 to 0.97. The test-retest reliability and the inter-rater reliability were high (ICC=0.99) for all domains. The MDFRS demonstrated moderate to high correlation with a range of functional rating scales. The confirmatory factor analysis supported a four-dimensional construct. The floor and ceiling effects were small and the responsiveness of various types of muscular dystrophies was well.

The MDFRS combines four domains to rate mobility, basic activities of daily living, arm function and impairment. The number of items of each domain is 9, 6, 7 and 11 respectively (Table 3). The scale offers much important information of muscular dystrophy such as the mobility ability, dependence of daily living, the arm function, and many impairment conditions. The arm function part of the MDFRS effectively conquers the disadvantages of the Brooke scale (Lue et al. 2006; Lue 2010).

Each item of MDFRS is scored on a 4-point scale (1-4), with 1 representing being unable to do the activity and is completely dependent; 2 needing assistance from another person, 3 is independent, without assistance from another person but movement or completion of an activity is slow, and 4 means no problem for the activity and can be done at normal speed. The impairment domain includes the items for measuring contractures and scoliosis, strengths, and respiratory function, and the scoring system was specially designed by the characteristics of the items.

In the mobility domain, the 9 items included measuring the ability of stair climbing, outdoor mobility, indoor mobility, transfers from bed to chair, wheelchair manipulation, standing from sitting, sitting from lying, rolling and changing body position in bed. The items of stair climbing, outdoor and indoor mobility can effectively rate the function of the initial stage of the disease, and the ability of the sitting from lying, rolling and changing body position in bed is needed to examine the condition of the patients with terminal stages of the disease, such as the patients with DMD.

Domains			
Mobility domain	Basic ADL domain	Arm function domain	Impairment domain
1 Stair climbing	1 Feeding	1 Managing objects over head	1 Severity of upper limb joint contracture
2 Outdoor mobility	2 Combing hair	2 Carrying objects	2 Severity of lower limb joint contractures
3 Indoor mobility	3 Brushing teeth	3 Cleaning table	3 Number of contracted joints in the upper limbs
4 Transfers from bed to chair	4 Dressing upper/lower parts of body	4 Writing	4 Number of contracted joints in the lower limbs
5 Wheelchair manipulation	5 Toileting	5 Turning books	5 Severity of neck contracture
6 Standing from sitting	6 Bathing	6 Picking up small objects	6 Strength of the neck
7 Sitting from lying		7 Managing objects over head	7 Strength of the trunk
8 Rolling			8 Scoliosis
9 Changing body position in bed			9 Orthopnea
			10 Sputum clearance
			11 Ventilator assisted

Table 3. Domains and Items of the Muscular Dystrophy Functional Rating Scale.

In the basic activity daily living domain, the 6 items included measuring the ability of feeding, combing hair, brushing teeth, dressing upper/lower parts of body, toileting and bathing. The bathing activity is the most difficult item, and the feeding and combing hair items are easy activities for patients with muscular dystrophy.

In the arm function domain, the 7 items included measuring the ability of managing objects overhead, carrying objects, clearing a table, writing, turning books, picking up small objects, and manipulating small objects. The items were designed to be more functional as needed for daily routine activities. The ability of managing objects over the head and carrying objects is useful to assess the better upper extremity function for patients with muscular dystrophy.

The part of impairment section of the MDFRS offers simple measurement methods for measuring the condition of the contracture and scoliosis, weakness of the head and trunk muscles to provide head control and sitting balance, and the condition of the pulmonary function. In the impairment domain, the 11 items included measuring the problem of severity of upper and lower limb joint contracture, the number of contracted joints in the upper and lower limbs, the severity of neck contracture, strength of the neck, strength of the trunk, severity of the scoliosis, and three respiratory problems such as orthopnea, sputum clearance ability, and the need to use a ventilator. These impairment items are all important symptoms and signs of the various types of muscular dystrophy, and decreasing the complication of contracture is the most important issue for management of such patients. At the end stage of the disease, vital respiratory care needs to be added, and the 3 items of impairment domain of the MDFRS could offer the general condition of the pulmonary function. Therefore, the assessment from the impairment domain could offer a lot of useful information for clinicians and caregivers to easily know the condition of the patients and provide better care for them at different stages of the disease.

The total scores of each domain sum up the scores of each item, therefore, the range of scores for 4 domains are 9-36 for the mobility domain, 6-24 for the basic activity of daily living domain, 7-28 for the arm domain, and 11-44 for the impairment domain respectively. The scores of each domain can be calculated as a percentage to represent the functional performance of a person compared to normal condition; the equation is as follows: (total scores-number of item) / full total scores and multiple 100. The % of mobility ability = (the sum of score from 9 item -9) / 36 *100; the % of basic activity of daily living ability = (the sum of score from 6 item -6) / 24 *100; the % of arm function ability = (the sum of score from 7 item -7) / 28 *100; and the % of impairment condition = (the sum of score from 11 item -11) / 44 *100.

7. Conclusion

In conclusion, various types of muscular dystrophy present differing speeds of disease progression with decreasing muscular strength in different patterns. Due to some disadvantages of the Brooke and Vignos grading scales applied to patients with muscular dystrophy, clinical application of these scales should be used with caution, especially in patients with slowly progressive muscular dystrophy. We suggest that the applications can be used in combination with MDFRS, which is a multi-domain instrument, a valid and reliable scale, capable of evaluating the various levels of functional status of different types of muscular dystrophy.

8. References

Bäckman, E. (1988). Methods for measurement of muscle function. Methodological aspects, reference values for children, and clinical applications. *Scand J Rehabil Med* Sppl 20:9-95.

Bohannon, R. (1988). Make tests and break tests of elbow flexor muscle strength. *Phys Ther* 68(2): 193–194.

Bohannon, R. (1999). Inter-tester reliability of hand-held dynamometry: a concise summary of published research. *Percept Mot Skills* 88(3): 899-902.

Brussock, C., Haley, S., & Munsat, T. (1992). Measurement of isometric force in children with and without Duchenne's muscular dystrophy. *Phys Ther* 72(2): 105-114.

Kendall, F., McCreary, E., & Provance, P. (1993). Muscles testing and function. 4th ed. Williams & Wilkins, Baltimore.

Kilmer, D., McCrory M., & Wright N. (1994) The effect of a high resistance exercise program in slowly progressive neuromuscular disease. *Arch Phys Med Rehabil* 75 (5): 560-563.

Lue, Y., Jong, Y. & Lin, Y. (1992). The strength and functional performance of patients with Duchenne muscular dystrophy based on natural history. *Kaohsiung J Med Sci* 8(11): 597-604.

Lue, Y., & Chen, S. (2000a). Strength and functional performance of patients with limb-girdle muscular dystrophy. *Kaohsiung J Med Sci* 16(2): 83-90.

Lue, Y., & Chen, S. (2000b). The strength and functional performance of patients with Facioscapulohumeral muscular dystrophy. Kaohsiung J Med Sci 16(5): 248-254.

Lue, Y., Su, C. & Yang, R. (2006). Development and validation of a muscular dystrophy-specific functional rating scale. *Clin Rehab* 20 (9): 804-817.

Lue, Y., Lin, R., & Chen, S. (2009) Measurement of the functional status of patients with different types of muscular dystrophy. *Kaohsiung J Med Sci* 25(6): 325-333.

Lue, Y. (2010). Muscular Dystrophy Functional Rating Scale (MDFRS) In: Registry of Outcome Measures. URL: http://www.researchrom.com/masterlist/view/199. Accessed 2011.7.20.

Mark, B., Martine, A., & Neil, A. (2003). Assessment and interpretation of isokinetic muscle strength during growth and maturation. *Sports Medicine* 33(10): 727-743.

Scott, E., & Mawson, S. (2006). Measurement in Duchenne muscular dystrophy: consideration in the development of a neuromuscular assessment tool. *Dev Med Child Neurol* 48(6): 540-544.

Stratford, P., & Balsor, B. (1994). A comparison of make and break tests using a hand-held dynamometer and the Kin-Com. *J Orthop Sports Phys* 19(1): 28–32.

Stuberg, W., & Metcalf, W. (1988). Reliability of quantitative muscle testing in healthy children and in children with Duchenne muscular dystrophy using a hand-held dynamometer. *Phys Ther* 68(6): 977-982.

Tiffreau, V., Ledoux, I., & Eymard. B. (2007). Isokinetic muscle testing for weak patients suffering from neuromuscular disorders: a reliability study. *Neuromuscul Disord* 17(7):524-531.

17

Motor Function Measure Scale (MFM): New Instrument for Follow-Up Brazilian Patients with Neuromuscular Disease

Cristina Iwabe[1], Anamarli Nucci[2],
Beatriz Helena Miranda Pfeilsticker[3] and Luis Alberto Magna[4]
[1]Faculty of Medical Sciences (FCM), Campinas State University (UNICAMP)
[2]Department of Neurology, FCM UNICAMP,
[3]Department of Neurology, FCM UNICAMP,
[4]Department of Medical Genetics, FCM UNICAMP,
Brazil

1. Introduction

Neuromuscular disorders include a variety of conditions that affect motor neurons (spinal muscular atrophy), peripheral nerves (neuropathy), neuromuscular junction (myasthenia gravis) or muscle fibers (myopathy) (1).

Myopathy is characterized by primary and generally irreversible skeletal muscle tissue degeneration, including genetic, inflammatory, metabolic or endocrine disorders and the different are charaterized by the muscle fibre type affected, mode of inheritance, age of onset and course of evolution (2,3,4).

The term muscular dystrophy has been used in cases of rapidly progressive myopathy as well as of slow progressive degeneration of muscle, such as myotonic dystrophy (2).

Myotonic Dystrophy (MD) is defined as the most common inherited myopathy in adults, with multisystemic involvement (cardiovascular, respiratory, nervous, visual, endocrine), autossomal dominant pattern and distinct clinical manifestations (2,5,6). Depending on the genetic trait, MD is classified as type 1 (MD-1), type 2 (MD-2) (7), or type 3 (8); being the type 1 the most common and the type 3, very rare.

The MD-1, described by Steinert in 1909, is caused by expansion of CTG nucleotides repeat in the region of the gene for dystrophy myotonic protein kinase (DMPK) on chromosome 19; over 35 and ranging from 80 to more than 4,000 repetitions in the affected individuals. This abnormal protein is responsible for the disability of muscle, cardiac and nervous cells, involving several systems (9).

This disease can be classified in: congenital, infantile, classic (age of onset between 10 to 50 years) and with minimal involvement (10). Usually the earlier the onset of symptoms, the greater the number of repetitions of the nucleotides (7,11).

The muscle involvement is the main clinical feature with variations in the degree of weakness (facial, neck and distal muscles of limbs), as well as myotonia. In the congenital form, the deficit is prominent at birth without myotonia. In the infantile form, weakness is relatively mild, and in adults form there is slowly progression of the symptoms (11).

In contrast to muscular dystrophy, the congenital myopathy is described as non-progressive or slowly progressive and rarely fatal disease. Among them is included the Congenital Fibre Type Disproportion (CFTD) (12). The CFTD is a congenital myopathy described by Brooke (13) as having generalized weakness, hypotonia at birth and slow progression of symptoms associated with abnormal histological predominance of type 1 muscle fibres, and smaller size of at least 12% than type 2. The patients have abnormalities such as congenital hip dislocation, foot deformities, kyphoscoliosis, ligament laxity, high palate and underweight (14,15,16,17).

The CFTD pattern suggests a autossomal dominant trait although sporadic recessive cases has been described (18,19,20,21). Distinct mutations in the gene that codes the α-skeletal muscle actin (ACTA1), selenoprotein N (SEPN1) and α-tropomyosin (TPM3) proteins were identified in some cases, but the molecular mechanisms that cause the disparity of the fibres are still unknown (22,23).

Individuals with CFTD show different degrees of weakness, more severe in the early stages of development, especially in the lower limbs (20). Generally they have a good prognosis, but in some cases they may be associated with respiratory (14,20) or cardiac (16,21) failures.

Considering the CFTD and MD-1, both have weakness as the main physical limitation (17,24,25) and the individuals become more and more dependent to achieve their routine activities. Rehabilitation programs must measure and maximize patients motor skills and optimizing their functionality.

 Now a days, several therapeutic techniques and other health professionals assessment tools can be used for patient selection, therapeutic monitoring and to establish prognosis for recovery (26).

 Generally, the evaluations are qualitative test, not allowing for the individual assessment of the recovery of the better patients (27). Currently, Medical Research Council scale (MRC) for measuring muscle strength is being used for clinical examination and patient follow-up however, it does not reflect the real abilities of each individual (28)There are several scales to measure function in neuromuscular diseases, including the Barthel Index (BI), Vignos scale and Motor Function Measure (MFM) (28).

The MFM have been developed and validated for neuromuscular diseases by the research group of the Department of Pediatric Reeducation L'Escale, Lyon, France.This is a more comprehensive, specific and functional scale, analyzing the function of the head, trunk, proximal and distal segments in several neuromuscular diseases (28).

The scale comprises 32 items, including static and dynamic evaluations, divided into three dimensions:

-    Dimension 1 (D1): a standing position and transfers, with 13 items
-    Dimension 2 (D2): axial and proximal motor function, with 12 items.

- Dimension 3 (D3): distal motor function, with seven items, six of which are related to the upper limbs.

Each item is graduated on a 4-point scale (scores 0 to 3), with the instructions detailed in the scoring manual, specific to each item. Score 0 - can not start the requested task or can not keep the starting position. Score 1 – initializes the item. Score 2 - partially performs the requested movement or fully realized, but imperfectly. Score 3 - completes the item, with controlled movement (normal).

In cases of tendon retraction or joint limitation, the individual is graduated as not presenting adequate strength to perform the movement, preventing them from receiving the maximum degree. The total score and each dimension are expressed in percentages relative to maximum score (96 points).

In 2008, Iwabe et al. (29) demonstrated the reliability of the Portuguese version's MFM (P-MFM), showing a high correlation intra and inter examiner results.

The aim of this chapter is to describe the validation of the P-MFM and its applicability to evaluate the motor function in muscular myopathy and dystrophy individuals.

2. P-MFM Validation

The population comprised a total of 65 patients, 37 male and 28 female, average 33.09 years (8-60 years), with laboratory findings confirming clinical diagnosis of congenital muscular dystrophy (n = 7), Duchenne (n = 5), Becker (n = 4), limb girdle (n = 4), facioscapulohumeral (n = 8), distal myopathy (n = 4), mitochondrial (n = 3), centrocore (n = 6), congenital fibre types disproportion (n = 1), myotonic dystrophy (n = 21) and spinal muscular atrophy (n = 2); outcome in the Neuromuscular Diseases Clinic of the Faculty of Medical Sciences, Campinas State University (UNICAMP).

Patients were evaluated according to the P-MFM, BI and Vignos scales. All evaluations were performed by the same examiner and BI questions were answered by the patient, or in some cases with the help of their parents.

Statistical analysis - the total scores and each of the three dimensions of P-MFM were correlated with Vignos scale and BI by the Spearman correlation coefficient, with significance level of 5% ($p < 0.05$).

It was observed that in P-MFM scale, both its three dimensions and total score, were correlated negatively and significantly with the Vignos scale, and correlated positively and significantly with the BI (Table 1).

P-MFM	Vignos scale	BI
Dimension 1	-0,858*	0,946*
Dimension 2	-0,852*	0,871*
Dimension 3	-0,671*	0,736*
Total	-0,894*	0,980*

* - $p < 0,001$

Table 1. Correlation between P-MFM, Vignos scale and BI.

Validation is defined as the ability of an instrument to measure a particular aspect, and for this it is necessary the correlation with other validate scales, and similar characteristics (30). Miller et al. (31) defined some factors for the scale's development and validation. The instrument must represent the function at the moment, following the patient's evolution over the time, and each individual serving as his own control.

The MFM was developed for this purpose, containing items easily implementable and understandable by patients from different age groups (6-60 years). This scale has the capacity of analyze the most important motor functions and deficiency in several neuromuscular diseases. It can measure the activity of the proximal and distal segments members; as well as the standing position and transfering at the moment and over time (28).

The capacity of MFM scale to analyze the various body segments and their mobility in all neuromuscular diseases, empathizes its use in research and clinical. To be applied in Brazil, it was necessary perform the validation process of the Portuguese version, considering that the scale item was approved in reproducibility and reliability (29).

In Brazil, there are only two assessment instruments validated for patients with dystrophy (32).

The P-MFM validation study used two functional scales, the BI and Vignos scale (33,34,35,36). BI and Vignos scale are clinical instruments often used to assess the level of functionality in neuromuscular diseases (35). These two scales were used in the study by Nair et al. (37), with Duchenne muscular dystrophy, showing to be a valid instrument for assessing the functional limitations in this patients.

Previous validation studies about functional neuromuscular diseases using the BI and Vignos scale (28,38,39) demonstrated the correlation between them. Studies analyzing the functionality of individuals with neuromuscular diseases after clinical or surgical treatment, or correlating it to other parameters, such as muscle strength using these same scales (40,41,42,43,44) established them as easy to use instruments.

In this study, we found a high significant correlation among the P-MFM, Vignos scale and BI, allowing for validation of the Portuguese version of MFM.

3. Applicability of P-MFM in family with CFTD, associated muscle magnetic ressonance

We studied members of a family with clinical and laboratory CFTD. They were evaluated for muscle strength (MRC scale) and motor function by the scale P-MFM (29) and were previously examined in the Neuromuscular Diseases Clinic through physical examination, serological and neurophysiological tests and muscle biopsy. One sample was taken from the biceps muscle from the father in a family. The obtained sample was fixed in isopentane and frozen in liquid nitrogen. Sections were stained with hematoxylin-eosin (H & E), Gomori trichrome modified (TRI) or oil red O and analyzed by histochemical techniques for nicotinamide adenine dinucleotide phosphatase, nicotinamide dehydrogenase tetrazolium reductase (NADH-TR), succinate dehydrogenase (SDH) and immunohistochemistry for slow and fast myosin, desmin and alpha B crystalline.

Muscle magnetic resonance imaging (mMRI) was performed in magnetic field of 2.0 Tesla, T1-weighted images in axial plane for the leg muscles from each patient, according to De Cauwer et al. (45).

Image data were analyzed quantitatively according to the degree proposed by Mercuri et al. (46) and modified by Nucci (47).

0 = normal appearance
1 = slight appearance of "moth-food", with sporadic areas of hyperintensity.
2 = moderate appearance of "moth-food" with related areas of hyperintense spaced, comprising less than 30% of muscle volume.
= 2.5 appearance of "moth-food" with moderate hyper spaced areas, comprising 30 to 60% of muscle volume.
3 = severe appearance of "moth-food", with numerous areas of confluence of hyperintense with muscle still present in the periphery.
4 = complete fatty degeneration, with replacement of muscle by connective tissue and fat.

The family pedigree is shown in Figure 1. It was not possible to examine patient's mother (I-1) and patient's uncle (I-2). Throughout the family's history, the patient's mother was indicated as asymptomatic, and the uncle as having the phenotype very similar with myopathy aspects.. Thus, I-2 was marked as affected in the pedigree.

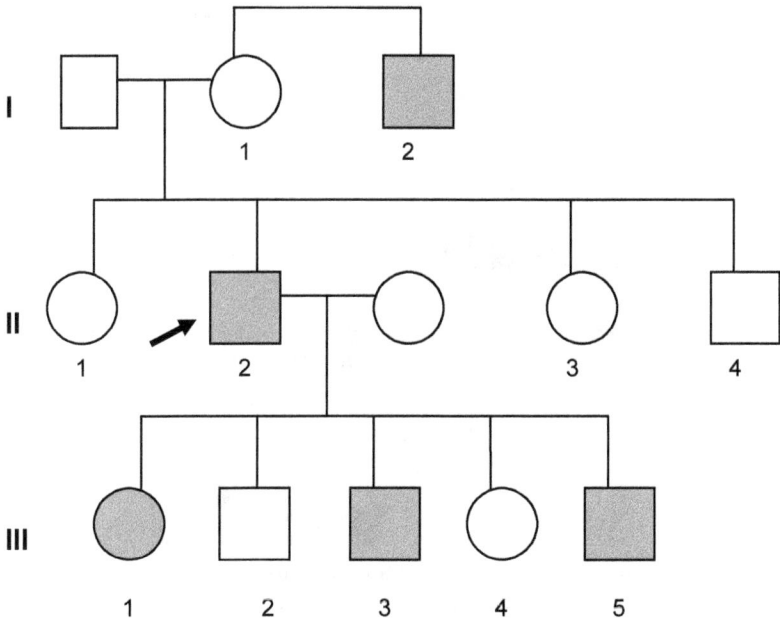

Fig. 1. Family pedigree. The grey figures are the affects cases. The white figures are the normal cases

CASE II -2 Male, 48-year-old with consanguineous parents, complaining about muscle weakness since childhood, considered a "sick child" due to limitations in physical activities and difficulty in gaining weight. The acquisition of motor milestones was delayed, just being able to walk around 5 years old. The initial clinical examination showed a collaborative and lanky patient (1.78 meters, 48 kg), with severe scoliosis dextro-convex compensate cervical, and high palate. A complex gait was observed due to the misalignment of the spinal cord and the tendency to walk with his feet fallen. The muscles stretch reflexes were hypoactive, but the cranial nerves, the cognition and sensibility were normal. The laboratory findings for creatine kinase (CK) showed 181 U / L (normal values below 170), and the study for motor and sensory nerves conduction were within normal limits. Electromyography (EMG) of the deltoid and biceps brachii showed the most potential of motor units with respect polyphasic, low amplitude and short duration, myopathy indicative,, despite the present right quadriceps were relatively normal. The electrocardiogram (ECG) and routine laboratory tests showed no abnormalities. The main morphologic abnormality in biopsy was a disproportion of the fibre types with small type 1

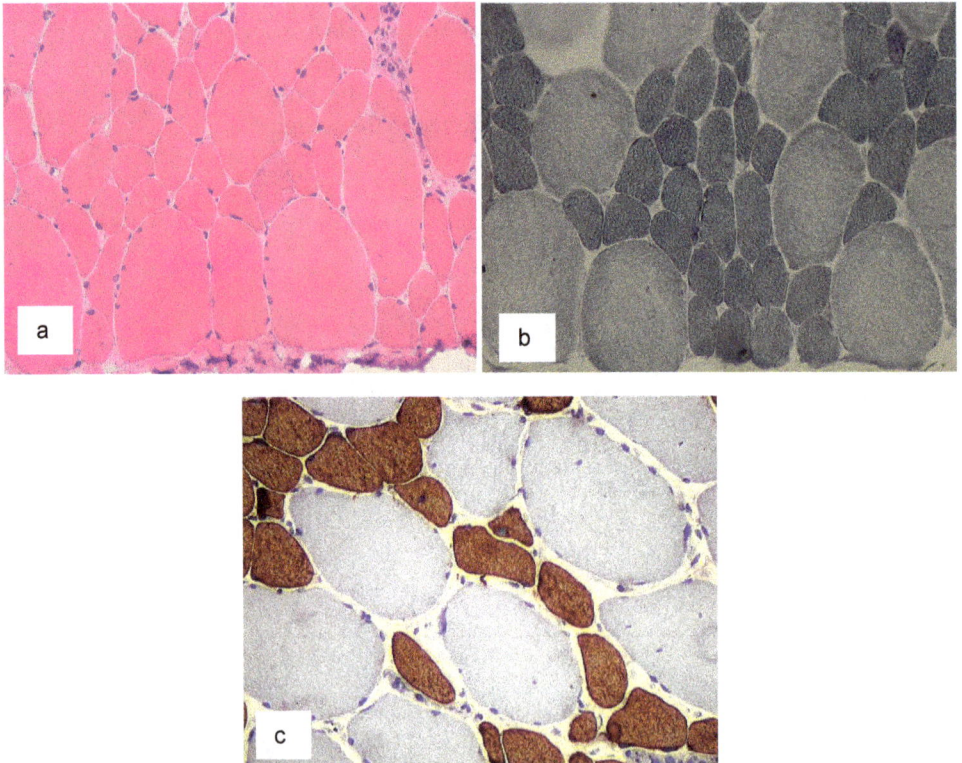

Fig. 2. a - H & E staining showing two populations of muscle fibres with different diameters average. b - NADH-TR staining where small diameter fibres show a higher oxidative activity (type 1) than the large fibres (type 2). c - Immunohistochemistry for myosin slow - small diameter fibres are positively stained for slow myosin fibres (type 1), in contrast to the larger fibres that are unmarked (type 2).

fibres (Figures 10 a-c). The electron microscopy showed neither central focus, minifocus, nemaline bodies nor mitochondrial alterations, also no protein deposits were observed.

The most significant data from the biceps muscle biopsy from case II-2 is illustrated in figure 2 c.

CASE III - 1 Female, 13 years old, daughter of the Case II-2, non-consanguineous parents. She was born at 40 weeks gestational age, 50 cm height, 2.670g weight, cesarean delivery for fetal distress, and a history of reduced fetal movements. The child presented a congenital hypotonia and delayed motor development, acquiring the standing posture approximately at 19 months of age with a clumsy posture. She did not gain weight like a normal child and physical activities were restricted. Like her father, she showed progressive deviation of the spine, and recently complained with pain in the dorsal region, especially during physical activity. On examination, the patient was a tall and thin child, with marked kyphoscoliosis, long face, high palate, atrophy muscle and global hypoactive muscle stretch reflexes. There were no motor deficits in the face or external ophthalmoparesis. CK values were between 65 to 73 U / L (normal below 145 U / L). Glucose, IgA, IgG and IgM, transaminases, and electrolytes were normal, but with a TSH value of 7.23 IU / ml (normal 4.5) and FT4 of 1.68 ng / dl (normal range). Sensory nerve conduction velocity (median, ulnar, radial and sural) and motor nerves (median, ulnar, peroneal and tibial) were within normal limits. EMG of deltoid, biceps, rectus femoris, tibialis anterior and gastrocnemius showed myopathic changes. The patient was doing physical therapy in 50-minute sessions per week in pediatric neurology ambulatory UNICAMP. At 15 years old she had an episode of severe pneumonia which complicated by fatal septicemia.

CASE III - 3. Male, 10 years old, third son of the case II -2. He was born at 38 weeks gestational age with cesarean delivery, and had a history of reduced fetal movements. The child presented a congenital hypotonia and delayed motor development to roll, sit and crawl, acquiring the standing posture around 11 months age, and unsteady gait around 2 years old. According to his parents, he used to present recurrent episodes of urinary tract infection, pneumonia and ear infections during childhood. In the first consultation, there was a decreased in motor performance, diffused muscle hypotrophy, scoliosis, high palate and hypoactivity of muscle stretch reflexes. There was no facial weakness or external ophthalmoparesis. Sensibility and cognition were preserved. Values of CK, glucose, IgA, IgG and IgM, transaminases, electrolytes, vitamin B12 and TSH were normal. The EMG test was not performed at the request of his father.

CASE III - 5. Male, 9 months of age, born after 38 weeks of pregnancy, cesarean delivery, and with a history of reduced fetal movements. He had a slight delay in motor development, and at clinical examination an evident hypotonia, with preserved muscle stretch reflexes. Laboratory findings revealed mild microcytic hypochromic anemia, CK of 89 U / L (normal 170 U / L) and TSH and T4 L-us normal. Clinical monitoring was suggested by over time. He was re-evaluated at 2 years and 6 months of age. At this time he was walking without support, with mild myopathic patterns. The muscle stretch reflexes were hypoactive, hypotonia clearly present and dextro-convex scoliosis and lumbar cord. For treatment physiotherapy was indicated. We did not evaluate him using the scale P-MFM due to this method is recommended for patients over 6 years.

Figure 3 a-c illustrate the data from the mMRI for cases II-2, III-1 and III3.

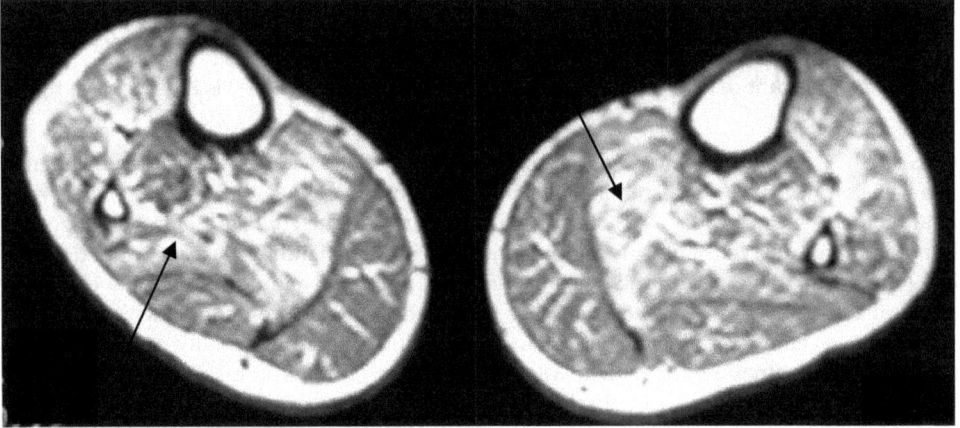

Fig. 3.a - Case II-2. mMRI, T1-weighted images and axial sections showing fatty infiltration of muscle compartments of the anterior, posterior deep and superficial leg, with greater involvement of the anterior and deep posterior compartment.

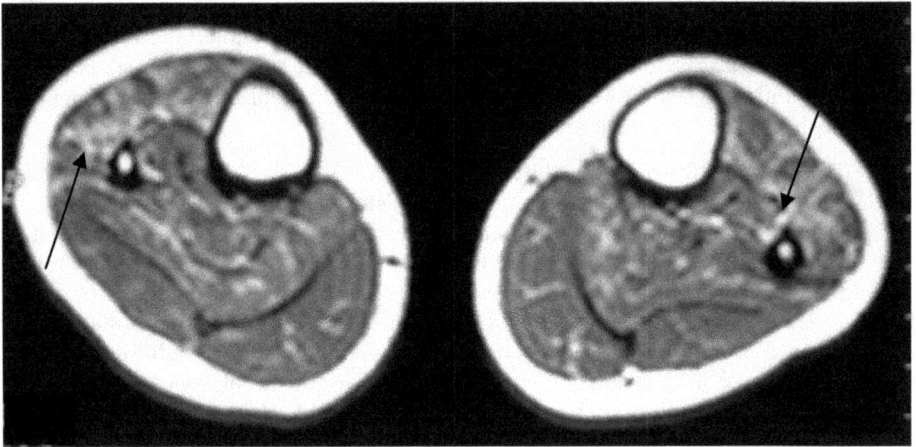

Fig. 3.b - Case III-1. mMRI, T1-weighted images and axial sections showing fatty infiltration of muscle compartments of the anterior, posterior deep and superficial leg with less alteration of the superficial posterior compartment. Note the symmetry condition.

Figure 4 represents the scores of each dimension and the total score of P-MFM in cases II - 2, III - 1 and III - 3, at different ages.

Different types of muscle fibres are present in the muscles of normal adults in a typical mosaic pattern, with ratio of approximately 1 / 3 of fibre type 1 (Figures 2a and 2b). The differentiation of the fibres occurs between the 22° week of gestation and the first year of life. At birth, the child had about 40% of type 1 fibre. The percentage of these fibres increased up to 60% in the first year of life and remained unchanged until adulthood. The sizes of type 1 and 2 fibres are almost equal in childhood, with little variability in relation to adults (75).

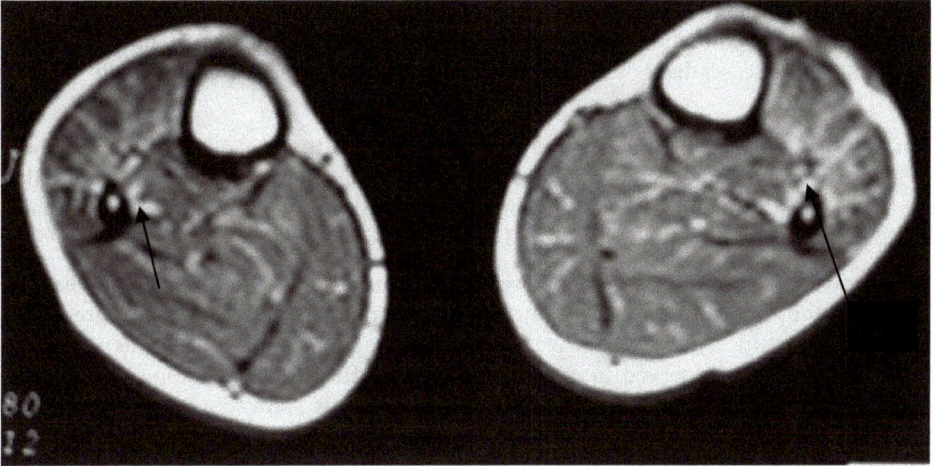

Fig. 3.c - Case III-3. mMRI, T1-weighted images and axial sections showing fatty infiltration of muscle compartments of the anterior, posterior deep and superficial leg with less alteration of the superficial posterior compartment. Note the relative preservation of muscle compared with the previous cases.

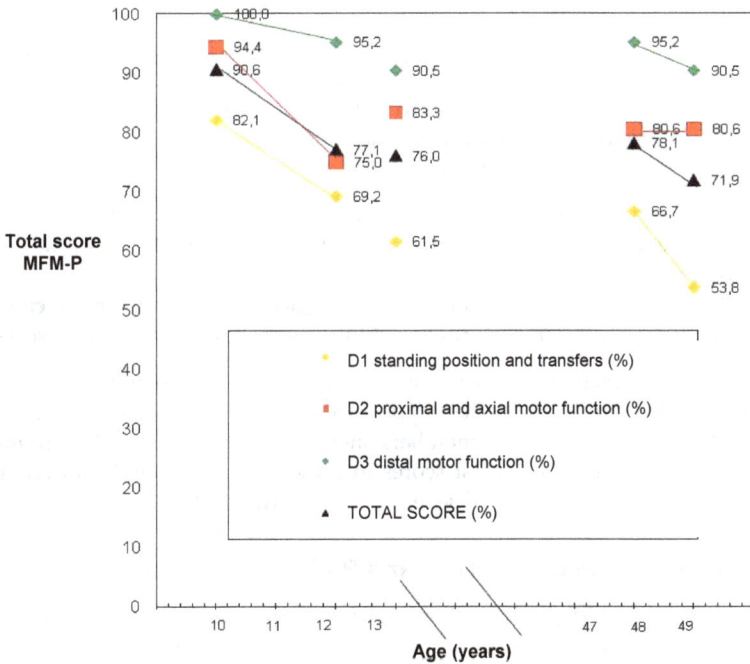

Fig. 4. Distribution of scores for each dimension and total score of the P-MFM from each patient. The evaluation at 10 and 12 years refers to case III-3, the evaluation at 13 years refers to the case III-1, and evaluation at 48 and 49 years to case II-2.

The mutation in the genes ACTA1 (22), SEPN1 (48) or TPM3 (23) express the morphological and histochemical alteration in CFTD (49). Since the first description of this disease, approximately 67 cases have been described (16), but just a few cases originally in Brazil (50).

Clinical characteristics of patients in the study were similar to those described in previously works, such as congenital hypotonia, delayed motor skills, kyphoscoliosis and high palate. Also data for additional tests as EMG myopathic pattern and CK levels are normal or slightly altered according to the literature (14,17,51,52,53,54).

The natural course of CFTD is in most cases characterized by slow progression of weakness, affecting mainly the lower limbs beginning at the proximal muscles and progressing to distal. However, in some patients weakness is widespread (16,17). The deterioration of muscle strength was observed in our patients, with difficulties to standing, walking and running. During assessment of motor function, all patients showed greater difficulties in activities related to standing position and transfers (Dimension 1) due to loss of muscle strength.

All the seven cases described by Sobrado et al. (17) had difficulty in activities like those described in our study (raising themselves from a chair or from the floor, walking or running on heels), in addition to muscle weakness in lower limbs (grade 3 to 4). These data agree with descriptions of Linssen et al. (55) in which cases presenting degree of muscle strength equal to 4, have functional limitations.

Some patients with CFTD have severe respiratory complications, as with the patient in the case III - 1. This condition could happen due to hypotrophy of type 1 fibres found in the respiratory muscles, including the diaphragm (14,16,20,22,48,49) or as a result of severe kyphoscoliosis, which progressively diminished lung capacity. Thus, it is important that patients be monitored for maintenance of a postural alignment and breathing function.

The mMRI is proposed as a useful method to study congenital and metabolic myopathy (56), although there are few publications using this technique in CFTD (17). In the current study, it was possible to qualitatively observe intense changes in distal segments of the lower limbs in all images of affected patients. These changes correspond to an increased leg muscle weakness with difficulties in performing activities according to the P-MFM scale.

The evaluation of muscle function by P-MFM associated with the examination of mMRI led to a full characterization and motor phenotype evaluation in these patients. The first evaluation using the P-MFM in family's members showed a co-occurrence of more intense abnormalities in the mMRI with the worst scores in standing position and transfer. There was also a correlation between the age and severity of the mMRI and P-MFM score.

4. Correlation between muscle strength and P-MFM in myotonic dystrophy

The study included a total of 21 patients, 10 males and 11 females, from 20 to 60 years old, with an average of 38.14 years, and with clinical-laboratory diagnosis of MD-1, outcoming the Neuromuscular Diseases Clinic Clinical Hospital of UNICAMP.

Patients were evaluated by MFM-P (29) and submitted to examination of muscle strength by MRC scale (1976) that includes 14 muscle groups of upper limbs (UL), 14 groups in the cervical muscles and lower limbs, trunk flexors and extensors. Muscles were grouped according to the segment's function.

Statistical analysis - The correlation of each of the three dimensions and the total score P-MFM, with the degrees obtained by the MRC scale in the muscle groups studied was made using Pearson's correlation coefficient.

Patients showed a variation in the degree of muscle strength from 2 to 4. In the distal muscle groups, such as flexors, extensors of the fingers and wrist extensors, the degrees of force were grade 2-4. And the proximal muscles strength varied from 3 to 4.

In the lower limbs, muscle strength ranged from grade 2 to 5. In distal muscles the strength varied from 2 to 4 and the proximal muscles strength ranged from grade 3 to 5. Also the evaluation of axial muscles showed strength ranged varying from grade 2 to 4.

The deficits found in patients were symmetrical in both the axial region and in the upper and lower segments.

To analyze the distribution of the total score and each dimension of the P-MFM scale values were arbitrarily classified as: mild (100 to 70%, independent patient), moderate (69.9 to 50%, partially dependent) and severe (<50%, dependent).

A higher number of patients presented lower scores (<50%) in activities related to P-MFM Dimension 1 (standing position and transfers) (Table 2).

Score	Dimension (score)			
	D1	**D2**	**D3**	**Total score**
Mild	4	18	20	12
(100– 70%)	(89,74 – 76,92)	(100 – 80,56)	(100 – 71,43)	(95,83 – 72,92)
Moderate	7	3	01	09
(69,9– 50%)	(69,23 – 53,85)	(63,89 – 58,33)	(57,14)	(66,67 – 54,17)
Severe	10			
(< 50%)	(48,72 – 25-64)	----	---	---

Table 2. Number of patients according to scores obtained in each dimension and total score of P-MFM

Analyzing the correlations between the degrees of upper limb strength in each dimension and total score P-MFM, we observed a significantly positive correlation between the proximal muscles and Dimension1 and Dimension 2, and correlation between the distal muscles and Dimension 3.

Similarly for lower limbs, we observed a significantly positive correlation between the plantar flexors and extensors of the hips strength with the scores of D1; and also between the finger extensors and dorsiflexors of the ankles strength with the scores of D2. The strength values of the finger extensors, dorsiflexors, ankle inverters and eversion were significantly positive correlated with the score of D3; and the plantar flexors, dorsiflexors, eversion ankles, and hip extensors strength were significantly positive correlated with the total score of P-MFM.

Analyzing the correlations between the neck and trunk strength, with each dimension and the total score of P-MFM, we observed a significantly correlation between the neck and abdominal flexor with D1; between neck flexors with the D3; and between neck flexors and abdominal flexor with total score.

The assessment of functional capacity and degree of muscle strength in patients with neuromuscular disease are essential aspects for their diagnosis and follow-up. Assistance in clinical decisions, treatment, prevention of any complications (like respiratory failure or retractions), indication of the type and intensity of exercise are important aspects to be considered (57,58).

The MD-1 shows a pattern of muscle weakness primarily affecting the facial muscles, neck flexors, and dorsiflexors of fingers. The proximal muscles may not show deficits or mild clinical signs (2,59,60). Lindeman et al. (59,61) showed that in MD-1 there is a great variability in degrees of strength in the affected muscle groups (62.63). The symmetric and progressive muscular weakness involves proximal muscles (64). The deficit predominantly distal and axial deficits, as well as the later weakness proximal segments was also demonstrated in studies by Whittaker et al. (60), Lindeman and Drukker (65) and Lindeman et al. (66). Similar topography of motor impairment was observed in this study, in patients with MD-1.

The strength graduated in 4 on the MRC scale, defined as the ability of active muscle contraction against moderate resistance, was correlated with a negative impact on the ability to perform functions like running, climbing stairs and walking (55,59,67,68,69,70,71,72).

In this study, we found a great variability in the degree of muscle strength with greater involvement in distal segments of the lower limbs, and motor skills assessed by the P-MFM and a greater activity limitation in the standing position and transfers. The positive correlations obtained between muscle groups and the dimensions of P-MFM were restricted, noting that the most significant one occurred between the groups with lower degree of strength of the distal segment (hand and foot) and D3.

According to Whittaker et al. (60) the weakness of flexors and extensors of fingers and wrist is the major cause of disability in DM-1. This early involvement of distal muscles allowed the correlation of these groups, especially with the D3. The proximal and axial body segments act as posture stabilizer factors to provide a stable basis for the distal movement (73). Considering that during the measurement of the scale items the subjects had trunk and limbs supported, they did not need an effective action from the muscles of the trunk and proximal limbs. So, it was possible to correlate specifically the strength of distal muscles with their respective activities.

Poor limitations in proximal muscle groups (extensors of the hip and shoulder) were observed in few activities (Dimensions 1 and 2) limiting other activities (60,65,66) in late stage of this disease.

The proximal muscular deficit can influence the performance function (64, 74, 75, 76.77, 78). According to Galassi et al. (79) and Linssen et al. (55) even when the weakness is predominantly in the distal limb segments, there is a bilateral proximal atrophy area in the computer tomography scans from patients with muscular dystrophy, also demonstrating the involvement of bilateral and proximal muscles, even when there is a clear manifestation of symptoms.

Lindeman et al. (59,61,76)and Aldehag et al. (80) correlated a specific muscle with a particular activity (like the quadriceps strength and standing up from a chair) in patients with DM-1, and found a positive correlation between strength and function. However Dawes et al. (81) found no correlation between muscle strength and function, when these activities were more complex.

Besides strength, other variables may be influencing the individual's functional ability, such as age (82), gender and weight (83). In our cases these variables were not considered because they were not included in the objectives.

So, it is important to analyze a large number of myotonic dystrophy patients to observe any correlation between strength and motor function.

5. Final considerations

The use of MFM proved to be an interesting tool in the study of the congenital myopathies as CFTD; although we were limited by time and sample size. The correlation of severe myopathy and mMRI data for smaller scale scores P-MFM, enables the use of a non-invasive diagnostic tool to study the course of myopathy diseases. They also indicate that both methods could be used in to analyse the results of pharmacological interventions and rehabilitation in these diseases.

The P-MFM has a high reliability and validity to be used as a tool for clinical diagnosis and monitoring of neuromuscular diseases, allowing the inclusion of Brazilian patients in international clinical trials. Thus, we can mention that:

1. The positive correlations between the BI, Vignos scale and P-MFM allowed the validation of P-MFM in Brazil.
2. The application of P-MFM could demonstrate the progressive dysfunction in two of the three members of a family with CFTD. The muscle magnetic resonance showed that the more severe the motor function, the worse were the changes in the image worst severe functional motor, the worst change images.
3. The application of P-MFM in MD-1 showed the predominance of distal myopathy, expressed by the lower scores of muscle strength correlating positively with the scores mainly in D3.

6. References

[1] Jensen MP, Abresch RT, Carter GT. The reliability and validity of a self report version of the FIM instrument in persons with neuromuscular disease and chronic pain. Arch Phys Med Rehabil. 2005; 86: 116-22.
[2] Harper PS. Myotonic dystrophy London: WB Saunders; 2001.436p.
[3] Otsuka MA, Boffa CFB, Vieira ABAM. Distrofias Musculares: Fisioterapia aplicada. Rio de Janeiro: Ed Revinter; 2005. p.2-28.
[4] Beenakker EAC, Maurits NM, Fock JM, Brouwer OF, Van der Hoeven J. Functional ability and muscle force in healthy children and ambulant Duchenne muscular dystrophy patients. Eur J Paediatr Neurol. 2005; 9: 387-93.

[5] Giorgio A, Dotti MT, Battaglini M, Marino S, Mortilla M, Stromillo ML et al. Cortical damage in brains of patients with adult-form of myotonic dystrophy type 1 and no or minimal MRI abnormalities. J Neurol. 2006; 253: 1471-7.
[6] Angeard N, Gargiulo M, Jacquette A, Radvanyi H, Eymard B, Heron D. Cognitive profile in childhood myotonic dystrophy type I: is there a global impairment? Neuromuscul Disord. 2007; 17: 451-8.
[7] Schara U, Schoser, BGH. Myotonic dystrophies type 1 and 2: a summary on current aspects. Semin Pediatr Neurol. 2006; 13: 71-9.
[8] Le Ber I, Martinez M, Campion D, Laquerriére A, Bétard C, Bassez G et al. A non-DM1, non-DM2 multisystem myotonic disorder with fronto temporal dementia: phenotype and suggestive mapping of the DM3 locus to chromosome 15q21-24. Brain. 2004; 127: 1979-92.
[9] Cho DH, Tapscott SJ. Myotonic dystrophy: emerging mechanisms for DM1 and DM2. Biochimic Biophysic Acta. 2007; 1772: 195-204.
[10] Brunner HG, Jennekens FGI, Smeets HJM, de Visser M, Wintzen AR. Myotonic dystrophy (Steinert's disease). In: Emery AEH, ed. Diagnostic criteria for neuromuscular disorders. 2° ed. Londres: Royal Society of Medicine Press; 1997. p 27-9.
[11] Kroksmark AK, Ekstrom AB, Bjorck E, Tulinius M. Myotonic dystrophy: muscle involvement in relation to disease type and size of expanded CTG-repeat sequence. Dev Med Child Neurol. 2005; 47: 478-85.
[12] North K. Congenital myopathies. In: Engel AG, Franzini-Armstrong C. Myology. United States of America: McGraw-Hill; 2004. p.1473-533.
[13] Brooke MH. Congenital fiber type disproportion. In: Kakulas BA. Clinical studies in myology. Proc of the 2nd Int. Cong on Muscle Diseases, Perth, Australia, 1971. Part 2. Amsterdam: Excerpta Medica (pub.) 1973. p. 147-59.
[14] Cavanagh NPC, Lake BD, McMeniman P. Congenital fibre type disproportion myopathy. A histological diagnosis with an uncertain clinical outlook. Arch Dis Child. 1979; 54: 735-43.
[15] Clancy RR, Kelts KA, Oehlert JW. Clinical variability in congenital fibre type disproportion. J Neurol Sci.1980; 46: 257-66.
[16] Clarke NF, North KN. Congenital fibre type disproportion – 30 years on. J Neuropathol Exp Neurol. 2003; 62: 977-89.
[17] Sobrido MJ, Fernandez JM, Fontoira E, Pérez-Sousa C, Cabello A, Castro M et al. Autosomal dominant congenital fibre type disproportion: a clinicopathological and imaging study of a large family. Brain. 2005; 128: 1716-27.
[18] Curless RG, Nelson MB. Congenital fiber type disproportion in identical twins. Ann Neurol.1977; 2: 455-9.
[19] Kula RW, Sher JH, Shafiq SA, Hardy-Stashin J. Variability of clinical pathological manifestations in familial fiber type disproportion. Trans Am Neurol Assoc. 1980; 105: 416-8.
[20] Sulaiman AR, Swick HM, Kinder DS. Congenital fibre type disproportion with unusual clinico pathologic manifestations. J Neurol Neurosurg Psychiatry. 1983; 46: 175-82.
[21] Bartholomeus MGT, Gabreels FJM, ter Laak HJ, Van Engelen BGM. Congenital fibre type disproportion a time-locked diagnosis: a clinical and morphological follow-up study. Clin Neurol Neurosurg. 2000; 102: 97-101.

[22] Laing NG, Clarke NF, Dye DE, Liyanage K, Walker KR, Kobayashi Y et al. Actin mutations are one cause of congenital fibre type disproportion. Ann Neurol. 2004; 56: 689-94.

[23] Clarke NF, Kolski H, Dye DE, Lim E, Smith RLL, Patel R et al. Mutation in TPM3 are a common cause of congenital fiber type disproportion. Ann Neurol. 2008; 63: 329-37.

[24] Fowler Jr WM. Management of musculoskeletal complications in neuromuscular diseases: weakness and the role of exercise. Advances in the rehabilitation of neuromuscular diseases. Physic Med Rehabil. 1988; 2: 489-507.

[25] Kurihara T. New classification and treatment for myotonic disorders. Internal Medicine. 2005; 44(10): 1027-32.

[26] Stteg AM, Lankhorst GJ. Screening instruments for disability. Critical Rev Phys Rehabil Med. 1994; 6: 101-2.

[27] Cacho EWA, Melo FRLV, Oliveira R. Avaliação da recuperação motora de pacientes hemiplégicos através do Protocolo de Desempenho Físico de Fugl-Meyer. Rev Neurocienc. 2004; 12(2): 94-102. Errata, 12(4):221.

[28] Bérard C, Payan C, Hodgkinson I, Fermanian J. A motor function measure scale for neuromuscular diseases. Construction and validation study. Neuromuscul Disord. 2005; 15(7): 463-70.

[29] Iwabe C, Miranda-Pfeilsticker BH, Nucci A. Medida da função motora: versão da escala para o português e estudo de confiabilidade. Rev Bras Fisioter. 2008; 12(5): 417-24.

[30] Masuko AH, Carvalho LBC, Machado MAC, Morais JF, Prado LBF, Prado GF. Translation and validation into Brazilian Portuguese of the restless legs syndrome rating scale of the international restless legs syndrome study group. Arq Neuropsiquiatr. 2008; 66(4):832-6.

[31] Miller DK, Malmstrom TK, Andresen EM, Miller JP, Herning MM, Schootman M et al. Development and validation of a short portable sarcopenia measure in the African American Health project. J Gerontol A Biol Sci Med Sci. 2009; 64A(3): 388-94.

[32] Silva MB, Asa SKP, Santa Maria NN, Zanella EM, Fávero FM, Fukujima MM et al. Análise dos instrumentos de avaliação na miopatia. Rev Neurocienc. 2006; 14(2): 29-43.

[33] Forst J, Forst R. Lower limb surgery in Duchenne muscular dystrophy. Neuromuscul Disord. 1999; 9(3): 176-81.

[34] Vondracek P, Bednarik J. Clinical and electrohysiological findings and long-term outcomes in paediatric patients with critical illness polyneuromyopathy. Eur J Paediatr Neurol. 2006; 10(4): 176-81.

[35] Jansa J, Pogacnik T, Gompertz P. An evaluation of the Extended Barthel Index with acute ischemic stroke patients. Neurorehabil Neural Repair. 2004; 18: 37-41.

[36] Tiffreau V, Viet G, Thévenon A. Pain and neuromuscular disease: the results of a survey. Am J Phys Med Rehabil. 2006; 85(9): 756-66.

[37] Nair KP, Vasanth A, Gourie-Devi M, Taly AB, Rao S, Gayathri N et al. Disabilities in children with Duchene muscular dystrophy: a profile. J Rehabil Med. 2001; 33: 147-9.

[38] Martinez JAB, Brunherotti MA, Assis MR, Sobreira CFR. Validação da escala motora funcional EK para a língua portuguesa. Rev Assoc Med Brás. 2006; 52(5): 347-51.

[39] Vandervelde L, Van den Bergh PY, Goemans N, Thonnard JL. ACTIVLIM: a Rasch-built measure of activity limitations in children and adults with neuromuscular disorders. Neuromuscul Disord. 2007; 17(6): 459-69.

[40] Werneck LC, Bonilla E. Dystrophin in the differentiation between Duchenne and Becker muscular dystrophies: an immunihistochemical study compared with clinical stage, serum enzymes and muscle biopsy. Arq Neuropsiquiatr. 1990; 48(4): 454-64.

[41] Werneck LC. Correlation between functional disability, age and serum enzymes in neuromuscular diseases. Arq Neuropsiquiatr. 1995; 53: 60-8.

[42] Thong MK, Bazlin RI, Wong KT. Diagnosis and management of Duchenne muscular dystrophy in a developing country over a 10 year period. Dev Med Child Neurol. 2005; 47(7): 474-7.

[43] Chen JY, Clark MJ. Family function in families of children with Duchenne muscular dystrophy. Fam Community Health. 2007; 30(4): 296-304.

[44] Brunherotti MA, Sobreira C, Rodrigues-Junior AL, de Assis MR, Terra Filho J, Baddini Martinez JA. Correlations of Egen Klassification and Barthel Index scores with pulmonary function parameters in Duchenne muscular dystrophy. Heart Lung. 2007; 36(2): 132-9.

[45] De Cauwer H, Heytens L, Martin JJ. Report of the 89th ENMC international workshop: central core disease. Neuromusc Disord. 2002; 12: 588-95.

[46] Mercuri E, Talim B, Moghadaszadeh B, Petit N, Brockington M, Counsell S et al. Clinical and imaging findings in six cases of congenital muscular dystrophy with rigid spine syndrome linked to chromosome 1p (RSMD1). Neuromusc Disord. 2002b; 12: 631-8.

[47] Nucci A. Miopatia a corpos hialinos. Estudo clinico-laboratorial e de ressonância magnética [Tese – Livre Docência]. Campinas (SP): Universidade Estadual de Campinas; 2006.

[48] Clarke NF, Kidson W, Quijano-Roy S, Estournet B, Ferreiro A, Guicheney P et al. SEPN1: associated with congenital fiber-type disproportion and insulin resistance. Ann Neurol. 2006; 59:546-52.

[49] Mizuno Y, Komiya K. A serial muscle biopsy study in a case of congenital fiber-type disproportion associated with progressive respiratory failure. Brain Dev. 1990; 12(4): 431-6.

[50] Levy JA, Alegro MSC, Lusvarghi ES, Salum PNB, Tsanaclis AMC, Levy A. Desproporção congênita de fibras. Atrofia de fibras tipo 1. Arq Neuropsiquiatr. 1987; 45(2): 153-8.

[51] Jaffe M, Shapira J, Borochowitz Z. Familial congenital fiber type disproportion (CFTD) with an autosomal recessive inheritance. Clin Genet. 1988; 33: 33-7.

[52] Vestergaard H, Klein HH, Hansen T, Muller J, Skovby F, Bjorbaek C et al. Severe insulin-resistant diabetes mellitus in patients with congenital muscle fiber type disproportion myopathy. J Clin Invest. 1995; 95: 1925-32.

[53] Sharma MC, Ralte AM, Atri SK, Gulati S, Kalra V, Sarkar C. Congenital fiber type disproportion: A rare type of congenital myopathy: A report of four cases. Neurol India. 2004; 52(2): 254-6.

[54] Na SJ, Kim WK, Kim TS, Kang SW, Lee EY, Choi YC. Comparison of clinical characteristics between congenital fiber type disproportion myopathy and

congenital myopathy with type fiber predominance. Yonsei Med J. 2006; 47(4): 513-8.

[55] Linssen WHJP, Notermans NC, Van der Graaf Y, Wokke HJ, Van Doorn PA, Howeler CJ et al. Miyoshi – type distal muscular dystrophy. Clinical spectrum in 24 Dutch patients. Brain. 1997; 120: 1989-96.

[56] Mercuri E, Pichiecchio A, Counsell S, Allsop J, Cini C, Jungbluth H et al. A short protocol for muscle MRI in children with muscular dystrophies. Eur J Paediatr Neurol. 2002a; 6: 305-7.

[57] Hogrel JY, Ollivier G, Desnuelli C. Manual and quantitative muscle testing in neuromuscular disorders. How to assess the consistency of strength measurements in clinical trials? Rev Neurol. 2006; 162 (4): 427-36.

[58] Cup EH, Pieterse AJ, Brook Pastoor JM, Munneke M, Van Engelen BG, Hendricks HT et al. Exercise therapy and other types of physical therapy for patients with neuromuscular diseases: a systematic review. Arch Phys Med Rehabil. 2007; 88: 1452-64.

[59] Lindeman E, Leffers P, Reulen J, Spaans F, Drukker J. Quadriceps strength and timed motor performances in myotonic dystrophy Charcot-Marie-Tooth disease, and healthy subjects. Clin Rehabil. 1998; 12: 127-35.

[60] Whittaker RG, Ferenczi E, Hilton Jones D. Myotonic dystrophy: practical issues relating to assessment of strength. J Neurol Neurosurg Psychiatry. 2006: 77: 1282-3.

[61] Lindeman E, Leffers P, Spaans F, Drukker J, Reulen J. Deterioration of motor function in myotonic dystrophy and hereditary motor and sensory neuropathy. Scand J Rehabil Med. 1995a; 27(1): 59-64.

[62] Murakami N, Sakuta R, Takahashi E, Katada Y, Nagai T, Owada M et al. Early onset distal muscular dystrophy with normal dysferlin expression. Brain Dev. 2005; 27: 589-91.

[63] Lamont PJ, Udd B, Mastaglia FL, Visser M, Hedera P, Voit T et al. Laing early onset distal myopathy: slow myosin defect with variable abnormalities on muscle biopsy. J Neurol Neurosurg Psychiatry. 2006; 77: 208-15.

[64] Mathieu J, Boivin H, Richards CL. Quantitative motor assessment in myotonic dystrophy. Can J Neurol Sci. 2003; 30(2): 129-36.

[65] Lindeman E, Drukker J. Specificity of strength training in neuromuscular disorders. J Rehabil Sc. 1994; 7: 13-5.

[66] Lindeman E, Spaans F, Reulen J, Leffers P, Drukker J. Progressive resistance training in neuromuscular patients. Effects on force and surface EMG. J Electromyography Kinesiology. 1999; 9: 379-84.

[67] Hosking JP, Bhat US, Dubowitz V, Edwards RH. Measurements of muscle strength and performance in children with normal and diseased muscle. Arch Dis Child. 1976; 51(12): 957-63.

[68] Milner Brown HS, Miller RG. Muscle strengthening though high resistance weight training in patients with neuromuscular disorders. Arch Phys Med Rehabil. 1988; 69(1): 14-9.

[69] Lue YJ, Chen SS. Strength and functional performance of patients with limb girdle muscular dystrophy. Kaohsuing J Med Sci. 2000; 16(2): 83-90 (abstract).

[70] Kelm J, Ahlhelm F, Regitz T, Pace D, Schmitt E. Controlled dynamic weight training in patients with neuromuscular disorders. Fortschr Neurol Psychiatr. 2001; 69(8): 359-66.

[71] Van der Kooi EL, Lindeman E, Riphagen I. Strength training and aerobic exercise training for muscle disease. Cochrane Database Syst Rev. 2005; 25(1): CD 003907.

[72] Stubgen JP. Limb girdle muscular dystrophy: an interval study of weakness and functional impairment. J Clin Neuromuscul Dis. 2008; 9(3): 333-40.

[73] Shumway-Cook A, Woolacott MH. Reach, grasp and manipulation: changes across the life span. In: Shumway-Cook A, Woolacott MH. Motor control: theory and pratical applications. 2ed. London: Lippincott Williams & Wilkins; 2001. p. 471-96.

[74] McFadyen BJ, Winter DA. An integrated biomechanical analysis of normal stair ascent and descent. J Biomech. 1988; 21: 733-44.

[75] Kotake T, Dohi N, Kajiwara T, Sumi N, Koyama Y, Miura T. An analysis of sit to stand movements. Arch Phys Med Rehabil. 1993; 74: 1095-9.

[76] Lindeman E, Leffers P, Spaans F, Drukker J, Reulen J, Kerckhoffs M et al. Strength training in patients with myotonic dystrophy and hereditary motor and sensory neuropathy: a randomized clinical trial. Arch Phys Med Rehabil. 1995b; 76: 612-20.

[77] Hedberg B, Anvret M, Ansved T. CTG-repeat length in distal and proximal leg muscles of symptomatic and non-symptomatic patients with myotonic dystrophy: relation to muscle strength and degree of histopathological abnormalities. Eur J Neurol. 1999; 6: 341-6.

[78] Kierkegaard M, Tollback A. Reliability and feasibility of the six minute walk test in subjects with myotonic dystrophy. Neuromuscul Disord. 2007; 17: 943-9.

[79] Galassi G, Rowland LP, Hays AP, Hopkins LC, DiMauro S. High serum levels of creatinekinase: asymptomatic prelude to distal myopathy. Muscle Nerve. 1987; 10: 346-50.

[80] Aldelrag AS, Jonsson H, Ansved T. Effects of a hand training programme in five patients with myotonic dystrophy type I. Occup Ther Int. 2005; 12(1): 14-27.

[81] Dawes H, Korpershoek N, Freebody J, Elsworth C, Van Tintelen N, Wade DT et al. A pilot randomized controlled trial of a home based exercise programme aimed at improving endurance and function in adults with neuromuscular disorders. J Neurol Neurosurg Psychiatry. 2006; 77: 959-62.

[82] Ikeda ER, Schenkman ML, Riley PO, Hodge WA. Influence of age on dynamics of rising from a chair. Phys Ther. 1991; 71: 473-81.

[83] VanSant AF. Life span development in functional tasks. Phys Ther. 1990; 70: 788-9.

Permissions

The contributors of this book come from diverse backgrounds, making this book a truly international effort. This book will bring forth new frontiers with its revolutionizing research information and detailed analysis of the nascent developments around the world.

We would like to thank Dr Arunkanth Ankala and Dr Madhuri Hegde, for lending their expertise to make the book truly unique. They have played a crucial role in the development of this book. Without their invaluable contribution this book wouldn't have been possible. They have made vital efforts to compile up to date information on the varied aspects of this subject to make this book a valuable addition to the collection of many professionals and students.

This book was conceptualized with the vision of imparting up-to-date information and advanced data in this field. To ensure the same, a matchless editorial board was set up. Every individual on the board went through rigorous rounds of assessment to prove their worth. After which they invested a large part of their time researching and compiling the most relevant data for our readers. Conferences and sessions were held from time to time between the editorial board and the contributing authors to present the data in the most comprehensible form. The editorial team has worked tirelessly to provide valuable and valid information to help people across the globe.

Every chapter published in this book has been scrutinized by our experts. Their significance has been extensively debated. The topics covered herein carry significant findings which will fuel the growth of the discipline. They may even be implemented as practical applications or may be referred to as a beginning point for another development. Chapters in this book were first published by InTech; hereby published with permission under the Creative Commons Attribution License or equivalent.

The editorial board has been involved in producing this book since its inception. They have spent rigorous hours researching and exploring the diverse topics which have resulted in the successful publishing of this book. They have passed on their knowledge of decades through this book. To expedite this challenging task, the publisher supported the team at every step. A small team of assistant editors was also appointed to further simplify the editing procedure and attain best results for the readers.

Our editorial team has been hand-picked from every corner of the world. Their multi-ethnicity adds dynamic inputs to the discussions which result in innovative outcomes. These outcomes are then further discussed with the researchers and contributors who give their valuable feedback and opinion regarding the same. The feedback is then collaborated with the researches and they are edited in a comprehensive manner to aid the understanding of the subject.

Apart from the editorial board, the designing team has also invested a significant amount of their time in understanding the subject and creating the most relevant covers. They scrutinized every image to scout for the most suitable representation of the subject and create an appropriate cover for the book.

The publishing team has been involved in this book since its early stages. They were actively engaged in every process, be it collecting the data, connecting with the contributors or procuring relevant information. The team has been an ardent support to the editorial, designing and production team. Their endless efforts to recruit the best for this project, has resulted in the accomplishment of this book. They are a veteran in the field of academics and their pool of knowledge is as vast as their experience in printing. Their expertise and guidance has proved useful at every step. Their uncompromising quality standards have made this book an exceptional effort. Their encouragement from time to time has been an inspiration for everyone.

The publisher and the editorial board hope that this book will prove to be a valuable piece of knowledge for researchers, students, practitioners and scholars across the globe.

List of Contributors

Mieko Yoshioka
Department of Pediatric Neurology, Kobe City Pediatric and General Rehabilitation Center for the Challenged, Japan

Jnanankur Bag, Quishan Wang and Rumpa Biswas Bhattacharjee
University of Guelph, Department of Molecular and Cellular Biology, Guelph, Ontario, Canada

Tomoko Yamamoto, Atsuko Hiroi, Yoichiro Kato, Noriyuki Shibata and Makio Kobayashi
Department of Pathology, Tokyo Women's Medical University, Japan

Makiko Osawa
Department of Pediatrics, Tokyo Women's Medical University, Japan

Jonathan J. Magaña
Genetics Department, Genomic Medicine Laboratory, National Rehabilitation Institute, Mexico

Bulmaro Cisneros
Genetics and Molecular Biology Department, CINVESTAV-IPN, Mexico

J.L. Anderson
Childrens Hospital, Westmead, Sydney, Australia

S.I. Head
School of Medical Sciences, University of New South Wales, Sydney, Australia

J.W. Morley
School of Medicine, University of Western Sydney, Sydney, Australia

Yuko Iwata and Shigeo Wakabayashi
National Cerebral and Cardiovascular Center Research Institute, Japan

Marie Féron
University of Nantes CNRS UMR6204, France

Karl Rouger
ONIRIS/INRA UMR 703, France

Laetitia Guével
University of Nantes CNRS UMR6204, France
ONIRIS/INRA UMR 703, France

Hao Shi
Department of Pharmacology, United States

Anton M. Bennett
Department of Pharmacology, United States
Program in Integrative Cell Signaling and Neurobiology of Metabolism, Yale University School of Medicine, United States

Nevenka Juretić, Francisco Altamirano, Denisse Valladares and Enrique Jaimovich
Centro de Estudios Moleculares de la Célula, Facultad de Medicina, Universidad de Chile, Santiago, Chile

Gustavo Ferreira Simões and Alexandre Leite Rodrigues de Oliveira
University of Campinas (UNICAMP), Brasil

Imelda J.M. de Groot, Nicoline B.M. Voet, Merel Jansen and Lenie van den Engel-Hoek
Radboud University Nijmegen Medical Centre, The Netherlands

Leigh B. Waddell, Frances J. Evesson, Kathryn N. North, Sandra T. Cooper and Nigel F. Clarke
Institute for Neuroscience and Muscle Research, Children's Hospital at Westmead and Discipline of Paediatrics & Child Health, University of Sydney, Australia

Toshio Saito
Division of Neurology, National Hospital Organization, Toneyama National Hospital, Japan

Katsunori Tatara
Division of Pediatrics, National Hospital Organization, Tokushima National Hospital, Japan

Eiji Wada, Namiko Kikkawa, Mizuko Yoshida, Munehiro Date, Tetsuo Higashi and Ryoichi Matsuda
The University of Tokyo, Japan

Arunkanth Ankala and Madhuri R. Hegde
Emory University, USA

Yen-Mou Lu
Department of Orthopedics, Kaohsiung Medical University Hospital, Kaohsiung Medical University, Kaohsiung, Taiwan

Yi-Jing Lue
Department of Physical Therapy, College of Health Science, Kaohsiung Medical University, Kaohsiung,
Taiwan
Department of Rehabilitation, Kaohsiung Medical University Hospital, Kaohsiung Medical University, Kaohsiung, Taiwan
Department and Graduate Institute of Neurology, School of Medicine, College of Medicine, Kaohsiung Medical University, Kaohsiung, Taiwan

Cristina Iwabe
Faculty of Medical Sciences (FCM), Campinas State University (UNICAMP), Brazil

Anamarli Nucci
Department of Neurology, FCM UNICAMP, Brazil

Beatriz Helena Miranda Pfeilsticker
Department of Neurology, FCM UNICAMP, Brazil

Luis Alberto Magna
Department of Medical Genetics, FCM UNICAMP, Brazil